Contents

Foreword

Travel is one of life's gifts. Yet once the bug has bitten, the condition can be permanent. This book is incredible – how I wish it had been available when I started my own travelling career. Mark Wilson has clearly worked overtime to write it and had tremendous enjoyment getting there.

As health services become ever more restrictive for the health professional or student, many look elsewhere for experience, teaching, greater personal responsibility and, let's be honest, fun. My own student elective, which took me from the comfort of London to Pakistan's remote and war-like North-West Frontier, started a process that continues to this day. India, Africa, Middle East, Far East, Central America, South America, Balkans . . . I could go on for pages. This year alone I have been to a dozen distant lands. Only last week I was in Lapland talking to the Finns.

I look at those who do not travel and my heart goes out to them. They are missing so much and frequently do not realize it. Character building and medical training are not all about reading huge tomes and wafer-thin journals. I interview a lot these days, dozens of CVs passing across my desk for the handful of posts a teaching hospital can offer. Everyone – almost – is highly qualified, matching the specification like a glove. How do I learn what the applicant is *really* like? Could I work with them? How will they react when under stress? I look for two things – personal interests and, wait for it, travel. They have never let me down. You only have to flick through these pages to feel a sense of excitement grow within your chest. What next? I want to be out there. I want to be everywhere. I want to journey to far-flung lands. Read this and I'll wager the travel bug will bite. Congratulations, Mark Wilson. You have done restless folk like me a gigantic service.

Richard Villar
Cambridge

Preface

Medicine, as a doctor, nurse, physio or student, is your passport to the world. We can turn up virtually anywhere around the globe, be welcomed and then be suddenly involved with the most important part of local people's lives, their health. There is probably no other profession that can offer this entrance into so many cultures. For this reason, if wanting to travel, doing it while working is a superb way of really experiencing life in another country.

All medical schools and many nursing schools have an 'elective' period offering a golden opportunity to undertake some training overseas. More and more qualified medics are taking time out of the normal career path to gain such experiences. However, whether studying or working, finding out about destinations can be difficult. You'll want to make sure you're going to the 'right' place for you. This book is designed to help.

Section 1 of this guide consists of three chapters giving advice on planning an elective, arranging work and organizing your own health requirements (both vaccinations and occupational) before departure.

Section 2 gives details about healthcare systems and hospitals in over 100 countries. If you know that you really want to work (play!) on a sunny tropical island, take a look at either the Caribbean or Pacific Island section. If you want developing world medicine, look in the Africa or Asia chapters. If it's hi-tech you're after, try the USA. Wherever possible, as much information about the hospital, its specialities and its social life and local activities (such as skiing or beaches) has been given. For elective students, there's some idea of accommodation costs. Medics can, of course, work in more than just hospitals. For the adventurers out there, other organizations, such as ski-patrols, NASA and the Royal Flying Doctor Service, are also listed at the end of their respective countries.

Section 3, 'The Appendix' is a valuable reference tool. If you want to work with an overseas organization rather than directly through a hospital, look under non-governmental organizations. This is a comprehensive list of agencies that provide aid overseas and require medics. A list of bursaries mainly for elective students in the UK is also given. Finally, details of embassies in Australia, the UK and the USA, as well as suggested vaccine requirements, are provided.

The countries that are popular and interesting have been the focus all along. In a similar fashion, interesting hospitals, even those with only 20 beds, may have more text than a hospital with 1000 beds. There is also more detail on countries where English is spoken or where translators are available.

The Medic's Guide is as up to date as possible at the time of writing, but of course hospitals and staff change. It has also sometimes had to rely on personal opinions. If you find things better, worse or in any way different, please let us know. Information on any hospitals not listed would also be greatly appreciated. There's a £200 prize, and you will of course get a mention in the next edition. Either fill in the coupon at the back of this book or e-mail us at updates@medicsworldwide.com Updates, lists of locum agencies and other information will also be provided on www.medicsworldwide.com

This information should give you some idea of where you would like to go and a taste of what medicine is like in that country. Everyone seems to benefit from time overseas. The patients benefit from some care they might otherwise not have had, and you benefit from what the experience teaches you. If you plan your trip well and choose a good destination, you will go a long way to insuring you have an interesting and enjoyable time. Remember, planning the trip is half the fun of it. Have a great time wherever your adventure takes you. If you do, please write and tell us.

MW
Whyalla, Australia
2000

Acknowledgements

There are many people who have helped contribute to this book. The medical schools of the universities of Edinburgh and Cambridge, UCH and the Middlesex and St Bartholomew's and the Royal London must be thanked for allowing me to look through their elective reports. Those whose elective reports proved extremely useful and those whose signatures I could read are named below. Thank you for writing interesting and detailed reports. You've made it a great deal easier for others to find out about places. There were quite a few names I couldn't read. I'm really sorry I haven't been able to include your name but thank you just the same. Thanks to the embassies and other medical schools in the UK that also supplied information.

A number of other people have also helped with the project: Dr Dennis D'Auria for co-authoring the Health section, Mr Alistar Wilson for the great careers advice, Stephen Miles, Hugh Montgomery, Mr Richard Villar, Safdar Naqui, Richard Hanny, Paco (sorry mate ... forgot your surname), Flynn Snell, Patrick Medd, Heather Le Cocq, Caphwin Laband, Mike Wells, Bip Nandi and Mr Paterson Brown for their enthusiasm. Dr Alan Hargens of NASA-Ames Research Center also has to be thanked for giving me a great start.

I must also express thanks to Fiona Goodgame and Sarah de Souza of Arnold for their extremely hard work in getting this off the ground. Thanks also to all those in production who have made it look nice and corrected my spelling!

Finally thanks to my family and Kelly for putting up with me whilst this was compiled. I'm sorry it took a bit longer than expected!

Naa Annan, Dominic Hennessy, Lleona Lee Cam, Abigail Turner, Susan Dowling, C L Hardie, Helen Dormand, Sian Fiend, Simon Brown, K Gardiner, Stephen Kelly, Jennifer Kitson, Helen Briggs, Duncan Bew, Nicola Finneran, Lisa Clampitt, Marko Kerac, Hammon, H Law, Eric Yeung, Matthew Bur, S Lam, Amrit Ray, Bip Nandi, Sophie Coutouvidis, Mark Latimer, Gwyn Carney, Julia Relf, Madhumita Bhattacharyya, Anu Mitra, Katherine McGlone, Debi Ray, Sophie Dean, Diana Flemming, Julie Hutchison, Owen Anderson, H Sultan, G Sittampalam, Paul McGarry, Steven Epstein, Richard Edwards, Edward Hall, James Orr, Balsit Chander, Tara Bharucha, Anna Kirby, Mohini Varughese, Wanaratram Nasreen Jaffer, Emma Meikle, G Sittampalam, Sarah Gorman, Kate Janessy, S Cooper, Barnaby Major, Paul Albert, J Cheeseman, Joe Hall, Sonia Saha, Sheen Khanduri, Vicki Billing, Simon Calvert, Roger Patel, Ruth de Newtown, Neil McNamara, Gordon Peters, Stephen Wilson, Alan Clark, Freya Garbutt, Emma Nichols, Matthew Outram, R Henderson, Derek Kelly, S Bennett, Richard Bramble, James Porter, Catherine Theodorion, Rosie Davis, Kayode Adeniji, Lorna McCavat, Michael Chapman, Katherine Rank, Lisa Lewry, Paul Simons, Robin Johns, Catherine Scrutton, Brinda Murthsamy, Peter Williams, Geoffrey Corbett, A Morgan, T Thomas, Sarah Andersen, Giles Becker, Charlie Huins, Anna Bever, Vicky Johnson, Fraser, Georgia Page, Sally Ann Gibbs, Catherine Mackman, Angela Bell, Shareen China, S Teo, K Fong, Chumbi Chumbier, P Albert, Agarwala Godbolt, Lionel Tan, K M Nicol, Angela Bell, Susan Cook, Brinda Muthusamy, Alison Stewart, Lisa Andrews, Andrea MeKee, John Woolmore, Judith Brown, C Lawthom, Helen Twydell, Priya Prasad, Sarah Wray, Roland Bunting, Lynn Brown, Mike Wallace, Stephen Kelly, Chris Butler, Kirsten Henderson, Sarah

Hichens, Rebecca Underwood, Topun Austin, Hariet Fraser, G Hamlin, Emma Smith, Ed Fitzherbert, Baird, Maggie Ford, John LeMaitre, Eiva Tremaras, G Brynes, Simon Robinson, Emma Chan, R A Cadogan, W Mason, C Warwick, Katherine Oliver, Abigail Walker, Anne Baird, Heather Jack, Kerri Davidson, Kirstie Nicol, Joe McDowell, Dawn Alison, Kai Ren Ong, Alistair Brooks, M A Buchanan, K Graham, K Riddle, Andrew Fry, Angus Brown, Kirsty Friendly, Elspeth Macsween, Sam Cole, Eiva Trewavas, J McMillan, Berenice Oxford, R Reynolds, Sarah Sankey, Mark Craig, G R Dunn, Stephen Nicol, S Coutts, S Gulathakuta, E Doyle, Andrew Evans, K Connolly, Emma Davidson, Kryshani Fernando, Victoria Ferrar, Clare Byne, Ellen Rawlinson, Andrew Richardson, Sally Watkinson, A Sobaki, Sola Sobaki, Robert Carter, M Choudhry, Mohammed Belal, Leigh Crutchfield, Hilary Stephens, S Brown, Graham Collins, Chris Lambert, Kate Jarony, K Blight, Jennifer O'Brien, Annalisa Payton, Mathew Clark, Helen Twydell, Matthew Clark, Hevs Le Cocq, Richard Stumpfle, Jane Henderson, Thomas Martin, Emma Davidson, K Connolly, Jovina See, Li Wee, Choo Chin Hong, Charmaine Foo, Edwin Cooper, Stanley, James Crawford, Emeline Dean, Simon Butcher, David Porter, Nicholas Park, S Petrie, G Whitfield, Andrew McGin, C McAdam, Andrew Bracewell, James Henderson, Pete Wilde, Kay Seymour, Greenwood, Sinclair Gore, Chris Watts, Kamillar Porter, Sweeney, Nicola Marks, Jane Heraghty, Anne Chan, Jeremy Reynard, M Oddy, Thomas Bate, Sabastian Stur, Anton Bungay, Kim Williams, Simon Clint, Mark Wilson, Simon Matthews, Kate Washington, C McAdam, Tracey Sims, A Ransen, R Waller, James Myerson, Kate Williamson, Anya Wechsler, Ed Moran, Jennifer Anderson, Nicky Henderson, Laura Townsend, Kate Hodder, Stephen Ward, Nick Burfitt, Natalie Heaton, Deborah Wake, Hirst, K Gardiner, Alistair Brit, Elizabeth Davies, Richard Baxter, Nicola Smith, Tracey Smith, Alex Hart, C Efthymiou, Mike Wells, Z Christie, F Saunders, Neil Abeysinghe, Rachel Bullock, J Philips, Rosie Peet, Philip Hammond, Sarah Al-Termini, Charlotte Davies, Philip Davies, Julia Rebstien, Lara Tate, David Banks, Kate Chester, Choong-Sian Fong O C J Thompson, Jasmin Hussein, Carolyn Cooke, Angharad Puw Davies, Sanjay Patel, Matthew Smith, Elizabeth Sapey, Ramani Moonesinghe, Michelle Lee, Rina Pancha, Stella Wong, Rachel Protheroe, Louise Tofts, Caroline Noakes, Eva Lew, Claire Plunkett, Vijai Ranawat, Mary Garthwaite, Adam Boyd, Hayley Barbet, Rosalind Tandy, Gareth Bashir, Russell Hawkins, Emily Watkinson, Helena Deeney, Anna Munday, Christina Thirlwell, Donna Gray, A Stanb, Ellis Hamilton, Mark Weatherall, Cathy Brice, Claire Mitchell, Baak Javid, Sarah Clark, Samantha Cole Haddon, Clare Cuckson, Eleanor Wood, Jonathan D'Souza, Stuart Benzie, Brain Chro-Kay, K T Porter, Sarah Lee, Claire G Harrison, Daniel Thurley, Lucy Meakin, Mark Braganza, Simon Harlin, Nick Haden, Charlotte Anderson, Paul Beirne, Paul Monks, Khan, Mohammed Ziaur Rahman, Samantha Stephen, Judith Littlejohns, Julia Maltby, Caroline H Costello, Hazel Wilkins, R Harisworth, Sarah Walmsley, Nicholas Conway, Suzanne O'Neill, Siobhan Whitley, Brian Lockey, Johanna Bell, Caphren Laband, Julian Harrold, Lawrence John, Clare McLaugh, Karen Julils, Elspeth Wise, Irene Chang, J Cheeseman, P Holmes, Andrew Douglas, Bryan Morland, Lindsey Smith, Lindsay Cosgrove, James Barry, B Choo-Kang, Jeanette Richard, C Harchie, Gordon Fetes, Jennifer Ketson, Karen Mitchell, Martin Chambers, Claire Neale, Stanley Chia, Yen-Ch'ing Chang Lee, Paul Kelland, Jonathan White, Rosie Davis, Kayode Adeniji, Lorna McCavat, Michael Chapman, Katherine Rank, Lisa Lewry, Paul Simons, Robin Johns, Catherine Scrutton, Peter Williams, Roger Alcock, Fiona Collins, J Mills, M Guttikonda, Fiona Black, Kirsten Henderson, David Bacon, Jon Biro,

Richard Griffiths, James Evans, Sarah Horn, Alison Stewart, Natasha Gilcrest, Sarah Gibson-Smith, Andrew Sykes, Roger Alcock, Marion Dimigen, Julie Baptie, Dominic Hennessy, Jeffrey Khoo, Peter Scholten, Amanda Clements, Julie Wood, Angela Luck, Patrick Fenny, Ruth Groves, Tim Caroe, Andy Curry, Helen Barker, Doug West, Georgia Libby, R Newell, Nick Green, Chin Whybrew, M Murray, Isabel Andrews, Beth Weatherley, Nicholas Brown, Tom Wright, P Crosbie, Lynsey McHugh, Edward Duncan, Kerry Gardner, Isabel Andrews, Emma Halliwell, Rachel Hoyles, Emma Wykes, Daniel Park, Jenny Dowler, Ambreen Kalhoro, Michael Hamblyn, Paul Barker, Bruce McManus, Joana Monjardine, Claire Neale, Monica Paris, Neil Abeysinghe, Ashlesha Dhairyawan, Anthony Cheesman, C A Mason, Zoe Astrouakis, K T Pother, Robert Henderson, M Sidery, Robin Johns, Morley, G Homill, M Cadamy, Jamie F Welch, Nicola Starritt, K Rice, Thereza Christopherson, Stephen Young, David Cairns, Amrit Ray, Stanley Chia, Andrew McDuff, Nilay Patel, Bobby Kumar, Maty Simpson, Serena K Ng, Paul Bishop, Bellemy, E Carling, Marcia Schofield, Sally Axelby, Adrian Cree, Jonathan Burns, Emma Spurrell, Andrew Sharp, Gavin Richard Speke, Megan Smith, Juliette Jackson, Mark Litchfield, Laurence Nunn, Kim Williams, Tom Konig, Natalie Morris and Luke Gompels.

I am grateful to Irene Wells, Jane Fox, Ann Coney, Ann Cassey, Vicky Ibrahim, Shazia Jamal, Maria Brolley, Fiona Oaks, Heather Roberts, Diana Walton, Jane Zuckerman, Pratiba from UCL and all the other elective co-ordinators in the UK who have helped.

Others I would like to thank are Mike Aratow, Sandy Green, Gita Murthy, Paul White, Ben Harrison, Catherine Walker, John Mathewson and Carrie Walker.

Section 1: Getting Ready

Planning Your Elective

The period you have for your elective can be the best and most rewarding time of your medical student years. It's a time when you have complete autonomy to travel anywhere and do whatever you want. With that in mind, you'll want to make the most of the trip. Organized planning and having the right contacts is therefore vital. This book is designed to give you a few tips on how to plan it, but more importantly, it gives you the contacts that can otherwise be very hard to come by. For those who don't yet know where they want to go, the ideas generated from these places may spark further investigation. There are a whole host of factors that you should consider in choosing where to go.

DO I HAVE TO GO TO A HOSPITAL?

Do not immediately assume that you have to go to a hospital for an elective. Most sensible Deans will see great potential if one of their students does, for example, research at NASA or forensic investigation in New York. You can push this further to diving medicine, joining a mountain rescue team or an emergency ski patrol. The world really is your oyster. Lists of such places are included in the 'Something different' sections of each chapter. Think about any hobbies or special interests you have ... can you squeeze them into your elective?

HOME OR ABROAD?

For some people, financial or personal constraints (or exam re-sits) may mean that they have to do their elective at home. DO NOT DESPAIR. There are still great opportunities to be had. If you're the academic type there'll be plenty of projects either at your home medical school or somewhere else. Think about what has really interested you. If you simply can't afford to go abroad, consider at least going somewhere different; for example if you're training in London, why not do a spell in Edinburgh or Dublin? Before you resign yourself to staying put, remember that there are plenty of travel awards for the taking. An award of only a few hundred pounds may well be enough to get you abroad and, if you pick a poorer area, the cost of living can be minimal. Whatever you do, do SOMETHING. It's never too late to organize an elective even if you have left it to the last minute or your original plans have fallen through.

DEVELOPED OR DEVELOPING WORLD HOSPITALS?

If you have decided on going to a hospital you need to consider what you want to get from your elective. Do you want space-aged hi-tech investigations that you may not get at home? If so, one of the large university or private hospitals in the Western world (especially the USA, Canada and Australia) would be a wise choice. This may also give a different kind of cultural experience showing how medicine can be with a big pot of money. Is it any better? At the other extreme you can try the more destitute developing world scene. Although you will learn nothing about positron emission tomography (PET), you will learn a great deal about common diseases and some that are rare back home. You will also be of more use to the hospital and more likely to be learning by experience than lectures. You may well find yourself sitting behind a desk with (or without) a translator on your first day and be expected to run a clinic. There is no quicker way to learn than this. Many students find this incredibly frightening at first; the patients trust you as they assume you're a doctor. DON'T PANIC. Most hospitals of this sort have very limited resources and therefore you'll only have access to a very limited weaponry with which to do harm! Make sure you have your Oxford Handbooks and the *BNF* to hand. Occasionally, things are very bad and students have found themselves the most-qualified (or least-unqualified) person around. In these situations you tend to learn how not to do things. Whether patients benefit in these situations is debatable, but it may be all they can get. Working overseas to be allowed to do things you could not do back home does pose some interesting ethical questions.

Also think about how much you need home comforts. If you're willing to rough it for a bit the experience developing communities offer can well make it worth your trouble. If you're on a tight budget, you may find you can live for next to nothing. If there is no way you can cope without a hairdryer or a McDonalds around the corner, try somewhere else. Along similar lines consider whether you want urban or rural life. If you are stuck in a bush clinic there may not be many clubs etc. at night. There may well be a great social life with other members of staff. If you need your Friday nights on the town, stay near cities.

There is one other tip if going to a developing country. It is sometimes the case that government run hospitals are underfunded, lack resources and have staff that may not be that interested in medical students. Missionary hospitals are also usually underfunded and lack resources. Usually though, they are more efficiently run, have staff that are trained overseas and often have a better social life. This book has therefore occasionally concentrated on such hospitals in areas where the government hospitals are not recommended. Wherever possible an idea of how 'Christian' they are is given so that you don't offend or feel awkward if it's 'not really your scene'. In general, most missionary hospitals and organizations are happy if you just 'respect those with Christian beliefs'; a few, however, require full participation.

As most medical schools give eight to twelve weeks for an elective it may well be worth trying both extremes of medicine.

ACTUALLY, I JUST WANTED A HOLIDAY:

Another very important consideration is what to do in your time off. If you are in a remote isolated place you may get incredibly bored unless the social life in the hospital is good. Under 'Elective notes' in the various sections, hints on how the social life runs and what there is to do nearby have been included. You can pick your hospital so that it is conveniently located next to a ski slope or beach. Remember that your elective is a big holiday as well. You may want to work for most of it and have a couple of weeks travelling. Alternatively, you may want to pop in the hospital for one day, get your forms signed then get out scuba diving. Whatever, think about where you want to go and how good the transport links from your hospital are. Where possible, how much work consultants expect has also been included.

FINDING OUT ABOUT PLACES:

Well you've begged, borrowed or stolen a copy of this book and this lists many places and gives ideas for electives outside of hospitals. Maybe, however, you still want something else. There are a number of places you can look for more information.

The Internet

The world-wide web is growing at a tremendous rate and is an excellent source of information, especially for the USA and Europe. Where available, web addresses have been included with hospitals listed in Section 2. A full list of American hospitals and some from other parts of the world is available on 'Hospital Web' (http://neuro-www.mgh.harvard.edu/hospitalweb.shtml).

If what you're looking for isn't there then try to use a search engine such as 'Yahoo' (www.yahoo.com) or 'AltaVista' (http://altavista.com). Using one of these methods you may well be able to find the name of a specialist in the field you want to study.

One big drawback of the Internet is it doesn't supply information on small hospitals, for example in Africa and on Pacific or Caribbean Islands. This book has therefore concentrated on such places. One useful site for developing world healthcare is run by the Medical Missionary Association (www.interdart.co.uk/mma/ovac/htm).

Don't forget to check www.medicsworldwide.com for updates on this book.

Previous reports:

Students in the years above your own will be able to recommend or warn you off certain destinations. Their advice can be invaluable. Ask them and look at their elective reports.

Hospital staff:

Consultants and other seniors tend to have buddies all over the world, especially in their field of interest. Ask if they can recommend people.

Organizations:

Many non-governmental organizations (NGOs) and missionary organizations (*see* Section 3: The Appendix) are happy to take students. That said, a few consider students to be a bit of a burden so don't get upset if they don't rush to accept your 'help'. The International Health Organization, Salvation Army, African Inland Mission (and other Christian organizations) are examples of those that have been very helpful in the past.

There are also organizations specifically for medical students.

The International Federation of Medical Students' Associations (IFMSA) (www.who.ch/programmes/ina/ngo/ngo-74htm) has previously helped with electives.

Europe (excluding the UK) is not a popular elective destination, presumably because of language barriers. The **European Medical Student Association** (EMSA, Club's Union, St Bartholomew's and the Royal London Hospital, Whitechapel, London E1. Tel: 020 7247 3185) has been set up to promote exchanges between European countries.

The **European Action Scheme for Mobility of University Students** (ERASMUS/SOCRATESE Programme) (UK Office, The University of Canterbury, Kent CT2 7PD www.ukc.ac.uk/ERASMUS/erasmus/) organizes exchanges (for a minimum of three months) between European universities. It is open to all subjects and even helps with funding. Countries involved include: Austria, Belgium, Cyprus, Czech Republic, Denmark, Finland, France, Germany, Greece, Hungary, Iceland, Ireland, Italy, Liechtenstein, Luxembourg, Netherlands, Norway, Poland, Portugal, Slovakia, Spain, Sweden, Romania, and the UK.

The World Health Organization has published a directory of medical schools though really this only gives addresses. Some of its information is now quite out of date.

The *Student BMJ* often has extremely good articles on electives in a number of countries, so keep an eye out there for more ideas.

CLIMATE:

You may have always had a burning desire to visit a particular country but find out what the weather is like at the time of year that you can go. For example, the Himalayas are incredibly beautiful and relatively warm in October, but at other times of the year they are bitterly cold and dangerous. Some of the hospitals listed in Canada are always in snow but certain times of the year are better than others. Ask at a student travel shop or look in the front of the Lonely Planet guide for that country. Also, remember that areas of large countries can vary tremendously. The coast of Australia is relatively cool compared to some of the deserts of its interior.

LANGUAGE:

Obviously it is vital that you can converse with both patients and the medical staff. Fortunately, English is often the language used to teach medicine even if it is not the local language. Also because of their education, many doctors in non-English countries (e.g. many parts of Africa) speak English. However, it is vital that you find out about this. In China and South America in particular you may get very stuck if no one speaks English. Do not be put off if locals don't speak English as there will normally be nursing staff or translators available. Even if that is the case, try to learn some of the language, the pleasantries and a few words such as 'Where does it hurt' . You will often get out what you put in. Some people will love to chat to you to improve their English. If no one speaks it you may get left by the wayside. Check the *BMJ* as courses in foreign languages are sometimes advertised (contact EMSA (see above) for more details).

SAFETY AND TO GO ALONE OR WITH FRIENDS?

If you're lucky enough to have friends, you may well want to go with them. This has some great advantages and a few disadvantages. The most important consideration is 'Are you going somewhere dangerous?' Many places, especially in areas of South Africa are really quite dodgy even for chaps travelling with a colleague. Seriously consider going with someone if you are planning to go as a lone female. On the subject of danger, try to avoid war zones. They may produce interesting stories but only if you're around to tell them. The other big advantage of going with someone is that it gives you someone to talk to, to share your experiences and generally have a good time with. Sharing travel costs (e.g. car hire) can also increase your spare cash. Problems may arise though if you fall out, if they want to go hiking while you'd rather be on the beach, if you discover they've been sleeping with your boy/girlfriend etc. Make sure they are good buddies before you go. Remember that death (of patients) is common in developing countries. If on your own this can be quite disturbing especially if you have no one to talk to.

Something you may not notice though is that with a companion you tend not get involved in the life of the local community as much as you would otherwise. You may not get quite the adventure or cultural experience you had hoped for.

With regards to safety, if you are in any doubt, contact the Foreign Office for advice (www.fco.gov.uk/travel). If going somewhere a little dicey, it is worth giving your home embassy in that country your details when you arrive so that if an emergency arises, they know where you are.

WHAT DISEASES WILL I SEE AND WHICH ONES CAN I CATCH!

Many Western countries will have the diseases you are used to seeing at home. They also tend to be quite safe from the point of view of what you can catch. If you want to see the things that are rare at home then developing world countries are the places to go. (*See Health Whilst Abroad* for more detail). Think carefully. Countries differ greatly. Nepal, for example, has TB and rheumatic fever, to name but a few, but is low in trauma and HIV. Some areas of Africa have been swamped with the complications of HIV and in some Zulu townships the prevalence is approximately 50%. The population you see in a hospital setting therefore has an even higher prevalence. Although this means you will see a wide variety of complications, you will see little done about it. These hospitals can only afford basic care with antibiotics and no more. The other consideration is risk to yourself. The needle-stick transmission rate is around 0.3%, that is incredibly low. However, the prospect of tests hanging over you if you sustain one can ruin your elective. ALWAYS USE PRECAUTIONS, including goggles. Some of these areas are very violent and so there is plenty of minor ops and suturing. Great experience, just be careful.

OK, I'VE DECIDED WHERE TO GO. HOW DO I APPLY?

APPLY EARLY. If you know what you want, write as soon as possible. Chances are someone else wants to go there too. If you want to join the Royal Flying Doctors, for example, you should probably apply during your first or second year at college. Even then, many associations now have links with Aussie medical schools and therefore can't take you. Some of the hospitals in Australia get booked up a year and a half in advance. Popular hospitals in other countries have similar waiting times.

If you have left it until the year of your elective, don't panic. Still apply. People drop out and places may still be available. For hospitals in developing regions it may not be so much of a problem, although slow postal services mean you should still leave plenty of time.

How do you get in touch? This book lists addresses, phone and fax numbers and where possible websites. Unfortunately, names of individuals have not been included, primarily to stop them getting bombarded with mail, but also because people move on at an incredible rate. You don't want your letter to get put in the bin simply because the addressee doesn't work there any more. The best advice is to try to find out the name of the medical superintendent or equivalent. Visiting the hospital website or a quick phone call can do this. Addressing your letter to a specific individual will increase the chances of getting a result. If this is too much effort, simply address the letter to the Medical Superintendent (for most developing country hospitals), the Chief Medical Officer (in Australia/NZ) or the Elective Co-ordinator or Admissions Organizer if applying via a University.

If the hospital is on the web, you may be able to find the name of someone in the speciality that you're interested in. Write to that individual directly. He or she may say that they would be happy to have you shadow/assist them. You can then write to whoever is in charge saying that Dr X has kindly offered me an opportunity to follow his work for Y weeks ... and you were writing to enquire about accommodation etc.

You may find while surfing the web that these people have e-mail addresses. Many people see it as more polite to receive a letter for a first correspondence. E-mail is almost like giving someone your home phone number. There is still something about opening a nicely presented letter (see below) accompanying a hard copy of a CV. The recipient will feel more guilt throwing it in the bin than he will dragging your electronic 10KB of text across the screen and onto the trash icon. Only use e-mail as a first means of contact if you are running short of time. For a similar reason, faxing should be saved for the second wave of attack. Include your e-mail address in your letter so that you can at least speed up a reply. If you're writing to many places in an attempt to get an answer from one it is usually cheaper to write than fax them all.

You've sent your letter but have heard nothing. For many areas it can take weeks or months to get a reply. Now you can start to fax and e-mail.

If you receive a reply then you **must** write back and confirm acceptance, or if you have had other replies, politely say that you have already accepted another offer. Never just forget it. They may be making plans for you and you are withholding someone else's elective place. By all means reply by fax/e-mail.

Miserable Medical Residence
London
Joe@st.cuthberts.ac.uk

Dr Jones
Medical Superintendent
The Tropical Island Hospital
Paradise

5th June 2000

Dear Dr Jones

I am a final-year medical student at St Cuthbert's Medical School in London. During this year of my course I have the opportunity to spend X weeks abroad discovering how medical practice differs from here. I have heard impressive reports from those that have previously visited your hospital and I am writing to ask if it would be possible for me to spend some time at the Tropical Hospital between X and Y, 2001. I really would appreciate the chance to study in Paradise.

Please find enclosed a copy of my CV and please do not hesitate to get in touch at the above address/fax number if you have any questions.

Thank you for your time in reading this letter.

With best wishes

Yours sincerely

Joe Bloggs

Sample covering letter

What if they don't speak English? Bear in mind that you're not going to get very far if you don't learn their language. If you want to write, say in Spanish, either get a Spanish friend to do it for you or visit http://babelfish.altavista.com/ This is an amazing translation service. Type in your letter in English and it will be translated. It may not be 100% correct, but the recipient will be glad you tried. You can then translate their reply using the same service.

BUREAUCRACY:

Do you need a visa to study or work at a hospital? The official lines for the various countries have been included at the beginning of each chapter. If you're from outside the UK you will have to enquire at the Embassy in your country for more detail (*see* Section 3: *The Appendix*). Having said that, you will get into most countries as a tourist. Obtaining a tourist visa is usually not difficult. Most hospitals won't check (or care) what kind of visa you have. However, this can be a dangerous ploy. The last thing you want is for the passport control not to let you in. This book is only allowed to give official advice and therefore the official advice is to get a visa if required. If you're happy to take a bit of a risk and say that you're just on holiday as you walk through … good luck. For many countries (especially in the developing world) you'll probably be fine. Be very careful in the USA and Canada, they may well require a medical as well as a visa. Hospitals there may also be keener to check for security reasons. Most places have a limit to the length of time a tourist may stay … make sure you're not going to exceed this. Landing cards often require an address for your stay in your destined country. Putting down a hospital is asking for questions. It is safer to get a visa.

FUNDING:

For most students, getting some cash is vital for their elective. There are many organizations that can help you out. BE ORIGINAL. A list of commonly used bursaries is included in Section 3: *The Appendix*. Drug companies receive thousands of letters. Although a few of these may produce results, most drug companies have specific funds that require applicants to write essays. It is still worth trying as this puts many people off. Other medical-related companies (there are thousands from nappy makers and baby food suppliers to those that make medical equipment) may well be worth approaching. If you can relate your elective to the company and state why they should sponsor **you** over any one else you immediately put yourself at an advantage. Canvass anyone and everyone. Offer a copy of your elective report on your return.

Your own institution may well have prizes and sponsor awards. If at Oxbridge, your college may be able to help a bit. If you went to a posh school they may have a bit of spare cash. Offer to give a talk about your trip when you get back.

Organizations such as Rotary Clubs and local churches are often keen to do a bit of fundraising for you. If taking money from Joe Public though you really should be doing an elective where you are of use rather than funding a trip to Bondi Beach. Offer to give a talk on your return.

Local companies may sponsor you (it has tax advantages for them). Apply to anyone you can link yourself with, from the local shops to the local brewery (after all, you've probably been funding them for the last five years).

You could also try making a bit of money. Can you sublet your room while you're away? Can you loan out your bike/computer etc?

Whatever, apply to as many people as you can and try to be different from the thousands of other letters they receive.

Some books that list organizations include: *The Directory of Grant Making Trusts* (Charities Aid Foundation), *The Grant Register* (Macmillan Press), *Educational Grants Directory* (John Smyth and Kate Wallace), *Sponsorship for Students* (CRAC/ Hobsons).

If you haven't already got one, you can also apply for a student loan (which unfortunately has to be paid back, usually over a five-year period from the April after graduation). Contact: The Student Loans Company, 100 Bothwell Street, Glasgow G2 7JD (Tel: 0800 4050100).

When applying for funding you should include a few items:

- A very nice (typed) letter introducing your application and reasons why it deserves funding
- A copy of your CV (see below)
- A copy of your research proposal if appropriate (see below)
- Ideally, a letter from your Dean confirming that you're not a fraud

RESEARCH:

You may be using your elective purely as a holiday, but if wanting help financially, wanting to win some prizes or even trying to produce a paper, a project can be an excellent plan. It can be anything from estimating HIV prevalence in an African village to high-tech research for NASA. Whatever, plan early. Often ethics committees need to be consulted and you'll want to work out a viable method for your investigation. Some organizations (*see* Elective bursaries) will reward you handsomely for your efforts. The Medical Research Council (20 Park Crescent, London W1 4AL. Tel: 020 7636 5422 www.mrc.ac.uk) has contacts all over the world.

You will want to write a detailed but brief research proposal that you can submit when applying for funding. It should not really be more than one side of A4 paper in length. Some important tips are:

- Have a good clear title
- Start with an Introduction/Abstract that demonstrates you've done some background reading ('It has been found that …')
- State clearly and precisely the aim(s) of your project (don't be over-ambitious)
- Outline your method, including the number of subjects you hope to use
- Outline how you will analyse your results
- Explain how what you may find will be of future use

Setting a proposal out in this standard 'scientific' fashion looks much more impressive (and hence more likely to get funding) than just stating a title in a letter.

YOUR CV:

By now you have probably written many CVs, possibly for your house jobs. Everybody thinks their CV is the best. In case you've never written one or want a few tips, below is an example of how to set one out. Sticking (or cutting and past-

Curriculum Vitae

Name: Joe Bloggs

Date of Birth (Age): 1st April 1980 (20)

Address: Miserable Medical Residence, London
e-mail Joe@st.cuthberts.ac.uk

Driving Licence: Full

Education: Dibelthwaite Comprehensive
St Cuthbert's Medical School, London

Exam Results:
GCSEs 5 Grade A, 4 Grade B
A levels Biology B, Chemistry B, Physics C

Medical Exams:
1st MB 54%
2nd MB 52%

Intercalated BSc:
Social Anthropology (2:2 wth Hons)

Papers/Abstracts:
One hundred and one uses for a chocolate teapot. Bloggs J, Snogs E. *Journal of Home and Garden* 1999; 13: 110–111

Previous Employment:
McDonalds restaurant summer job 1997–1999

Hobbies and Non-academic Achievements:
Fly-fishing and Blue Peter badge (1997)

Referees: Dr Dean, The Dean, St Cuthbert's, London
Dr Do Little, Dept of Social Studies, St Cuthbert's, London

ing if really good on computers) a photo will also make your CV more appealing (unless of course the rear end of a camel is more attractive!).

WHAT SHOULD I TAKE?

Without stating the obvious: passport, tickets, clothes and a toothbrush. However, there are things that you may not think of both for yourself and, if going to a remote area, for the hospital.

For the hospital and staff:

- British National Formularies. You've probably collected loads of these by now. Ever looked in one? You will need to now. If going to a developing country take all the copies you have no matter how out-of-date. You will make instant friends with the sister and clinic staff if you give them a new supply.
- Any slightly out-of-date textbooks that you're not going to use would also go down well.
- Drugs/supplies. You may be asked to bring a few supplies out. It's a very nice gesture to offer. If it's just a couple of boxes of gloves it shouldn't be a problem. For medications a bit more planning is necessary. Ask the hospital to send you a letter requesting exactly what they need. Keep this safe so you can produce it if any problems are encountered at customs. If they see a letter from their own country they will be more sympathetic than if they see a scrap of paper signed by one of your mates. Equipment for Charity Hospitals Overseas (ECHO), Ullswater Crescent, Coulsdon, Surrey CR5 2HR Tel: 020 8660 2220. Fax: 020 8668 0751 (e-mail cs@echohealth.org.uk) can give plenty of advice on what is legal/illegal to take out.
- Sunday newspapers/magazines. If you know that there are missionaries/ex-pats who have been out of touch for years where you are going, you will guarantee friendships if you bring them news from home.

For yourself:

- The (Cheese and Onion) *Oxford Handbook of Medicine* and the *Handbook of Specialities* ± the mini Kumar and Clarke. Wherever you go, these are vital, especially if you are going to be in a clinic on your own. Your own *BNF* will help as well.
- Stethoscope (obviously).
- Gloves and goggles. Most hospitals, even the most primitive, have these. However, some don't. If in any doubt take your own. If you have any allergies to gloves, take some you know you're OK with.
- White coat. Some places may expect you to bring your own. In others shorts and t-shirts are the dress. Take it just in case.

Other handy 'traveller's' items:

- Padlock (± chain) to secure your bag to roofs of buses
- A thin plastic sheet for dirty hostel beds
- Swiss Army knife
- Torch
- Sunscreen/lip balm
- Attack alarm for women
- Camera, notebook/diary (especially if you have to write a report when you get back)
- An old passport (hand it over in hotels rather than your real one)
- A First Aid kit (*see 'Health Whilst Abroad'*)

TOP TIP: You may be worried about losing your passport/visas etc. A cunning idea is to scan them into a PC and e-mail them to yourself as attachments. Then, if the worst does happen, even if all your bags go missing, you will still be able to get copies by walking into any Internet café.

INDEMNITY INSURANCE:

Once you've been offered a place you'll need to think about medical indemnity insurance to cover any 'mistakes' you make. For many people, especially those going to developing countries, this isn't a major issue. It will, however, be a problem in America, Canada and possibly Israel (which has the world's second highest litigation rate). You should ask your destination whether cover is provided automatically or whether you can purchase cover through them. Ask your defence union. The MDU and the MPS for example will cover most destinations, though not the USA or Canada. They can recommend brokers. The MDDUS has just started to provide some cover in the US. Obviously, this area is changing and you must contact your union for advice. Further medico-legal matters are included under the relevant country.

TRAVEL ARRANGEMENTS AND COSTS:

This is the fun part. With everything confirmed you can then go down to the travel agent and book your flights. Remember that discounts are available for students (as if you'd forget). Shop around. And don't forget travel insurance.

You should now be ready to go. Before you leave it may just be worth phoning or faxing your destination to make sure they are still expecting you. You've done all the hard work ... now go and enjoy yourself.

Working Overseas

More and more doctors and other health professionals are taking time out of the normal career path to work abroad. There are many reasons for this. An obvious one is to escape the pressures and strains of working back home, but this should by no means be a primary reason since, chances are, you'll have to come back one day. The vast majority of people want to travel to experience medicine in another culture. As medics, we are in a unique position. We can turn up virtually anywhere in the world, be welcomed and then be suddenly involved with the most important part of local people's lives, their health. There is probably no other profession that can offer this entrance into so many cultures.

Very early planning is extremely important in taking time out. Just going on a whim is asking for trouble. That said, if you want to work abroad and have found yourself without a job, there are a number of agencies that can arrange work in Australia and New Zealand with just a couple of months' notice. Reciprocally, locum work in the UK is usually abundant for visiting medics. You will get far better jobs though if you sit down and plan your trip.

If you are reading this you are obviously at least toying with the idea or working abroad. There are some questions though you need to ask yourself.

SHOULD I TAKE TIME OUT FROM THE NORMAL CAREER PATH?

You will get plenty of advice from seniors in your field. This typically ranges from 'I wouldn't do that … it's a competitive world you know' to 'Excellent idea – go for it'. Whose advice should you take? At the end of the day, both can be good or bad. It will depend on what you do and how well you sell yourself. You can guarantee it will be a topic of conversation at any interview and will help them remember you.

A very good piece of advice from a senior London A&E consultant is 'Go down the pub with a pen and paper. Have four or five pints, not enough to get drunk, but enough to get merry and honest with yourself. Then write down the five things you MUST do in your life.' If travel is one of them … read on.

WHERE SHOULD I GO AND DO I WANT PAID OR VOLUNTARY WORK?

WHERE and WHEN to go should be considered together. For your elective you probably know if you want a developed or developing world setting. This time you have to consider the need for paid work. If you need pay then you're probably looking at going to a developed country. Remember though that developing countries are often extremely cheap to live in and, if going through an organization, living expenses are sometimes provided for. You should ask yourself what you want to get out of this trip. Most specialities have obvious advantages for either setting. What would you enjoy and benefit from most? If wanting to do invasive cardiology, a trip to a high-tech speciality hospital may help your career more than listening to heart murmurs in Africa. If obstetrics is your forte, the frequency of complicated deliveries in a Third World setting may well be more use. If planning a trip for six months to a year there is no reason why you can't work in two or more places.

WHEN SHOULD I GO?

This is a very important consideration. If you're without a job then now is probably as good a time as any, although even locum work abroad can take a couple of months to set up (e.g. visa and medical requirements).

If you're sensible and planning it carefully bear the following points in mind. The earlier you go the less ties you have (mortgages, partners, children etc.) but the less experienced you are and hence the range of jobs available is less. The later you go, the more ties you'll have and you may well get trapped on a rotation.

Once qualified you could travel immediately. However, it is extremely difficult to get a clinical job anywhere if you haven't even registered in your own country. It really is probably a bad idea to travel in your pre-reg year.

Many people go before their first SHO job. This is a good time as you're not on a rotation and, as said above, probably don't have much to sort out at home. You still have to ask yourself 'How much use am I and where could I work?'. Some agencies in Australia and New Zealand require a minimum of three years' postgraduate work (and in Canada they often want some O&G and/or paeds work). Do not let this put you off. If you plan things well, going at this point can be very much to your advantage. Some organizations are now offering work that can actually count back in the UK. This means you can travel to Australia, do a six-month casualty job and have it count towards MRCP/MRCS etc. on your return. Make sure with the Royal College that they will recognize it before you confirm, but this is an excellent way of killing two birds with one stone. You may, however, be looking for something a bit different. You would imagine that developing countries would be grateful for any help available and, indeed, individual hospitals usually are (and hence writing directly will often give very positive results). NGOs and other agencies are often a little more picky however. They usually get a number of applicants and will take those with the most experience. Overall though, with a decent plan, this is a reasonable time to travel. Try to get a job for your return before you go (see below).

After the first SHO job (usually A&E) is another common departure time. The added experience just one SHO job gives makes you instantly more 'sellable', but remember, many agencies want those at the end of their SHO years. For example, ship's doctors are usually required to have a minimum of two years' experience as well as at least ALS or ATLS (posts are advertised in the *BMJ*). Apart from this, much of the advice is similar to that above.

In between SHO and Registrar posts is an excellent time to go, but if waiting till then, remember you may have ties. An irresistible job may also quash your ideas and you may have to postpone travelling for some time. The experience you have at this stage (especially if you have some O&G and paeds under your belt) makes you valuable everywhere. Locum agencies in Oz and NZ will snap you up as will NGOs and other organizations. This is currently a popular time for UK doctors to go as many people are waiting for Callman numbers and travelling (as well as research) can obviously help. The only problem is continuing to apply for numbers and jobs whilst you're away. You will obviously have to keep in close contact with someone at home who can check mail etc.

HOW DO I FIND OUT ABOUT AND APPLY TO PLACES?

This book has addresses and information on hospitals and other institutions as well as NGOs. You have a number of choices.

Applying directly to hospitals:
This is especially relevant if you want to go to a developing country, but many smaller hospitals, for example, those in rural Canada and Australia, are desper-

ate for people and will also welcome direct applications. This approach is ideal if looking for work for less than six months' duration. The main disadvantage is that you'll need to organize your own visa, registration, malpractice insurance and medical certificate where appropriate. Check hospital websites as this is commonly being used as a way of advertising jobs. When writing to a specific hospital try to address someone personally as this will give you a much better chance of a favourable reply. You can look on the web to find a suitable name or ring and ask for Personnel. For developing countries and small rural hospitals in Canada, Australia and New Zealand, you really want the name of the medical superintendent. As already said in 'Planning your Elective', you should include a covering letter stating why you want to work there and a detailed copy of your CV. Write as early as possible, especially for work in developing countries as the mail can take weeks. Try to include a fax number or e-mail address so they can respond quickly.

Let someone else do the work: You can let an agency find you work. This can either be a NGO if you want to do voluntary work, or a locum-type agency if you need paid work. This approach may give you less choice about the precise destination and agencies will usually only arrange contracts for six months or longer.

Non-Governmental organizations (NGOs): There are many different agencies that offer healthcare to those in need all over the world. Many are listed in the appendix. Some are missionary-based but most are based on apolitical and secular principles and receive funds from charity donations. Some run permanent hospitals, some provide relief aid where and when it is needed. You will almost certainly find a charity that would be grateful for your services in the area you are wanting to go. Be aware though that some NGOs can be quite choosey. If they have to go to the trouble of providing some preliminary training, organizing visas, accommodation etc. they will probably ask for at least a minimum of six months' commitment. Many now ask for around two years. Do not be disappointed if they do not appear grateful if you offer to work for a few weeks. For short-term work you may be best to apply to a specific hospital. Note that Médecins du Monde (UK) and VSO now take people for as little as three months. If it's disaster relief work you're after, an agency really is the only way. Although the work is usually voluntary most agencies cover expenses and some also give an allowance while you are away.

Medical Employment Agencies: For paid work, there are many agencies that advertise in the *BMJ* and equivalent journals. For Australia some can do virtually all the organization (including flights). Remember though that they often only have places that Australians don't really want to work in. They are usually remote. This may be great if you want an outback experience, but be wary of committing to a great deal of time if you don't know what the place is like.

If there's nothing in this book and you don't want to apply through an agency, look on the web. DoctorsNet and other medically related sites often advertise posts. http://neuro-www.mgh.havard.edu/hospitalweb.shtml is a very useful website that lists many hospitals around the world. Unfortunately, it does not help if you are looking for a hospital in a developing country that is not on the web. Asking colleagues in your hospital if they have any contacts and looking through previous medical students elective reports are other sources. The International Health Exchange (*see* The Appendix) produces a magazine that advertises jobs around the world. Visit www.medicsworldwide.com and look under 'Planning your Elective' for more ideas.

CONFIRMING A POST:

If you get an offer of work, either paid or voluntary, you must write back and accept or cancel it. If you have any concerns about a post, you can discuss it with the BMA (if a member), but there is little they can do to enforce 'working conditions' etc. since it is outside the country. If you want a post to count towards postgraduate exams, make sure you enquire with the appropriate Royal College before accepting it.

HOW WILL I JUSTIFY IT AT INTERVIEW AND WHAT ABOUT A JOB ON RETURN?

It's an excellent idea if you can get a job to return to before you go (hence the VERY early planning). They will obviously want to know what your plans are. If you can't get a job you will have to bear in mind that you will either have to come home early to try to get one, be able to apply from abroad or be willing to do locum work. Whatever, at some point someone is going to ask you about your trip. They are going to want to know why you are going/why you went. 'I didn't like Great Yarmouth' and other negative reasons should definitely not be mentioned. Emphasize the gains. Say that although you realize medicine is highly competitive, you are not wanting to race up the career path. State that you wanted to gain wider experience beforehand that you could then use in your later work. Remember, interviewers are usually not so bothered about acaedemic qualifications at interview, but rather the qualities of people they would enjoy working with. The kind of qualities that working abroad can enhance. Try to have some interesting stories from your time abroad or a good plan if you have not yet gone. So long as it is not obviously a huge holiday, most forward-thinking consultants see overseas work as a big plus.

FUNDING:

This may or may not be an important issue. If you have savings and have a paid job to go to there should be few problems. NGOs will often provide a small allowance. If you are doing something entirely voluntarily, your finances may be stretched. A number of grants are available (*see* 'Elective Bursaries' in the Appendix) even for those who are qualified. Further details of other grant bodies can be found in *The Directory of Grant Making Trusts, The Grant Register* (Macmillan Press), *Educational Grants Directory* (John Smyth and Kate Wallace), *Sponsorship for Students* (CRAC/Hobsons). You can also write to local companies, clubs and your church. If you're not earning (e.g. working for an NGO or just volunteer work) you can save yourself £140 by telling the BMA you're a 'medical missionary' getting free membership for a year. See the section on 'Funding' in 'Planning your Elective' for more ideas on how to raise cash. Money can still be paid into a superannuation fund while you're away. Some NGOs now pay into it and employers abroad should also be able to.

MEDICAL REQUIREMENTS:

Many countries require that an overseas doctor has a medical before practising. This is especially true of developed countries such as Canada and Australia. Details are given under the relevant country. A medical can usually be arranged through your GP, but you may be able to get the relative components done by hospital mates. For example, a CXR report, an HIV (± syphilis) test and Hep. B titre level are sometimes required. See 'Your Health Whilst Abroad' for information on how to organize this.

INDEMNITY INSURANCE:

Your current provider may well cover you for work abroad in many countries (sometimes at no extra cost). A definite exception will be for those wanting to work in the USA or Canada. For both of these, the MDU, MPS and MDDUS (in the UK) can recommend insurance brokers (see the relevant country). You must contact your provider if wanting to work anywhere abroad to ensure that they cover you, and to get advice if they don't. If they do cover you, ask for a letter confirming this and take it with you as it may be required when you arrive. For example, the MPS and MDU have reciprocal arrangements with most government hospitals in Australia and New Zealand whereby you are automatically covered. This does not however include private or GP work.

MEDICAL REGISTRATION

The requirements to register as a medical practitioner vary greatly. In the USA for example you have to sit a series of exams. In some Third World countries you probably don't even need to register. If going through a locum agency or NGO your registration should be sorted out for you, but if going directly you will need to contact the appropriate medical council for that country. As much information as possible has been included under the respective countries in Section 2 (and visit www.medicsworldwide.com).

WHAT TO TAKE:

Apart from the obvious travel items for yourself you might also want to consider taking:

For the hospital and staff:

- Spare *BNF*
- Any unused textbooks
- Drugs/supplies (*see* Planning your elective
- Newspapers/magazines

For yourself:

- The *Oxford Handbook of Medicine*/ Specialities and any books relevant to what you will be doing (e.g. tropical medicine)
- Medical equipment (e.g. stethoscope, ophthalmoscope etc.)
- Gloves and goggles if there's a chance they might not be provided. If you have an allergy to some types of glove make sure you take your own

Other handy items include:

- Padlock (and chain) to secure your bag to bus roofs
- A thin plastic sheet for dirty hostel beds
- Swiss Army knife
- Torch
- Sunscreen
- Attack alarm for women
- An old passport (hand it over in hotels rather than your real one)
- First Aid Kit (*see* Your Health Whilst Abroad)

A top tip is to scan in your passport/visas/degree certificates and e-mail them to yourself before you go. That way if all your bags get nicked, you can still get copies by walking into any internet café.

Have a quick flick through the Planning your Elective section as quite a bit is still relevant for planning work. If everything is organized well you should have few problems and you can start looking forward to a wonderful time ahead. The final job is to organize your flights (use an under-26 card if you can) and travel insurance. Give your destination a call before you leave to make sure they're still expecting you. Good luck!

Your Health Whilst Abroad

The main reason for travelling with medicine (apart from the holiday) is to see things that you don't see at home. This can be anything from weird tropical diseases and herbal medicines to trauma. Under each country is a list of the common causes of death, but in this section an outline of infectious diseases and other conditions that can affect you is given. Although these conditions are rare in most of the Western world, some are common in developing countries. It's good to see them, but try not to catch them. Hence read through the diseases and if you're going somewhere it is prevalent, get vaccinated. This does require some planning a few months before you go, as you can't always have all your jabs at once. It can also add quite a lot to your expenditure if you get them from a specialist travel clinic. The occupational health department of your hospital should be able to help and can usually get them for you free or at cost price. If you're friendly with your GP and he knows that you are a poor underpaid junior doctor (or an unpaid student) you may also get them free.

For your own health it is simplest to divide your needs into:

- What you need to do before you go
- What you need while you're away
- What you need to do when you get back.

Another occupational health issue is what will the host country require from you to work in one of their hospitals. For most developing countries no medical is needed. Where information is available, any specific requirements have been included under the relevant country.

If you are planning to travel with medicine, either working or as a student, get some official documents sorted before you go. Ideally the following test results/vaccinations should be drawn up and validated on a single document on official hospital or medical school notepaper. They should be signed and stamped by the college medical adviser or GP and preferably bear an official validating stamp. You may need to show:

- Hep. B status (indicating the titre level),
- A list of vaccinations you have had (with dates)
- A chest X-ray report from the last six months
- A statement of your good health.

A number of countries also require an HIV test before you can work. In the UK taking such a test can create problems, as when you tick 'Yes' to 'Have you had an HIV test?', insurance companies take it as a marker for risk behaviour. They don't appreciate that it was done as part of your work and by having a (negative) test, you are less of a risk for them. Up-to-date guidance is available from the national AIDS trust. If you have all the above you should have little trouble with occupational health departments in most countries (but see Canada which is an exception).

Most of the next section is written for those travelling from the UK but requirements are similar no matter what your home country.

WHAT TO DO BEFORE YOU GO:

Your own health:

Once you've decided on your destination, the first thing to do consider is 'Do I have a condition that means I should not go there?' If you've had your spleen removed it can be extremely dangerous to go to countries where pneumococcus or malaria are common. If you have asthma is it well-controlled? If you have a severe attack (possibly triggered by a strange environment) will your inhalers be enough or can you get to a (decent) hospital? Are you epileptic and would having a seizure put you in danger?

If you have any condition that may in some way be a problem discuss it with your GP/occupational health department before you go. This is vital. It may well invalidate your travel insurance and you may end up in a bad way and not able to get home.

It's also worth going to the dentist if you'll be away for a while or if you're planning to go diving (the expansion of air bubbles in a tooth cavity on surfacing can be agony).

If travelling from the UK make sure you have adequate travel insurance or if going to an EU country, get form E111 from the Post Office giving you free/reduced cost emergency treatment.

Is the country safe?

Political situations are always changing and watching the news is simply not enough. It is obviously a good idea to avoid wars, but in some areas political struggles and fighting have been going on so long that they no longer attract any attention. The Foreign Office can give advice (www.fco.gov.uk/travel/). Also ask anyone you know who has recently been there. Alternatively, ask the hospital you are going to.

Vaccinations:

About three months before your departure you need to consider what vaccinations you may require. A brief list is given in Section 3, but it is vital that you get up-to-date information. The list is only a guide. There are a number of up-to-date sources: *Doctor*, *Practice Nurse*, *MIMS* and *Pulse* magazines, your GP or your occupational health department. The Medical Advisory Service for Travellers (MASTA) a unit in the London School of Hygiene and Tropical Diseases (Keppel Street, London WC1E 7HT. Tel: 020 7631 4408) can also give advice. They not only give vaccine requirements but also a summary of the political stability of the country. Prerecorded health advice is available from the London Hospital for Tropical Diseases (0898 345081) or Liverpool School of Tropical Medicine (0891 172111). Another useful source is the Internet, though the question of reliability has to be raised. One good site is the Center for Disease Control based in Atlanta (www.cdc.gov). This is updated regularly but tends to be a little overprecautious (e.g. only drink bottled water in the UK). From here there are links to other sites.

TROPICAL DISEASES THAT HAVE VACCINES:

Yellow fever:

A viral disease transmitted by the mosquito in African and South American forests. The disease is usually confined to monkeys but 'jungle' yellow fever occurs when an infected mosquito infects a human. Although this is bad news for him there is also a real danger that he can then act as a host that transmits to mosquitoes that usually feed on humans. Once a cycle has been established in humans, 'urban' yellow fever is said to exist. Countries such as India (see chart) do not have yellow fever, but they do have a ready supply of mosquitoes to transmit it. It is for this reason that they require a certificate stating that you have been vaccinated if you are coming from a country that does have it. The vaccine is only given in yellow fever centres (ensuring vaccine storage, administration and certification is carried out correctly) so that an internationally valid certificate is given. A list of centres is included in the Department of Health publication *Health Information for Overseas Travel*, but your friendly occupational health department or GP should be able to point you in the right direction. The vaccine is a single live attenuated vaccine and the certificate is valid between 10 days and 10 years after it is given. Countries where yellow fever is currently a problem include: Angola, Benin, Burkina Faso, Congo, Gabon, Gambia, Ghana, Guinea, Liberia, Nigeria, Sierra Leone and Suda in

Africa; Bolivia, Brazil, Columbia, Ecuador, French Guiana and Peru in South America.

Typhoid fever:
Since typhoid is spread faecal–orally, risk obviously increases as hygiene decreases. This varies within a country (from the top five-star hotel to the student flea-pit) and also varies between individuals. In most areas of Europe, America, Canada and Australia hygiene will be fine, but if going anywhere where there may be doubt get vaccinated (it's a single i.m./s.c. injection requiring boosts every three years.)

Hepatitis A:
Like typhoid, Hepatitis A is transmitted faecal–orally and hence is more common where hygiene is poor. Two types of immunizations are possible, the active vaccine (conferring immunity for 10–20 years after two doses six months apart) and passive immunoglobulin (protecting for up to six months). These should be considered if visiting areas with reduced hygiene.

Hepatitis B:
Medics (including students), nurses and others who are at risk in the UK should already have been vaccinated and have had their antibody titres checked. It is vital to ensure you are up-to-date on this. A booster is normally required after five years. Enquire with your occupational health department. Areas of extremely high risk include Africa, Malaysia, Thailand, the Pacific Rim and Aboriginal and Maori clusters in Australia and New Zealand.

Meningococcal A and C:
Epidemics of meningococcal A are common in Africa between the Sahara and Egypt down to Malawi and Zambia. Areas of India, Nepal, Pakistan and Bhutan are also at risk. It's usually a problem in the first six months of the year. If staying there for any length of time it is well worth getting vaccinated. It is mandatory if going to Saudi Arabia during the Haj. It's a single injection requiring a booster approximately every five years.

Rabies:
Still a major problem in many countries. Australia, New Zealand, the UK and the Antarctic are rabies-free. Epidemiologically, it is divided into 'urban rabies' (transmitted through rabid dogs/cats) and wild rabies where a reservoir of disease is maintained in foxes, skunks, bats etc. Once clinically symptomatic, death is inevitable. If travelling where rabies is a problem and immediate post-exposure treatment is not available, pre-exposure treatment should be considered. This consists of two injections four weeks apart. If a booster is then given a year later, up to three years' cover is gained. Note: if taking chloroquine, it may cause problems. If you are bitten you still need treatment. Prophylaxis just buys you time and lowers the dose of the treatment needed.

Japanese B encephalitis:
Endemic in Asia and the Pacific Islands, Japanese B encephalitis is spread by culicine mosquitoes that normally live on rice paddies. Monsoons can cause epidemics. It occurs between North-east India throughout South-east Asia and the Far East. Pigs and birds are the main hosts. High fever, headaches and meningism with a 40% mortality occur in humans. A two-dose vaccine (one to four weeks apart) is available.

Tick-borne encephalitis:
Transmitted by ticks in the forests of Scandinavia, central and eastern Europe. You are at risk if doing lots of walking/camping. You should wear long trousers and insect repellent. If bitten, a post-exposure immunoglobulin is available in high-risk areas (get it within four days). If contact with long grass is unavoidable a two-component vaccine can be used.

Tuberculosis:
All tuberculin-negative school children should have a BCG by the age of 13. If

unvaccinated and travelling to an area of increased risk (Asia, Africa, Central and South America and the Pacific Rim) immunization (if tuberculin negative) should be seriously considered.

Some diseases that have vaccines that are rarely given include the following.

Cholera:
The vaccine is very poor and now not available in the UK. Just watch what you drink in Africa, tropical Asia, South and Central America.

Plague:
Occurs mainly in India, some parts of Africa and South America. Vietnam has quite a problem at the time of writing. However, unless contact with rodents is unavoidable it is very unlikely you will need vaccination.

VACCINES YOU MAY NEED BOOSTED:

Polio:
If not boosted in the last 10 years.

Tetanus:
If not boosted in the last 10 years.

Diptheria:
Although this is part of the routine childhood immunization programme, some adults may not be immune. Diphtheria is common in overcrowded areas, especially Africa, Asia, eastern Europe, Russia and Central and South America. If working in such areas vaccination or booster (if not boosted in the last 10 years) should be considered.

SOME DISEASES WITH NO VACCINES:

Malaria:
Around 12 UK travellers a year die from malaria. Up-to-date lists of the malaria status of different areas are available from the Malaria Reference Laboratory, London (020 7636 8626), Glasgow (0141 946 7120) and Liverpool (0151 708 9393). Remember that malaria status can change in different areas within a country.

There are three components to preventing malaria:

- Avoid being bitten by *Anopheles* mosquitoes
- Use the correct chemoprophylaxis (YOU MUST TAKE IT AS INSTRUCTED)
- Seek medical help as soon as possible if you develop a fever

Avoiding bites: *Anopheles* mosquitoes tend to bite indoors and at night. Wear long sleeves and trousers where possible and use a good insect repellent. More than 15% but less than 30% Deet is recommended, but some people get a reaction to it (test a bit first). Mosquito nets impregnated with parmethrin and mosquito nets over windows are recommended. Using an insecticide around the room in the evening will help further.

Chemoprophylaxis: Countries (and areas within) are divided into three categories with three different prophylactic regimens. In any category, start prophylactics (bar mefloquine) a week before departure to ensure no allergy to the medication and continue it for four weeks after returning. If using mefloquine, it needs to be started three weeks before departure to ensure no side-effects.

The advice in the table at the end of the Appendix is only a guide. You must check up-to-date information.

Current regimens are as follows but do check for up-to-date information (try www.vnh.org/malaria):

- *Regime A:* For areas where *P. falciparum* has not yet been found to be chloroquine resistant a once weekly dose of chloroquine (500 mg salt, 300 mg base) alone is recommended. It's usually well-tolerated especially if taken with meals.
- *Regime B:* Where chloroquine-resistant *P. falciparum* exists, mefloquine (250 mg salt, 228 mg base) once a week is recommended. Those with a

past history of seizures, psychiatric disorders or cardiac conduction defects should not take it.

- *Regime C:* Doxycycline (100 mg/day starting a couple of days before arrival) can also be used where there is chloroquine resistance. Some people, however, get GI side-effects and/or thrush. It should also be noted that it reduces the effectiveness of the OCP.

Remember, even with prophylactics, malaria is still possible and if you develop a fever seek medical attention (this can be up to a year after return). The fevers with malaria usually present with severe shaking and sweating. You feel quite well between them. If in doubt assume it is malaria and get to a hospital. In the mean time take quinine (600 mg = two tablets) three times a day for three days and doxycycline (100 mg) daily for seven days at the same time. Fansidar (a single course of three tablets all at once) is an alternative but fails occasionally (especially in East Africa).

HIV:
HIV is probably the biggest concern to medics abroad. It has become a huge problem reaching prevalences of 60% or higher in some areas of Africa. Avoiding transmission through sexual intercourse is hopefully fairly easy. For most, the real concern is from needle-stick injuries or receiving blood products if you become ill. It is important to remember that needle-stick transmission is reported to only be in the region of 0.3%. However, a needle-stick injury in an area of 60% prevalence with no one to talk to and no occupational health procedures can destroy an elective (it is thought that one UK doctor has died from HIV that he probably contracted while on elective in Africa in the early 1980s). A number of medical schools have now banned students going to places such as Africa for this reason. This is a shame, as a great deal can be learned from such places. Many people go to South Africa to see trauma. Unfortunately, this is probably the department where you are most likely to get a needle-stick injury. Think seriously before you go. Will you just act as an observer? When you arrive you may be the only medical person around and have no choice but to get on with stitching someone up. Are you willing to take the risk? The only advice possible is to ALWAYS USE UNIVERSAL PRECAUTIONS on everyone. Always wear gloves (double) and mask; always wear goggles (splashes get around glasses); always wear a plastic apron under a gown in theatre (you'll never find a waterproof gown in an African hospital and you won't be pleased when you undress to find blood, amniotic fluid etc. soaked through to your skin); always take extra care with needles and when assisting in theatre always keep your hands out of the way.

Some things such as goggles and gloves should be provided, but often they are not. If in doubt take some with you.

It is very difficult to get accurate information on HIV rates. A table of countries and percentage prevalence is simply not possible and fairly meaningless. Within a country rates vary massively and it is often small villages that have high levels, whereas the average in the country may be low. For this reason, wherever possible, an estimate of the prevalence at hospitals with high risk has been included rather than just a blanket X% for the country.

So if you've done all the above and you are fit and vaccinated, the next thing you need to do is pack a medical kit. It should include most of the things you are likely to need for your own health whilst away. Components are listed in the next section.

WHILST YOU'RE AWAY:

Whilst away you should take precautions not to become ill and know what to do if you do.

Precautions to prevent illness:
All the advice below is common sense, but it can be so easy to forget.

Trauma: With all the concern about vaccines, you may think you are safe once you've had them all. Sadly, you cannot be vaccinated against the common serious condition travellers get. You are far more likely to be involved in some form of trauma than you are to catch dengue fever. Be constantly aware of this and do things to protect yourself. Even if local customs are not to wear cycle helmets or seatbelts, it is still obviously safer to do so. If the bus has bald tyres, a smashed windscreen and a driver who is drinking, don't get in it. It's never worth it.

If a disaster does happen try to avoid blood transfusions unless life-threatening blood loss demands it. For some areas of particularly high risk you may wish to consider taking some cannulae, a giving set and plasma expander (see below).

Travellers' diarrhoea: Expect to get diarrhoea if going to India or where hygiene is not 100%. There are a number of things you can do to avoid it though:

- Try only to eat hot foods or fruit that you actually peel yourself
- Avoid salads, fish and meat unless you're entirely sure of their source
- You are best to boil water or use chlorine tablets or iodine drops in all water you drink. Alternatively, use bottled water but be careful if in any doubt of its authenticity. Famous (bottled) fizzy drinks are usually OK. (Say 'No' to ice cubes in drinks)
- Avoid milk and its products
- Remember foods such as coconut can provide a lot of fluid (for much less cost) that is safe. Maintain a high intake of fluids if it's hot or you have diarrhoea. (See 'Your Medical Pack' later in this chapter for more details of oral rehydration therapy (ORT)).

Swimming: Whilst on the subject of water, make sure any water you swim in is safe, both from drowning and from schistosomiasis (common in Africa). Either stick to swimming pools or the sea.

Sunburn: As on any holiday, wear high-factor sunscreen and try to stay in the shade if you're the type that burns easily.

STDs: Try to avoid collecting venereal diseases! They are very common in tropical areas. The locals may also want to kill you for messing with their people. (This is actually an important point. In some parts of KwaZulu-Natal in South Africa, just looking at a girl (not in any kind of admiring sense) can cause great aggravation.) The risk of death in overseas travellers is ten times higher from HIV than malaria (*BMJ* 1990; 301: 984–5). It is patronizing to tell medics to be careful and advising use of condoms should really not be necessary. Just remember, alcohol can make you forget.

Acute Mountain Sickness (AMS): AMS can occur in anyone at altitudes over 2500 m. It is far more likely to occur if no time has been spent acclimatizing and you have flown in or climbed too quickly. It is thought to occur because low oxygen tensions at altitude cause electrolyte changes which favour fluid retention. This is evident as peripheral, and more concerning, cerebral and pulmonary oedema. Symptoms usually occur within the first 12 hours of arrival and disappear over a few days if you climb no further. Occasionally it develops over a few days and worsens. Over 50% of people get it if trekking above 4000 m. The symptoms are headache, nausea, vomiting, fatigue, dizziness, sleep disturbance and anorexia. Of course, all these can occur with the flu or if pissed. Always however assume it is AMS and do not go any higher. Some divide AMS into benign and malignant. The above symptoms are the benign part. It can then worsen as oedema accumulates further causing breathlessness, dry cough (becoming productive with pink frothy sputum), severe headache, vomiting, irritability, drowsiness, and finally unconsciousness. AMS can and does kill even at 3000 m. For the benign symptoms it is best just to wait at that altitude. If they worsen, or any of the malignant symptoms develop get down as fast as possible. Get urgent help. Drug treatments are always secondary. Preventative measures include:

- Slow, graded ascent, each night above 3000 m should be no higher than

300 m than the last, with two rest nights every 1000 m. Sleep lower than the greatest height reached that day.

- Drink plenty of fluids and avoid alcohol
- Don't use sedatives
- Drug prophylactics that are sometimes recommended include acetazolamide 250 mg b.d. or dexamethasone (not as effective) 4 mg q.d.s.

The *High Altitude Medicine Handbook* (Pollard and Murdich, Radcliffe Publication, 1998) is vital reading for those working at high altitude.

YOUR MEDICAL KIT:

Things to obtain for your own medical kit and what they should be used for. Like on the ads, 'always read the label' before using any of the following.

For gastrointestinal problems:

Loperamide (trade name Imodium): Useful for diarrhoea, although the most important thing to do is keep yourself hydrated. It is useful to relieve pain if nothing else. Take two tablets with the first loose stool and then one for every subsequent one.

Dioralyte: Or other rehydrating mixture, especially if diarrhoea is severe.

Antibiotics: If you note blood with the stool or develop a temperature, a short course of ciprofloxacin should do the trick. If diarrhoea continues (especially if it may be amoebic or giardiasis infection) with nausea, frothy stools and lots of wind metronidazole would be a wise choice.

Cyclizine or prochlorperazine: May help if nausea and sickness is a major problem.

Oral rehydration therapy (ORT): Put one 5 ml teaspoon of salt with eight teaspoons of sugar in one litre of CLEAN drinking water and take 1–2 cups with each loose motion.

For allergies/insects:

Chlorpheniramine: (For example, Piriton) or promethazine is handy for most allergies, including those to insect bites. It also helps in motion sickness. It can make you drowsy, but this can also be an advantage if the itchiness is keeping you awake.

Insect repellent: (And often a net) are essential. *See* malaria. If you're really prone to being bitten, 'after-bite' type remedies are available.

For throat/skin infections:

Augmentin (Or doxycycline) is handy for a bad sore throat, most chest infections and skin that has become infected secondary to bites or sores. Combinations of amoxycillin with flucloxacillin can also be used.

For trauma/pain:

Analgesic: (aspirin or paracetamol or codeine/paracetamol combination). Note the latter can make you drowsy and bung you up ... handy when you've finished the loperamide.

Bandages and plasters: Handy for blisters.

Syringes and cannulae: These are for the adventurer who is going places you really don't want to be getting ill. Areas with high HIV and hepatitis levels are not areas to have accidents. Although taking your own cannulae may protect you from contaminated needles, it won't help you much if it is being used to give you infected blood. If you really are going to take such risks, a bag of gelofusin or similar may be a good idea (although the chances are if you need it, you're not going to be in a fit state to set it all up).

General things:

- Sunscreen
- Water purification tablets/iodine drops
- Scissors ± tweezers
- Antiseptic cream/Fucidin ointment

Elective medical packs are available from Trebova Medical Student and Junior Doctor Supplies, 7 Burton Close, Gustard Wood, Wheath Hampstead, Herts AL4 8LU. These include some syringes, Sterets™, cannulae, suture kit,

Steristrips™, triangular bandages, pins and scissors. You may be able to obtain these from your school or occupational health department. You are well-advised to carry a letter (get a qualified friend to sign it) stating that you are a medical student or doctor caring medical supplies in case of any trouble with customs.

WHEN YOU RETURN:

It's not over yet. If taking malaria tablets continue them for another four weeks and keep an eye out for anything unusual. If you feel there is anything wrong, a persisting cough or occasional fever go down to your occupational health department as soon as possible. They can arrange a tropical screen.

FURTHER READING:

- *ABC of Healthy Travel*
- The infectious diseases chapters in *The Oxford Handbook of Medicine*.
- *The High Altitude Medicine Handbook* (Pollard and Murdich, Radcliffe Publication, 1998)
- *Good Health, Good Travel: A guide for backpackers, travellers, volunteers and overseas workers* (Ted Lankester, Hodder & Stoughton, 1995).

Section 2: Destinations

AFRICA

Botswana

Population: 1.5 million
Language: English
Capital: Gaborone
Currency: Pula
Int Code: +267

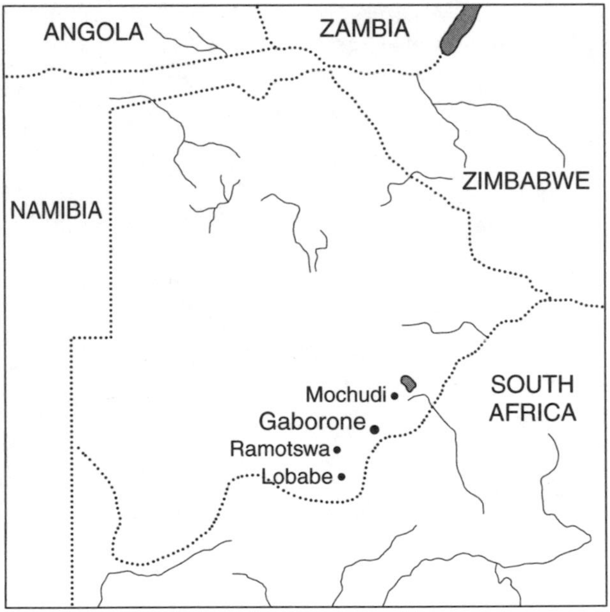

Botswana's population is mainly located in the eastern grasslands where diamonds provide a relatively stable economy. To the west lie the Kalahari Desert and the Okavango delta. Many areas are prone to drought.

✪ Medicine:

Primary healthcare in terms of protection against drought as well as adequate nutrition and basic health needs are the main objective at present. The doctor:patient ratio is a staggering one per 5150. The big killers are infectious diseases, TB and other pneumonias as well as heart disease. WARNING: The HIV prevalence is very high. Botswana has no medical schools.

◎ Climate and crime:

The warmest times are November to March, but June and July have the lowest rainfall. Generally, crime rates are low. Diamond smuggling and robbery are the common crimes.

Gaborone

Princess Marina Hospital

PO Box 258, Gaborone, Botswana.

The hospital: Princess Marina hospital is the main government-run hospital of Botswana and therefore receives referrals from many district hospitals. The staff are multi-national and they are often using Botswana as a stopping point on their way to somewhere else.

O Elective notes: They tend to be friendly and willing to teach and let you perform procedures. Most of the medical wards are filled with AIDS and TB patients. The paediatrics team is particularly keen to teach.

Deborah Relief Memorial

Mochudi, Botswana.

The hospital: Is a district hospital about 70 km from the city.

Balmete Luteran Hospital

Box 6, Ramotswa, Botswana.

The hospital: A mission hospital that is very popular. Apply early.

The Gambia

Population: 1.1 million
Language: English
Capital: Banjul
Currency: Dalasi
Int Code: +220

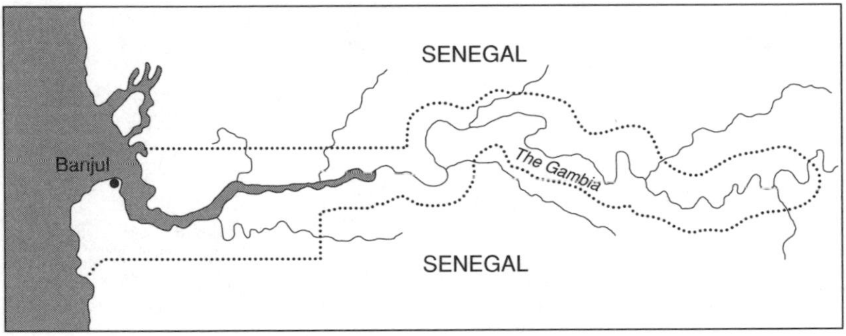

Gambia is a beautiful and interesting (if a little narrow!) country with lovely beaches situated on the west coast of Africa. Sixty-five per cent of its GDP comes from agriculture. From Banjul it is possible to arrange trips to Senegal. It is not a popular elective destination and most voluntary work has to be arranged through NGOs.

✪ Medicine:

Basic medical services are available to most of the population; however, neither medical care nor medicines are free. There is a vast shortage of doctors (only one for every 12,000 people) and a quarter of state doctors work in the main hospitals in the capital.

➲ Visas and work permits:

The Gambia is not a popular destination for elective students and hence no reliable information regarding the absolute necessity for a visa is available. Contact the embassy for up-to-date information on this and the need for work permits.

The Royal Victoria Hospital

Banjul, The Gambia.

The hospital: This is one of the main hospitals in the capital. There are many unusual conditions. They also arrange field trips.

MRC UNIT

Fajara, PO Box 273, Banjul, The Gambia, West Africa Fax: 495919/496513.

The MRC unit is principally for research, although it does have a small 40-bed hospital.

O Elective notes: This is great if you want to do research (for funding help *see* Wellcome Trust under 'Grants'), but there is little clinical exposure and you shadow on ward rounds. There is, however, good teaching. The beach is very close. You are better going to the Royal Victoria if you want procedures. Limited places available at the MRC and it is popular … apply early.

Ghana

Population: 18 million
Language: English
Capital: Accra
Currency: Cedi
Int Code: +233

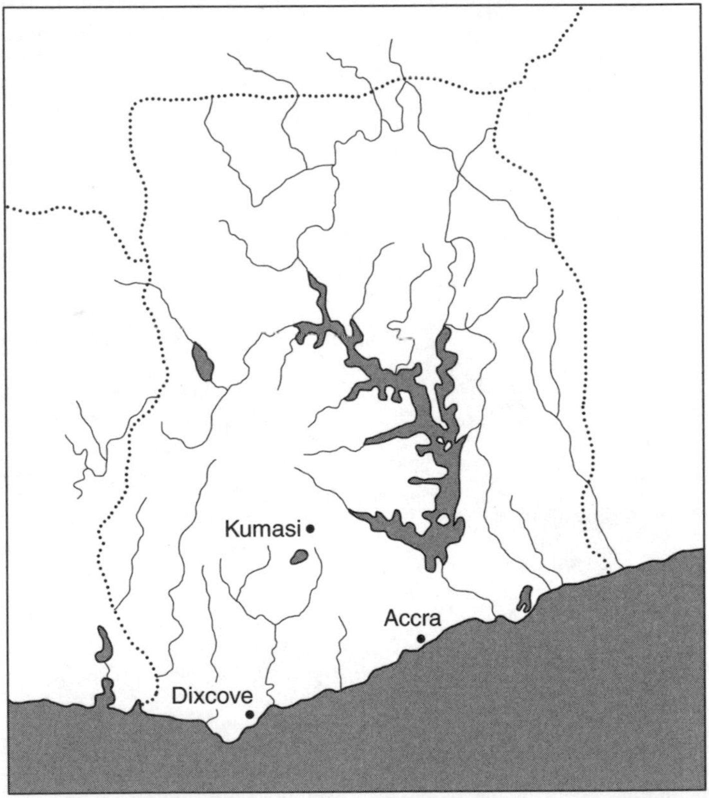

Ghana gained independence from the UK in 1957 and subsequently came under intermittent military rule. In 1992 democratic elections were held. Although not a popular tourist destination, it does have some beautiful beaches and coastal forts. The Ghanaian people are extremely polite and kind (although this can change if they want to sell you something!). Ghana is an excellent country to travel round in, being very safe and almost entirely unexposed to tourism (although this means that things like travellers cheques are difficult). It is politically stable now (unlike many of its neighbours) and there is no major tribal division. The people are exceptionally friendly and curious

about Westerners and problems with police and officials are rare. However, the roads are dreadful and all forms of transportation fairly erratic and uncomfortable. There are also supply problems for all non-domestic products, although Ghanaian food and beer are good. In the North the Mole Game Reserve has elephants, antelope and baboons. The Akosombo Dam, Lake Volta and the railway to Kumasi are all worth seeing. It is worth getting a multiple entry visa as this also allows you to visit the Cote d'Ivoire and Burkina Faso.

✪ Medicine:
Infectious diseases are very common, although public hygiene improvements have been of great benefit. Malaria, TB and gastroenteritis are seen regularly. Because of the economic situation, resources are universally scarce and patients often have to pay for treatments (even bags of saline). In addition to the hospitals below there may be a new hospital in Tamale soon.

MEDICAL SCHOOLS AND TEACHING HOSPITALS

Ghana has two medical schools.

University of Ghana Medical School

PO Box 4236, Accra, Ghana.
This is the oldest and main medical school and is situated in the capital which lies on the coast. One of its teaching hospitals includes:

Korle-Bu Hospital

K-Bu, Accra, Ghana.
The hospital: Korle-Bu is the largest of the teaching hospitals in Ghana. Like most state hospitals, resources are limited. It is pretty run down and hence some students have preferred Kumasi (*see below*).
O Elective notes: Since it's a teaching hospital there are well-organized tutorials and other students about. Good for practical experience.
Accommodation: Costs $50/week.

University of Science and Technology

School of Medicine, University Post Office, Kumasi, Ghana.
This is the only other Ghanaian medical school and is situated inland in Ghana's second biggest town. It uses:

Komfo Anokye Teaching Hospital

Kumasi, Ghana.
The hospital: Komfo Anokye Hospital is a teaching hospital in Kumasi. All the specialities are here, but community health gives an excellent opportunity to see rural Ghana. Many of the diseases seen at the KA are poverty or malnutrition-related and the expense and difficulty of getting to hospital makes late presentation universal. There are a lot of strange tropical diseases.
O Elective notes: The amount of support available on the ward is also very limited and there are many post-op problems rare to the West. There are a number of European doctors who give advice on everything, from where to change money to where to get football tickets. Kumasi itself is a beautiful city in the rainforest region of Ashanti, with woodcarving and weaving being commonplace and a number of hotels and bars. It is well-sited for travelling to other parts of Ghana. KA is a very good choice of hospital since Korle Bu in Accra is very run down and the capital is pretty unattractive. Similarly, district hospitals are often incredibly isolated.
Accommodation: There are about 35 students in their sixth (final) year who all live in an excellent hostel (with elective students) built a few years ago, with security, laundry and meals provided. The hospital is within Kumasi town, but the rest of the university is on a large campus about three miles outside town, with a supermarket, bars and a (very green) Olympic-sized swimming pool.

A RURAL HOSPITAL:

Nana Hima Dekyi Hospital

Dixcove, PO Box 5, Ahanta West, Western Region, Ghana.

The hospital: Nana is a 50-bed hospital encompassing general medicine, surgery, paeds, O&G and psychiatry. Ward rounds in the morning are followed by outpatients and surgery in the afternoon. Lots of malaria, typhoid and other infectious diseases. Rural clinics are run from here. Again, there are severely limited resources, to the extent that running water is sometimes not available. Dixcove itself is a colourful fishing village and food is excellent.

❍ **Elective notes:** It's busy with quite a bit of responsibility, although there is always supervision.

Accommodation: There is a local hotel, but previous students have been able to stay with staff.

Kenya

Population: 29 million
Language: Swahili
Capital: Nairobi
Currency: Kenya shilling
Int Code: + 254

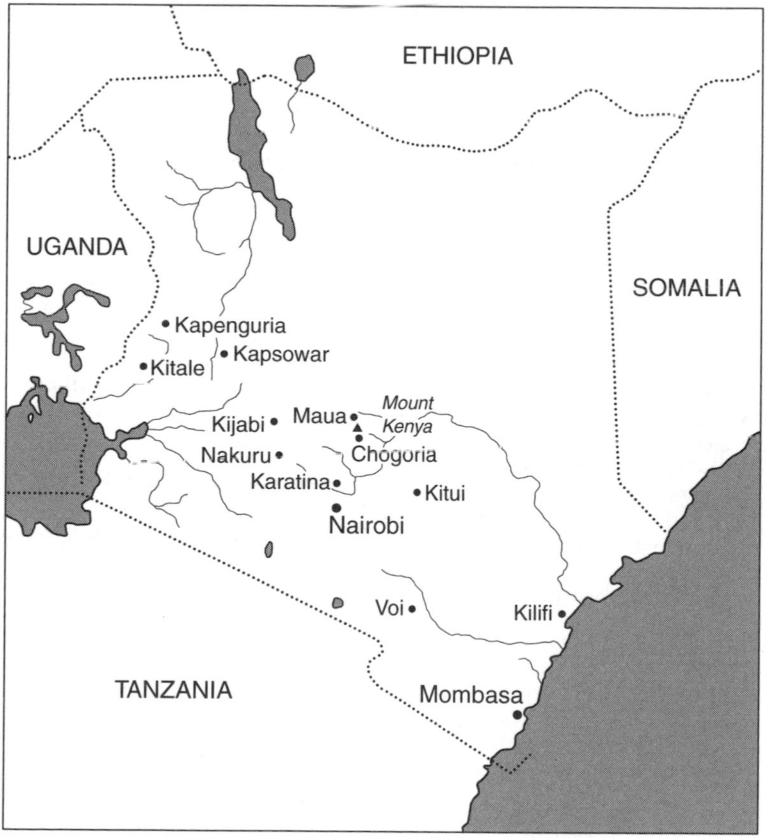

Kenya, situated in the east of Africa with the equator running through it, is probably best known for its game parks and coffee. Since its independence from the UK in 1963, tourism and agriculture (in the east) have become the country's mainstay. Recently there has been trouble with political and tribal violence. There's plenty to do: Climb Mount Kenya ($250 for porter, maps and meals over five days), visit Mombasa (the coast) and go on safari. Most people only speak Swahili (or a form of it), but English is understood in the capital.

⊕ Medicine:
Both state and private healthcare institutions exist across Kenya. The state system has become very run down with limited resources and, as wealth disparities between rich and poor grow, poverty-related diseases are increasing. Some people who work have a minimal private insurance scheme through their employer. The private institutions are mainly charity and mission-run hospitals. These tend to provide a better standard of care even though resources are as, if not more, restricted. In either, patients usually have to pay a small fee to be seen and/or the cost of medications. Most touring medics go to the mission/charity hospitals (even if they are not religious in any way) as they can get more involved, they are usually more hospitable, and there are usually other Westerners around. For these reasons, this chapter will tend to concentrate on these. Infectious diseases such as malaria, chest infections and gastroenteritis are common. HIV has become a major problem. It is estimated that HIV prevalence in Nairobi is around 11%, and 8% in rural areas. There is only one doctor per 10,150 of the population.

Note: Where stated, some hospitals are linked to the African Inland Mission (2 Vorley Road, Archway, London). They run four hospitals and 45 dispensaries in total across Kenya. You can apply for electives/work places through them. They require you to complete a form confirming you are a Christian.

➲ Visas and work permits:
Since the UK has introduced visas for former commonwealth countries, Kenya has reciprocated. You now need to get a visa costing £35.

A useful address: **Public Health Office, Ministry of Health, Medical Officer of Health, PO Box 438 Nyambene, Kenya.**

Note: Be careful in Kenya if you're a female travelling alone … you are regarded as a second-class citizen … always cover your legs at least to the knees.

Nairobi

University of Nairobi

Department of Medicine, Kenyatta National Hospital, PO Box 19876, Nairobi, Kenya.
Founded in 1967 this is the only medical school in Kenya. It uses a number of hospitals, but the principal one is:

Kenyatta National Hospital

PO Box 20723, Nairobi, Kenya Tel: 726300 Fax: 725272.
The hospital: A government-run teaching hospital providing care for the poor. Many patients are too poor to pay for their medications. It caters for most specialities (including cardiothoracic surgery) and has resources such as a CT scanner (even though it often does not work). Tropical medicine is big. HIV, malaria, TB and typhoid are common.
❍ Elective notes: As a teaching hospital there are formal lectures and tutorials (in English). It's handy if you know Swahili. Lots of procedures and signs. Taxis are expensive but safer than buses. Don't go around Downtown at night.
Accommodation: Stay at Nairobi Youth Hostel; basic, but only a five-minute walk from the hospital.

The Aga Khan Hospital

PO Box 30270, Nairobi, Kenya.
The hospital: Built by charitable donations, it serves both insurance populations (the rich and poor). It has departments in medicine, surgery, ortho, neuro, paeds, O&G and A&E.
❍ Elective notes: Is well set up for elective student and can offer time in any of the above.
Accommodation: Not available to elective students. The YMCA offers cheap flats for £50–80/month.

HOSPITALS OUTSIDE THE CAPITAL:

Chogoria

PCEA Chogoria Hospital

PO Box 35, Chogoria, Kenya Tel: 0166 22620 Fax: 0166 22122 e-mail: chogoria@africaonline.co.ke

The hospital: Chogoria is a 200–300 bed mission hospital situated on the slopes of Mount Kenya, about five hours (200 km) north of Nairobi. It has two surgical, two medical, paeds and maternity wards as well as outpatients, ophthalmic, dental and community health departments. It is very well-run by African standards, relying on patients' fees and charity. Drugs are always available. There are lots of tropical diseases – malaria, leprosy, TB, rheumatic heart disease, heart failure, nephrotic syndrome and HIV (prevalence approx 10% in surrounding area). There are usually six to eight doctors from all over the world as well as Africa. The nursing staff kindly translate.

O Elective notes: Elective students spend their first week with a doctor and then are set free, being first on-call and prescribing. You do your own ward rounds, outpatient consultations, lumbar punctures, paracentesis, bloods (be careful), catheterizations and assist in theatre. Lots of signs and few investigations. The doctors are all very relaxed and supportive which all goes to make this a fantastic elective. Write to them very early as they only take two students at a time.

Accommodation: Great – a small cottage for two students with cooker, fridge, bath, flushing loo and there's a swimming pool on the staff compound.

Kapenguria

West Pokot District Hospital

PO Box 63, Kapenguria, Kenya.

Kapsowar

AIC Kapsowar Hospital

PO Box 68, Kapsowar, Kenya (linked to African Inland Mission).

The hospital: A mission hospital (and the cheapest for patients to attend) in the Rift Valley. It is very rural. There are three doctors with midwives and nurses from the West.

O Elective notes: There is a 1:4 on-call rota for students. You can have as much responsibility as you are happy with but back up is always available. Rural clinics are also run. You are supposed to apply through the AIM.

Accommodation: Provided in a very nice house with mod-cons.

Karatina

PCEA Tomotomo Hospital

Private Bag, Karatina, Kenya.

The hospital: In a rural area 80 miles north of Nairobi. It is government-run and has 180 beds. Patients pay a small fee for treatment. There are usually around three doctors and it is very busy. Lots of TB, malaria, HIV and p.v. bleeding due to illegal abortions.

O Elective notes: It is busy and medical students help is greatly appreciated. There is a 1:3 rota for on-call. There are plenty of practical procedures and there is always someone to help. Highly recommended.

The Presbyterian Mission Hospital

Tumu Tumu, PO Karatina

e-mail tumutumu@africaonline.co.ke

Kijabi

Kijabi Medical Centre

PO Box 20, Kijabe, Kenya (linked to Africa Inland Mission).

The hospital: A 208-bed general hospital in rural Kenya, one hour's drive from Nairobi. It is at 7500 ft overlooking the Great Rift Valley. The site also has a church, schools and Bible college. One hundred and twenty-five patents are seen in the OPD a day and a mobile clinic offers women's and children's care to villages 12 times a month. There is a casualty, O&G, paeds and general medical, and surgical male and female wards. Student nurses are trained here to recognize common diseases and run rural dispensaries. A small fee is charged to patients for services. Trauma, HIV, malaria, TB, diabetes and hypertension are common.

O Elective notes: There are usually a couple of students from Nairobi Univer-

sity medical school and it is a well-established elective destination. On-call is every third night and you are very well supported by staff. Note, this is a very Christian setting, Bible study in the mornings, lots of discussion with patients about God and literature given to them at the end of consultations. Language here is Kiku. The nurses translate for you.
Accommodation: Available with cooker, fridge and washing machine (US$5 (372.65 KES) day).

Kikuyu

PCEA Hospital

Kikuyu, PO Box 45, Kenya Tel: 154 32412
Fax: 154 32413
e-mail pceagenhosp@maf.org

The hospital: Has female and male, paeds wards, an orthopaedic clinic and casualty. Inpatients have to put a deposit of 5000 KSH (£50) down to ensure that they pay for investigations at the end. Guards with clubs allegedly ensure they don't escape. HIV and TB are common. Most doctors are Kenyan or from the US.
○ **Elective notes:** Students are on call two to three times a week with the on-call doctor.
Accommodation: Provided.

Kilifi

Kilifi District Hospital (The Wellcome Trust's Kemri Costal Unit)

PO Box 230, Kilifi, Kenya.

The hospital: Kilifi District Hospital is a medium-sized general hospital. It is also home to the Wellcome Trust's Kemri unit which carries out extensive research into malaria (especially in children) in East Africa (works in conjunction with Oxford University). Here you can either do a lab-based project and/or clinical work. In paediatrics at least there is a great deal of interesting pathology. Most illness is related to malaria, gastroenteritis or malnutrition. There is less HIV than in other parts of Kenya. The Wellcome Trust runs an eight-bedded paediatric intensive care unit equipped to Western standards. This contrasts markedly with the poor facilities in the rest of the hospital. The maternity unit has no running water and no obstetrician working there regularly. The British doctors doing research help out. Kilifi itself is a small seaside village situated 19 km north of Mombasa. It sits directly on the Indian Ocean and has a population of about 1000.
○ **Elective notes:** The staff are friendly, but do expect you to do a bit of work. There are a few procedures to do and patients to present at unit meetings. On the whole though, life is pretty relaxed. The beaches are spectacular, you can scuba-dive or hop up to Watamu or down to Mombasa at weekends. Integrate yourself with the friendly locals or the VSO workers if you're looking for drinking buddies. The social life has very good reports. This elective is repeatedly thoroughly recommended.
Accommodation: A flat right in the middle of the village (approx £1.50 (178.11 KES)/night).
Grants: Look for The Wellcome Trust under 'Bursaries'.

Kitui

Mutomo Hospital

The Sisters of Mercy, PO Box 16, Mutomo, Kitui, Kenya Tel: Mutomo 16.

The hospital: Established by an order of Irish nuns in 1964. It now has 130 beds and a major and minor operating theatre. It is run by seven sisters and two doctors. Malaria, AIDS (10% prevalence in blood donors) and leprosy are common.
Accommodation: Provided.

Maua

Maua Methodist Hospital

PO Box 63, Maua, Nyambene, Kenya
Tel: 0167 21003/21107 Fax: 0167 21121
e-mail linmaua@maf.org

The hospital: Maua Methodist Hospital is a 200–300 bed hospital serving a large, widespread rural community in the eastern foothills of Mount Kenya at

6000 ft. It has male, female, paeds and maternity wards. Like many mission hospitals it is greatly overcrowded (especially maternity and during dysentery season) and lacking funds. Patients pay 85 shillings (about £1, but one shilling buys a banana) to be seen. Malaria, dysentery, machete wounds, leprosy, HIV, rheumatic fever, malnutrition and parasitic worms are the order of the day. Maua is a relatively violent area and there is a high incidence of serious trauma. There are rural clinics (petrol permitting).
O Elective notes: This is a popular elective destination (35 students a year). Medical students are integral to the running of the hospital, as the doctors are unable to cope with the workload. Some students have not found the nursing staff particularly helpful. However, the students from the nursing college and other medical students are friendly. The medical experience is great as students are first on call at night and take outpatient clinics (a cross between A&E and a GPs surgery). There's little back up from the doctors. Although there's quite a bit of it, Maua is not a great place to do trauma as the HIV rate is high and nurses do all the suturing (they're better than you at it and you're more useful diagnosing and prescribing). The night rota is an inaccurate 1:3. A couple of students have said they felt they learned little and were taken for granted. There are plans to make an elective here a minimum of eight weeks. If that is the case, think seriously before going as it can be hard work. The hospital would like students to play a part in the religious side of the hospital, but this is not compulsory. Smoking and alcohol are prohibited within the hospital grounds.
Accommodation: Provided with the other students.

Mombasa

St Luke's Hospital
PO Box 16, Kaloleni, Mombasa, Kenya.
The hospital: A 150-bed missionary hospital run by one doctor. It is very busy with limited facilities. Many beds are shared between two or three patients. Cholera epidemics, malaria, tetanus and HIV (~40% prevalence in some villages) are common. Lots of interesting tropical medicine. Kaloleni is 50 km outside Mombasa. There are a few shops in the village.
O Elective notes: Learn by doing and observing rather than direct teaching. It can get quite stressful.
Accommodation: Very basic (water collected from rainwater tank). There's intermittent electricity and a gas cooker. It's clean and comfortable.

Nakuru

Provincial General Hospital
PO Box 71, Nakuru, Kenya.
The hospital: The referral centre for the Rift Valley province with medical, surgical, paeds, O&G, TB and neonate wards. There is a large outpatients and casualty. They are very short of resources and staff. Common diseases include malaria, TB and HIV (over half the inpatient population is HIV positive).
O Elective notes: Students are welcomed. The amount of 'hands on' is up to you. Most is observing. Students have no on-call duties.
Accommodation: Elective students need to stay at the Carnation Hotel in the centre of town. You can go and explore the Rift Valley, but it can get very lonely if you are on your own.

Nyans
Nyans District General Hospital, Nyans, Kenya.

Via Kitale
The District Hospital, Kapenguria, PO Makutano, Via Kitale, Kenya.
The Catholic Mission Hospital, Otrum, Via Kitale, Kenya.

Voi
Moi Hospital, PO Box 18, Voi, Kenya.

Lesotho

Population: 2.1 million
Official Languages: English and Sesotho
Capital: Maseru
Currency: Loti
Int Code: +266

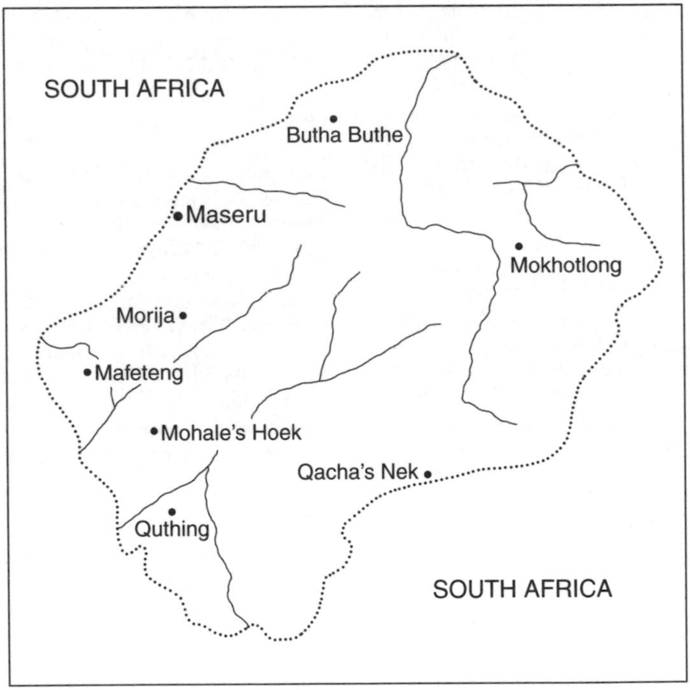

Since Lesotho is entirely surrounded by South Africa, it is entirely dependent on its neighbour for transport links to the rest of the world. It is a mountainous and beautiful country and the new highland water scheme aims to generate electricity for export. Its military rule ended in 1993; however, it is still a very poor country as its health statistics show. It is not a common elective destination. There are no medical schools.

✪ Medicine:

Health standards are generally poor with low life expectancy and high infant mortality. Both private and government-run hospitals exist (*see below*). There is also a flying doctor service, but this does not cover the highlands adequately (only 13,300 people live in the capital Maseru). The leading causes of mortality are: tuberculosis, parasitic diseases and malnutrition. Doctor:population ratio is a staggering 1:18,600.

➲ Visa and work permits:

Citizens of Australia, western Europe (including the UK) and most of the world do not need a visa to enter Lesotho. However, citizens of the USA, India, Pakistan, China and the Far East do. For them a single entry visa costs £5 (valid for three months). For more information and information regarding work permits write to the High Commission.

To obtain a licence to practise contact: The Lesotho Medical, Dental and Pharmacy Council, PO Box MS 726, Maseru. You need your diploma and a certificate of good practice from your previous employer.

A useful address: The Principal Secretary, The Ministry of Health, PO Box 514, Maseru 100, Lesotho Tel: 314404 Fax: 310467.

GOVERNMENT HOSPITALS:

Botsabelo Hospital, Private Bag A149, Maseru 100, Lesotho Tel: 312353.
Butha Buthe Hospital, PO Box 514, Maseru 100, Lesotho Tel: 4602210.
Leribe Hospital, c/o PO Box 514, Maseru 100, Lesotho Tel: 400305.
Machabeng Hospital, PO Box 8, Qacha's Nek 600, Lesotho Tel: 950229.
Mafeteng Hospital, c/o PO Box 514, Maseru 100, Lesotho Tel: 700208/700377.
Mohale's Hoek Hospital, PO Box 337, Mohale's Hoek 800, Lesotho Tel: 785210/785292.
Mohlomi Mental Hospital, PO Box 540, Maseru 100, Lesotho Tel: 313744.
Mokhotlong Hospital, PO Box Mokhotlong, Maseru 100, Lesotho Tel: 920360.
Queen Elizabeth II Hospital, PO Box 122, Maseru 100, Lesotho Tel: 312501.
Quthing Hospital, PO Box 3, Quthing 700, Lesotho Tel: 750213/750203.
Teyateyaneng Hospital, PO Box 514, Maseru 100, Lesotho Tel: 500272.

PRIVATE HOSPITALS:

Maluti Seventh-Day Adventist Hospital, PO Box MG11, Mapoteng, Lesotho Tel: 540203.
Maseru Private Hospital, Private Bag A58, Maseru 100, Lesotho Tel: 313261/313260 Fax: 310142.
Scott Hospital, Hospital Road, Private Bag Morija, Lesotho Tel: 360209.
St Joseph's Hospital, PO Roma 180, Lesotho Tel: 340206.

DEFENCE HOSPITAL:

Makoanyane Military Hospital, Private Bag A166, Maseru 100, Lesotho.

Madagascar

Population: 15 million
Languages: Malagasy and French
Capital: Antananarivo
Currency: Malagasy franc
Int Code: +261

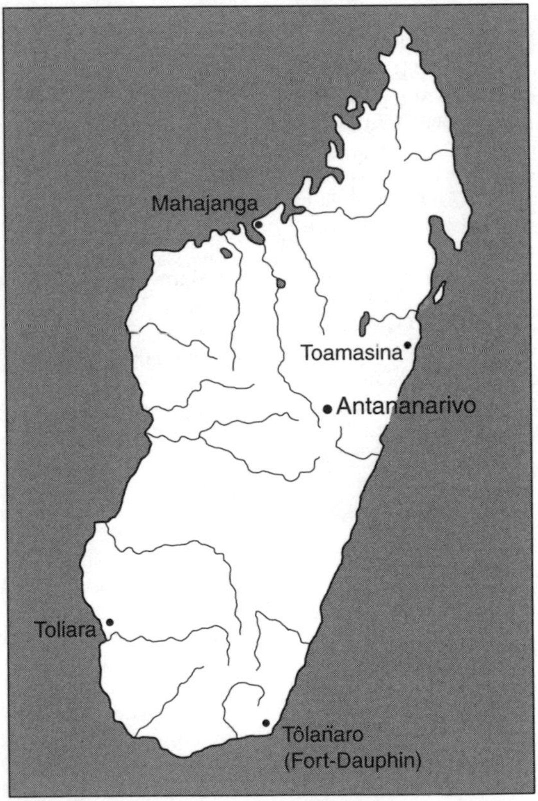

Madagascar is the third poorest country and the fourth largest island in the world (twice the size of the UK). The people are fantastically hospitable. Outside of the hospitals there are wonderful beaches (beware of sharks) and scenery. This can be a real adventure ... the odd cyclone and some amazing wildlife. It now has a multiparty democracy. French is spoken widely and is the usual language of hospital work so a bit of knowledge is essential. Malagasy has 12 completely different dialects. Have a go!

✪ Medicine:

A highly inefficient and under-funded state healthcare system can't cope and private hospitals have now been set up for those with any money. Infectious diseases such as malaria are extremely common. There have been outbreaks of bubonic plague in recent years. It is thought that there is only one doctor per 8100 patients. HIV is not a major problem and hence, if you're worried about needle-sticks, it's a good place for Third World medicine without the high risks. Only 3% of the population is over 65; therefore there's effectively no geriatrics.

➲ Visas and work permits:
Enquire with the embassy as it is not a common elective destination and no clear information is available. At present, to work you need to register with the Ordre de Médecins, Place Charles Renel, Antaninandro, Antananarivo. Some special arrangements exist with France.

◎ Climate and crime:
Madagascar has a tropical coast, temperate inland and near desert south. Cyclones are pretty common. Crime is not a major problem but is rising.

Note: To arrange electives here it is best to write in French. Try to enclose an international pre-paid reply coupon as most hospitals are really strapped for cash.

MEDICAL SCHOOLS AND TEACHING HOSPITALS:

Université D'Antananarive
Faculté de Médecine, BP 375, Antananarivo 101, Madagascar.
This is the principal medical school of Madagascar (founded in 1962). They can arrange electives in their main teaching hospital:

Befelatanana General Hospital (Hôpital Général Befelatanana)
PO Box 2097, 101 Antananarivo, Madagascar.
The hospital: Is the state run public hospital and the teaching hospital. The hospital provides free service and the patients are very poor. It has very restricted facilities. Drugs and even soap are in short supply. Rheumatic fever, TB, malaria and nephrotic syndrome (secondary to traditional drug use) are all common. The doctors have amazing dedication.

Mahajanga

Université de Madagascar
Faculté de Médecine, Etablissement d'Enseignment supérieur des Sciences de la Santé, Ambodrona, Mahajanga, Madagascar.
This is the only other medical school.

Hopitaly Loterana Antanimalandy
BP 653, Mahajanga-401, Madagascar.
The hospital: A Lutheran hospital about 8 km out of town. Due to the very poor conditions there is a great deal of pathology to be seen.
Accommodation: Difficult to arrange. Previous visitors have made friends with the local Lutheran missions and obtained accommodation through them.

Fort-Dauphin

Hopitaly Loterana Manambara
BP 108, Fort-Dauphin (614), Madagascar.
The hospital: Manambaro Lutheran Hospital is a small (50 bed) mission hospital with four doctors in a small fairly isolated village. Specialities include medicine, surgery, paediatrics and O&G. It can be a bit quiet, so do a bit of everything. Common illnesses include malaria, schistosomiasis, typhoid, diarrhoea and dehydration. Equipment is limited although there are ECHO, ECG and X-ray facilities. French is not spoken widely here. You will need a translator. Don't expect to improve your French at all.
O Elective notes: A normal day consists of ward rounds at 7.30 am, a couple of operations and outpatients in the afternoon. There is obviously not much to do in the local vicinity, but at weekends you can get out into the nearby town of Fort-Dauphin which is beautiful.

Accommodation: Provided in a guest house (£3 (31,817 MGF) a night) with a cook/housekeeper.

Toliara

Centre Hospitalier Regional (Hôpital Principal de Toliara)

Toliara, Southern Madagascar.

The hospital: is a relatively attractive hospital with some new equipment. It is fairly busy. Common conditions include typhoid, hepatitis, rheumatic fever, malaria, malnutrition and recently plague.

O Elective notes: It has previously been difficult to arrange. They usually welcome you in, however. All ward rounds are in French so some knowledge is ideal. Procedures can be done in A&E. There are some beautiful beaches close by.

Tamatave

Hôpital Principal de Toamasina

Toamasina, Madagascar.

The hospital: In Tamatave (the country's largest port with a population of 100,000), a mile north of the town centre (right on the beach). It runs like a small DGH with X-rays and ECHO. It has 400 beds with a two-tier system of care.

O Elective notes: You can do medicine, surgery, O&G, A&E or Radiology. There's a huge range of conditions to see: typhoid, malaria, TB and schistosomiasis are the bread and butter. Take any books you don't want and *BNFs*. There is a sandy beach near by but don't swim (sharks). Write to the Medécin-Chef.

Malawi

Population 11 million
Languages: Chewa and English
Capital: Lilongwe
Currency: Malawian kwacha
Int Code +265

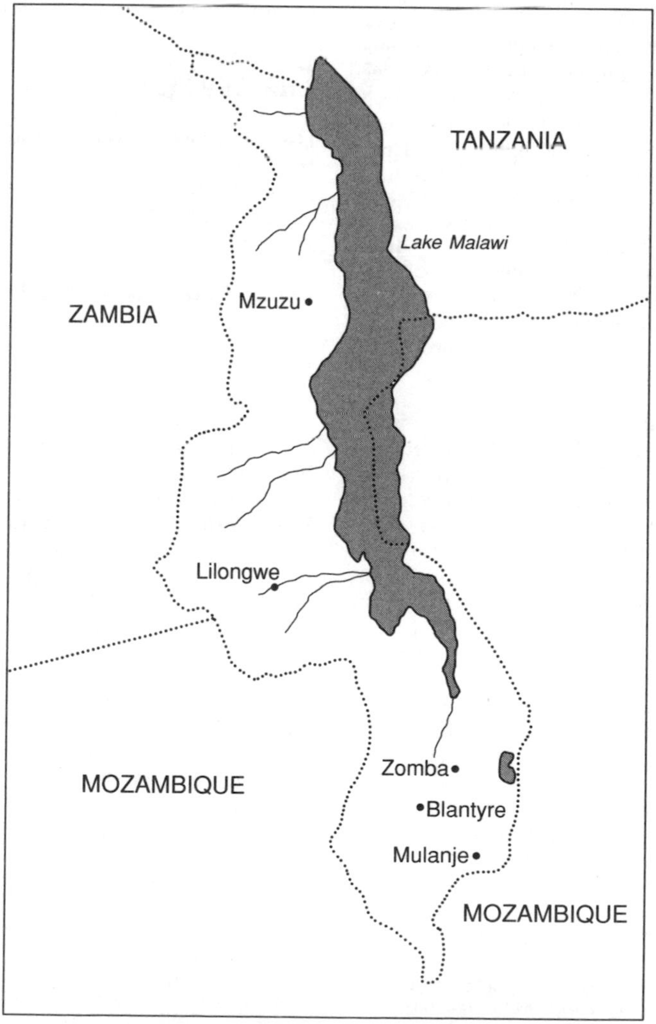

Until the early 1990s Malawi has been under the dictatorship of Dr Hastings Banda, a GP who practised in the UK and then went back to his own country and proclaimed himself president for life. It was a harsh time for the people: imprisonment without trial and other human rights abuses were common. Since 1994, however, democratic elections have been held. The country itself is beautiful. It's most prominent feature, Lake Malawi, supports a sizeable fishing industry.

Medicine:
It has a pretty poor record with one of the lowest life expectancies (42 years) and highest infant mortalities. Over half of children under five are short for their age but a massive vaccination campaign and combat malnutrition programme is beginning to work. Infectious diseases are common. HIV prevalence in some areas is thought to be over 30%. It has been estimated that there is only one doctor per 50,000 people. Prior to the change in government there were no medical schools. These are now being set up.

Visa and work permits:
British passport holders do not require a visa to visit Malawi. If staying longer than three months or from a country that does require a visa, a visitors permit (approximately £25) is required. To get a temporary employment permit for working in a hospital/voluntary organization contact the High Commission. It is usually quite easy.

Climate and crime:
The rainy season is in the winter (December–March). This is also when it's hottest. It's a pretty safe country to travel in. Hitchhiking is fine if there are a couple of you. Note for women: showing your knees can make people think you're a bit of a slapper.

USEFUL ADDRESSES:

Ministry of Health, PO Box 30377, Capital City, Lilongwe, Malawi Tel: 783 044 Fax: 744 943.

National AIDS Control Programme, PO Box 30622, Lilongwe 3, Malawi Tel: 781 344 Fax: 784 227.

Lilongwe

Lilongwe, the nation's capital has recently set up a health sciences school and uses the Central Hospital.

Lilongwe School for Health Sciences, PO Box 30368, Capital City, Lilongwe 3, Malawi Tel: 720 911.
Lilongwe Central Hospital, PO Box 149, Lilongwe, Malawi Tel: 721 555.

Blantyre

University of Malawi College of Medicine

Private Bag 360, Chichiri, Blantyre 3, Malawi Fax 674 700.
Founded in 1994 this uses:

Queen Elizabeth Central Hospital

PO Box 95, Blantyre, Malawi.
The hospital: The main referral centre for southern Malawi and the largest hospital in the country. It is also the main teaching hospital for the College of Medicine (located in the University building opposite). Nurses, midwives and clinical officers are also taught here. It is very run-down and desperately short of funds. There are six paeds wards and there may be three or four children to a cot. At the time of writing it had one of the two orthopods in the entire country. Many rare things are common: malaria, TB, kwashiorkor and marasmus, HIV, typhoid, Burkitt's lymphoma, osteosarcoma, KS, hippo and crocodile bites. HIV prevalence is near 100% on the TB wards and 50% on the general wards. It is also very common on the paeds wards though patients are often sent home to die.
Elective notes: There's plenty to see and assist in. Teaching has been excellent but may vary depending on the consultants who are there now. A friendly hospital and highly recommended.

Another hospital in the region is: **Adventist Health Services** PO Box 951, Blantyre, Malawi.

Mulanje

Mulanje Mission Hospital

PO Box 45, Mulanje, Malawi.

The hospital: A small hospital (set up in the early 1900s by Scottish ministers) in a Presbyterian mission at the foot of Mulanje Massif (3000 m+). There are four doctors (recently all Dutch, but all hospital work is done in English). There is a great deal of O&G, general medicine and surgery, but not many opportunities for practical procedures. There are a total of 146 beds in female, male, maternity, paeds, TB and private wards. Morning prayers and songs are in Chichewa. There are also village clinics. Malaria, TB, pneumonia and malnutrition as well as AIDS are common. The HIV prevalence around Mulanje is about 30% which means that approximately three-quarters of hospital patients have AIDS-related illnesses.

O Elective notes: This place gets fairly booked with elective students so apply well in advance. Mulanje has some VSO workers in it … go to the nightclub for a laugh. There is a sports club. Some people have felt that a month is adequate here. Mulanje District Hospital is a lot more modern and bigger, but government-run.

Accommodation: Very good (including cook/cleaner) in a guest wing of the mission at a cost of £40 (2963.73 MWK)/ month.

Mzuzu

St. John's Hospital

PO Box 18, Mzuzu, Malawi.

The hospital: A 216-bed mission hospital in northern Malawi. It is divided into male, female, paediatric, isolation and maternity wards with a busy OPD. It admits from all over north Malawi. It is a friendly hospital and well-staffed by African standards.

O Elective notes: There's lots of responsibility and procedures but you're well supported. You can go to any department. At weekends relax in town or on Lake Malawi. Try to go with someone as it can get a bit lonely in the evenings.

Accommodation: For two is in a little flat for around £50 (3704.98 MWK) month.

Nkhoma

Nkhoma Hospital

PO Bag 48, Nkhoma, Malawi Tel: 722799 Fax: 723090.

e-mail: nkhoma@mlw.healthnet.org

The hospital: Has 220 beds run by four doctors. TB, HIV, malaria, cholera, malnutrition and O&G complications are common. It is a very rural setting with limited investigations (X-ray always broken) and hence it is a great place for clinical skills. Outreach clinics are also run.

O Elective notes: It's well organized and has friendly staff who teach well. Lots of gross pathology and procedures. Highly recommended. Apply early as it books up very rapidly. It is quite isolated. Take a book/friend. It is a mission town but not being religious is not a problem, just no big swinging nights. Access to e-mail is available.

Accommodation: Lovely guesthouse is provided 40 MWK/day (50p). Bring a mosquito net.

Zomba

Zomba General Hospital

PO Box 21 Zomba, Malawi Tel: 523 195.

Mauritius

Population: 1 million
Language: English
Capital: Port Louis
Currency: Mauritian rupee
Int Code: +230

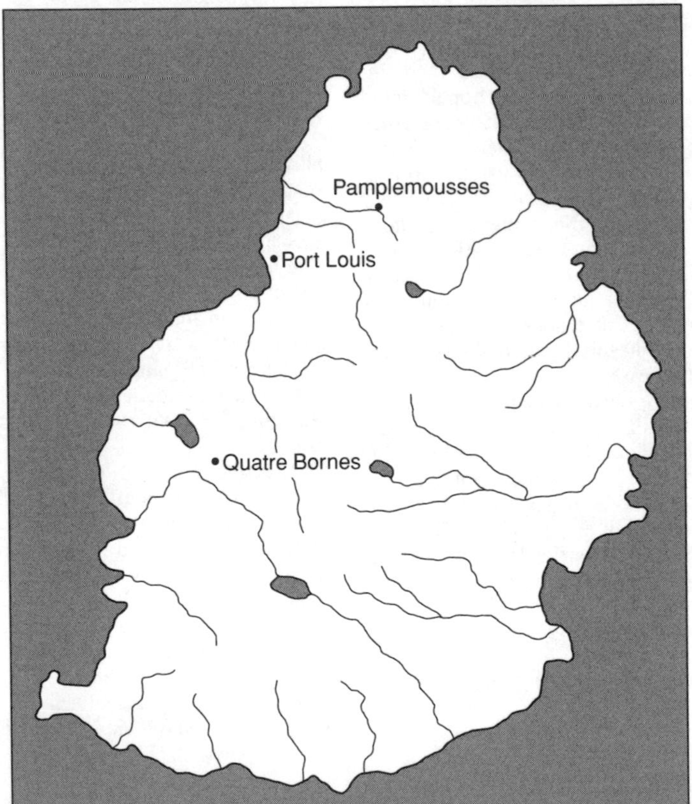

Mauritius is a small beautiful volcanic island in the Indian Ocean, hot with beautiful white beaches and coral reefs. Unfortunately it is terribly overpopulated which has led to extreme social variation – obscenely wealthy living very close to the very poor in slums and shanties. The population consists of Indian, Afro–Mauritian, Chinese and French–Mauritian, each with their own culture, religion and cuisine. The economy is based on sugar, textiles and tourism. Since independence the government has promised

a certain standard of healthcare for all. Despite Mauritian love for bureaucracy, improvements have been occurring. Language is officially English, but in reality it's mainly Creole (based on French). Being able to speak French helps a lot. There are lots of watersports, including scuba diving (especially on the west coast).

⊕ Medicine:
Mauritius has a healthcare system that is free to all. In the primary setting are 'dispensaries' (a cross between a chemist and GP). There are also private doctors for the rich. Either of these can refer to hospital. There are three main Government hospitals on Mauritius. The Sir Seewoosagur Ramgoolam National Hospital (SSRN) in the northern district, the Jetto in the capital, Port Louis, and the Victoria in Quatres Bornes. The SSRN is the biggest. Many pathologies today are due to the westernization of Mauritius. Big medical problems include diabetes hypertension, NIDDM, heart disease and alcoholism (and hence trauma). Rheumatic fever and diarrhoea and vomiting are also common conditions in paediatrics.

◎ Climate and crime:
Climate is subtropical with the warmest months being January and February. Crime rates are extremely low.

To do an elective in Mauritius you are best to write to: The Elective Co-ordinator, Ministry of Health, Emmanuel Anquetil Building, Port Louis, Mauritius. They can sort the rest out. You may be asked to see the Co-ordinator on arrival in which case take some smart clothes. Also, have a letter from the Co-ordinator with your passport as often the customs chap doesn't understand why you are spending so long in Mauritius.

Port Louis

AG Jeetoo Hospital
Port Louis, Mauritius.
The hospital: Is in the capital, very overcrowded, busy and not very well-organized. Notes are in English (and doctors speak it) but patients speak Mauritian Creole. There's plenty of rheumatic fever, alcohol-related problems and heart disease.
O Elective notes: The staff are very friendly and translate in clinics (which can seem like a conveyer belt). It's not a complete holiday; you have to do a reasonable amount of work.

Pamplemousses

Sir Seewoosagur Ramgoolam National Hospital
Pamplemousses, Mauritius.
The hospital: The SSRN was built in 1968 as part of an independence agreement with the British. It is the largest hospital in Mauritius. It has busy large clinics and all major departments. The contrast between the rich and poor can be seen in the SSRN where high-profile operations, such as heart and renal transplants, are carried out while patients may be two to a bed or on a mattress on the floor. The paeds unit, for example, has only one peak-flow meter. Birds and dogs are free to roam the wards.
O Elective notes: Most of the consultants are British- or French-trained and keen to teach. There are lots of patients to see and as much 'hands on' as you like. There is plenty of time off to do as you wish. This is probably a better elective if you really want a holiday.
Accommodation: A list of apartments is provided; however, the north west is the happening area and apparently renting a flat in Grand Baie is better. Try to book in advance as entering Mauritius without a booking can be difficult.

Quatre Bornes

Victoria Hospital
Candos, Quartre Bornes, Mauritus.
The hospital: Is a very busy government-run converted army barracks, but is a major hospital for the region. It is understaffed but has a wide range of

facilities. It also contains the Princes Margaret Orthopaedic Centre.

O Elective notes: Some great clinical signs but as it's so busy it can be difficult keeping up on ward rounds. Lots of NIDDM and hypertension. Staff are very friendly and teaching good.

Accommodation: Not provided.

Namibia

Population: 1.5 million
Language: English
Capital: Windhoek
Currency: Namibian dollar
Int Code: +264

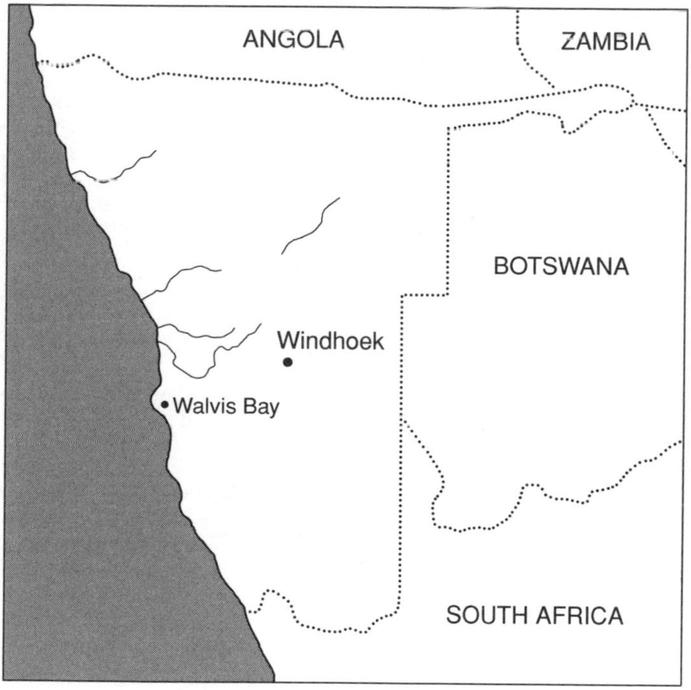

Namibia is a land of amazing contrast, from desert on the coast and in the east to green farmland in the north, mountain ranges in the centre and Fish River canyon in the south. There is also great diversity in culture with influence from the original San Bushmen and the European and South African colonial invasion. There are many local dialects (e.g. Ovambo, Nama, Damara) but the nurses in each area are fluent in these and translate.

✚ Medicine:
Namibia is a vast country, making health provision awkward. All major areas have hospitals. To be seen in a government hospital the patient pays N$9 (about £1) which entitles them to any care they require. Family practitioners in cities are inaccessible for most of the population. In remote rural areas there are clinics as it may take days to walk to the nearest

hospital. Most of the doctors are Namibians, who have trained abroad, or South Africans. Windhoek is the referral centre for the whole of Namibia. If the service can't be provided there the patient either has to be transferred to South Africa or wait until the specialist does his annual visit. Basic hygiene is still a big issue with many areas not having safe water. Infectious diseases are very common. HIV has become a major problem across the country.

➲ Visa and work permits:
For stays of up to three months British citizens do not require a visa. If officially studying or working you will need to get a letter of acceptance/employment from the institution you are visiting and the High Commission will then issue the appropriate permit.

Note: At the beginning of 1998, the Namibian Ministry of Health said that foreign medical students would only be allowed in the capital, Windhoek. Contact the High Commission.

HOSPITALS:

Katatura State Hospital

Harvey Street, Private Bag 13198, Windhoek Tel: 61 203911 Fax: 51 221332.

The hospital: Is part of the Windhoek Medical Complex, including the Windhoek Central Hospital (which admits some private patients), a TB hospital and a psychiatric hospital. Katatura (entirely state-run) has 16 wards for medicine, surgery, paeds, trauma and O&G. There is also an OPD/Casualty. In A&E a triage nurse refers directly to the relevant speciality. TB, malaria, HIV and malnutrition are common diseases. It has been estimated that between 20% and 30% of babies born are HIV positive. As it is the referral centre for the entire country many unusual conditions are also seen.

Accommodation: Provided free in the doctors' residence at the central hospital. There is also a large swimming pool and barbecue on site. It is very sociable. The lively town centre (with shops, cinema and restaurants) is about a mile away.

Mediclinic, Heliodoor Street, Eros Park, PO Box 9819, Windhoek Tel: 61 222 687 Fax: 61 220 027.
Rhino Park Day Hospital, Hosea Kutako Drive, PO Box 8177, Bachbrecht, Windhoek Tel: 61 225434 Fax: 61 225431.
Rhino Catholic Hospital, 92 Stubel Street, PO Box 157, Windhoek Tel: 61 237 237 Fax: 61 236 416.

Nigeria

Population: 112 million
Language: English
Capital: Abuja
Currency: Naira
Int Code: +234

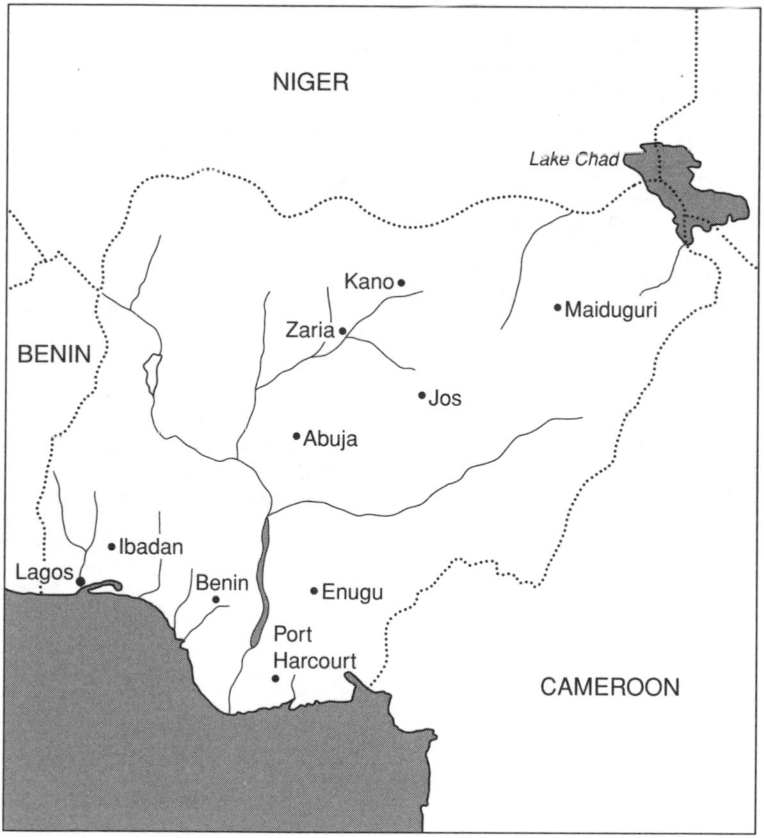

Nigeria gained independence from the UK in 1960. Since then it has had a number of military governments which has had dire consequences on what was one of Africa's most productive countries. There is now a great deal of poverty. The country itself has desert in the north and dense rainforest in the south.

✪ Medicine:

Healthcare is very poor and really only available to those living near cities. As a result, infectious diseases, including yellow fever, malaria, yaws and trachoma are commonly seen.

➲ Visas and work permits:

To do an elective in Nigeria you will need a visitor's visa. This requires a passport (valid at least for six months), a completed visa application form (IMM 22), a letter of invitation from Nigeria addressed to the Visa Section, Nigeria High Commission accepting full immigration/evidence of sustaining self whilst in Nigeria, a return ticket and a fee if appropriate. Allow at least five working days for your visa to be processed.

To work as a medical practitioner you have to register with the Nigeria Medical Council, Private Mail Bag 12611, Plot PC 13, Idowa-Taylor Street, Victoria Island, Lagos. You'll need a work permit and may be asked to sit the Nigeria Medical Council Assessment Examination.

Useful address: Federal Ministry of Health, Block 4A, (301–99) Third Floor, New Federal Secretariat Complex, Shehu Shagari Way, PMB 83, Garki Post Office, Abuja, Nigeria Tel: 09 5234590.

SOME OF THE MAIN MEDICAL SCHOOLS:

Ahmadu Bello University, Faculty of Medicine, Zaria, Kaduna
Bayero University, Faculty of Medicine, Kano
University of Benin, College of Medical Sciences, Private Mail Bag 1154, Benin City, Bendel
University of Ibadan, College of Medicine, Ibadan, Oyo
University of Jos, Faculty of Medical Sciences, Private Mail Bag 2084, Jos, Plateau
University of Lagos, College of Medicine, Private Mail Bag 12003, Idi-Araba, Lagos
University of Maiduguri, College of Medical Sciences, Maiduguri, Borno
University of Nigeria, College of Medicine, Enugu, Anambra
University of Port Harcourt, College of Health Sciences, Port Harcourt, Rivers

Ecwa-Evangel Hospital

PMB 2009, Jos, Plateau State, Nigeria.

The hospital: Is a 160-bed mission hospital and teaching hospital for GP residents (many lectures). The staff are very welcoming and medicine, surgery, O&G and paeds can be practised. There is also a busy OPD. It's a good place to see Christian Medical Evangelism in action. Most of the trainees are from JUTH-Jos University Teaching Hospital, but the seniors are missionaries from all over the globe.

Accommodation: A comfortable house is provided.

Vom Christian Hospital

PMB 06, Vom, Via Jos, Plateau State is another mission hospital in the same area.

Seychelles

Population: 73,000
Language: Creole
Capital: Victoria
Currency: Seychelles rupee
Int Code: +248

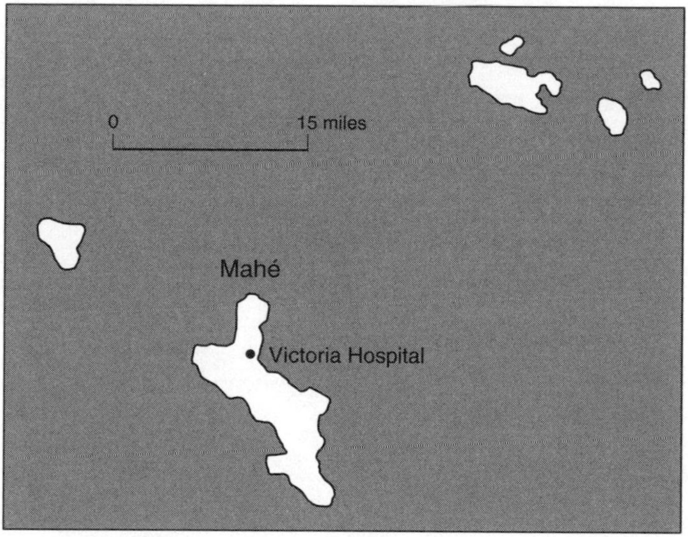

Fancy medicine in paradise? The Seychelles are a group of 115 islands in the Indian Ocean. Formally a British colony, it has had democracy since 1993. There are beautiful beaches, excellent diving sites (including diving with whale sharks in June–August) and a very relaxed lifestyle. Be warned though, the main economy is tourism and this is an incredibly expensive place to visit (£4 for a drink).

✪ Medicine:

The government provides a free state healthcare system mainly employing a few ex-pat doctors and local nurses. Western diseases (cardiovascular, heart and cancers) are the common pathologies.

◎ Climate:

Hot (not surprisingly). It rains quite a bit between November and February.

Victoria Hospital

Ministry of Health, PO Box Mont Fleuri Road, Victoria, Mahé, Seychelles.

The hospital: This is the main hospital. Reports say that despite the good funding, the relaxed lifestyle leaves something to be desired about the efficiency. There are good surgical and medical departments.

○ Elective notes: If it's hands on experience and teaching you want it is best to look elsewhere. The anaesthetic department is keen, however. If you want a very relaxed time with sunny beaches then this is the place. Community medicine (with a local GP) has received very good reports (arrange through the Ministry of Health).

Accommodation: Has previously been provided by the Ministry of Health.

South Africa

Population: 42 million
Languages: English, Afrikaans and nine separate African languages
Capitals: Pretoria, Cape Town and Bloemfontein
Currency: Rand
Int Code: +27

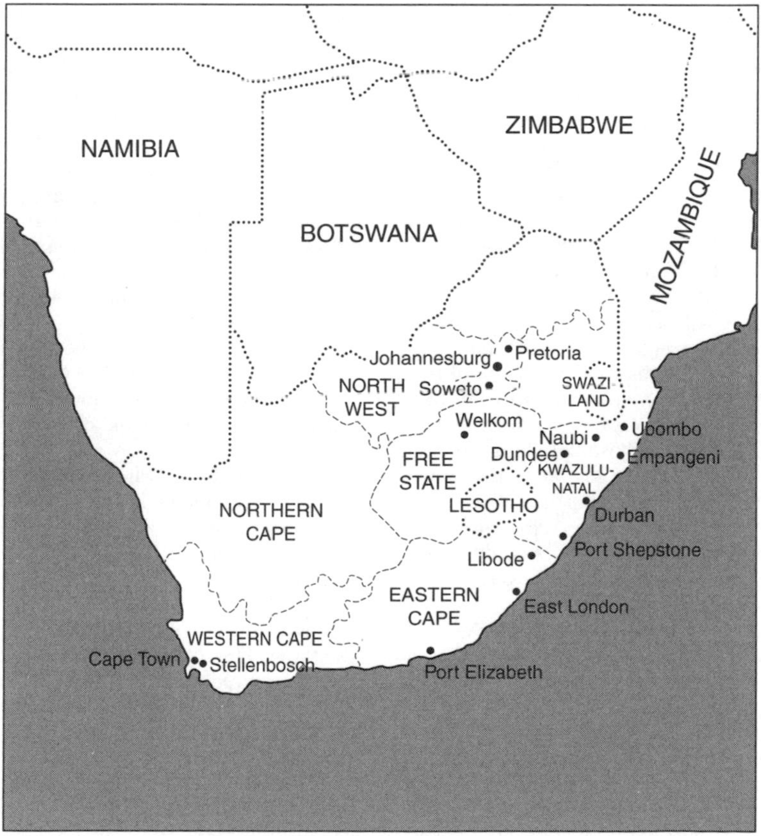

In 1994 the 80 years of apartheid and white minority rule was over. This has given a new-found freedom to so many of the natural population. It has, however, meant that many whites have decided to leave the country. It will be a test of the government to see if it can maintain the country's economy during this change. The land itself has many natural

resources (diamond and gold mining) and some beautiful countryside, the Drakensburg Mountains and the Garden route for example. Many students go here as it is renowned for violence and trauma and hence it can offer great experience in Emergency departments. You may think that the place would be becoming more peaceful with the change in politics. The opposite is true. Many poor and unskilled people now have just enough money to buy a gun (available for a few pounds) and these have replaced traditional fighting weapons.

✪ Medicine:

It is often described as Third World medicine in a First World setting. Until 1990, medical care in South Africa could be segregated into that for whites (good, very high-quality Western-style care) and that for blacks (much more of a Third World situation). Indeed, the incidence of diseases still reflects this divide. Infectious diseases (especially HIV and TB) are extremely common in Zulus. Two hundred of every 1000 children die before the age of five. Western diseases of ageing are in the domain of the white people. There has been a huge push to try to improve the health of rural folk. This has involved plans from basic sanitary care to immunizations and the building of new hospitals. Junior doctors are now forced to do three years' compulsory internship to ensure that they work in rural areas (where there is a shortage of doctors). Many don't like this and hence leave the country for greener pastures.

Two points about South African medicine have to be stressed. Trauma and violence are common. This is great if it's your speciality. It is not great if you happen to be actually experiencing it. Many people who have been there will say that stressing this point is just scare-mongering, they never saw any trouble. Indeed, most tourist areas are pretty safe. Chances are though that if you're going to a hospital, it's not in a tourist area. In years gone by, the worst that could happen is a threat with a knife of *nob keri*. You could run away. You can't run away from a gun. For this reason it is not illegal to jump red lights at night. Try not to look too much like a tourist. Road traffic accidents (especially amongst Zulu taxi drivers who also have taxi wars) are also common. These problems are really only confined to certain areas, mainly in KwaZulu-Natal, Johannesburg and townships near Cape Town. Speak with someone who has been there recently.

HIV also has to be mentioned. A number of UK medical schools have now banned students from going to South Africa unless they sign a disclaimer. This is a real shame as it is a wonderful place to see a great deal of medicine. The concern is over the risk of getting a needle-stick injury. Again it depends on location. Some areas have HIV rates below 10%, others as high as 50%. There are a number of options. You can refuse to do any exposure-prone procedure, though remember that may be difficult if they have taken you on to help them out. You should (as you would anywhere) always use universal precautions (*see* 'Your Health Whilst Abroad'.) Remember that the seroconversion rate from needle-sticks is very low (<1%) but it will absolutely destroy your elective if you have the prospect of tests on your return.

Note: South African students have their summer holiday during November–December. This means only elective students on wards … can be fun, can be lonely.

➲ Visas and work permits:

Most EU, US, Australian and NZ citizens do not require a visa to visit South Africa for up to 90 days. The Embassy states that *students going on elective are required to obtain a work permit* for which a letter of acceptance from the institution is needed. This rip-off costs £90 (R500). Many students don't bother with it and say they are going on holiday (which indeed many of them are). In recent years, however, it has been enforced more rigorously. If going to a University hospital you definitely will need it. The official line is to get a visa … you don't want your elective ruined. Obtaining a work permit for paid employment will also cost £90.

A useful address: **Department of Health,** Hallmark Building, Proes St, Pretoria 0002 Tel: 12-312-0000.

Climate and crime:

It can get very hot (35°C+) in January and February and quite cold in winter (June–August). With regards to crime, see above. Avoid townships and heed local advice.

The Western Cape

CAPE TOWN:

An amazing city with lots to do, including Table Mountain, beautiful beaches, diving, surfing, climbing, penguins at Balder's Bay, Stellenbosch (winery), Cape Point, skydiving, great restaurants and clubs. Hire a car (£13/day) if over 23 and go down the Garden Route. It is relatively cheap to eat out (£5 for a three-course meal and a couple of beers).

University of Cape Town

Faculty of Medicine, Anzio Road, Observatory Cape Town 7925 Tel: 021 406 6911 Fax: 021 478955.

For electives apply to all the UCT hospitals via the University but note, most elective places are filled up to a year in advance. Processing of applications can take several months. You may well be best writing to your destination first and saying 'Dr X has said I can work with him …' If organized through the university there is a fee for administration. This costs 600R (£100) (has been increasing) and then you have to pay to register with the South African Medical and Dental Council (SAMDC) giving you permission to practise in the country and covering you for malpractice. Write to Mrs Jackie Esterhuizen, (Elective Officer Medfac@medicine.uct.ac.za) at the above address for a form. Note, UCT also runs a Student Health and Welfare Community Organization (SHAWCO). This consists of UCT students and a doctor going out into townships to run clinics. Previous elective students have found it an excellent experience and it may be worth enquiring about.

Groote Schuur Hospital

Anzio Road, Observatory 7925, Cape Town.

The hospital: A huge hospital serving a large segment of Cape Town and the townships. All specialities are here. It has a Level One trauma unit which is busy seeing 35,000 cases a year, half are deliberate acts and half are penetrating trauma. It's mainly gunshots, stabbings and car accidents (the latter make up only 20%). There is an acute arm – admitting and stabilizing trauma patients and a surgical arm – performing acute and subacute procedures on them. Common trauma includes thoracic such as stabbed hearts, neck trauma, abdominal and vascular injury. The hospital spends 1,000,000R a year on security to stop gangs coming in to finish the job. There is a high incidence of HIV (15%). There is also an excellent neurology and cardio-thoracic department.

O Elective notes: Apply at least year in advance if wanting to do trauma. It is popular with Australian, German, Dutch and British students (excellent social life). It's good for trauma with many practical procedures (chest drains and central lines) and there's a good lecture programme (two hours (optional)/day). There are however lots of UCT students who have preferential treatment. Reports say that the head of department is VERY strict … you do not manage any patients without senior consultation and you must be present (to work) when you are supposed to. Medical pathology includes TB, AIDS and rheumatic fever. Cardio-thoracic surgery is good as the students have a rota system giving plenty of time off; however ward rounds start at 7 am. There are 22 languages used in the area, not a problem unless you are doing psychiatry where it really does limit you to being an observer.

Accommodation: The Lodge, 36 Milton Road, Observatory, Cape Town (021 448 6536) is a good place to stay (£3/night). It seems like all medical students stay here (and some people have left because of this and questions of security). Nelly (the owner) is friendly and handy if you're going to Namibia or Zimbabwe. They can also arrange cheap car hire. The Green Elephant Hostel (two-minute walk) is also good. Some people have preferred Sunflower Stop, Main Road, Greenpoint (Tel: 021 434 6535 Fax: 6801) which is nearer the beaches and waterfront.

Victoria Hospital

Private Bag x2, Wynberg, Plumstead 7800, Cape Town.

The hospital: A small (160-bed) state hospital in a leafy suburb of Cape Town (20 min by car from the centre). It has medical, surgical, O&G and paeds wards as well as a fairly busy trauma department. Repeatedly it has been described as very friendly.

❍ Elective notes: University of Cape Town students are attached here, though not to the casualty. There are quite a lot of gunshots but most major trauma is seen at the Groote Schuur. Groote Schuur, however, has a very large number of students ... here there are only elective students. Many people have said this is a better place for practical experience as you get taken on as an important member of the team.

Red Cross Children's Hospital

Klipfontein Road, Rondebosch 7700, Cape Town.

The hospital: Is the largest paediatric hospital in South Africa and has a huge range of conditions spanning those of the First to Third Worlds. Common conditions include HIV, TB, malnutrition, asthma and meningitis. It sees the acute paediatric emergencies in Cape Town. They can then be referred on for supportive care. It has very specialized departments, from paediatric cardiology to surgery.

❍ Elective notes: Working for the Red Cross requires quite a bit of dedication and responsibility. When working, a full day's work is expected. It makes you very confident in your clinical skills. Thoroughly recommended.

Accommodation: Stay at Nelly's (*see* Groote Schuur Hospital).

Somerset Hospital

Private Bag, Green Point 8051, Cape Town
e-mail somhosp@ilink.nis.29

The hospital: A medium-sized public hospital located by the V and A waterfront, an area with excellent nightlife. It is lacking in facilities and trauma makes up a large part of the surgical workload (stabbings and gunshots). There are medical, surgical, paeds and O&G departments. Malnutrition, TB meningitis, gastroenteritis and HIV-related disease is common in paeds. There are three busy paeds wards. Acute paeds is seen at the Red Cross Hospital not here.

❍ Elective notes: Teaching on ward rounds (8 am) is excellent and it is relaxed as to how much you put in. A R30 admin charge is requested. A highly recommended elective.

Accommodation: In the nurses home, about ZAR360/month (£13/week) and basic (no catering facilities).

GF Jooste Hospital

Manenberg Road, Manenberg 7767, Cape Town Tel: 021 691 7962 Fax: 021 691 7962.

The hospital: Is in the Cape Town townships in the area of the Cape Flats (20 min drive from Cape Town). It is a secondary referral centre and has a trauma unit, male, female, HDU and surgical wards totalling 180 beds. There is a great deal of penetrating trauma seen in A&E. HIV rate in patients is thought to be 50%. This is a dangerous area (the security guard is behind bulletproof glass and you have to go though a metal detector in the reception). There is incredible poverty in the townships.

❍ Elective notes: You will need transport as public transport isn't safe. Some of the junior doctors don't want to be here: they are forced to do their two years' community service. Consultants, however, are excellent. Plenty of opportunities for practical procedures such as chest drains. Go with friends to spread cost of car hire and for safety.

Princess Alice Orthopaedic Hospital

White Road, Retreat 7945, Private Bag X13, Tokai 7966, Cape Town.

The hospital: A relatively small hospital with six wards of a dozen beds. It carries out all the elective orthopaedic surgery for the Cape in two theatres. It also has a large rheumatology department.

Stellenbosch University

Tygerberg Campus, PO Box 19063, 7505 Tygerberg.

This is very much the Afrikaans' University. Many German elective students go here. Surgery is popular with them as it is less work than in Germany and once done, they don't have to do it at home. The university is quite a way out of Cape Town (30 minutes on train … don't do it after dark). Write to the Elective Student Officer at the above address.

Accommodation: Usually provided in the elective student residence.

Tygerberg Hospital

Private Bag x3, Tygerberg 7505 Fax: (021) 931 1451.

The hospital: Part of the University of Stellenbosch but is some way from it and also some way from Cape Town. It is a very Afrikaans hospital which can cause language problems. Violence here is incredible, stabbings, gun shots and accidents being the run of the mill.

O Elective notes: Incredibly busy in the Trauma unit. Loads of assisting in theatre. Ward rounds are sometimes in English, sometimes in Afrikaans and there's not that much to do in the local area. You need to get into Cape Town.

JOHANNESBURG AND PRETORIA:

Some people will say this is overstated but Johannesburg IS VERY DANGEROUS. *Elective students get mugged here. If you can live in fear you will learn loads and the opportunities are immense. Once inside the hospitals everything is fine, but be careful if going out alone. Try to make friends with a local who can show you the sites. Despite all this J'burg is a good base for getting up to Krugar National Park and Pretoria. Pretoria, on the other hand, is the base of the Government, safer and much more pleasant.*

University of the Witwatersrand Medical School

7 York Road, Parktown 2193 Johannesburg Tel: 011 6447 1111.

Write to the Electives Officer here to get an elective at the J'Burg Gen or the Bara, and visit www.wits.ac.za

Johannesburg General Hospital

Jubille Road, Parktown, Johannesburg.

The hospital: Is huge (but not as big as the Bara) (1800 beds) with the Medical School next door. It has a very busy trauma department with helicopter service.

O Elective notes: Students become very much part of the ER team and there are plenty of opportunities for procedures. The South African students have a two-week trauma attachment and elective students can attend their lectures. For plastic surgery this is a great experience and there are plenty of opportunities for 'hands on' work.

Accommodation: Available at the Johannesburg College of Education residences for ZAR40 (about £6)/day. There's a large outdoor pool.

The Chris Hani Baragwanath Hospital

PO Bertsham 2013, Soweto, Johannesburg Tel: 011 647 1111 Fax: 011 643 4318.

The hospital: Is part of the University of the Witwatersrand and is massive. It has 4000 beds serving the three to four million people in Soweto. It is like no other hospital. The Surgical Pit in the ER is world renowned for the amount of trauma seen. It is like working in a war zone. HIV is thought to be around 15%.

O Elective notes: This is a very very dangerous area. Once inside the guarded hospital you are safe. The medicine seen is very impressive. The final-year students (and yourself) basically do the job of a house officer. You must try to spend some time in the Surgical Pit. There are many local and elective students. Say hello to everyone and you'll get loads out of it. Students get to do lots of procedures while the big boys remove the bullets. Fifty per cent of patients have stab/gunshot wounds. It is very popular with German students. An elective here comes extremely highly recommended if you are interested in a trauma career.
Accommodation: can be arranged through the University which supplies a list of private houses and hostels. Account for around £5/day.

Pretoria Academical Hospital

Private Bag 169, Pretoria 0001.
The hospital: Is the main government hospital in Pretoria and has a good quality of medicine. It is situated next to the medical faculty. The main conditions are TB, malnutrition and HIV. The staff are friendly and, although it tends to be an Afrikaans area, everyone speaks English.
O Elective notes: Elective fees are around £125, half payable in advance. It's busy and you'll see loads. The local students are friendly and will help you out. Paeds ward rounds start at 7 am. There are plenty of opportunities for procedures. Pretoria is nicer and safer than J'burg but still don't walk around alone, especially at night.
Accommodation: Good quality and close to the University (£150 (1564ZAR/ month).

KwaZulu-Natal

KwaZulu-Natal as its name implies is a predominately Zulu area of South Africa. It has a great deal to offer. The Drakensburg Mountains, a number of National Parks, St Lucia wetlands, Cape Vidal, some excellent diving and water sports, as well as the City of Durban. Beware though, some areas are pretty dodgy.

DURBAN:

A multi-cultural city that is not (yet) as dangerous as Johannesburg. There is a pleasant coastal area to the city; however there are areas that are dangerous. Take local advice seriously and drive with doors locked at night.

University of Natal

Faculty of Medicine, Student Affairs,
Box 17039, Congella 4013 Tel: 031 260 4248/260 4377 Fax: 031 260 4410.
They can arrange electives in Durban and in Natal, but most people write direct to the hospital.

King Edward VII Hospital

PO Box Congella, Durban, KwaZulu-Natal.
The hospital: The main teaching hospital in Durban. Before the end of apartheid it was a blacks only hospital with Indian medical students. Today still the vast majority of patients are Zulu.
O Elective notes: This is a superb place to study trauma. Often, both emergency trauma theatres are running throughout the day with little or no elective surgery. Gunshots, stabbings and car accidents are the common conditions. Lots of practical experience.

Addington Hospital

Durban, KwaZulu–Natal.
The hospital: Has a big trauma and orthopaedics department.
O Elective notes: Highly recommended if you're into ortho/trauma.

McCord Zulu Hospital

28 McCord Road, Overport 4065, Durban 4001.
The hospital: A Christian mission hospital serving the African and Asian communities of Durban. It has 278 beds and an extremely busy outpatients department. Despite this the staff are

friendly and there is a relaxed atmosphere. Over half the patients on the wards are HIV positive.

O Elective notes: Elective students can do whatever speciality they feel like when they get up in the morning. There are no formal academic teaching sessions, but much can be gained from practical experience. In surgery they'll teach you to perform circumcisions, lumbar punctures, insert chest drains, drain liver abscesses and suture. Do as much or as little as you wish. You can get out to do clinics at rural hospitals in Natal if you wish. McCord is now charging £350.00 (3000R) for the privilege of doing an elective here.

Accommodation: And food is cheap and provided by the hospital.

RURAL KWAZULU-NATAL:

Ngwelezana Hospital

P Bag X20021, Empangeni, 3880, KwaZulu-Natal Tel: 942311.

The hospital: Ngwelezana is a township approximately 7 km from Empangeni (300 km from Durban) and the hospital serves this township. The population is Zulu; very few speak English. It has 800 beds with about 40 beds per ward. There is a great deal of trauma in this violent eye-opening area. If doing orthopaedics, you get a wide range of experience, a couple of days a week in theatre, a couple of days on the wards and a day in outpatients. HIV prevalence is thought to be 14% in the general population and 25% in the inpatients. The O&G experience is superb (200 deliveries a week, no privacy and no analgesia), but there is obviously a lot of blood contact. Be VERY careful.

O Elective notes: You can choose to do what you want when you get there depending on what other students are doing. Empangeni itself is beautiful and there is a free Commonwealth pool for you to use opposite the hospital. There is also a cinema and several restaurants. Doctors are friendly and regularly arrange weekends away and barbecues. However, some have not found this to be their cup of tea as you are very isolated without a car.

Accommodation: Was in flats nearby where the doctors live but is now often in a house on the opposite side of town. Expect to pay ZAR600 (£90)/month.

Mseleni Hospital

PO Sibhayi 3967, KwaZulu-Natal,
Tel: 035 574 1004 Fax: 035 5741 0126.

The hospital: Mseleni is a mission hospital (established in 1908, although 1959 before the first doctors came) situated in the bush in KwaZulu-Natal approximately 80 km from Empangeni. The hospital has 120 beds and up to 200 patients covering general medicine, surgery, paediatrics, O&G, infectious diseases and orthopaedics. In 1999 there were nine doctors (two British, one American, one German and five South African). Nursing staff are predominantly Zulu. Ward rounds are in English and Zulu nurses translate for non-Zulu-speaking doctors. As well as the six wards there is a busy outpatients (seeing 100 people/day) (patients pay R4 (60p)), two operating theatres, a maternity block and facilities for X-ray, ultrasound, haematology, microbiology and biochemistry. Specialized clinics visit the hospital and mobile clinics from the hospital go out into the bush. HIV is endemic and TB and bilharzia are common. Malaria, worm infections, malnutrition and gastroenteritis are other common pathologies. Mseleni joint disease is a form of osteoarthritis confined to the local area and associated with a genetic collagen defect. Hip and knee replacements are required at an early age and to this end an orthopaedic surgeon visits once or twice a month. Clinics (by plane) are also carried out from here.

O Elective notes: It's a good opportunity for responsibility and practical procedures in a lovely setting. Very friendly docs. Lake Sibhayi (with crocs and hippos) is close by and there is a good sports complex. It's quite remote (1½ hours from nearest tarmac road).

Take a mosquito net. Repeatedly highly recommended. Still has a mission hospital feel to it. This hospital is linked to the Africa Evangelical Fellowship (6 Station Approach, Borough Green, Sevenoaks, Kent TN15 8AD, UK)
Accommodation: Is free as is the (somewhat predictable) canteen food.

Benedictine Hospital

PBX 5007, Nongoma 3950, KwaZulu-Natal Tel: 0358 310221.
The hospital: A rural hospital with around 750 beds. Wards consist of male and female medical and surgical, O&G, paeds, TB, psychiatry and ITU.
O Elective notes: Some have had a fantastic time here. There is a large paeds department (burns and gastroenteritis) and community clinics in a 4X4. There is lots of orthopaedics and C-sections. Nearby hospitals include Empangeni (Ngwelezana Hospital) and Hlabisa.
Accommodation: A real problem. Because of this it may be better to apply to another hospital.

The Charles Johnson Memorial Hospital

P/Bag X5503, Nqutu, KwaZulu-Natal 3135 Tel: 034 2711900 Fax: 034 2710234.
The hospital: Has approximately 400 beds. It is in an entirely Zulu area. It has male and female medical and surgical wards, obstetrics and a large paediatric department. Currently, the friendly doctors are mostly Cuban, although the Superintendent is from Mozambique. Common things include malnutrition, TB and HIV. It is estimated that there may be an HIV prevalence of up to 45%.
O Elective notes: There is responsibility to do rounds and outpatient clinics, but there is always good support. There are rumours that the area around the hospital is VERY dangerous. (The hospital has barbed wire fencing all around it and gun checks on the gates.) Going to the market is safe, but check before you go. Highly recommended but it's advisable to go with someone.
Accommodation: A good bungalow and food is provided free.

Bethesda Hospital

PB X602, Ubombo 3970, KwaZulu-Natal.
The hospital: Ubombo is a settlement in the Lebombo mountains, Maputoland about 320 km east of Durban. Methodist missionaries started the hospital in the 1930s. The Provincial Department of Health now operates it though there are usually Western doctors here. It has 245 beds serving 100,000 people. Ubombo is 15 km on a dirt track up a hill from the larger town Mkuze (on the main road from Durban). It is high and malaria is not a problem here unlike the valley below. It has a Post Office and general store. The doctors don't really specialize (although there are male, female, isolation, paeds and maternity wards) but there is usually a surgeon. Patients pay ZAR4 (60p) to visit the busy outpatients. Most of the population are Zulus. HIV prevalence is around 30% in some areas. Malaria, schistosomiasis, TB and STDs are also common. Tuesday is flying day when small villages are reached by light aircraft.
O Elective notes: Responsibilities include doing rounds and clinics. The flying involves flights over Mkuze Game Parks and is beautiful. This is an excellent elective as it gives some responsibility and an opportunity to see many conditions. Some have found it difficult to get to. It is best to go with a companion.
Accommodation: About £2/day (ZAR20).

Mosvold Hospital

PO Box X2211 Ingwavuma, 3968 KwaZulu-Natal Tel: 0355 9191 22 Fax: 0355 9191 33.
The hospital: A rural hospital with the basic specialities and friendly staff. The HIV rate is very high (60%+ on the wards). Medicine, surgery, paeds, O&G and anaesthetics specialities can be done. TB and malaria are common. There is a busy outpatients and rural clinics (reached by car/plane). The actual hospital is on top of a mountain so there's no malaria. Locals speak only Zulu, nurses translate. The nearest big town is Mkuzi.

O Elective notes: You're only limited by how much you want to get involved. There's responsibility with good support and opportunities in theatre. Staff are friendly and will see sites with you. You really need a car. Repeatedly highly recommended. Excellent game parks near by (Mkuzi/Hluhluwe) and Mozambique. Go to Sodwana bay for diving.
Accommodation: And food are provided free, though a donation should be made. Advised to bring a mosquito net. Local market stocks basic foods.

Edendale Hospital
Postbag X509, Plessislaer 4500, KwaZulu-Natal Tel: 0331 954 370.
The hospital: Serves the local township and is busy with a large amount of trauma, TB and HIV. Medicine, surgery, paeds, O&G and anaesthetics are the specialities.
O Elective notes: There's plenty of pathology and doctors are keen for students to get procedures done. It's also very sociable but a car is essential to get out.
Accommodation: And food are both basic but free.

St Mary's Hospital
3601 Mariannhill, Kwazulu-Natal.
The hospital: A small rural hospital about 20 km from Durban. Its 300 beds provide paeds, O&G, medicine and surgery services. The doctors are not specialists but can work on any ward. A great deal of trauma (RTAs and violence) is seen here. Very serious trauma gets referred to Durban.
O Elective notes: Plenty of opportunity for procedures. It is an isolated town so a car is ideal. There are usually no other students so going with a friend is advised.

Emmaus Hospital
Private Bag x16, Winterton 3340 Tel: 036 4881570 Fax: 036 4881156.
The hospital: Has 150 beds with five wards (male, female, materity, paeds and TB) and is situated in the Drakensburg Mountains. The outpatients functions as a GP/A&E department. There are rural clinics and surgery is done one morning a week. Patients are all Zulu. It is not wildly busy so not the best if you're wanting stabbings and gunshots.
O Elective notes: There is a friendly group of eight doctors from Europe and South Africa. English is the common language. You can choose what you want to do. It is isolated so a car is advisable.
Accommodation: Free in the new nurses' home. Meals cost £1 (ZAR 10)/day.

Dundee Municipal Hospital
Dundee, KwaZulu–Natal.
The hospital: Dundee (population 150,000) is a small, mainly middle-class town close to the Drakensburg Mountains. The hospital has private (which still means mainly white) and government wards. The private are as good, if not better than those in the West. There are 250 beds in the government part. Most medical, surgical and obstetric procedures can be carried out by one of the four doctors working there, but serious cases are transferred to Peitermaritzberg. The doctors also run the town's GP service.
O Elective notes: There is a great deal of freedom to do what you want.
Accommodation: Normally available.

Murchison Hospital
Private Bag 701, Port Shepstone 4240 KwaZulu-Natal.
The hospital: A rural mission hospital with 250 beds in a very poor area of KwaZulu-Natal. It's 120 km north of Durban and 15 km from Port Shepstone. It has a small casualty, two paeds wards, a maternity and two combined medical and surgical wards. There is a small operating theatre. HIV is a major problem. It is estimated that 40% of the hospital population are infected, 27% in the community. TB is also rife. A hospice team visits the terminally ill in their homes (mainly AIDS-related). There are peripheral clinics.
O Elective notes: They are very welcoming to students and you are free

to rotate round and do what you want. The staff are friendly, encourage you to do practical procedures and often invite you round for dinner. The surrounding countryside is beautiful and there are great beaches in Port Shepstone. The staff offer lifts but your own transport is ideal.
Accommodation: And meals are provided free in the nurses' home (make sure you like rice).

Provincial Hospital
P Bag x5706, Port Shepstone 4240.
The hospital: The main hospital for the area south of Durban.
O Elective notes: It has no students of its own and does not receive many elective students. Because of this there isn't the 'student fatigue' that you get at teaching hospitals. The staff are friendly and will let you do as much or as little as you wish. There's no library, but there is a fully stocked, reasonably priced bar. It is situated half a km from the coast in an area packed with surfing/fishing beaches, golf courses, tennis courts and rugby fields. This elective won't suit those wanting city life and may not be pleasant for those who object to spending lots of time with white conservative South Africans.
Accommodation: Cheap, basic but wonderful. The rooms have a balcony and overlook the Indian Ocean.

Marguzi Hospital
P Bag 301, Kwangwanase 3973.
The hospital: Marguzi is a rural hospital, miles from the nearest city. The population is entirely black South Africans and there is plenty of TB, HIV, bilharzia, worms, malaria and marasmus. For South African standards, the trauma load is very small. Travelling outside the town is difficult without a bike or car. There are many game reserves close by and the beach is about 16 km but there is no road. Mozambique is 16 km away.
Accommodation: In the hospital with the other doctors. They form a tight-knit, family group, but it can get a bit lonely.

The Eastern Cape

EAST LONDON:

Is a city on the south coast between Cape Town and Durban. It is close to some very nice beaches (if you have a car) and is small enough to be very friendly. There are some nice pubs and clubs and diving is popular.

Frere Hospital
Private Bag x9047, East London 5200.
The hospital: Is pretty busy and the patients reflect the conditions outside. Every night there are stabbings and RTAs. Diseases tend to be almost Third World, with HIV being a major problem. Translators translate Xhosa to English.
O Elective notes: Try to go with someone or go out with Frere students as it can be a bit dangerous at night.

Cecilia Makiwane Hospital
Mdantsane, Private Bag X13003, Cambridge, East London 5207 Eastern Cape Tel: 0403 6182134 Fax: 0403 611158.
The hospital: A fairly run down general hospital 25 km from East London in Mdantsane (South Africa's second largest black township). Major specialities are catered for. Lots of TB, HIV, malnutrition, diabetes mellitis, and poverty problems (including trauma).
O Elective notes: It's very much 'have a go' medicine in a supportive environment.
Accommodation: Usually available somewhere.

PORT ELIZABETH:

Port Elizabeth is a pretty town on the South Coast of South Africa. It is a pleasant drive through the Garden Route to Cape Town.

Dora Nginza Hospital
Private Bag X11951, Algoa Park, Port Elizabeth 6005 Tel: 041 406 4201 Fax: 041 644683.
The hospital: An impressive new hospital with the major specialities

(medicine, surgery, paeds and O&G). It is in the heart of a township where poverty and crime are major problems. Common conditions include HIV (++), TB, pneumonia and trauma.

O Elective notes: It's pretty short on facilities and hence some students have found that, although they have seen a fair bit, procedures and drug treatments might not be that appropriate at home.

Accommodation: On site you can get fairly lonely. King's Beach Backpackers (R210–270/week (around £30)) is in Port Elizabeth and near the beach.

St Barnabas Hospital

PO Box 15, Libode 5160, Eastern Cape Tel: 047 555 1010.

The hospital: St Barnabas is a small (approx 200-bed) rural hospital in the heart of the Transkei (a former 'independent' black homeland created during apartheid). There are normally around six doctors and six wards, male, female, maternity, paediatric, TB and outpatients/casualty. The doctors rotate round. TB, HIV and malnutrition are commonplace.

O Elective notes: You can go anywhere you want and visit rural clinics. The doctors are friendly but it can get a bit lonely if you're on your own.

Accommodation: Is in a singles quarter in the hospital grounds and is free.

Kiriman Hospital

Main Road, P/Bag 910, Kiriman 8460.

The hospital: A busy government-funded rural hospital with one medical and one surgical ward. Clinics occur daily from 11 am to 5 pm. TB, AIDS, hypertension and diabetes are very common. The nurses are happy to translate.

O Elective notes: Recently the two doctors have been Cuban and keen to teach and encourage practical procedures.

Accommodation: Available at Moffat Mission.

SOMETHING DIFFERENT:

Ernest Ppenheimer Hospital

Welkom (part of the Anglo-American Corporation of South Africa Ltd., PO Box 61587, Marshaltown 2107).

The hospital: Deals with the acute medical and surgical problems of the 100,000 employees of this big gold and diamond conglomerate. It is in Welkom, a purpose-built gold mining town. There are many admissions due to industrial accidents. The life here is very Afrikaans but the miners speak Sootoo.

Phelophepa Mobile Health Care Train

Transnet Park, 8 Hillside Road, Parktown 2193, PO Box 72501.

The train: This is a train that travels around the country at weekends and then sets up a clinic for the following week. It has 12 carriages, each with a different role. There is a health clinic, eyecare clinic, dentist, pharmacy and X-ray carriages as well as living quarters. It is run by nursing, dentistry and ophthalmology students under the supervision of their tutors. There is a minimal fee for treatment but it is very busy and serves a very worthwhile purpose to the communities it visits.

O Elective notes: Write to the senior manager at the above address. They may only be able to take you for a week whilst stationary.

Swaziland

Population: 900,000
Languages: Siswati and English
Capital: Mbabane
Currency: Lilangeni
Int Code: +268

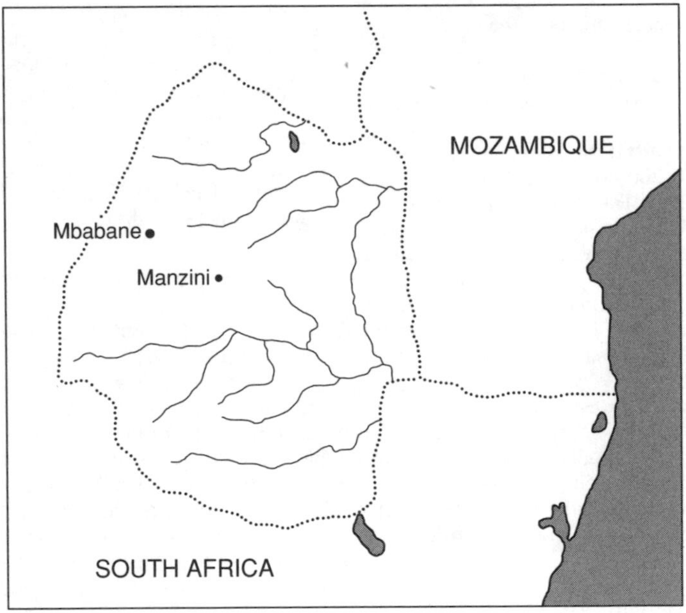

Swaziland is a very small country populated by friendly people with strong cultural and traditional beliefs (including witch doctors) and a powerful monarchy led by King Mswati III. Dry season is from May to October (20–25°C) getting cooler at night, but there are no mosquitoes. In the summer the place buzzes with them. To get around you'll need to hire a car or use the 'kombi' vans. It's easy to get to Mozambique and South Africa.

✚ Medicine:
There is no Health Service and there are no medical schools. Healthcare therefore relies on a few mission and a few government-run hospitals (*see* Section 3: The Appendix for organizations that run these.) Infectious diseases, AIDS/HIV, TB, STDs, malnutrition and diarrhoea are all very common.

An example of a mission hospital that has taken a number of students in the past is:

Manzini

Manzini is the industrial hub of Swaziland … not exactly pretty. There is a small cinema and a few restaurants, though it's best not to go out late at night if you don't want to get stabbed, robbed etc. Hire a car and get out into the bush.

Raleigh Fitkin Memorial Hospital

PO Box14, Manzini , Swaziland.

The hospital: The hospital is very busy, 60 paeds beds and 70 for general medicine. The O&G ward has around 20 deliveries a day. Outpatients runs throughout the day. It has strong Nazarene church connections: no smoking, drinking or 'cohabitation'. Females in trousers and wild jewellery are also completely unacceptable. Apart from these rules it's very friendly.

O Elective notes: You'll be consulting alone, but the other doctors are close at hand. You'll need a Swazi person to translate. You're expected to be first on call on a 1:3 rota. You are given a great deal of responsibility and practical experience. This is great if you swim rather than sink.

Tanzania

Population: 29.7 million
Languages: English and Swahili
Capital: Dodoma
Currency: Tanzanian shilling
Int Code: +255

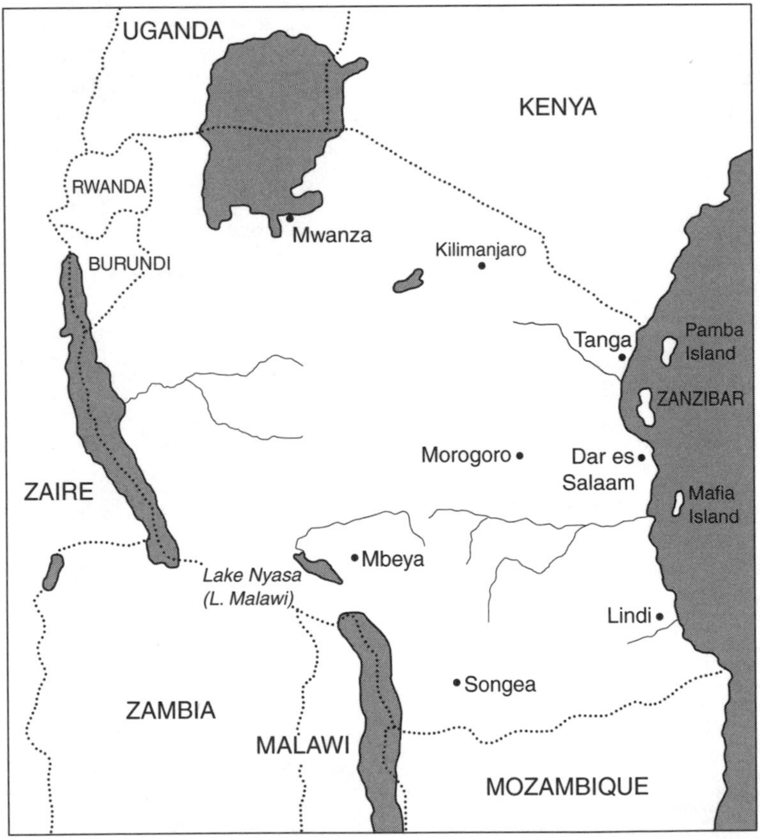

On the East African coast, Tanzania comprises the mainland and a number of small islands such as Zanzibar and Tanganyika. There is a great variety of scenery from the coastal lowlands to the volcanic highlands and the Great Rift Valley.

The highlands are home to Mount Kilimanjaro, Africa's highest peak. Tanzania is famed for its wildlife. Herds of wildebeest, zebras, lions, cheetah and hyenas are in abundance. The beaches are beautiful and the cities friendly. If you want an exotic island break then visit Pemba or Mafia. These are not yet overrun by tourists. Tanzania has a long history. One of the oldest human remains (1.75 million years old) was found here recently. The various African tribes (mainly Masai from Kenya) inter-married with trading Arabs 2000 years ago forming a new people with their own language, Swahili. Tanzania later became a German territory but was surrendered to the British after World War I. Tanzania then became independent in the 1960s. After you've climbed Mount Kilimanjaro head to the north: for Ngorongoro Crater (the largest unbroken caldera in the world), Olduvai Gorge, Serengeti, Arusha, Tarangire and Lake Manyara National Parks. Then go south: Selous Game Reserve, Mikumi, Ruaha and Udzungwa Mountains National Parks. Other places to visit are: Katavi, Gombe, Rubondo Island and Mahale Mountains National Parks, Lake Victoria and Tanganyika. Don't forget Zanzibar!

✪ Medicine:

Basic medical care is state-funded, although there are also a number of Christian missions. Rural areas are served by local clinics. Despite relatively good medical care, diarrhoea, respiratory diseases and malaria are still big killers. HIV is increasing and is around 20% in rural regions. Most hospital work is done in English (e.g. ward rounds and notes) but the majority of patients speak only Swahili.

◎ Climate and crime:

The coastal areas are hot and humid with an average daytime temperature of 30°C. The central plateau has hot days and cool nights. The hills below the northern highlands are pleasant between January and September with temperatures around 20°C. The area around Mount Kilimanjaro is warmest between December and March (22°C). For the whole country, October to February is the hottest and March to May the wettest. Crime levels are low, although theft is rising in Dar es Salaam.

➲ Visas and work permit:

A visa is needed. For up-to-date information visit: http://www.tanzania-online.gov.uk or e-mail Balozi@tanzarep.demon.co.uk Alternatively, contact the embassy.

THE MEDICAL SCHOOL:

Muhimbili University College of Health Sciences
Office of the Principal, PO Box 65001, Dar es Salaam, Tanzania Tel: 15302-6 e-mail dfmed@much.ac.tz
They can organize electives, for example in Mbeya Consultant Hospital. Only around 50 Tanzanian students enrol a year and there is a high drop-out rate. This makes Tanzania very short of doctors.

GOVERNMENT HOSPITALS:

Muhimbili Medical Centre
PO Box 65000, Dar es Salaam, Tanzania Tel: 051 150939/1500816.

Kilimanjaro Christian Medical Centre
PO Box 3010, Moshi, Tanzania Tel: 00255 57 54263/52291 Fax: 055 54381.

Bugando Hospital
PO Box 1370, Mwanza, Tanzania Tel: 068 40610.

Mbeya Referral Hospital
PO Box 419, Mbeya, Tanzania Tel: 065 3576.
The hospital: A large (by Tanzanian standards) referral hospital in south-west Tanzania. It is a teaching centre for clinical assistants (who do a similar job to junior doctors). Common pathologies are malaria, pneumonia, meningitis, malnutrition and sickle cell disease. HIV is also very common.
O Elective notes: They don't often get students so it's up to you what and how much you want to do. If you stay around you can end up running wards. There is good support. The doctors don't really get out much. Lake Malawi/Nyasa is only a couple of hours away by car.

Mbeya itself is a busy town with a small ex-pat community of coffee buyers, NGO workers and missionaries.

Mnazi Mmoja Hospital

PO Box 338, Zanzibar, Tanzania Tel: 00255 54 31071.

The hospital: Zanzibar is a beautiful place … sun, sea, sand, palm trees … however, the hospital is a bit disorganized. It is government-run and underfunded so most of the doctors spend their time in private practice. Despite this, the staff are very friendly and helpful and there are interesting clinics to attend.

O Elective notes: A surgical elective is especially recommended here (the main surgeon is very efficient and helpful). There's also acupuncture and the chance to go on outreach clinics.

Hindu Mandal Hospital

PO Box 581, Dar es Salaam, Tanzania Tel: 00255 51 110237/110428.

Agha Khan Hospital

PO Box 2289, Dar es Salaam, Tanzania Tel: 00255 51 114096.

Nachingwea District General Hospital

Nachingwea, Lindi, South Tanzania

The hospital: With 179 beds, was built in 1952 principally as a TB centre. It is government-run (with two doctors) and resources are scarce. Malaria, anaemia, pneumonia, meningitis and diarrhoea are the common causes of death. Infant mortality is high (124/1000) and under-fives 209/1000. There is a busy outpatients/ A&E, a theatre, an X-ray machine and very basic lab facilities. There is an AIDS department.

O Elective notes: The hospital has long-standing links with St Andrews Church, Stapleford, Cambridge and hence Cambridge students. There is plenty to see and do.

Accommodation: And food are provided in the teacher training college.

Teule District Designated Hospital

Muheza, Tanga Region, Tanzania.

The hospital: Recently designated a district hospital. Currently it is run by an amazing British doctor. Its 260 beds are usually at 150% capacitance catering for its catchment of 250,000. Muheza itself has a population of 30,000 and lies 35 km from Tanga and 350 km from Dar es Salaam. It has nine wards: two medical, two surgical, two paeds, one maternity, one isolation and one diarrhoea. There is theatre, ITU, X-ray and delivery suite. There is also a mobile clinic. Malaria is the biggest problem, with TB, typhoid, dysentery and meningitis. HIV prevalence is around 17%. The hospital is partly government-funded but still receives overseas aid. It was originally an Anglican Mission hospital (in a Muslim area) and still receives help from the church. Patients pay 2000 shillings (about £2) for a week in hospital. That's a week's income. This covers food and medicine, but X-rays etc. are extra. There are a couple of doctors, a surgeon and a number of assistants. There is a nurse and midwife school of 120 students. The local language is Kiswahili.

O Elective notes: You are very much needed here. From day one you may well find yourself doing ward rounds alone. There are opportunities to go to rural dispensaries. It can get lonely … try to go in pairs. There are daily prayer meetings. Try to learn a little Swahili. Highly recommended.

Accommodation: Basic but only £2 (2543 TZS)/month.

MISSION HOSPITALS:

Berega Mission Hospital

Berega, Morogoro, Tanzania.

The hospital: A 120-bed mission hospital established in the 1890s. It is often described by Paul White in the 'Jungle Doctor' series. Most of the locals are subsistence farmers. Berega has a population of only a few hundred but the hospital covers a vast population of 200,000 (some have to walk for two days to get there). There are male and female, paeds and O&G wards and recently community health services. Most diseases are infectious: malaria, pneumonia, gastroenteritis, skin infections and worm infestations. Conditions in the hospital (run by a Tanzanian, a couple of Australians and a British doctor at the time of writing) are very poor. Patients often have to share beds, families live under them and provide nursing care and food (only 15 nurses in the hospital). There is a bucket of water in the corner for washing. The flying surgeon visits occasionally. The electricity generator is switched on if the theatre is needed. Some lab facilities (including HIV testing) are available. The HIV rate in those donating for blood transfusion is 13%. In paeds there is measles, malnutrition, burns and fractures. The community health team is trying to immunize them. There are lots of complicated deliveries (the normal ones don't come in). The nearest phone box is 50 miles away and post relies on a weekly visit to Morogoro (135 km south).

O Elective notes: An excellent if somewhat isolated elective.

St Anne's Hospital

PO Box 2, Liuli (via Songea), Tanzania (connected via USPG charity).

The hospital: Liuli is a small village on the Tanzanian side of the banks of Lake Malawi with the Livingstone Mountains behind it. It is very remote; when the road is washed away in the wet season, the only way to it is by boat. The hospital is an Anglican mission hospital established in 1906, rebuilt in the 1970s but still very shabby. There are 100 beds (20 female, 20 male, 20 paeds, 23 maternity and 17 isolation) but many more patients. It serves a population of 100,000 with very limited resources. Common rare diseases include: malaria (especially with the lake), TB, HIV, typhoid and meningitis. Schistosomiasis occurs but not that commonly as there are no reeds in this area of Lake Malawi.

O Elective notes: Your help is very much appreciated, e.g. taking clinics. There are plenty of procedures in theatre.

Accommodation: Available in a guest-house. A cook costs £20 (25,439 TZS)/month.

St Francis Hospital

Kwo Mkono, Handeni District, Tanzania.

The hospital: Another mission hospital.

Uganda

Population: 22 million
Language: English
Capital: Kampala
Currency: New Uganda shilling
Int Code: +256

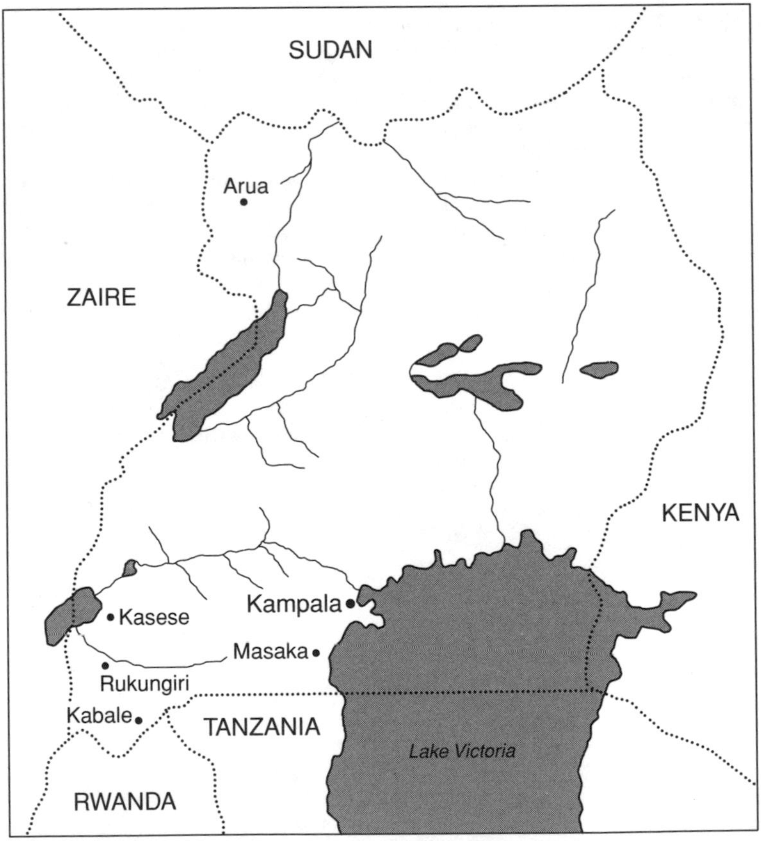

Since democracy in 1986 Uganda has had good economic growth. However, some areas are still very poor and, especially in the north, rebel attacks and ambushes still occur. Uganda is a former British colony and 80% Christian. The official language is English but it's really only in cities.

⊕ Medicine:
Fifty per cent of healthcare in Uganda is provided by NGOs. Mission hospitals rely on charity aid, some money from the government, the church and small fees paid by patients. Government hospitals provide free care. By the end of 1997,

52,000 cases of AIDS had been reported with an estimated 1.5 million HIV positive. It is thought that 30% of the urban and 15% of the rural populations are positive. Be VERY careful if doing procedures. Other infectious diseases, especially malaria, measles and gastroenteritis are also very common.

SOME MISSION HOSPITALS:

Kisiizi Hospital

PO Box 109, Kabale, Uganda Tel: 00 871 761 587 164 Fax: 00 871 761 587 166 (this is a satellite phone and very expensive).

The hospital: A medium-sized (200-bed plus floor space) rural mission hospital (founded in 1958) over an hour from the main road through south-west Uganda. It is usually run by around four British and Ugandan doctors and has maternity (900 deliveries/year), surgical, medical, paeds, SCBU and isolation wards and two operating theatres. The A&E/OPD commonly sees malaria (occasional epidemics), HIV medicine, pneumonia, rheumatic fever, malnutrition, trauma (secondary to alcohol), diabetes, meningitis, STDs, trauma and alcohol-related disease. The hospital has basic lab facilities, X-ray and ultrasound. There are community visits to local villages and a newly developed AIDS programme (including AIDS orphans programme). Patients have to pay for care here but a scheme of community health insurance is being set up. A nursing school has just opened.

O Elective notes: Whilst there be prepared to work fairly hard and have a fair bit of responsibility, although it's fairly flexible when you want to go. You'll have clinics and ward rounds to do. The staff (mainly Western doctors, currently a British surgeon and GP) are keen to teach and support during practical procedures. There are medical students (elective and Ugandan) most of the year. Kisiizi is very Christian (Chapel 8 am every morning) but no one holds anything against non-Christians so long as they are sympathetic to their beliefs. There are beautiful walks in the nearby hills and a hospital football team. Alcohol is frowned upon. Kabale, the nearest town, is over two hours away (30 miles). It has been described as a great experience and very friendly. It is a very popular elective destination. Plenty to do near by: Lake Bunyonyi, Kisoro (Mgahinga National Park with gorillas), Queen Elizabeth National Park. Take 'Angel Delight' (*not* banana flavour!) and Sunday newspapers to make friends.

Accommodation: Provided for students in a guesthouse at £10 (23,982 UGX)/week.

Note: This can be arranged through the Mid-Africa Ministry (MAM) 157 Waterloo Road, London SE1 8UU Tel: 020 7261 1370 Fax: 020 7401 2910. They will send a lot more information about the place.

Kagando Hospital

Private Bag, Kasese, Uganda Tel: 00256 41 267462 (the Mission Aviation Fellowship in Kampala ... they can radio a message to Kagando, no phone there) Fax: 00256 41 241413 (the Uganda Protestant Medical Bureau which can also radio the hospital).

The hospital: A missionary hospital of 220 beds with some government funding. It is very much part of the community of Kagando and situated near Kasese and the Rwenzan Mountains (mountains of the moon) in western Uganda. It serves a population of 380,000 and is run by three to four physicians, two surgeons and two anaesthetists. There are also Ugandan House Officers. There is a wide variety of pathologies. Cholera, TB and malaria are common. There are also major problems with a rebel versus government war with families being displaced and children even being burned. This puts great restrictions on travel outside the hospital. It has also caused more malnutrition and surgically there are many casualties from gunshots, burns and mines.

O Elective notes: It is a Christian hospital and accordingly there is a prayer service at 8 am. You can see patients on your own in OPD but there is always

support. There is much to see and the area is very beautiful with mountains and woodland. Overall, recommended, but enquire about safety regarding rebel activity before you go.
Accommodation: Very good (approx £4 (9593 UGX)/day including cleaner and cook … this money helps to fund Ugandan medical students).

Nyakibale Hospital

PO Box 31, Rukungiri, Uganda.

The hospital: An ex-mission hospital with about 300 beds and a large maternity wing. It is in south-west Uganda, close to the Zaire border and about 400 km from Kampala. It's a 20-minute walk to Rukungiri (a small town). Around four Ugandan doctors (± Westerners) who are very welcoming usually run it. The hospital provides medical, surgical, ortho, paeds and O&G services. There is a large OPD and primary healthcare programme. Common diseases include malaria, HIV, typhoid and meningitis. Despite an HIV prevalence of ~15%, malaria still causes twice as many deaths.
O Elective notes: The surrounding countryside is beautiful.

Kuluva Church of Uganda Hospital

PO Box 28, Arua, Uganda.

The hospital: A rural hospital. Malaria, malnutrition with gastroenteritis, TB, HIV, pneumonia and meningitis are on the menu.
O Elective notes: Students normally do a 1:3 rota and have a great deal more responsibility than in Western hospitals. Can be organized through the Africa Inland Mission, London (*see* p. 38).

Masaka Hospital

PO Box 18, Masaka, Uganda Fax (in local Post Office) 481 20514.

The hospital: Has the basic specialities (medicine, surgery, paeds, O&G). It's basic healthcare in a friendly hospital.
O Elective notes: It's up to you how much you do. A car is ideal so you can get out to national parks.

Zambia

Population: 9.5 million
Languages: English, Bemba and Nyanja
Capital: Lusaka
Currency: Zambian kwacha
Int Code: +260

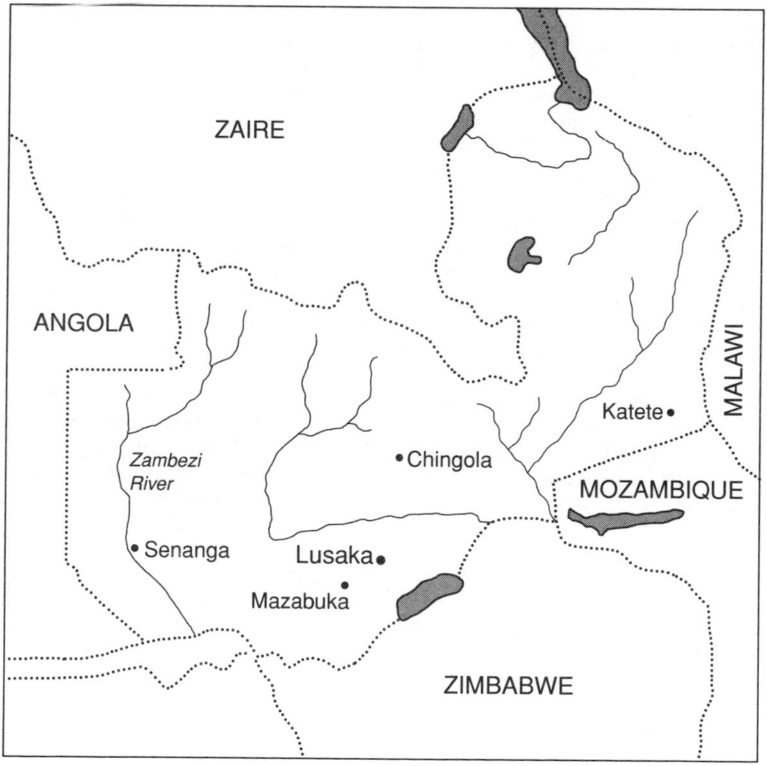

Zambia is a large landlocked country. It gained independence from the UK in 1964, and since has been one of Africa's poorest nations. The situation's not improving. Previously it had a large copper industry, but since prices dropped this has reduced drastically. The largest bank note is 500 kwacha (worth about 30 pence). People live in small villages in mud huts and the economy is now based on subsistence farming. With all that said, it is a beautiful country with very friendly people. There is a police system but corruption is rife. There are half a dozen languages with many dialects but the official language is English and staff in hospitals usually translate.

⊕ Medicine:
Healthcare is based on a government scheme like the British NHS. This was fine when the copper industry was booming, but since it collapsed healthcare has fallen apart. Currently, the government is trying to give more money to local areas so that they can decide their own priorities. In the western province the Dutch have stepped in to try to provide primary healthcare. Rarities that are common include: malaria, TB, schistosomiasis (be careful if you go swimming), syphilis, Burkitt's lymphoma, sickle cell, osteomyelitis, meningitis and trauma. HIV is rife with an estimated prevalence of between 30 and 60% depending on location. Like much of Africa, culture states that the more partners a man has, the higher his position in society. This with the fact that traditional healers commonly treat with escarification increases transmission. Zambia has 11,300 people per doctor and the University of Zambia only trains around 100 per year. They are, however, training clinical officers. They have three to four years basic medical training and do the jobs of junior doctors.

There are a number of mission hospitals listed below. For more information contact: **Christian Missionary Association of Zambia,** PO Box 8085, Woodlands, Lusaka, Zambia.

THE MEDICAL SCHOOL:

The School of Medicine at Zambia University

PO Box 50110, Lusaka, Zambia.

They can recommend places and help with electives. The main teaching hospital is:

University Teaching Hospital

PO Box 50110, Lusaka, Zambia.

The hospital: The main hospital in Zambia and has all major specialities. The staff (and patients) are incredibly friendly; however, morale is low as resources have been limited for so long. There is a great deal of HIV, malnutrition, tropical and infectious diseases (malaria, TB).

○ Elective notes: English is widely spoken though it is handy to know a little Nyanja. Some teachers have been excellent and there is a great deal of pathology. You are made to feel useful.

Accommodation: That provided by the University (HS$1/day) is pretty appalling. You may be able to arrange something when you get there.

St Francis' Mission Hospital

Private Bag 11, Katete, Zambia.

The hospital: Is situated 500 km north-east of Lusaka, although it is actually another 5 km from the town of Katete (population 10,000). It is a DGH serving 165,000 people from a wide area. It has 365 beds forming male, female, surgical, paeds, maternity, TB wards as well as an outpatients, SCBU and isolation units. It is a very busy hospital run by six doctors who specialize in everything from ophthalmology to surgery. There are three operating theatres, an AIDS department and it has ultrasound and X-ray facilities. By Zambian standards the hospital has good facilities but they are very low on many drugs and don't stock expensive ones. It has a very good reputation (John Cairns, author of *Primary Surgery* worked here for years) and people come from the University to study for the FRCS. Rural outreach clinics are often held.

○ Elective notes: A great deal of pathology to see and you get a good deal of opportunity to run clinics with help whenever needed. Nurses take blood so the only exposure-prone procedures are in theatre (goggles provided). Although it's a Christian (Catholic and Anglican) mission there is no pressure to get involved. There is a football team to try to join.

Note: They are very keen that you spend your ENTIRE elective (at least 45 days) with them. You work every weekday and Saturday mornings. Lake Malawi is three hours away and there is also a game park. It is advisable to go with someone so as not to get lonely.

Accommodation: Provided for around £5 (23,316 ZMK) per night, including full board and laundry and Katete has a Barclays Bank.

Mpanshya Mission Hospital

Lusaka, PO Box 32789, Zambia.

The hospital: A 100-bed General Hospital 200 km from Lusaka serving 600,000 people over a very wide area. Three Polish nuns (of the order of St Charles Borromeo) run it. There is some funding from the Zambian government (£380/month), the rest is from charity. Facilities are very basic. There is no mains electricity, no telephone and only a limited range of drugs. It has a male, two female, a paeds and maternity ward, an isolation unit and OPD. There is one doctor and his clinical officer. Big problems are malaria, TB, HIV, pneumonia, malnutrition and gunshot wounds. Satellite clinics are also run. The local culture has a very high pain threshold. Women give birth in silence.

O Elective notes: Medical students are very welcome as it gives the doctor (and his clinical officer) a bit of a break as you can see patients at night. If the doctor is ill, you have to see the patients. It can be hard work but the staff are very friendly and appreciative and make sure you are OK. This is popular with students from Poland, NZ and Ireland.

Accommodation: Provided in a guest-house.

Chikankata Hospital

Private Bag S-2, Mazabuka, Zambia.

The hospital: A Salvation Army Mission Hospital with 250 beds, 130 km south of Lusaka (local language is Tonga). The nearest town, Mazabuka, is 60 km away. Five doctors work at the hospital, mostly Western volunteers. Basic investigations and X-ray are available. There are general medical and surgical wards, male and female TB, paeds, labour, gynae, and mother and baby wards. There is also an ICU and ward for terminally ill patients with HIV. It has two operating theatres. Facilities are not bad but drugs are in short supply. HIV, leprosy, malnutrition, malaria are the order of the day. There are also outreach clinics to attend. Consultations cost about 6p.

Elective notes: Lots to see and do and well-recommended.

Accommodation: Available (previously around £100 (466,325 ZMK)).

Senanga District Hospital

Senanga, Western Province, Zambia Tel: 260 7 230022.

The hospital: The largest and busiest district hospital in Senanga (one of the largest districts in the western province). It is on the Zambezi River about an hour south of Mongu, 10 hours west of Lusaka. South, a dirt road leads to Namibia, Botswana and Victoria Falls. Within the district, 23 rural health centres provide basic care with Senanga being the referral centre. Senanga itself (population 10,000) has a few shops, a Post Office and the hospital. The hospital is well-run and very busy. The basic specialities are catered for.

O Elective notes: Students get to take responsibility for one or two wards and help with on call. There are opportunities in outpatients and theatre as well as any projects they are interested in. It is a lot of work, but the Dutch doctors are very friendly and there are plenty of trips to sites such as game parks, Victoria Falls and Botswana. The town has running water, electricity, a phone line, bus service and e-mail. Don't send heavy things to them as they have to pay postage at the other end. Fax or e-mail are the best ways to get in touch.

Accommodation: Provided.

A couple of other hospitals are:

Kabompo Rural District General Hospital
PO Box 140046, Kabompo, Zambia.
Mpongwe Mission Hospital
PO Box 90096, Luangshya, Zambia.

SOMETHING DIFFERENT:

Zambia Consolidated Copper Mines Ltd

Nchanga Division, South Hospital, PO Box 10063, Chingola, Zambia.

The hospital: ZCCM Ltd is a mining company that funds the North and South hospitals in Chingola. It is free for employees, although there is a private facility as well. Medicine, surgery, paeds and O&G are all available.

O Elective notes: This elective is popular with Belfast students as one of the consultants is from Belfast.

Accommodation: Available in the nurses' home.

Zimbabwe

Population: 11.3 million
Language: English
Capital: Harare
Currency: Zimbabwe dollar
Int Code: +263

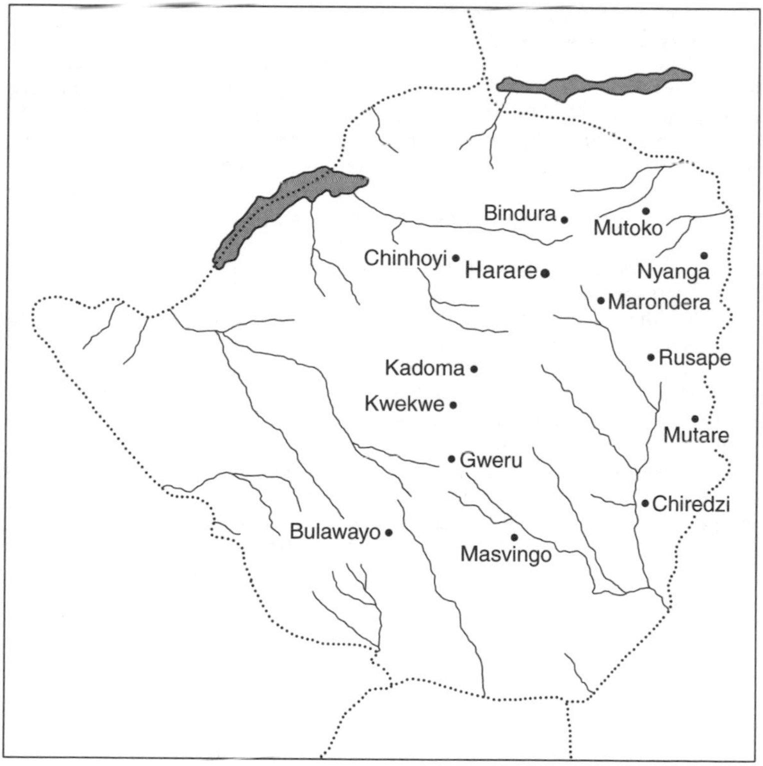

Zimbabwe borders Botswana, Mozambique, South Africa and Zambia and is famed for possessing the Zambezi River which goes on to form the Victoria Falls. Since Zimbabwe's independence from the UK in 1980 clashes between the two ethnic groups the Ndebele (known as the Matabele, making up 15%) in the south and the Shona (known as the Mashona, making up 80%) in the north has been a problem. It reached a height in the mid-1980s and riots and clashes have become a serious problem in the new millenium. Tourism was growing as there are a number of attractions. Safaris in the many national parks, the Victoria Falls, the Kariba

Dam, the Great Zimbabwe ruins near Masvingo and World's View in the Matopo Hills. In recent years, action/adventure trips have become more popular, such as white water rafting, bungee jumping and climbing. Public transport is pretty poor and buses always break down. Food is, however, cheap. There's widespread use of English, but Shona and Ndabele are used amongst locals. A note for girls going to rural areas: don't wear trousers (wear below-knee skirts); it is not the local custom as 'prostitutes wear trousers'. In the cities it's OK. Check with the Foreign Office before you arrange an elective/work here.

✪ Medicine:

Health services are free for those who earn less than Z$400/month (about £26) but the quality is poor due to the lack of staff and resources. Most districts in Zimbabwe have government-run hospitals and a mission hospital. Since independence from the UK in 1980 there has been a high priority on developing primary healthcare, especially in rural areas although the government has a pretty poor track record, especially on its slow reaction to AIDS. Despite HIV, the population is still growing at 3.5% per annum. In adults aged less than 45 the seroprevalance of HIV is thought to be around 60% with 80–90% of the hospital population being infected. (Government statistics say 30% general prevalence, but it is thought by doctors to be a lot more.) Antenatal HIV rates in Gwanda district have risen from 17% to 33% over the last five years. There is a real taboo about AIDS and the health services are no where near tackling the problem. There is so much denial that it even has another name – New Serology (NS) positive. It is particularly bad in rural areas as husbands go to cities to get work, use prostitutes and then return to their wives. Zimbabweans come to hospital late after visiting a traditional healer (the Nyanga). They encourage sex with a virgin as a cure for AIDS and also perform escarification which probably transmits it. Malaria and TB are also very common. There is a severe shortage of doctors and the newly qualified ones often leave the country.

◎ Climate and crime:

Due to the high altitude, Zimbabwe is actually cooler than you might expect for a tropical country. It is wettest between November and March, but drought is also common. October to April are the warmest months. Crime is mainly a problem of urban areas. Murder rates are 17 per 100,000 and drug-related crime is increasingly a problem. It is a very safe area to visit for tourists.

➲ Visas and work permits:

British passport holders do not require visas to visit Zimbabwe (for less than three months) but they do require permits to do official study or work. Applications for student permits should be forwarded to: The Chief Immigration Officer, Department of Immigration, P Bag 7717, Causeway, Harare, Zimbabwe. They will require:

- A statutory fee of US$80 or the equivalent in any foreign currency
- A letter from the institution of affiliation
- Certified photocopy of birth certificate
- Documentary proof of accommodation
- Two passport-sized photos
- Radiological certificate if duration is in excess of six months

The University and the Immigration department states that you need a student permit to do an elective. Most medical students get away with saying they are visitors if not going through the University. Even if going through the University, many still don't bother. If doing this make sure you state that your purpose of visit is tourism. For working, once it is confirmed in Zimbabwe, the prospective employer applies for a work permit on your behalf.

Note: Some students have been told that you need to register with the University wherever you are doing your elective for a fee of US$200 dollars. If going to a rural hospital the money stays at the

University and the hospital sees none. Instead, make a donation when actually there. You may have to pay it if going to a hospital in Harare or the Mipilo in Bulawayo.

Handy address:

The High Commission of the Republic of Zimbabwe, Zimbabwe House, 429 Strand, London WC2R 0SA Tel: 020 7836 7755 Fax: 020 7379 1167.

Harare

Harare is the capital and a convenient base to tour the eastern highlands.

THE MEDICAL SCHOOL:

University of Zimbabwe Clinical School

Parirenyatwa Hospital, PO Box A 178, Avondale, Harare, Zimbabwe.

Write to the Electives Secretary, Electives Office at this address. Some students have had no problems but others have not been impressed by their organization. They can arrange electives in Harare and country hospitals but charge US$200 for the privilege. There have also been reports of students who have arranged electives with peripheral hospitals only to arrive there (with letters of conformation) to be told that they weren't expected. This has even led to students having to go home. If you do organize your elective through them get letters of confirmation and ring your destination to ensure they expect you. To add insult to all this, some people have been asked to get a chest X-ray to ensure you don't have TB! (Chances are you will have by the time you get back!)

GOVERNMENT HOSPITALS:

Parirenyatwa Hospital

Box CY 198, Causeway, Harare, Zimbabwe Tel: 4 79491.

The hospital: A government-run teaching hospital. It was initially the 'white' hospital, whereas the Central was the 'black'. There is no division now. It is big with lots of up-to-date equipment, including CT scanner (although lack of funds may mean things don't work). Most specialities are catered for (medicine, surgery, A&E, neuro, plastics to name a few). Practical experience is limited. Some medicine is very similar to typical Western medicine. Malaria and HIV (up to 50% prevalence) are common. Ward rounds are in English.

O Elective notes: Apply through the University (see address above). By applying through them you join their own student groups. This can mean you don't get to see or do much. Students are expected on ward rounds, to attend outpatients and tutorials. Plastics is recommended as there are no other students. No shortage of gloves (double-glove for everything). You may be able to get out to Rusape and do some minor surgery. Socially, if you find a few friendly local students, it's pretty good.

Accommodation: Available in the medical residency opposite the main entrance to the hospital, but space is limited (Z$31 (£1.20) a night, apply early). There are many local and elective students so the place is quite lively. A backpackers place around the corner (Possum Lodge) costs Z$50 (<£2) per night. Harare has many good places for eating and drinking, but get out to the rest of the country.

The Central Harare Hospital

Lobengula Road, ST 14 Southerton, Harare, Zimbabwe Tel: 4 664695/0.

The hospital: Originally the 'black' hospital it now has no division. It is in the more industrial part of town. It does have less facilities than the Parirenyatwa, but does have nearly all the same specialities (including A&E). It is the other teaching hospital. Conditions seen are very similar to those at the Parirenyatwa and are often AIDS-related.

O Elective notes: A number of students have said that the Central offers a better elective experience with a wider range of pathologies; however, the clinical school and students are based in the Parirenyatwa.

Harare Hospital, Lobengula Road, ST 14 Southerton, Harare, Zimbabwe Tel: 4 664695/0.
Sekuru Kaguvi Hospital, Milton Avenue, Box CY, Causeway, Harare, Zimbabwe Tel: 4 726121.
The Montague Clinic, 135 J. Chinamano Avenue, 5th Street, Harare, Zimbabwe.
The Avenues Clinic, PO Box 4880, Harare, Zimbabwe
Secretary for Health and Child Welfare, Box CY 1122, Causeway, Harare, Zimbabwe Tel: 4 730011.

Bulawayo

Is the country's second largest city, but seems to be stuck somewhere in the 1950s. Old buildings and old cars line the streets. The language here is Ndebele and the people are very friendly. Bulawayo has three main hospitals: the United Bulawayo Hospital (the central), Mpilo and the Mater Dei (a private hospital).

Mpilo Central Hospital

Vera Road, Box 2096, Bulawayo, Zimbabwe Tel: 9 72011/9.

The hospital: Large and very busy. It is understaffed, overcrowded and commonly runs out of drugs but by African standards it is quite well-run. The care given is very good. Most major specialities are provided. HIV is common with up to 90% of patients admitted being HIV positive (according to recent reports).

O Elective notes: Time is spent on the wards, in outpatients and visiting outlying hospitals. On occasion they have to visit Victoria Falls hospital (a short plane trip) which has 200 beds and is run entirely by nurses and one doctor. On-call is twice a week. People have found this a very enjoyable elective. There's currently a British consultant who is an excellent teacher. Take gloves as they are not always available on wards.

Bulawayo Central Hospital

United Bulawayo Hospitals, PO Box 958, Bulawayo, Zimbabwe.

The hospital: An urban state-run hospital. Diseases seen are typical for Zimbabwe and possibly a bit more complicated as it is a referral centre. Unlike more rural hospitals there is no drug shortage and it is well-equipped. UBH has an A&E, medical and surgical wards (including orthopaedics and paeds), operating theatres, radiology and outpatients. There is also an infectious diseases unit. The OPD is very busy.

O Elective notes: Reports say that it has been pretty disorganized in the past. It has a modern ICU and CT scanner but sometimes things like glucometers can't be found. Lots of procedures in A&E and assisting in theatre. Surgery is recommended. There are opportunities to fly to rural clinics.

Accommodation: Usually someone puts you up. If not there are youth hostels in town.

St Francis, Box 8256, Bulawayo Tel: 9 63411.
Ingutsheni Hospital, 23rd Avenue, Belmont East, Box 8363, Belmont, Bulawayo Tel: 9 66463/72420.
Nervous Disorders Hospitals, Box 949, Bulawayo Tel: 9 60021/62328.
Lady Rodwell Maternity Hospital
Robbie Gibson Hospital
Richard Morris Hospital
Ministry of Health and Child Welfare, Box 441, Bulawayo Tel: 9 62914 Fax: 9 79891.

GWERU

General Hospital, Box 135, Gweru Tel: 5451106/51301 Fax: 54 2406.
Birchenough Maternity Hospital, Box 59, Gweru Tel : 54 2399.

Mutare

Zimbabwe's fourth largest city, situated in a valley surrounded by mountains.

Mutare Provincial Hospital

PO Box 30, Mutare, Zimbabwe Tel: 20 64321.

The hospital: A 250-bed hospital on the outskirts of town and is the referral centre for the whole of the eastern highlands. Common conditions include malaria, TB, AIDS, kwashiorkor, schistosomiasis, STDs, rheumatic fever and CCF. Presentations are usually late due to ignorance and the fact that to see a doctor costs a whole week's wages.

O Elective notes: Lots of practical procedures and rare diseases.
Accommodation: Free in the nurses' home. The town centre is 15 minutes away for food.

Sakubva District Hospital, Box 3039, Paulington, Mutare, Zimbabwe Tel: 20 64204.
Marange Rural Hospital, PO Odzi, Zimbabwe.

OTHER HOSPITALS:

Kwekwe
Kwekwe General Hospital, Box 39, Kwekwe, Zimbabwe Tel: 55 2333/7.

Masvingo
Masvingo General Hospital, Box 114, Masvingo, Zimbabwe.
Ngomahuru Hospital, P Bag 9028, Masvingo, Zimbabwe.

Rusape
Rusape General Hospital, PO Box 10, Rusape, Zimbabwe.

Marondera
Marondera General Hospital, Box 20, Marondera, Zimbabwe.
Chiota Rural Hospital, Box 20, Marondera, Zimbabwe.

Chinhoyi
Chinhoyi General Hospital, PO Box 17, Chinhoyi, Zimbabwe.

Bindura
Bindura Provincial Hospital, PO Box 260, Bindura, Zimbabwe.

MISSION HOSPITALS:

Mtshabezi Mission Hospital
P Bag M 5212, Bulawayo, Zimbabwe.
The hospital: 120 km south-east of Bulawayo in the Gwanda district. Founded in 1951 by the American Evangelical church, Brethren in Christ. Funding is from the Ministry of Health, although it receives four to five times less than government-run state hospitals. One doctor runs 110 beds, including male, female, paeds, TB, antenatal, surgical, labour wards and outpatients. There are 17 nurses and 11 nurse aids. A surgeon from UBH visits once a month. The hospital's catchment is an 80–100 km radius containing 17,000 patients but many come from outside this area. AIDS has become a severe problem and has increased the number of patients greatly. It is the most common cause of failure to thrive in paeds. The OPD is very busy. An extensive system of rural clinics are also visited from here. They provide immunizations, women and children services and advice to small nurse-run hospitals.
O Elective notes: There is an open-air chapel service in the morning (attendance not expected but appreciated) followed by ward rounds (which you gradually do yourself) then outpatients. Loads of 'hands on' experience in OPD (plastering, I&D) and theatre. There's beautiful countryside around the hospital though not much to do.
Accommodation: Should be available somewhere in the hospital.

Bonda Mission Hospital
Box T7903, Mutare, Zimbabwe.
The hospital: A small, very friendly hospital in the beautiful eastern highlands. It is a well-run though overcrowded mission hospital in a rural area. Malaria, TB, abscesses and HIV are common.
O Elective notes: This is a very pretty area and comes highly recommended.

Note: They only take two students at a time so book in advance and it is best to book with a friend.

Murambinda Mission Hospital
P. Bag 625, Buhera, Zimbabwe.
The hospital: Buhera is the second poorest district in Zimbabwe. The hospital was established in 1968 by a group of Catholic nuns. It's about a three-hour drive south-east of Harare. It is both a mission hospital and also government-run. It has 120 beds (and floor space). One wing is O&G, the other wing caters for everything else. There are usually three doctors here (often two from the UK). In addition they visit rural clinics. It has X-ray facilities and a midwifery

school. TB, malaria, malnutrition, gastroenteritis and AIDS are commonly seen. It is thought that approximately 40% of antenatal patients are HIV positive and up to 70% of inpatients. A home-based care programme has been established with the role of educating people and caring for HIV patients. There is a busy OPD (nurses translate). Drug shortages are a major problem.

O Elective notes: There are usually a maximum of two elective students but the University of Zimbabwe also uses it. You can tag onto anything you like. Lots of hands on experience in theatre (most things under local, but there is a nurse trained in general). Very friendly. Highly recommended.

Accommodation: A two bed bungalow is provided (approx Zim$100/week). Murambinda is a medium-sized town but has no banks (Mutare, two hours away is the nearest).

Mutambara Mission Hospital

PO Box 90, Nhedziwa, Manicaland, Zimbabwe.

The hospital: Mutambara is a small Methodist mission 80 km south of Mutare with 1500 people. There is a hospital and school on site. The hospital itself has 120 beds (but 200 patients) and family (who may have the same disease) sleep on the floor. It has very limited resources and investigations such as X-ray are often broken. Drug shortages are another major problem. HIV prevalence in patients is thought to be around 60%.

O Elective notes: It is a very close-knit community which is very friendly and welcoming. The staff are very stretched so you will have your own clinic. Plenty of practical procedures as well. Take gloves. Highly recommended. There is a morning chapel service you are welcome to attend.

Accommodation: Previously students have stayed with local families.

Tshelanyemba Mission Hospital

P Bag, Maphisa 5703, South Matabeleland, Zimbabwe.

The hospital: Tshelenyemba is a Salvation Army mission complex 150 km south of Bulawayo with schools, a midwifery training centre and (no surprises) a chapel. It serves around 30,000 between Tshelenyemba and the Botswana border. The hospital has about 100 general and 20 maternity beds. There is also a shelter for women more than 37 weeks pregnant. One doctor runs everything, the wards, OPD, surgery and is on-call 24 hours a day, seven days a week. The nurses, however, are very experienced and admit patients and run clinics. Common diseases include: malaria, TB, STDs and AIDS (HIV prevalence is around 70% in adults, 30% in paeds). Rural clinics are also conducted within a 30 km radius.

O Elective notes: If it's procedures you want you should be following the role of the nurse rather than the doctor! When the doctor's away students find themselves running the show and are often the anaesthetist in operations. There is a service everyday at 7.30 am. There are also prayers before meals and before operations (while the patient is awake!). You don't have to be in any way Christian to go here. Recommended but not if going alone as there is not much to do outside. You may not learn a great deal about treatments but you will see a great deal of unusual conditions.

Accommodation: Provided in a hut which is in good condition with (occasionally) flushing loo.

Luisa Guidotti Hospital

PO Box 201, Mutoko, Zimbabwe.

The hospital: A catholic mission hospital owned by the Archdiocese of Harare and partly aided by the Zimbabwe government. It was founded in 1966 by Luisa Guidotti. She was accused of helping terrorists and was gunned down by the Rhodesian Guard Force. The hospital has 160 beds for a population of 130,000 in the Mutoko district. Wards include male (acute cases and HIV), female, maternity, paeds and two TB isolation wards. There is also an OPD and casualty. A number of small rural clinics refer to here. The hospital is run by one doctor. There are many cases of AIDS here and the hospital does its best to care for them.

Elim Mission Hospital

PO Box 2007, Nyanga, Zimbabwe Tel: 29 8 516.

The hospital: Has seventy-five beds and is 90 km north of Nyanga, forming part of a mission compound. It is in tribal highlands of north-east Zimbabwe. Staff and drug shortages are common. Conditions are like everywhere else in Zimbabwe. TB, HIV, rheumatic fever, meningitis, snake bites and burns are seen.

O Elective notes: Excellent signs and teaching. However, it is very isolated (don't go alone). Although it is a mission hospital, the doctor there at the time of writing is not Christian so don't worry if it's not your thing. After a couple of weeks settling in you do your own clinics and ward rounds. There's no electricity.

Songati Baptist Hospital

P Bag 735, Kadoma, Zimbabwe.

The hospital: A busy but friendly mission hospital. HIV is the major problem.

O Elective notes: Great, but expect to work very hard. There's quite a bit of responsibility. HIV prevalence is very high (think hard as you can't really go and not help out with things). The doctors are friendly and can be asked at any time. It is a mission hospital and therefore .they prefer Christians, but it doesn't matter.

Rusitu Mission Hospital is another popular mission hospital in the eastern highlands of Zimbabwe. It has links with the Christian Medical Fellowship. To do an elective here you need to get in touch with the CMF (*see* Section 3: The Appendix); they may interview you and then you have to sign to confirm you are a Christian.

SOMETHING A BIT DIFFERENT:

The Hippo Valley Health Centre

PO Box 1, Chiredzi, Zimbabwe.

The hospital: In an unusual situation. In the 1930s a project was undertaken to dam tributaries of the Save and Runde rivers. This has provided agricultural land and now the Hippo Valley Company (a large Anglo-American corporation) has set up in Chiredzi (450 km from Harare). It farms sugar cane and employs 40,000 people. The area has supermarkets, schools and hospitals. The hospital serves the workers through the company insurance scheme. Despite its corporate backing it is still a busy hospital run by only five doctors. HIV is estimated to be prevalent in 30% of the workforce. Education is the main weapon being used. Malaria, TB, Kaposi's sarcoma, rheumatic fever, meningitis, malnutrition and syphilis are also common. Sector and peripheral clinics run by nurses (which the doctors visit) refer here. The hospital has male (16 beds), female (five), and paeds wards as well as an OPD.

O Elective notes: You are encouraged to do your own OPD with a translator. Excellent if you want a well set up hospital in a Third World rural setting. No need for gloves but take spare *BNFs*. No white coats.

Accommodation: Can be arranged at the Hippo Valley Country Club (costs around £7/night, including breakfast for two sharing, but is very comfortable with golf course, pool, bar, tennis and squash courts.

ASIA

Bangladesh

Population: 120.4 million
Language: Bengali
Capital: Dhaka
Currency: Taka
Int Code: +880

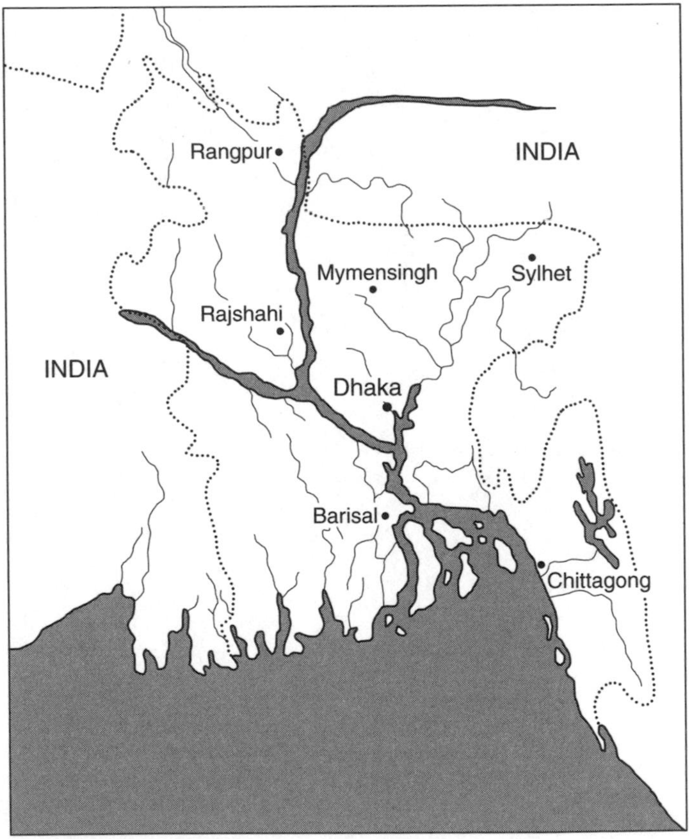

Bangladesh borders India and Burma and to the south has the coastline of the Bay of Bengal. Although most of the country consists of fertile alluvial plains, the north is mountainous. Bangladesh has had a troubled past, both politically and from natural disasters. Knowing some Bengali will obviously be an advantage, although many in the hospitals speak English. It is not a particularly common elective or work destination.

O Medicine:
Bangladesh has severe health problems. There are many reasons for this, but staff and resource shortages and the repeating demand caused by natural disasters are the main ones. Over the last decade, rural health and birth control have taken priority. This has reduced the population growth rate from 23% 15 years ago to less than 3%.

➲ Visas and work permits:
A visa is required to visit Bangladesh, as is a work permit if intending to do more than voluntary work. Contact the embassy.

Notes for the visitor: Friday is the day off … they work all the others.

◎ Climate and crime:
Up to two-thirds of the country can become flooded in the monsoon season (March to October). During this time, water levels can rise to 20 feet above sea level. As well as the heavy rain, the melting snow of the Himalayas causes the Ganges, Meghna and Jamuna rivers to swell and flood the delta where they converge. Cyclones can build in the Bay of Bengal and can be particularly devastating (killing 140,000 in 1991). Crime has been rising, but severe penalties are curbing it.

MEDICAL SCHOOLS IN BANGLADESH:

Each has its own associated hospitals:
- **Chittagong Medical College,** Chittagong
- **Dhaka Medical College,** Dhaka
- **Mymensingh Medical College,** Mymensingh
- **Rajshahi Medical College,** Rajshahi
- **Rangpur Medical College,** Rangpur
- **Sher-e-Bangla Medical College,** Barisal
- **Sir Salimullah Medical College,** Dhaka
- **Sylhet Medical College,** Sylhet

Language of instruction in most institutions is English. You can write to one of these to ask for an elective in its teaching hospital, but most people write directly to a hospital.

Dhaka

Dhaka, the capital is becoming a rapidly developing, heaving metropolis with lots to see and do (e.g. the old forts from the British Raj and many shops). Many of the foreign embassies have small cinemas and social clubs for you to meet fellow travellers. The weather is best around Christmas.

Only some of the hospitals listed provide accommodation, but hotels in Dhaka cost around £6/day. Try to make friends with some Americans as the American Embassy supposedly has some good facilities.

The International Centre for Diarrhoeal Diseases Research, Bangladesh (ICDDR, B)

Mohakhali, Dhaka, Bangladesh.

The centre: The ICDDR, B was established by the Bangladesh government in 1981 as a successor to the former Cholera Research Laboratory. It's the world centre for diarrhoea. It receives some funding from the Bangladesh government, but most is from foreign governments. It is a place to see every type of diarrhoea: acute watery diarrhoea … persistent diarrhoea … invasive diarrhoea. Lots of pooh and lots of causes.

O Elective notes: The hospital itself is (surprisingly!) clean and there is good teaching. This elective has been highly recommended a number of times.

Accommodation: Has been available before.

Institute of Postgraduate Medicine and Research

Dhaka, Bangladesh.

The hospital: Very large with all faculties of medicine and surgery. It mainly caters for training of postgraduates. It is claimed that it has some of the best departments in Bangladesh. Despite this, due to the economic situation, some

investigations that would be routine in the West are not done. There's much more emphasis on clinical skills.
O Elective notes: Presentations are in English but ideally you should speak Bengali.
Accommodation: Not provided.

Bangladesh Institute of Research and Rehabilitation in Diabetes, Endocrine and Metabolic Disorders (BIRDEM)

Bangladesh

Ibrahim Memorial Diabetes Centre, 122 Kazi Nazrul Islam Avenue, Dhaka 100, Bangladesh.
The hospital: Unique in treating almost exclusively diabetic patients. It houses all departments and manages diabetics who develop illnesses either as a result of diabetes or otherwise. It is a centre for research and a WHO Collaborating Centre for diabetes. As well as the common IDDM and NIDDM that we see in the West, there is the tropical form of diabetes called 'malnutrition-related diabetes mellitus' (MRDM).
O Elective notes: The people and doctors are very friendly. They are busy, but make time to teach.
Accommodation: And living is cheap ... total costs (food and accommodation) should no be more than £100 (8061 BDT)/month.

Dhaka Shishu Hospital

Shar-e-Bangla Nagar, Dhaka-1207, Bangladesh.
The hospital: The main children's hospital in Dhaka.
O Elective notes: It's interesting, but not much in the way of practical skills or responsibility.

Centre for Rehabilitation of the Paralysed

PO CRP, Chapain, Savar, Dhaka, Bangladesh.
The hospital: Has both an inpatients (mainly orthopaedics/plastics) and outpatients department specializing in spinal cord injuries. It is well-organized but there is a lack of equipment.
Accommodation: Previously available in the hospital grounds.

Heed Bangladesh Kamalganj Project

Keramatnagar (near Srimangal), Moulvibazar, Bangladesh. Contact the Leprosy Mission (TLM, Goldhay Way, Orton Goldhay, Peterborough PE2 5GZ Tel 01733 370505.)
The project: Responsible for TB and leprosy control in the whole Sylhet division in Bangladesh. They have a TB/leprosy hospital and many field clinics.
O Elective notes: The staff are friendly and have good English and the tea gardens and jungle nearby are beautiful. It's excellent if you want to be a leprosy expert. The area, however, is pretty isolated.
Accommodation: In the project guesthouse, costs around £3/day.

China

Population: 1.2 billion
Language: Mandarin
Capital: Beijing
Currency: Yuan
Int Code: +86

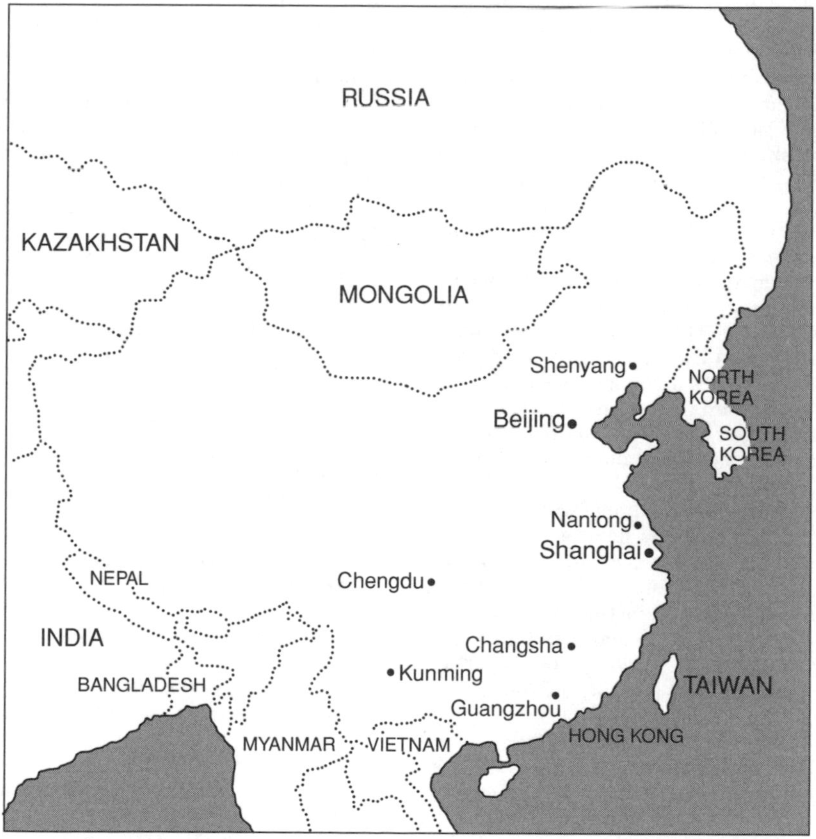
RUSSIA
KAZAKHSTAN
MONGOLIA
Shenyang
NORTH KOREA
Beijing
SOUTH KOREA
Nantong
Shanghai
NEPAL
Chengdu
INDIA
Changsha
Kunming
BANGLADESH
TAIWAN
Guangzhou
HONG KONG
MYANMAR
VIETNAM

China is a huge country with mountains bordering the north (the Tien Shan Mountains) and south-west (the Tibetan plateau). Two-thirds of China's vast population lives in the low-lying eastern region of the country. Ninety-three per cent of the population are Han Chinese. Of the remaining 92 million, many are of minorities such as the Tibetans, Mongolians and Muslim Uygurs. They inhabit disputed border areas. These small groups do not face the one-child policy that the Han Chinese do as otherwise

they would soon become extinct. Tourism has increased over the last decade with the relaxation of immigration control. The Great Wall, the Terracotta army and the Forbidden City are popular tourist attractions. It is very difficult to get an elective or medical work in Tibet as the Chinese do not want you to see what they are doing to the people.

✪ Medicine:

Traditional Chinese medical treatments are still very widely used. A number of medical schools specialize in this. However, Western medicine has also become accepted and a number of institutions practise both. With Communism, all have had access to relatively high standards of medical care. However, in recent years an economic gap has started to form a split between public and private practice. Attempts to curb families to one child only have had limited success. City hospitals tend to be extremely busy and some are very large, commonly having more than 1000 beds. China has 114 medical schools and no attempt to list them will be made here. China is not a common destination for the Western medic, probably because of language and political reasons. The major centres, and places of interest are below.

Languages: In some of the central teaching hospitals there will be doctors who can speak some English. Very few patients will be able to. Further out there is a high chance that no one will speak any English at all and therefore a little knowledge of Mandarin or the appropriate language is highly advisable.

➲ Visas and work permits:

For all types of Chinese visas the following are required: one completed application form, a passport photo and a passport with blank pages. Then you need the following. For a **Tourist Visa** you need travel information, including return airline ticket and itinerary. For a **Student Visa** (where necessary) you should present the application form for international students (JW-201 or 202 form) issued by the Ministry of Education of China and a letter of admission from a Chinese University /College. A **Work Visa** requires a letter and an employment permit from the Ministry of Labour or the State of Foreign Experts of China.

Note: British passport holders enjoy six-month visa free treatment for Hong Kong only for the purposes of tourism or short-term business. For other nationalities ask the Visa Officer or phone 020 7436 1248. Allow three days for visas to be processed.

For travel to Tibet: contact the Tourist Bureau of Tibet (Fax: 891 6334632) to obtain approval before applying for a Chinese visa. They will send an itinerary of where you are allowed to go and charge you for this 'tour'. (*See* Section 3: The Appendix for embassy addresses or visit the web site http://www.chinese-embassy.org.uk)

◎ Climate:

Being a vast country, there is a great range of weathers. In general, the north around Beijing is fairly arid, the south being warmer but wetter.

Beijing

Formerly Peking, China's capital has a huge population (19 million) and is a busy centre for commerce and industry.

Peking Union Medical College Hospital

Chinese Academy of Medical Sciences,
Dong Dan, San Tiao, Beijing 100730, China
www.pumch.ac.cd

The hospital: The Peking Union Medical College and its hospital are in the heart of Beijing. It stands as one of the foremost medical institutions in China, with 900 beds catering for every speciality. Over 3000 outpatients are seen a day. The Department of Internal Medicine, especially the specialities of endocrinology and rheumatology, is considered to be the best in China. The hospital was established in 1921 by the

Rockfeller Foundation, USA, and it continues to retain an American tradition in its organization. The standards of clinical practice are very high with MRI, angioplasty and transplant procedures being performed. However, these all depend on patients' financial abilities.

O Elective notes: The amount of clinical material to be seen is exceptional as it acts as a tertiary referral centre, and even if a disease has only 0.0001% incidence, they'll be plenty of it in China.

Accommodation: Not provided by the hospital. Hotels are costly and hostels are basic. Best if you have friends you can stay with. Transport around the city is cheap and easy by bus and taxi.

Beijing Medical University

38 Xue Yuan Road, Beijing, Post: 100083, China www.bjmu.edu.cn

Founded in 1912 the BMU is a comprehensive and leading medical university in China situated in the north-west suburb of Beijing. It is huge (1500 professors) and affiliated with eight teaching hospitals. Three hospitals are incorporated as colleges of clinical medicine.

The First Affiliated Hospital (the First College of Clinical Medicine). Originally founded in 1915 the hospital, with very up-to-date facilities, has 42 wards providing 1136 beds and an outpatients department seeing 5000 patients per day. It is a centre of excellence both for clinical care and research. As well as being a tertiary referral centre, it also runs a special primary care office for local people. It is renowned for its excellence in renal, cardiovascular and oncological diseases. It has an outpatient acupuncture department treating sciatica, headaches, tinnitus etc. It has six very active research institutes. It is quite a way out of Beijing and a slog to get to.

The Peoples' Hospital at Beijing Medical University www.phbjmu.edu.cu/ is effectively the second affiliated hospital. It too has a number of specialities.

The Third Affiliated Hospital. The hospital was founded in 1958 as a general hospital and in 1987 the Beijing Medical University decided to set up its third college of clinical medicine in it. It has 945 beds and all major medical and surgical specialities. Some interesting departments include the department of traditional Chinese medicine and the central sterilization room. It has the national departments of sports medicine. There are four research centres, including sports medicine, laser medicine and plastic surgery.

There are a number of other affiliated hospitals (the sixth is concerned with mental health); contact the University for more.

O Elective notes: Write to the Foreign Students Office at Beijing Medical University, Beijng 100083. You need to fill in forms four months in advance and there is a cost of US$400/month. Although many doctors speak some English, if you can't speak Mandarin you won't be able to clerk patients. Electives here come recommended.

Accommodation: Provided in the foreign students building at very cheap rates. Food is also cheap.

Beijing College of Traditonal Chinese Medicine

Beijing, China.

The medical school: Was founded in 1956 and has 700 beds. It uses both Western and traditional medicines with obvious emphasis on the latter.

Guangdong

In the south-east of China, Guangdong is becoming a centre for foreign investment and hence industry is growing.

Guangzhou College of Traditional Chinese Medicine

San Yuan Li, Guangzhou, Guangdong Province, China.

The hospital: Combines traditional Chinese medicine with Western medicine. It is one of only two hospitals like this that are centrally funded.

Hunan

This area of China is mainly agricultural.

Hunan Medical University

Hunan, Changsha, China.

The medical school uses the three main hospitals: Xiang Ya Hospital, one of the oldest hospitals of Western medicine in China (founded 1906) now has 1085 beds and sees 2000 outpatients a day. It has many areas of speciality, including organ transplantation. The Second Affiliated Hospital of Hunan Medical University (Remin Road, Changsha) was founded in 1958 and has 1200 beds. Both of these hospitals pride themselves on their strict, hardworking reputation. There is also a third affiliated hospital.

Liaoning

Most of the north-east of China is sparsely populated. Liaoning is the exception. It is a booming city receiving a great deal of investment.

China Medical University

92 North Road, Heping District, Shenyang, Liaoning. PR 110001, China Tel: 24 238 63731 Fax: 24 387 55391 www.cnu.edu.cu

Initially a mobile medical school (founded in 1931) following the red army, it settled in its present place in 1948. It has all major departments, including stomatological, nursing and a very large forensic department. There are three teaching hospitals and eight general hospitals associated providing 6000 beds. It has a number of research centres, including brain, cancer and paediatrics. Instruction is in English and Chinese.

Jiangsu

Jiangsu is a state just north of Shanghai.

Nantong Medical College

19 Qixiu Road, Nantong, Jiangsu 226001, China Tel: 513 5517191 Fax: 513 5517359.

This medical college, at the end of the Yangtze River, uses 34 teaching hospitals and is associated with a nursing school (in the First Affiliated Hospital).

Shanghai

Shanghai is very overcrowded (population 12.5 million). Previously it has had an important role in the formation of the Communist Party; now, like much of China, it to is gearing up as a manufacturing city.

Rui Jin Hospital, Shanghai Second Medical College

197 Rui Jin ER Road, Shanghai, China.

The hospital: Rui Jin hospital is surprisingly well equipped. The wards are crowded and there is the great opportunity to see traditional Chinese medicine combined with Western practice. There is a great deal of pathology to be seen.

O **Elective notes:** There are acupuncture and herbal clinics for you to attend if you wish. The staff are very friendly and visiting students have been treated very well. Most doctors speak English and all the medical students are expected to learn either English or French. A number of ward rounds and teaching sessions are conducted in English. Try the street food markets, the Jade Buddha temple and visit the areas around Shanghai.

Accommodation: is basic and hygiene standards are Chinese, not Western. There are rats and cockroaches to keep you company and no electrical appliances (e.g. no fridge). The shower can only manage dribbles. However, it's very liveable due to the large number of friendly visiting medical students (mainly from Taiwan, Malaysia or other parts of south-east Asia and Africa). They know where the parties are.

Sichuan

Chengdu in west China is a busy town and the gateway to China for people who travel via Tibet.

West China University of Medical Science

Chengdu, Sichuan 610041, China.

The University/hospital: The University is central in Chengdu and is reported to be the third-largest medical school in China. The University hospital has most specialities and knowledge is similar to Western standards. However, facilities are limited.

O Elective notes: Fees are charged to do an elective here, at least $400/month. However, accommodation is provided and it is a very cheap place for food and travel (you can survive on less than £20/week). English classes are part of the medical school curriculum so students can speak it (though may be shy). Rent a bike from the Traffic Hotel (10 yen/day) to get around. The students are very friendly. You can organize electives through the WaiBan (Office for International Co-operation) at the above address.

Accommodation: Provided in a foreign guesthouse within the University (luxury ... own bathroom, TV, telephone).

Yunnan

Kunming City is the capital of Yunnan Province which is the most south-western province in China bordering Burma, Laos and Vietnam. In China it is known as the 'city of eternal spring' because of the pleasant weather all year round.

Kunming Medical College

84 Western Renim Road, Kunming, Yunnan 650031, China.

The hospitals: Kunming uses a number of hospitals. In all conditions are fairly poor. Relatives stay day and night and hence provide many of the patients' needs. The second Affiliated Hospital (Kunming Medical College, Kunming, Yunnan 65010) has a specialist hepatobiliary and pancreatology department.

O Elective notes: It seems a bit odd. Nurses take blood and give i.v. drugs while medical students change dressings. That said, there is plenty to do in theatre and outpatients.

Accommodation: Provided by the medical college. It has good facilities, but also cockroaches (the doors lock at 11 pm so make sure you're back!). Food is cheap. A reasonable meal should cost Y1.20 (10p).

Hong Kong

Population: 6 million
Languages: English and Cantonese
Capital: Victoria
Currency: Hong Kong dollar
Int Code: +852

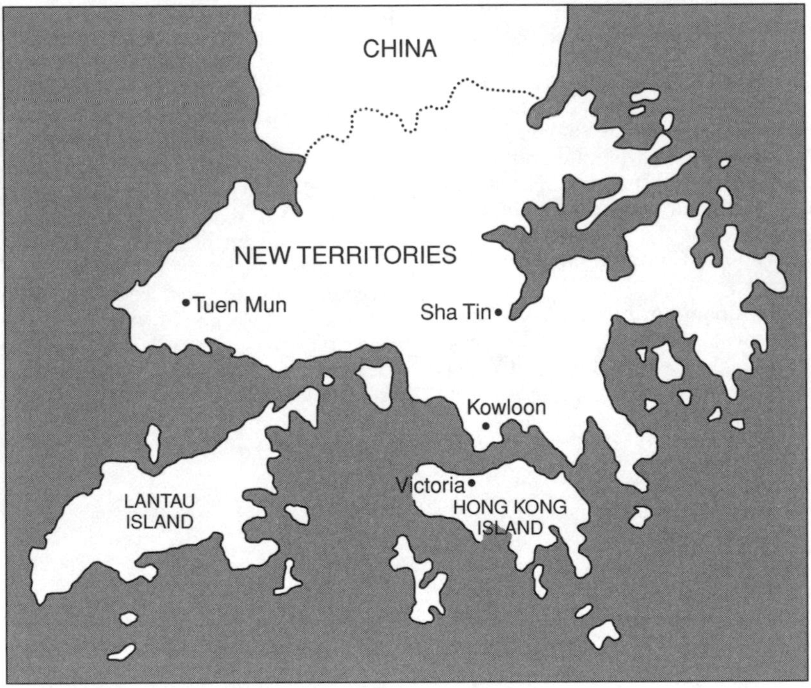

Since the hand-back in 1997, Hong Kong has become a 'Special Administrative Region' of China. The area itself comprises Hong Kong Island, Kowloon and the New Territories. It is a financial and trade centre and despite its hand-back, this should not change. What may change over the coming years are the (currently British) names of hospitals and places. Hong Kong is a multicultural society and there is plenty to do and buy (shop 24 hours a day!). There are even night markets that open at 10 pm. Currently, all lectures and meetings in hospitals are in English. However, the local language is Cantonese and so having some knowledge of this is essential for getting the most out of contact with local patients.

Medicine:

The state provides subsidies for medical care so patients only have to pay a fraction of the cost of hospital treatment.

Emergency and maternity/paediatric care is given entirely free. There is no public GP service though private hospitals and private GPs are popular. Since this is a highly Westernized part of Asia, Western diseases (cardiovascular and cancers) are common causes of mortality.

➲ Visas and work permits:
This is currently changing. British citizens are allowed to enter Hong Kong without a Chinese visa, although a permit may soon be required. As for other nationals, contact your local Chinese Embassy.

UNIVERSITIES AND ASSOCIATED HOSPITALS:

The University of Hong Kong

7 Sassoon Road, Pok Fu Lam, Hong Kong
Tel: 2819 9296 Fax: 2855 9742
www.hku.hk

Hong Kong University Medical School is in the western part of Hong Kong and the Queen Mary Teaching Hospital is across the road. It was founded in 1911. It is a large medical school admitting 170 students/year. Apply here (to the electives supervisor) to do an elective in one (or more) of its affiliated hospitals. You will probably find yourself attached to some Hong Kong students and may have to move around hospitals with them. It's all well-organized. They require a letter from your Dean saying that he/she approves your proposal. You can then select one of the following options: medicine, surgery, paediatrics, obstetrics, gynaecology, orthopaedics, psychiatry, radiology or general practice (must speak fluent Cantonese for GP).

You can apply to one or more for a total of no more than eight weeks. Some departments will not accept elective students during their elective periods and exams:

- Medicine: December, January, February and May
- Paediatrics: January, February and mid-July to mid-August.

No fee is charged. It is not the University's responsibility to find accommodation (which is possible at hostels or the YMCA, but note Hong Kong is expensive; best to see if you've got any relatives or friends there). It can occasionally find accommodation in the Madam SH Ho Residence for Medical Students, 6C Sassoon Road (write directly if desperate). If accommodation can't be organized they may not take you. Bring a white coat. Chaps need to wear a tie and chapesses need to wear a dress. Jeans and t-shirts are a definite no-no. APPLY AT LEAST 12 MONTHS IN ADVANCE.

Queen Mary Hospital

102 Pok Fu Lam Road, Hong Kong.

The hospital: A large, acute, modern teaching hospital for the University of Hong Kong. Established in 1937, it provides most specialities.

❍ Elective notes: If you select surgery you can choose between a number of specialities, e.g. ENT, upper GI, vascular etc.; however, in doing this you isolate yourself from most other students and so you're better off going for medicine where most of the other students are. Ward rounds start at 7 am and there is another at 5 pm. During the day there is theatre to visit (all ops are filmed and shown on overhead monitors for you to see) and clinics to attend. In medicine there are ward rounds and teaching in the mornings and in the afternoon you go out to peripheral hospitals ... the other students make sure you get there. There may be up to 15 students in one clinic with just one patient. It's not the best way to learn. Paeds has some interesting cases: Kawasaki disease, for example, is much more common.

Accommodation: When available, it has been universally described as poor but is right opposite the hospital. Do anything to avoid it. Stay with family/friends if you have them.

Princess Margaret Hospital

Lai Chi Kok, Kowloon, Hong Kong.

The hospital: A district general hospital in eastern New Territory serving approximately one million people in the western part of the Kowloon Peninsula. It is a busy, crowded (45 beds per ward, 1000 in total) hospital and, although ward rounds and meetings are in English, the local population only speaks Cantonese. It has the only infectious diseases centre in Hong Kong.

Other hospitals associated with the University of Hong Kong:

- **Grantham Hospital** (near Ocean Park) is where the first heart–lung transplant in Hong Kong was done. Big place for cardiology.
- **Queen Elizabeth Hospital,** the largest in Hong Kong with 2500 beds serving the entire population of the Kowloon Peninsula. It is a general hospital.
- **The Ruttonjee Hospital**, good for respiratory medicine.
- **The Duchess of Kent Hospital,** Sandy Bay, on the western part of Hong Kong, is a paediatric hospital for the mentally handicapped. It's in a very picturesque setting.

The Chinese University of Hong Kong

Faculty of Medicine, Shatin, New Territories, Hong Kong.

The main hospital used is the Prince of Wales. Apply to the above for the application forms. Specialities you can choose include: general medicine and surgery, O&G, paeds, A&E, orthopaedics and psychiatry. They make it their policy NOT to provide accommodation and the cheapest hotels are around £20/night. You really do need friends or relatives to go here. Alternatively, if in a crowd, you can try to share a hotel room (e.g. Regal Riverside). It's not cheap (£290/month each if sharing with two others). HAGGLE.

Prince of Wales Hospital

30–32 Ngan Shing Street, Sha Tin, New Territories, Hong Kong Tel: 2632 2211 www.ha.org.hk/pwh/greeting.html

The hospital: One of the two major teaching hospitals for the Chinese University of Hong Kong and the regional hospital for the eastern New Territories. It is large (1400 beds) and has a new Children's Cancer Centre which receives paediatric oncology patients from most of Hong Kong. There is a busy A&E.

Elective notes: You blend in with the local students attending their tutorials. You can do what you want. Local students will translate when talking to patients. Teaching is in English.

OTHER HOSPITALS IN HONG KONG:

Castle Peak Hospital

15 Tsing Chung Koon Road, New Territories, Hong Kong Tel: 2456 6289 Fax: 2455 9330 www.ha.org.hk

The hospital: Opened in 1961 and is a massive 1741-bed psychiatric hospital. Every branch of psychiatry imaginable is here: child, adolescent, psychogeriatrics and forensic to name a few. It has close links with community units.

St Teresa's Hospital

327 Prince Edward Road, Kowloon, Hong Kong Tel: 27119111 Fax: 27119779.

Tuen Mun Hospital

Tsing Chung Koon Road, Tuen Mun, New Territories, Hong Kong Tel: 2568 5111 Fax: 2455 1911 www.ha.org.hk/tmh/

The hospital: Completed in 1990 and has 1606 beds. It is an acute hospital serving the north-west region of the New Territories.

Tun Wah Group of Hospitals

12 Po Yan Street, Sheung Wan, Hong Kong Tel: 2859 7500.

The hospitals: Tun Wah is a charity (that receives government funding) established since 1870. It has set up a number of hospitals to care for the poor and needy throughout Hong Kong.

India

Population: 16 billion
Official Languages: Hindi and English
Capital: New Delhi
Currency: Rupee
Int Code: +91

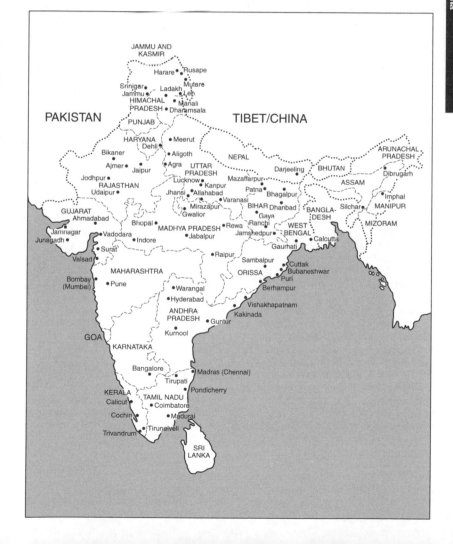

India is huge. It also is a land of great diversity. The landscapes and lifestyles in India contrast considerably from the highly polluted bustle of Delhi to the tranquil and spectacular Himalayas. It is also the second most populous country after China with a great deal of poverty and this is reflected in the medicine seen. There is a subtle division between south (more vegetarian) and north (more omnivore) which stems back to 1000BC when the original Indian civilization was pushed south by invaders from central Asia. There are 18 official languages in India and, as a result of this, English is still commonly used, especially in politics and bureaucracy (and by most doctors). Hindi is the main other language, but varies tremendously in different regions, again keeping English in use especially in Tamil Nadu and Himachal Pradesh.

A number of organized missions and charities run projects and hospitals in India. Some are listed in the NGO section in Section 3: The Appendix. The Emmanuel Hospital Association (808/92, Nehru Place, New Delhi 110019, India) runs a number of missionary hospitals across India. The Salvation Army also run many hospitals. Contact their HQ in your home country (in the UK 101 Queen Victoria St, London EC4P 4EP).

✪ Medicine:

The government does provide a health service, but this only stretches to one doctor and two healthcare workers per 2000 and is very restricted in resources. Malnutrition is still common and contributes to an infant mortality of 80 per 1000. Infectious diseases, especially respiratory, diarrhoeal and malaria are also big killers. Oral cancers (due to the habit of chewing betel quids) are much more common. Because of the difficulty accessing healthcare in some regions, many diseases present at a very late stage. Rheumatic fever affects 1% now, but many more in the past; therefore, there are lots of heart murmurs. Multi-drug-resistant TB is a growing problem, mainly due to patients wanting to avoid the social stigma of TB by stopping treatment as soon as symptoms cease. Because of this stigmata it is often referred to as 'Koch's disease'. To tackle this the WHO now makes anti-TB drugs freely available to anyone with AFB-positive sputum. In addition, to ensure compliance, a directly observed therapy (DOT) regime is employed where patients return to the clinic three times a week to be observed to swallow their medication.

The population is still rising rapidly despite desperate attempts to kerb it with policies such as forced sterilization and a campaign of giving away transistor radios in exchange for sterilization. What is really needed is education. Literacy is around 50% but varies dramatically between different castes (an Indian form of class system). The castes consist of the *Brahmins* at the top (priests) with *Kshatriyas* (soldiers and administrators) and *Vaisyas* (artists and business types) below. The *Sudras* are the lowest of the low . . . the peasants and toilet-cleaners. Between these four castes, the average wage turns out to be Rs 12,000/year, about 70 p/day.

To Western eyes India can seem a very unfair society. As well as the caste system (which has rituals to keep them all separate), women get a particularly rough deal. Fifty per cent of them have had their marriages arranged for them by the age of 20 and with that the bride's parents have to pay a sizeable dowry (e.g. if marrying a doctor they can expect to pay around £15,000). This involves loans, and families are plunged into poverty for years as they try and pay it off. Because of this, female infanticide is not uncommon. In some areas it has reached a population average of 45% female, 55% males and so 'sex determination' units have been banned; however, abortions still occur after illegal ultrasound clinics. Women who do get married then become very much the underdog in the relationship. Many are subjected to physical and mental abuse and bride-burning continues. The government-run hospitals tend to be overcrowded and inefficient. There are Christian and charity-based hospitals which are also overcrowded but run much better. These are probably the better places to go for experience on electives (and, if you become ill, better places to be treated). There are a number of private hospitals. Only a few are listed here as they are on the web and aren't used much for electives/temporary work. You may think that in India they would be grateful for all the help they could get (see a couple of appendectomies and then start doing them sort of thing). This is generally not the case as India has many of its own juniors. You will, however, get much more stitching and assisting experience than normal in a Western teaching hospital.

Not surprisingly, India has thousands of hospitals and over 100 medical schools. A comprehensive list is not possible here. The main institutions are listed and examples from each region given.

➲ Visas and work permits:
A three-month visitors' visa is available from the Embassy. A work permit is required for anything more than voluntary work.

Note: If planning an elective you are advised to organize things early (at least six months to a year in advance) as post is slow and India is renowned for unnecessary bureaucracy. The vast majority of students get in with just a visitor's visa, but some (on a pretty random basis) have found they required permission from the government and Ministry of Health of India which itself can take six months. Occasionally, hospitals have found that before they can confirm a place they have to apply to the Indian Government for permission to have a student visitor observer. Once that's through they then have to get specific permission to have an elective student! Another example of the paperwork is the need to have your passport to buy a train ticket.

◎ Climate and crime:
Climate varies tremendously from the north (hot, but occasionally cool especially in the Himalayas) to south (very hot). Beware of going in May (the heat may kill you) or after September in the monsoon season (when malaria probably will).

Delhi

Delhi consists principally of Old and New Delhi. The smaller Old Delhi contains much of the Islamic heritage and is separated from the larger New Delhi in the south by Connaught Place, an area of offices, banks and government buildings as well as some cheap accommodation. New Dehli was set up by the English and was completed in 1911. Overall, Delhi is a busy, heavily polluted city with a great deal of history. Some love it … others can't wait to get out. Some of the many things to do include train rides to Corbett National Park, the Taj Mahal and Jaipur.

MEDICAL SCHOOLS AND TEACHING HOSPITALS:

All-India Insitute of Medical Sciences (AIIMS)

Ansari Nagar, New Delhi 110029, India Tel: 11 661123 or 11 686 45851 Fax: 11 686 26630.

The hospital: AIIMS, located in the capital (30 minutes' bus ride from the centre), is India's premier teaching hospital and medical research institution. It is a tertiary referral centre and is where Indira Gandhi was brought after her assassination. Even if a disease has a prevalence of 0.01%, India will have 10,000 cases of it and many of them will be seen at the AIIMS. It is not government-run, but does receive some funding from the government. Patients (not in the A&E department) pay a Rs.10 (approximately 20p) registration fee, after which all consultation and staff fees are free, although medications and equipment have to be paid for. It is well-equipped by Indian standards with its own (working) X-ray machine. The A&E is a busy department with four teams doing a four-day rotating cycle. The doctors are friendly, speak good English and are happy to teach. However, the patients only speak Hindi and therefore a good grasp is necessary to be able to take a history. There's plenty of experience, e.g. trauma, TB, meningitis, cardiac arrests and drug-induced psychoses. You set your own timetable, so (if you have any sense) there's plenty of time to explore Delhi and surrounding areas. Departments which are quieter than A&E may be better if you don't speak Hindi as the doctors will have more time to explain things (although some students have found them very hierarchical). Between January and June they offer rural placements.

Accommodation: If you want to be where it's happening with a lot of foreign travellers, the central youth hostel is a good bet, but not at all cheap at £10 (694 Rs)/night. However, it's clean, has good facilities and one bus takes you straight to AIIMS in 25 minutes. AIIMS will send you a list of local guest houses/B&Bs, claiming to cost about £20 (1400 Rs)/week. Most are considerably more expensive or really a challenge to live in. The Upkar Guest House has been highly recommended. It's cheap (£3 (210 Rs)/night single, £4 (280 Rs)/night double), clean and has good toilets and showers. As you come out of AIIMS (main entrance) cross the busy main road, walk left for about 400 m into the shopping area and there is a small alley on the right before the Indian Oil House (on the left). It is in Yousef Surrai near the Post Office. The canteens in the student hostels provide good Indian and Chinese food at bargain prices.

OTHER MEDICAL SCHOOLS:

College of Medical Sciences, University of Delhi, Ring Road, New Delhi 110029, India.
Government Medical College, Maharishi Dayanand University, Rohtak 124001, India.
Lady Hardinge Medical College, University of Delhi, New Delhi 110001, India Tel: 11-343728.
Maulana Azad Medical College, University of Delhi, New Delhi 110000, India Tel: 11-331-9271.

OTHER HOSPITALS:

St Stephen's Hospital

Tis Hazari, Old Delhi, India.

The hospital: St Stephen's is a large general hospital founded by British missionaries to provide subsidized healthcare for working-class Indians in north Delhi. Churches in the UK initially funded the work, but it is now predominantly funded by cross-subsidy from private practice and money from the Overseas Development Agency. The hospital employs guards armed with large sticks (called *Latti's*) to marshal the endless patients into outpatients. The patients are usually very poor and there is a lot of noise and bustle. Wards are much the same as clinics except the patients are better-behaved.

O Elective notes: Good reports of theatre work. All the doctors speak English and they're a pretty jovial bunch. Language barriers can be a bit of a problem.

All India Blind Relief Society f2 Lajpat Nagar, New Delhi 110024; Willingdon Hospital, New Delhi 110001, India.
Amar Heart Centre, S357 Pnch Shl Park, New Delhi 110017, India.
Batra Hospital and Medical Research Centre, 1 Tughlakabad Institution Area, Mehraula Bbd Road, New Delhi 110062, India.
Deen Dayal Upahdyay Hospital, Harinagar, New Delhi 110064, India.
Delhi Child Health Centre, Fountain View, B Ram Road, 24 Darya Ganj, New Delhi 110002, India.
Dr Ram Manohar Lohia Hospital & Nursing Home, New Delhi, India Tel: 331 1621.
Escorts Heart Institute & Research Centre, Okhla Road, New Delhi 110025, India.
Hamdard Research Clinic & Nursing Home, 2/3a Ali Road, New Delhi 110001, India.
Kasturba Hospital, Near Jama Masjid , New Delhi 110002, India.
Lady Hardinge Medical College & Hospital, P Kuin Road, New Delhi 110001, India.
Lajpat Nagar Hospital, Laj Nagar, New Delhi 110024, India.
Lala Ram Sarum Hospital, Sri Aurobindo Marg, New Delhi 110030, India.
Lok Nayak Jai Parkash Narain Hospital, Jawarhal Nehru Marg, New Delhi 110002, India.
National Chest Institute, Sitaram Jiwarajka Hospital, Gautam Nagar, New Delhi 110049, India.
Nature Cure Hospital, Jawahar Nagar, New Delhi 110007, India.
New Delhi Tuberculosis Centre, JI Nehru Marg, New Delhi 110002, India.

Orthopaedic & Trauma Accident Clinic, 71 Ring Road, Laj Nagar III, New Delhi 110024, India.
Roshan Lal Bajaj Memorial Hospital & Medical Research Institute, 1C/D Guru Gs Marg, New Delhi 110005, India.
Safdarjang Hospital, Safdarjang, New Delhi 110016, India.
Sri Moolchand Khairati Ram Hospital and Ayurvedic Research Institute, Laj Nagar III, New Delhi 1100024, India.
St Luke's Clinic, 70 Vasant Marg, Vasant Vihar, New Delhi 110057, India.
University College of Medical Sciences & GTB Hospital, Sgagdara, Delhi 110095, India Tel: 11-228 0208.

Punjab and Haryana

Originally this area was just the Punjab, and was severely affected by the great divide in forming the border with Pakistan. Political unrest has persisted and only in recent years has it been safe to visit. Amritsar was the capital, but it's a bit too close to Pakistan for comfort. Apart from the Golden Temple there's not a lot to do in the city itself. Chandigarh has been built to be the new capital. Haryana was formed during another split in 1966. You have to go through it to get north from Dehli.

MEDICAL SCHOOLS AND TEACHING HOSPITALS:

The Christian Medical College and Hospital

Punjab University, Ludhiana, 141001, India.
The hospital: A 600-bed joint mission and government-run hospital with its own medical school. It is linked to the British Medical Fellowship.

The Postgraduate Institute of Medical Education and Research

Sector 10, Chandigarh (VT), Haryana, India.
The hospital: The PGI is a 1000-bed tertiary referral hospital serving Chandigarh and areas of Himachal Pradesh, Punjab and Haryana. It has a reputation as a centre of excellence and is advanced by Indian standards. Patients pay Rs 10 (20p) for a consultation and a similar fee per day in hospital. They also have to supply/pay for their medications, needles and dressings. Relatives do most nursing duties. It is busy with many different pathologies.

OTHER MEDICAL SCHOOLS:

Dayanand Medical College and Hospital, Punjab University, Ludhiana 141001, India.
Government Medical College, Punjab University, Patiala 147001, India.
Guru Govind Singh Medical College, Punjab University, Faridkot 151203, India.
Medical College, Guru Nanak Dev University, Amritsar 143001, India.

OTHER HOSPITALS:

Macrobert Hospital

Chariwai District, Gurdaspur, Punjab, India.
The hospital: Is run by the Salvation Army and has 110 beds providing general medical and surgical needs. Outreach eye clinics are also run. It has a small nursing school.

Escorts Hospital and Research Centre

Neelam Bata Road, Faridabad 121 001, Haryana, India.
The hospital: A private hospital and very well-equipped (e.g. CT scanner) 20 miles south of Delhi. It has all major specialities, including neurosurgery and intensive care. Tropical diseases (TB, malaria, typhoid and meningitis) are all pretty common. It's Third World medicine, but this hospital has the facilities to do something.
O Elective notes: Lots to see, but few patients or nurses speak English and not much responsibility for students. Great if you speak Hindi.
Accommodation: A guesthouse is nearby (£3 (210 Rs)/night) but hospital accommodation may be available.

Ajit Prasad Jain, Civil Hospital, Rajpura, Patiala, Punjab, India.
Christian Medical College & Hospital, Ludhiana, Punjab, India.
ESI Hospital, Ludhiana, Punjab, India.
Guru Nanak Mission Hospital, Jalandhar, Punjab, India.
Kdirhna Charitable Hospital, Model Town, Ludhiana, Punjab, India.
St Joseph's Hospital, Rani Col Camp, Hoshiapur, Punjab, India.

Maharashtra (including Mumbai (Bombay))

Mumbai is the financial centre of India with a large manufacturing industry and the world-famous 'Bollywood'. Its prosperity, however, also attracts migrants hopeful of a richer life. This has meant the slum areas have grown. The result is a diverse, vibrant city with an odd mixture of rich and poor in an unusual Victorian setting. Maharashtra itself is a large and prosperous state. The coast has plenty of beaches and small fishing villages. In the north are many buddhist caves such as the Ajanta and Ellora caves.

MEDICAL SCHOOLS AND HOSPITALS:

Armed Forces Medical College, University of Pune, Pune 411001, India.
BJ Medical College, University of Pune, Pune 411001, India.
Dr Vaishampayan Memorial Medical College, Shivaji University, Golibar Maidan, Sholapur 413003, India.
Government Medical College, Marathwada University, Aurangabad 43100, India.
Grant Medical College, University of Bombay, Byculla, Bombay 400008, India.
Indira Gandhi Medical College, Nagpur University, Central Avenue Road, Nagpur 440018, India.
Lokmanya Tilak Municipal Medical College, University of Bombay, Sion, Bombay 400022, India.
Mahatma Gandhi Institute of Medical Sciences, Nagpur University, Sevegram, Wardha 442102, India.
Medical College, Nagpur University, General Hospital, Nagpur 440001, India.
Miraj Medical College, Shivaji University, Miraj 416410, India.
Seth GS Medical College, University of Bombay, Acharya Donde Marg, Parel Bombay 400012, India.
SRTR Medical College, Marathwada University, Ambajogai 431517, India.
Topiwala National Medical College, University of Bombay, Dr AL Nair Road, Byculla, Bombay 400008, India.

Sion Hospital

Bombay, India.

The hospital: One of four large government-funded hospitals in Bombay serving the population of 14 million. It is very busy and situated next to Dharvi, the largest shanty town with many hundreds of thousands of people. (Dharvi itself has its own WHO-funded primary care hospital.) Even as a shanty town it's expensive. A house can cost £20,000 so many can't even afford to live here and are forced onto the streets. There is no sewage system and so faecal–oral infections are common. Illiteracy and malnutrition are also highly prevalent. Sion hospital is very large with most specialities. It provides a basic service free but if patients can 'afford' they get better investigations and the drugs they really need.

PD Hinduja National Hospital

Veer Savarkar Marg, Mahim, Mumbai, India
Tel: 445 1515.

The hospital: A large hospital with most specialities, including cardiology, nephrology and ICU. As with much of India, there is a great deal of TB and malaria seen.

O Elective notes: There are no other students. Staff are friendly and provide good teaching.

OTHER HOSPITALS IN MAHARASHTRA:

Jamkhed Hospital

Jamkhed, Ahmed Najar District, Maharashtra, India.

The hospital: Forty beds over three wards (one O&G and two general). The OPD sees around 100 patients/day. It is very rural and outreach clinics are run in local villages. Minor ops (no general anaesthesia unless surgeon visits) can be done. Rare cases commonly seen include TB, malaria, snakebites (++), trauma and dowry burning. Asthma is also quite a problem. There are plenty of doctors so not much responsibility is given to students. Currently there's not a high incidence of HIV here.

Richardson Leprosy Hospital

Miraj 416410, Sangl District, Maharashtra, India.

The hospital: Is run by Leprosy Mission International and is a tertiary referral centre covering 330,000 with reconstructive surgery, ophthalmology and dermatology. It has 120 beds and a very busy OPD. It is the HQ of the government leprosy survey. It can, however, get a bit specialized but they have links with nearby general medical hospitals. It is a friendly place and a good base in India.

Mure Memorial Hospital

Nagpur 440001, Maharashtra, India.

The hospital: A 120-bed mission hospital providing general and maternity services.

O Elective notes: Work is pretty hard here, but there is plenty to see.

NM Wadia Hospital

283 Shukrawar Peth, Pune 41102, India.

The hospital: A 200-bed missionary hospital providing all general medical, surgical, maternity and ophthalmological services.

Catherine Booth Hospital

Ahmedangar, Maharashtra, India.

The hospital: A 350-bed, Salvation Army-run hospital providing all basic medical, surgical, O&G and orthopaedic needs.

Acworth Leprosy Hospital, Wadala, Bombay 400031, Maharashtra, India.
B Nanavati Hospital, Swami Vivekanand Road, Vile Parle, Bombay 500056, Maharashtra, India.
BAI Jerbai Wadia Hospital for Children, Acharya Donde Marg, Bombay 400012, Maharashtra, India.
BCJ Santa Cruz General Hospital, Swami Vivekanand Road, Bombay 500054, Maharashtra, India.
BYL Nair Hospital, near Bombay Central Railway Station, Bombay 400008, Maharashtra, India.
Bhatia General Hospital, Chikalwadi, J Dadajee Road, Bombay 400017, Maharashtra, India.
Bombay Trust Hospital, Antop Hill Road, Bombay 400031, Maharashtra, India.
Breach Candy Hospital (& Nursing Home), 60 Bhulabhai Desai Road, Cumbella Hill, Bombay 400026, Maharashtra, India Tel: 022 363 2657.
Cama & Albess Hospital, Mahapalika Marg, Bombay 400001, Maharashtra, India.
Chinchpada Christian Hospital, Chinchpada, Maharastra, India. A mission hospital linked to the Emmanuel Hospital Association (see introduction).
Kasturba Hospital, Sane Guruji Marg, Bombay 400011, Maharashtra, India.
KB Bhabha Hospital, Bandra, Bombay 400050, Maharashtra, India.
King Edward Memorial Hospital, King Edward Road, Bombay 400012, Mahahashtra, India.
Lokmanya Tilak Municipal General Hospital, Sion, Bombay 400022, Maharashtra, India.
Mansadevi Tulsiram Municipal General Hospital, Mulund, Bombay 400080, Maharashtra, India.
Mental Hospital, Thane, Bombay 400064, Maharashtra, India.
Municipal Eye Hospital, Kamathipura, Bombay 400008, Maharashtra, India.
Municipal General Hospital, Rajawadi, Ghatkopar, Bombay 400077, Maharashtra, India.
New Hospital for Women, M Permanand Marg, Bombay 400004, Maharashtra, India.
Nowrojee Wadia Maternity Hospital, King Edward Road, Bombay 400012, Maharashtra, India.
Osteopathic Clinic, Dunkeld, JM Mehta Road, Bombay 400006, Maharashtra, India.
Petit Bomanjse Dinshaw Parsee General Hospital, B Desai Road, Bombay 400026, Maharashtra, India.
Raonibai Watumull Sanatorium, 120 Savarkar Marg, Bombay 400016, Maharashtra, India.
Ram Kunvar Charitable X-ray Institute, Dnayaneshwar Mandir Road, Bombay 400002, Maharashtra, India.
Saifee Hospital, 15 Karve Road, Bombay 400001, Maharashtra, India.
Sk Patil Arogya Dham, Daftary Road, Bombay 400064, Maharashtra, India.
St George's Hospital, P D'Mello Road, Bombay 400001, Maharashtra, India.
Seth AJ Bankerbihari Mun, ENT Hospital, Napier Road, Bombay 400001, Maharashtra, India.
Sir Hurkisondas Nurrotumdas Hospital, Prathnasamaj, Bombay 400001, Maharashtra, India.
Wanless Hospital, Miraj, Maharashtra, India.

West Bengal (including Calcutta)

Calcutta, once the Indian capital, conjures thoughts of Mother Teresa and desolate slums. Initially a prosperous town from jute-production, it was plunged into poverty with Partition which divided the mines from the refineries. Since then it has suffered a number of influxes of refugees. It is an amazing city that attacks the senses and can be quite trying. Within India it is known as a centre for arts and culture as well as being a thriving metropolis (the noble laureate Rabindranath Tagore and the film director Satyajit Ray came from these parts). To turn back the clock it is trying to change its name back to its original, Kalikata. It's a huge experience. Most hospitals won't provide accommodation; try Sudder Street in central Calcutta which is where all the foreign travellers head. The northern end of West Bengal is another extreme with quiet serenity in the tea plantations of Darjeeling and the Himalayan foothills.

MEDICAL SCHOOLS AND TEACHING HOSPITALS:

Nilratan Sicar Medical College and Hospital (NRS)

138 Acharya JC Bose Road, Calcutta-1, India.

The hospital: One of the largest in India and a government-run teaching hospital. It provides care for the very poor and is very overcrowded with poor facilities. Cats and goats roam freely around and there is no limit to the number of patients that can be squeezed in. Lots of tropical diseases. The staff however are very knowledgeable and have excellent clinical skills.

O Elective notes: Good teaching with the local students. Being able to speak Bengali is a BIG plus. Very few patients speak English and the staff are too busy to translate. Try to go to a private hospital in Calcutta to see the difference.

The Ramakrishna Seva Pratishtan (RKSP) Hospital

99 Sarat Bose Road, Calcutta 700 026, India Tel: 33 475 3636/37/38/39 Fax: 33 475 4351.

The hospital: The RKSP is a charitable hospital, but is also recognized as a post-graduate training institute by the University of Calcutta. It has an educational unit with reasonable library and some organized seminars/lectures. Patients have to pay for their own drugs, venflons, pacemakers etc. and hence this prevents the poorest being treated here. Surgery is a luxury beyond the means of most people.

O Elective notes: Some of the surgeons can give excellent teaching. Being able to speak Bengali is an obvious advantage. Again, as is common in India, because of the hierachical system, don't expect any more responsibility than in a Western hospital.

Accommodation: The hospital has a list of local accommodation.

Institute of Opthalmology, Calcutta Medical College

Calcutta, India.

The hospital: State-run and busy. Only the very poor come here. Beds are very close to each other, no curtains and there are only two or three nurses to cover several wards. Each operating theatre has two or three tables. Many of Calcutta's own students study here.

Accommodation: Not provided.

North Bengal Medical College

PO Sushruta Nagar, Darjeeling Pin: 734432, West Bengal, India Tel: 0353 75201 Fax: 0353 450285.

The hospital: A large teaching hospital. It is very busy with most specialities. Lots of unusual pathologies. The hospital is pretty dirty and crowded. Villagers come from miles to get to here.

O Elective notes: Highly recommended for surgery, but it is hard work.

Accommodation: Provided on campus for Rs 10/week (8p) and food = Rs100 (£1.50/week).

North Bengal Poly Clinic

Nivedita Road, Pradhan Nagar, Siliguri, 734403 West Bengal, India Tel: 0353 433120.

The hospital: Fairly large with all major specialities.

O Elective notes: Good teaching from friendly staff. Patients all speak Bengali.

Advanced Medicare and Research Institute

Calcutta, West Bengal, India.

The hospital: Is privately run and some patients here speak English. The contrast to government hospitals is incredible. It is like a Western hospital. Patients have to pay £5/night here, but that can only be afforded by the well-off.

OTHER MEDICAL SCHOOLS:

BS Medical College, University of Calcutta, Bankura 711303, West Bengal, India.

Calcutta National Medical College, University of Calcutta, Calcutta 700014, West Bengal, India.
Medical College, Burdwan University, Burdwan 713101, West Bengal, India.
Medical College, University of Calcutta, Calcutta 700012, West Bengal, India. (This is the oldest and largest medical college in Calcutta.)
RG Kar Medical College, University of Calcutta, Calcutta 700004, West Bengal, India.

OTHER HOSPITALS:

Belle Vue Clinic, 9 Loudon Street, Calcutta 700016, West Bengal, India.
Calcutta Nursing Home, 231/I Lower Circular Road, Calcutta 700020, West Bengal, India.
Kumup Sankar Ray TB Hospital, Jadavpur, Calcutta 700032, West Bengal, India.
Marwari Relief Society Hospital, 392 U Chitpur Road, Calcutta 700007, West Bengal, India.
Matri Mangal Pratisthan, 51 U Chitpur Road, Calcutta 700007, West Bengal, India.
MN Chatterjee Memorial Eye Hospital, 295/1 Acharya P Chander Road, Calcutta 700009, West Bengal, India.
North Howrah Hospital, 22 Guha Road, Ghusuri, Howrah, West Bengal, India.
Park Nursing Home, 4 Victoria Terrace, Calcutta 700017, West Bengal, India.
Paschim Banga Samaj Seva Samity, Baranagar Hospital, 282 Madjid Bari Lane, Calcutta 700055, West Bengal, India.
Woodlands Nursing Home, Alipore, Calcutta 700027, West Bengal, India.

Karnataka

Previously known as Mysore, Karnataka has both historic temples, ruins and natural beauty (especially the beaches). It is a major producer of silk, coffee and spices and its capital, Bangalore, is growing at an incredible rate with its high-tech industries. It is now the fifth largest city in India and extremely 'Westward' for India with an almost 'pub culture'. Hampi, a 500-year-old deserted city, is eight hours by train, 12 hours by bus and one hour by plane (£67). The main language is Kanada and the predominant religion is Hinduism.

MEDICAL SCHOOLS AND TEACHING HOSPITALS:

St John's Memorial College Hospital/St John's Medical College

Sarjapur Road, Bangalore 560034, South India.

The hospital: St John's is a large (900-bed), private, Catholic teaching hospital and tertiary referral centre situated in the south of the city. Both the outpatients department and the inpatient wards are incredibly busy. Guards man the wards to ensure no outsiders climb into a bed to be fed. Many patients have to leave hospital mid-treatment as their finances run out. Overall, it's all fairly disorganized. However, by Indian standards, it is well-equipped and does excellent research. There are facilities for cardiac catheterization and CT scanning and recently they have done their first heart transplant.

❍ Elective notes: It is a popular choice for elective students. You are encouraged to rotate around as many departments as possible, but are really given free rein as to what you want to do. The doctors are friendly and helpful. There are trips into the surrounding villages with the community outreach health team giving a great insight into village and slum life. Many of the students there are Catholic sisters who train specifically for a life dedicated to working in slums. There's no real integration with the Indian students; however, there are usually a few elective students there at any one time (usually 10–15). As Bangalore has become more Western, so have the diseases, e.g. MIs, diabetes and asthma. HIV is increasing (about five cases/day). There are many opportunities for minor procedures. Most people speak English and it's pretty easy to get around and away from. You have to pay £70 to work here. Overall it's a good gentle introduction to India and a good place to explore India from, although not a good place to see *Indian* medicine.

Accommodation: Cheap (Rs 50 = £1–£3/night) and adequate (*en-suite* toilet and basin) and the food not bad. The are usually other British/American elective students there, so the social life is pretty good. There are many restaurants (KFC, Pizza Hut, Wimpey) up to the five-star hotels. An evening out (five-star) with food and drinks costs Rs

150–700. There's a café on Brigade Road with e-mail and Internet access.

Kasturba Medical College/Hospital, Mangalore University

Manipal, India.

The hospital: One of the largest teaching hospitals in Karnataka with many services. A wide range of pathology is seen. Electives here have been well-recommended.

Accommodation: Has been available previously.

Cheluvamba Hospital for Women and Children (Krishna Rao Hospital)

Mysore 570001, Karnataka, India.

The hospital: A government hospital that treats very poor patients from Mysore. It is a teaching hospital for the state-run medical school with 600 beds and most specialities (e.g. plastics). Although the staff are very good, they perform this service with a shortage of drugs and in poor conditions. There is only one nurse per ward. Malnutrition, gastroenteritis, rheumatic fever and TB are all common. There's a busy outpatients and busy paeds ward.

Manipal Academy of Higher Education

Manipal, Karnataka 576119, India.

The hospital: A large teaching hospital with all major specialities. Manipal itself is a university town on a hill. The location is beautiful and there are plenty of sporting activities. Highly recommended for students.

Accommodation: The school has supplied rooms for Rs100/day.

Al-Ameen Medical College, Athani Road, Bijapur 586108, Karnataka, India Tel: 22472. (Established in 1984 and affiliated to Rajiv.)
Bangalore Medical College, Bangalore University, Bangalore 560001, Karnataka, India Tel: 812 601544.
Gandi Health University, Bangalore and Karnataka University Dharwad. (It has 100 students/year.)
Government Medical College, Gulbarga University, Bellary 583101, Karnataka, India.
Jadadguru Jayadeva Murugarajendra Medical College, Mysore University, Davangere 577004, Karnataka, India.
JLN Medical College, Karnataka University, Poona Bangalore Road, Nehri Nagar, Belgaum 590010, Karnataka, India.
Karnataka Medical College, Karnataka University, Hubli 580020, Karnataka, India.
Mahadevappa Pampure Medical College, Gulbarga University, Gulbarga 585105, Karnataka, India.
Mysore Medical College, Mysore University, Mysore 570001, Karnataka, India. (This is the oldest in Mysore.)

OTHER HOSPITALS IN KARNATAKA:

Church of South India Hospital

2 Col Hill Road, Chikballapur 562101, Karnataka, India Tel: 08156 72269.

The hospital: An overcrowded, self-funded 175-bed hospital in Chikballapur, a small town 60 km north of Bangalore. It gives a wide range of experiences with good general medical, surgical, O&G and paediatric cases daily. Five consultants and a few juniors run the show. Rural clinics are run three times a week. Pathology present includes: malaria, leprosy, typhoid fever, burns, CCF, liver failure, snake bites, bull gores and many normal and complicated deliveries. Diagnostic aids and medication are, unsurprisingly, lacking. Few of the patients speak English; however, all the doctors and nurses do.

O Elective notes: Currently run by a Scottish trained surgeon who'll turn his hand to anything. His surgery starts at 6.30 am so take an alarm clock. There are three weekly trips to treat patients in the community. Chikballapur (population 40,000) is a very quiet and peaceful place with Bangalore just 1½ hours away by bus. From there, the rest of India can be explored.

Accommodation: Has previously been available for about £1 (Rs 70) a day.

Holdsworth Memorial Hospital

Mysore City, Mysore, Karnataka, India.

The hospital: A 300-bed mission hospital. It has basic specialities and a heavy maternity load.

Jaya Vijayam Tribal Hospital

Virekananda Ginjana Kalyana Kenda, BR Hills 571441, Mysore District, Karnataka, India.

The hospital: This hospital was set up for the local tribes who until 15 years ago moved through the forests of the wildlife sanctuary. It has attempted to provide good medical care while preserving the traditional plant medicine knowledge the locals have. There is a very high incidence of sickle cell disease, TB and obstetric complications.

Manipal Hospital

98 Ruston Bagh, Airport Road, Bangalore, Karnataka, India Tel: 80 526 6646 Fax: 080 526 6757

The hospital: A large private hospital. Lots of excellent facilities and pathology to be seen.

O Elective notes: This is a very friendly place and electives here have been recommended.

Accommodation: Can be arranged.

Anath Ayurvedic Centre

3/89 Bull Temple Road, Bangalore 560 019, Karnataka, India.

The hospital: Practices ayurvedic medicine, a 4000-year-old traditional medical culture based on the holy scriptures of Hindu texts. It has specialities such as surgery, paeds and O&G but its diagnoses and treatments are very different using herbs, oils and powders. It is very popular. Visit herb gardens and see it used in general practice.

AB Shetti Hospital, Mangalore, Karnataka, India.
Baptist Mission Hospital, Bebal, Bangalore, Karnataka, India.
Bowring and Lady Curzon Hospital, Shivaji Nagar, Bangalore, Karnataka, India.
ESI Hospital, Indiranagar, Bangalore, Karnataka, India.
ETCM Hospital, PO Box 4, Kolar, Karnataka 563101, India. (A mission hospital run by the Emmanuel Hospital Association.)
National Institute of Mental Health & Neuro Sciences, PO Box 2979, Hosur Road, Bangalore 560029, Karnataka, India.
St Martha's Hospital, Nrupathunga Road, Bangalore, Karnataka, India.
Victoria Hospital, KR Market, Bangalore, Karnataka, India.

Tamil Nadu (including Madras (Chennai))

Chennai (formerly Madras) is a large city and compared with other Indian cities is clean and quiet. It has a large business and manufacturing industry contributing to its wealth, although as a tourist destination it does not have many 'sites'. Tamil Nadu State as a whole is the least-influenced area of India by outsiders. The Muslims didn't get very far into it and the British haven't left much of a mark either. It is predominantly vegetarian as a result and in some areas alcohol can be difficult to obtain. Pondicherry is the exception as it has had a strong French influence since the eighteenth century.

MEDICAL SCHOOLS AND TEACHING HOSPITALS:

Christian Medical College and Hospital Vellore, University of Madras

Ida Scudder Road, Post Box 3, Vellore 632004, Tamil Nadu, India Tel: 416 22603
http://cmch-vellore.edu/

The hospital: A missionary hospital with a medical school. It is the biggest hospital in south India with 1700 beds and has specialities such as cardiothoracic and plastic surgery. People come from all over India to be seen here. It is very highly regarded. It was founded by an America lady, Dr Ida Scudder, and trains male and female doctors and nurses. It offers care regardless of income, race or religion. Malnutrition is common (but it is mainly male children that get brought to see the doctor).

O Elective notes: The staff are friendly and you can do rounds, clinics or join CMC student teaching. Not great for hands on, but you will learn a lot as teaching is excellent. Due to the language problem, the doctors take the history then point out things to you. Language barriers (Tamil and Hindi) can restrict what you get out of it. They also don't like you wandering off in the week. Weekends are free. It's Third world medicine in an almost First World hospital. There is a small charge for electives here. The Community Health and Development Department (CMC Vellore, Tamil Nadu) is excellent for getting to study paediatrics and experience India's culture.

Accommodation: The college gives a list of hostels that you must write to directly. Some students have had basic accommodation in the hospital (less than £1/day). You will be expected to share in that. Very recently new accommodation has been built.

Sri Ramachandra Medical College and Research Institute

I Ramachandra Nagar, Porur,
Madras/Chennai 600 116, Tamij Nadu, India
Tel: 4828027-29 Fax: 44 4827008
http://205.216.249.36/srmc/
e-mail srmc@hostindia.com

The Medical School is deemed a university and uses the Sri Ramachandra Hospital.

The hospital: A non-profit making organization with 1050 beds in the suburbs of Madras. It caters for city and rural folk. Many advanced specialities, such as neuro and cardiothoracic surgery, transplant and advanced trauma services, are provided. Approximately 2000 outpatients are seen each day and given free consultations, investigations and prescriptions. Rates for inpatients are from Rs1 to Rs150. It has CT and MRI facilities. A great deal of tropical medicine is seen in rural patients.

O Elective notes: It is very friendly and you'll see more pathology than you thought possible. The hospital itself is partly private (300 beds) so there's not much hands on experience, but the teaching is superb. Surgery has been highly recommended. A special 'tropical medicine' elective programme has been set up. Full details and application form are on their web site. Unfortunately they charge $500 for the privilege.

Accommodation: Free, but you'll have to confirm this in advance.

Chingleput (or Chengalpattu) Medical College, University of Madras, Chingleput 603001, Tamil Nadu, India.
Coimbatore Medical College, University of Madras, Coimbatore 641014, Tamil Nadu, India Tel: 422-574375.
Jawaharlal Institute of Postgraduate Medical Education and Research, University of Madras, Pondicherry 605006, Tamil Nadu, India. (This is a large institute that comes recommended.)
Kilpauk Medical College, University of Madras, Madras 600010, Tamil Nadu, India.
Madras Medical College, University of Madras, Madras 600003, Tamil Nadu, India.
Medical College, Madurai University, Madurai 625020, Tamil Nadu, India.
Stanley Medical College, University of Madras, Madras 600001, Tamil Nadu, India Tel: 44 513311.
Thanjavur Medical College, University of Madras, Thanjavur 613001, Tamil Nadu, India.
Tirunelvelu Medical College, Madurai University, Tirunelveli 627002, Tamil Nadu, India.

OTHER HOSPITALS:

Christian Fellowship Hospital

Oddanchatram, Anna District, Tamil Nadu 624619, India.

The hospital: The CFH is a mission hospital in rural Tamil Nadu. It is very popular for electives and voluntary work, hence the detail below. It is subsidized and attracts patients from miles around. They come to queue in their hundreds at the outpatient clinics. Very few lab tests are available. This results in clinicians with excellent clinical skills. Oddanchatram is a semirural area about 120 km from Madurai, the south Indian city most famous for its huge Meenakshi temple, silk and cotton. It has an interesting history. In the late 1940s, a group of Christian medical students from Miraj decided to venture into the poverty-stricken village. In 1955 one doctor, one nurse and one paramedic came to work here permanently, setting up in a bamboo hut. Many patients came and it quickly grew to become a 40-bed hospital. In 1958 the hospital moved to new premises when a patient offered five acres of land and a builder offered his services for free. The hospital now has 270 beds and an average of 800–1000 outpatients a day. CFH is entirely self-sufficient, accepting no outside funds from mission societies or other organizations. Patients have to pay for all tests and treatments, but it is entirely at the doctor's discretion to allow concessions for those who genuinely are financially restrained. Despite this, poverty is still a problem. Many diabetic patients can't afford their insulin and so complications become a problem. A number of open-air clinics are performed in surrounding villages. They tackle education, housing, water and nutrition as well as starting cottage industries such as basket weaving. Common conditions include gastroenteritis and malnutrition in children, treated with the WHO strategy of basic oral rehydration. Following that successful campaign, they are starting another for lower respiratory tract infections. Primary healthcare workers in villages are trained to count a child's respiratory rate using an hourglass and act accordingly. It is taking off and effective. TB is also very common, diagnosed often on clinical grounds. Compliance with treatment is a common problem. Women are encouraged to have sterilization immediately after the birth of their second child in an attempt to reduce the population growth.

O Elective notes: Students are expected to see and treat patients on their own, an excellent way to learn medicine. There is good teaching within the hospital itself as well, especially the intensive care unit. The staff are very friendly and involve you in their postgraduate programme. However, because it is a rural hospital, there is very little to do in the evenings. The hospital is well served by buses and it is a great place from which to explore the south of India. Overall, it's an excellent place to learn, but take some good books. Once you've learnt a bit of Tamil you can examine patients very quickly. All the doctors speak English.

Accommodation: Provided, but very basic.

Government General Hospital

Indiragandi Nagar Road, Madras 60002, Tamil Nadu, India.

The hospital: The major general hospital in Madras.

Institute of Thoracic Medicine

Chetput, Chennai, 600031, Tamil Nadu, India.

The hospital: Good for chest disease and infectious/tropical medicine.

CSI Rainy Hospital

Royapuram, Madras 60021, Tamil Nadu, India.

The hospital: A 170-bed mission hospital providing all basic specialities.

Catherine Booth Hospital

Nagercoil 629001, Tamil Nadu, India.

The hospital: A 350-bed Salvation Army hospital situated on the tip of India providing all general medical and surgical needs.

MV Diabetes Specialties Centre

35 Conran Smith Road, Chennai 600086, Tamil Nadu, India Tel: 826 3038/828 2657.

The hospital: A specialist centre for diabetes.

Accommodation: Provided free.

Arignar Anna Govt Hospital of Indigenous Medicine, Arumbakkam, Madras 600029, Tamil Nadu, India.

ESI Hospital, 37 Madhavakkam Tank Road, Madras 600023, Tamil Nadu, India.

Govt Chest Institute & TB Training Centre, Spur Tank Road, Madras 800031, Tamil Nadu, India.

Govt Kasturba Gandhi Hospital for Women and Children, Madras 600005, Tamil Nadu, India.

Govt Kilpauk Medical College & Hospital, PH Road, Madras 600010, Tamil Nadu, India.

Govt Ophthalmic Hospital, Egmore, Madras 600008, Tamil Nadu.

Govt Royapettah Hospital, Madras 600014, Tamil Nadu, India.

Govt TB Sanatorium, Tambaram, Madras 400047, Tamil Nadu, India.

Govt Thiruvoteswarar TB Hospital, Konnur High Road, Otteri, Madras 600012, Tamil Nadu, India.

Gremaltes Hospital, Shannoy Nagar, Chennai is excellent for leprosy and skin diseases. They also run rural clinics.

Institute of Child Health & Hospital for Children, Halls Road, Madras 600008, Tamil Nadu.

Raja Sir Ramaswamy Mudaliar's Lying-In Hospital, Kamraj Road, Madras 600013, Tamil Nadu.

Stanley Hospital, Old Jail Street, Madras 600001, Tamil Nadu.

Tuberculosis & Chemotherapy Centre, Spur Tank Road, Madras 600031, Tamil Nadu, India.

Kerala

Kerala is a beautiful narrow strip of India in the south-west corner that is separated from the rest of India by dense forest. This has protected it from land invasion and enhanced its use of the sea. It has a large maritime as well as agricultural industry. International influence has created an area of well-educated (nearly 100% literacy) and relatively well-off Indians.

MEDICAL SCHOOLS AND TEACHING HOSPITALS:

Kottayam Medical College, University of Kerala, Gandhi Nagar, Kottayam 686008, Kerala, India.
Medical College, Calicut University, Calicut 673008, Kerala, India. (This is the largest with over 2000 beds.)
Medical College, University of Kerala, Pattom Palace PO, Trivandrum 695011, Kerala, India. (This is the oldest.)
TD Medical College, University of Kerala, Aleppey 688005, Kerala, India.

OTHER HOSPITALS:

Lal Memorial Hospital

Asan Nagar, Maddayikonam Irinjalakuda, Trichur Kerala, India.

The hospital: Lal Memorial Hospital is in a small town about two hours' drive from the nearest big city (Trivandrum). It is a small general hospital with departments in medicine, surgery, obstetrics and gynaecology, paediatrics, ENT and ophthalmology. It is run by a charity and is very basic, but there are plenty of opportunities to learn. They never have local students and therefore the doctors are very keen to teach and help.

Accommodation: Provided free in the hospital grounds where most of the doctors and nurses live. This is very sociable … you won't have a minute to yourself. The surrounding area is magnificent and typically rural India. There is an elephant next door in the local timber yard!

Mar Kurilose Mission Hospital

Anjoor, PO Thozhiyur – 680520, Trissur Dt, Kerala, India.

The hospital: Built in 1976 by the Malabar Independent Syrian Church. It is three minutes' walk from St George Cathedral (the church's headquarters) in Thozhiyur, a small town near the west coast of south India. It is financed completely by the church. It has 25 beds and employs one consultant and two junior doctors. Most of the medical consultations are for hypertension and diabetes. Heart disease is therefore a major problem. TB, typhoid and malaria are also seen. Women in Kerala are well-informed about childbirth risks; therefore most want hospital births. Perinatal and maternal mortality rates are low (comparable to Western rates) and Caesarean section rates are 10–20%. Education about family size is rigorous (sterilization offered after second child). Psychiatric complaints are very common, especially among the young women – commonly their husbands go off to work in the Gulf leaving them with the family. Depression is treated with simple antidepressants. Any psychosis is still managed by the church, the priest removing the demons.

Holy Cross Hospital, Cheriakadau, Cochin, Kerala, India.
Iruvella Medical Mission, Tirunelveli, Kerala, India Tel: 473 630144.
Josgiri Hospital, Tellicherry, Cannanore, Kerala, India.
Sree Chitra Tirunal Institute for Medical Sciences & Technology, Truvabdryn 695011, Kerala, India.
St Mary's Hospital, Kattakada, Trivandrum, Kerala, India.

Goa

Unlike the rest of India, the Portuguese influence is still very evident here. Roman Catholicism is still a major religion and there are more churches than temples. It is famed for its idyllic beaches, although this has made it a bit of a tourist trap. This in turn has made it a rich area with relatively good healthcare and education. It is also a much fairer society towards women.

THE MEDICAL SCHOOL:

Goa Medical College and Ribandar Hospital, University of Bombay

Ribandar, Panaji 403001 (or Bambolim 402202)

The hospital: A very busy teaching hospital with many students about (founded 1963, 700 beds).

O Elective notes: Very didactic teaching and not much in the way of hands on. Students translate though.

OTHER HOSPITALS:

Asilo Hospital Mapusa, Rajvedda, Mapusa, Goa, India.
Dr Fernando Menezes Hospital, Rai Salcete, Goa, India.
Goa Dental College & Hospital, PO Bambolim, Goa, India.
Rebello Hospital, Madel, Margao, Goa, India.
Salgonkar Medical Research Centre, Vasco da Gama, Goa, India. Tel: 0834 512524.
Shri Kamaxi Nursing Home, Shiroda 403103, Goa, India.
Sirsat Hospital, Tiska, Ponda 403401, Goa, India.
Usganonkar Hospital, Sadar, Ponda 403401, India.

Gujarat

On the west coast, Gujarat has ancient temples, tribal villages and is home to the Asiatic lion. There are also some beautiful beaches at Diu and Mandvi.

MEDICAL SCHOOLS:

BJ Medical College, Gujarat University, Ahmadabad 380016, Gujarat, India Tel: 272 376074.
Government Medical College, South Gujarat University, Surat 395001, Gujarat, India Tel: 261 41596
Government Medical College University of Baroda, Sayiji Gunj, Baroda Vadodara 390006, Gujarat, India Tel: 265 451594.
MP Shah Medical College, Sauashtra University, Jamnagar 361001, Gujarat, India.
NHL Municipal Medical College, Gujarat University, Ellis bridge, Ahmadabad 380006, Gujarat, India Tel: 272 76275.

OTHER HOSPITALS:

Sheth Vadilal Sarabhai General Hospital and Sheth Chinas Maternity Hospital

Ellisbridge, Ahmadabad, Gujarat 380006, India.

The hospital: The VS Hospital is a fairly large hospital seeing the poorer communities of Ahmadabad. Most facilities are available, but the conditions are poor with wards holding 80 patients plus relatives and pigeons. Some equipment, including gloves and needles, are recycled. The language can be a problem: although the notes and teaching sessions are in English, the signs are in (and most people only speak) Gujarati.

O Elective notes: The staff are friendly and you'll get to perform procedures on your own. The VS receives very few elective students, but they are fairly well set up for them. You are encouraged to go to theatre; however, you may be behind six other heads. Ahmadabad ('the Manchester of the east') is a friendly, safe place; however, there is little to do with alcohol being prohibited (but available for tourists).

Note: Between April and August it can get very hot (47°C). Also, if you're Caucasian, prepare to be stared at a lot.

Accommodation: Cannot be provided and it can be difficult to arrange.

Emery Hospital

Anand 388001, Gujarat, India.

The hospital: A 200-bed mission hospital with all basic specialities.

Accommodation: Has previously been provided for students.

Bhagat Nursing Home, Valsad, Gujarat, India.
Dr DM Gandhi's Hospital, Bardoli, Surat, Gujarat, India.
Dr JK Patel's Hospital, Vadodara, Gujarat, India.
Dr Johar Thakkar's Hospital, Veraval, Junagadh, Gujarat, India.
Dr KM Shah Hospital, Laldarwaja, Ahmadabad, Gujarat, India.
Dr NG Savsani's Hospital, Junagadh, Gujarat, India.
Dr Sakaruta Neducak & Surgical Hospital, Saraspur, Ahmadabad, Gujarat, India.

India

ESI General Hospital, Surat, Gujarat, India.
MV Rajda Charitable Hospital, Jamkhambhalia, Jamnagar, Gujarat, India.
St Mary General Hospital, Gomtipur, Ahmadabad, Gujurat, India.

Himachal Pradesh

This beautiful area extends from the foothills of the Himalayas high up to the Tibetan plateau. It differs greatly from the rest of India in its climate, altitude and religion. Tibetan Buddhism is the mainstay here. This is reflected in the practice of Tibetan as well as Western medicine. Shimla in the south is a very pleasant town with great colonial influence. Dharamsala is an old British Hill station, but now better known as the home to the Tibetan government in exile and the Dalai Lama. It is in the Himalayan foothills and has beautiful views. Many Tibetan monks are here, giving it a very unusual feel for India. It is a pleasant and popular place for electives and volunteers and hence both a Tibetan and Western Institute are listed below. To the north are yet more impressive landscapes. Manali in the Kullu Valley is not so attractive since it has been overrun by tourism, especially honeymooning couples. (It does however grow some of the finest marijuana in the world apparently.)

MEDICAL SCHOOLS:

Himachal Pradesh/Indira Gandhi Medical College

Himachal Pradesh University, Simla 171001, Himachal Pradesh, India Tel: 177 77820.

Tibetan Delek Hospital

Gangchen Kyishong, Dharamsala 176 215, Dist. Kangra, Himachal Pradesh, India.

The hospital: The hospital is run by the Tibetan community but serves the needs of the Tibetans, Indian people and Westerners living in the area. Although Tibetan-run, the doctors are mainly unpaid Western volunteers. There is a long-stay TB ward and much of the outreach work is also focused on TB treatment. There are about 20 inpatient beds for adults and children and daily or twice daily outpatient clinics, including a weekly antenatal clinic. The medicine practised here is Western style. There is also a torture victims unit on site (for new refugees from Tibet).

O Elective notes: There is a real sense of community at the Delek. Everyone cooks and eats together on the roof of the doctors' accommodation. There is plenty of medicine to get involved in and procedures such as draining abscesses, and ascitic taps to do. The hospital, and the two listed below, are up in the mountains. Many travellers come via here to see the Dalai Lama or to learn Buddhism. This elective gives an excellent insight into 'Third World medicine' and also the plight of the Tibetan people, their religion and culture.

Men-Tsee-Khang

Tibetan Medical and Astrological Institute of HH the Dalai Lama, Gangchen Kyishong, Dharamsala 176 215, Dist. Kangra, Himachal Pradesh, India.

The hospital: This is the institute for the preservation and further investigation into Tibetan medicine. It has a number of clinics all over India (and now throughout the world) that continue to practise Tibetan medicine. It has a clinic on-site and also one just up the road in Macleod Gange. The staff are incredibly friendly and if you fancy tasting medicine from a very different culture, this is highly recommended. Most of the time is spent in outpatients clinics. There are no beds here, although the Delek Hospital (for Western medicine) is right opposite.

Accommodation: Provided occasionally, but there are plenty of cheap guesthouses.

The Medical Dispensary

Geden Choeling, Nunnery, PO Macleod Gange 176219, Dharamsala, Dist. Kangra, Himachal Pradesh, India (run by Association un Dispensaire pour Dharamsala, Angigonda, 5 Bordeaux St Augustin 33035, Bordeaux, France).

The clinic: A drop-in clinic seeing relatively minor complaints in the local community.

○ Elective notes: Excellent teaching and plenty of opportunities to do minor procedures and, if busy, see patients independently. An elective here has been highly recommended.
Accommodation: There are plenty of guesthouses, but accommodation has been provided in the past.

Lady Wellington Hospital
Manali, Kullu, Himachal Pradesh 17131, India.
The hospital: LWH is a mission hospital in the foothills of the Himalaya with 40 beds and a busy outpatients run by about four doctors. Manali itself is a nice, but touristy town.
○ Elective notes: It's busy and there are plenty of minor procedures. Lots of superb trekking up to Lahaul or Ladalch. There are usually two medical students here. It can be hard work (on-call three nights/week) and some people have not enjoyed it, whereas others have got stuck in and loved it. There are outlying clinics. You don't have to be Christian, but do respect it.
Accommodation: Pretty squalid and dirty.

Bihar

Although Bihar is a holy area for Buddhists, Hindus and Jains, it also seems to be cursed. It suffers great floods and its inhabitants are among the poorest and most illiterate in India. Violence and crime are also commonplace compared to the rest of India. Watch your belongs if travelling through.

MEDICAL SCHOOLS AND TEACHING HOSPITALS:

Anugrah Narain Magadh Medical College, Magadh University, Bodhgaya, Gaya 823001, Bihar, India.
Darbhanga Medical College, LN Mithila University, Laheriasarai 846001, Bihar, India.
Mahatma Gandhi Memorial Medical College, Ranchi University, PO Mango, Jamshedpur 831001, Bihar, India.
Medical College, Bhagalpur University, Bhagalpur 812001, Bihar, India.
Nalanda Medical College, Magad University, Bodhgaya, Patna 800001, Bihar, India.
Patliputra Medical College, Ranchi Uinversity, Dhanbad 826001, Bihar, India.
Patna Medical College, Patna University, Patna 800004, Bihar, India.
Rajendra Medical College, Ranchi University, Ranchi 834001, Bihar, India.
Sri Krishna Medical College, Bihar University, PO Umanager, Muzaffarpur 842001, Bihar, India.

OTHER HOSPITALS:

St Luke's Hospital
PO Hiranpur, District Sahebganj, Bihar 816104, India Tel: 06435 8262.
The hospital: St Luke's is a mission hospital in north-east India. It is the largest hospital in the area and serves one of India's poorest and most backward areas. It has 100 beds and deals with general medicine and surgery, orthopaedics, O&G and ophthalmology.
○ Elective notes: A typical day consists of a ward round, outpatient clinic and theatre. There's plenty of pathology and tropical diseases to see – TB, malaria and kala-azar. Normally there are around three doctors, all of whom speak English and conduct ward rounds in English. There is some good teaching and there is often the opportunity to assist in theatre and perform minor procedures. You can do any speciality you like. Village clinics are also run.

Note: It is important to consider which season you will be visiting in. In the monsoon season (June–September) most people stay working on the paddy fields despite their illness. They are happy to give you time off to travel. Highly recommended (repeatedly). Apply early. There's not much to do in the evenings, but it is easy to visit Darjeeling (ten hours away), Calcutta (six hours), Nepal and to travel around India from the hospital. Although the doctors speak English, few patients do and this can be a problem.
Accommodation: Provided in the hospital at around £3 a day.

The Duncan Hospital
Raxaul, Champaran District, Bihar, India.
The hospital: A 200-bed mission hospital with general medial, surgical and O&G specialities.

Nav Jiwan Hospital
Satbarwa, Bihar, India.
A mission hospital run by the Emmanuel Hospital Association.

Uttar Pradesh

In the north Uttar Pradesh has the foothills of the Himalayas while the south has vast plains that often flood forming the basin of the Ganges. Hinduism is the religion and there are many holy places, especially Varanasi on the banks of the river Ganges. It also contains Agra, home to the Taj Mahal. For wildlife there is the Corbett Tiger Reserve. Uttar Pradesh is the most populated region of India.

The Director General for the region is at Medical and Health Services, Lucknow, Uttar Pradesh, India.

MEDICAL SCHOOLS:

Baba Raghav Das Medical College, Gorakhpur University, Gorakhpur 273013, Uttar Pradesh, India.
GSVM Medical College, Kanpur University, Kanpur 208001, Uttar Pradesh, India.
Institute of Medical Sciences, Banaras Hindu University, Varanasi 221005, Uttar Pradesh, India Tel: 542 310483.
JLN Medical College, Aligarh Muslim University, Aligarh 202002, Uttar Pradesh, India Tel: 571 28894.
KG Medical College, University of Lucknow, Lucknow 226001, Uttar Pradesh, India.
LLRM Medical College, Meerut University, Meerut 250001, Uttar Pradesh, India.
MLB Medical College, Kanpur/Bundelkhand University, Khansi (Jhansi) 284128, Uttar Pradesh, India.
MLN Medical College, University of Allahabad, Lowther Road, Allahabad 211001, Uttar Pradesh, India Tel: 532 601983.
SN Medical College, Agra University, Agra 282002, Uttar Pradesh, India Tel: 562 63913.

OTHER HOSPITALS:

Mahanagar Civil Hospital
Lucknow, Uttar Pradesh, India.
The hospital: In Lucknow (population 5,000,000), was originally a small dispensary set up by two doctors. It now has 35 doctors, 30 inpatient beds, four GP clinics, an outpatients, O&G, respiratory medicine, paeds, ortho and family planning. Facilities are very limited. Patients pay Rs 2.00 (4p) on arrival in the hospital. TB, malaria, typhoid, leprosy, tropical pulmonary eosinophilia and asthma are common. No one knows the degree of HIV.

Mahila Women's Hospital
Mirazapur, Uttar Pradesh, India.
The hospital: Is in a small town east of Lucknow with 62 beds of two obs and two gynae wards. It caters for a large rural population of Hindu and Muslim women. There are 3000 deliveries a year. The wards are crowded. Abortion here is legal up to 20 weeks. This hospital does not do ultrasound scans. However, some go to private hospitals (Rs 300 = £6 for a scan), find out the sex and if female then ask for an abortion.

Kachhwa Christian Hospital
Kachhaw, Uttar Pradesh
and
Landour Community Hospital
Mussoorie, Uttar Pradesh, India.
Are mission hospitals run by the Emmanuel Hospital Association.

St Mary's Hospital
Patna, Uttar Pradesh, India.
The hospital: A 360-bed hospital funded privately and located in the small town of Patna near Dehli. As it is private, you can see and examine patients, but you will not be allowed to do any procedures. However, the staff are keen to teach. There is a wide range of conditions, infectious diseases being the most common.

Asopa Hospital

Gailana Road, Agra, Uttar Pradesh, India.
The hospital: A general hospital. There are plenty of tropical diseases. Patients don't speak English. Agra is a pretty ugly place but it does have the Taj Mahal.
Accommodation: A hostel near the hospital costs Rs 300/night.

Madhya Pradesh

Lying in the centre of India, this huge state is mainly dry desert. It has mainly Hindi tribal people with most of the tourist attractions being in the north near Delhi. It has numerous Hindi temples and in the centre the forested Kanha National Park where Kipling's The Jungle Book *was set.*

MEDICAL SCHOOLS:

Gajra Raja Medical College, Jiwaji University, Gwalior 474003, Madhya Pradesh, India.
Gandhi Medical College, Bhopal University, Bhopal 462021, Madhya Pradesh, India.
JLN Medical College, Ravi Shankar University, Raipur 492001, Madhya Pradesh, India.
Medical College, Jabalpur University, Jabalpur 482001, Madhya Pradesh, India.
MGM Medical College, Indore University, Indore 452001, Madhya Pradesh, India.
SS Medical College, AP Singh University, Rewa 486001, Madhya Pradesh, India.

OTHER HOSPITALS:

Padhar Hospital

PO Padhar, Dist. Betul, Madhya Pradesh 460005, India.
The hospital: Padhar is a small village (population of about 300 people) in southern Madhya Pradesh (about 180 km south of Bhopal). The nearest town (with a phone) is Betul, 20 km away with a population of 30,000. The hospital was founded in 1939 by Reverend Moss, an English missionary, who was not a doctor at the time – he spent several years there using a medical textbook to diagnose and treat patients before he was persuaded to go to Medical School (in India) and become a doctor. Since then, the hospital has grown and now has about 250 beds and a busy outpatients. It serves an area of 300 km diameter. It employs 15 doctors covering general medicine, surgery, obstetrics and gynaecology, ophthalmology and radiotherapy. It also runs outreach clinics. It is run by the Evangelical Lutheran Church (ELC), which also has several other projects based in Padhar, working with the people in the local villages. Although this means that most (but not all) the staff are Christian, the vast majority of the patients are Hindus and Muslims from the surrounding villages and religion does not play a part in the day-to-day work apart from 'morning devotion' which is at 8 am each day. Despite donations from the ELC making the hospital well-equipped with facilities such as endoscopy and ultrasound, the hospital does expect patients to pay for at least part of their treatment. About 60% of the general medical work involves TB, but hypertension, angina and diabetes are also common.
O Elective notes: The doctors are trained in and speak good English. The patients, however, speak Hindi and this is the language of consultations. The doctors are willing to translate. This is highly recommended as a very Indian, unspoilt elective.
Accommodation: In the 'Big Bungalow', a guesthouse run by the hospital for foreign visitors. It's very comfortable with hot showers, electricity, all meals cooked for you and even a guard at night (cost, about Rs 300 (£3) per night). Hire of the jeep and driver to Betul is £3.

Chhatapur Christian Hospital

Chhatapur, Madhya Pradesh
and

Lakhnadon Christian Hospital

Lakhnadon, Madhya Pradesh, India
Are missionary hospitals run by the Emmanuel Hospital Association.

India

Rajasthan

Rajasthan is a beautiful area in north-west India, full of colour and immense history. Famed for its Rajiput warriors, there are numerous forts and museums.

MEDICAL SCHOOLS:

Birla Institute of Technology and Science, Pilani 333031, Rajasthan, India.
Dr SN Medical College, University of Rajasthan, Jodhpur 342003, Rajasthan, India Tel: 291 31987.
Jawaharlal Nehru Medical College, University of Rajasthan, Ajmer 305001, Rajasthan, India Tel: 145 22842.
RNT Medical College, University of Rajasthan, Udaipur 313001, Rajasthan, India Tel: 294 23613.
Sardar Patel Medical College, University of Rajasthan, Bikaner 334003, Rajasthan, India Tel: 151 23443.
Sawai Man Singh (SMS) Medical College, University of Rajasthan, Jaipur 302003, Rajasthan, India. (This is the largest and oldest medical school in the area.)

Jammu and Kashmir

This area is highly dangerous with the Pakistan conflict. Don't go there.

MEDICAL SCHOOLS:

Govt Medical College, Jammu University, Bakshi Nagar, Jammu 180001, India Tel: 191 46824 (founded 1972).
Govt Medical College, University of Kashmir, Srinagar 190010, Kashmire, India Tel: 194 73562 (founded 1959).

Andhra Pradesh

This east coast state, high on the Deccan plateau, is one of the poorest and most underdeveloped areas in India. It has a strong Muslim influence and has attractions such as the Golconda Fort and Qutb Shahi tombs. Like all proper poor areas it gets more than its fair share of tropical storms and floods.

MEDICAL SCHOOLS:

Andhra Medical College, Andhra University, Vishakhapatnam 530001, Andhra Pradesh, India.
Gandhi Medical College, Osmania University, Basheerbagh, Hyderabad 500001, Andhra Pradesh, India.
Guntur Medical College, Nargarjuna University, Guntur 522001, Andhra Pradesh, India.
Kakatiya Medical College, Osmania University, Warangal 506002, Andhra Pradesh, India (founded 1959).
Kurnool Medical College, Sri Venkatesvara University, Kurnool 518001, Andhra Pradesh, India.
Medical College, Sri Venkatesvara University, Tirupati 517501, Andhra Pradesh, India.
Osmania Medical College, Osmania University, Hyderabad 500001, Andhra Pradesh, India.
Rangarya Medical College, Andhra University, East Godavary District, Kakinada 533003, Andhra Pradesh, India.

OTHER HOSPITALS:

The CSI Campbell Hospital

Jammalamadugu, Cuddapah District, Andhra Pradesh, India Tel: 8560 70218.

The hospital: A 320-bed mission hospital. Most pathology is infectious disease, such as TB and leprosy, but O&G and orthopaedics are also catered for.

Assam

Assam in the north-east grows much of India's tea, produces oil, and has the rare horned rhinoceros, but be careful if going there. There is a great deal of strife between the United Liberation Front wanting Assam's independence and the Indians. The Bodo community is also getting in on the violence.

MEDICAL SCHOOLS:

Assam Medical College and Hospital, Dibrugarh University, Dibrugarh 786002, Assam, India.
Gauhati Medical College, Gauhati University, Gauhati 781001, Assam, India.
Silchar Medical College and Hospital, Gauhati University, Ghungoor, Silchar 788001, Assam, India.

Manipur

Manipur also high in the north-east, has a craft and agriculture industry. Violent struggles are also commonplace and so again it is another area to avoid.

MEDICAL SCHOOLS:

Regional Medical College, Gauhati University, Imphal 795001, Manipur, India.

Orissa

Orissa is a predominantly rural area with poor but friendly people. There is usually the odd cyclone, flood or drought to make sure they stay poor. For the visitor there are temples in Bhubaneswar and a beautiful beech in Puri.

MEDICAL SCHOOLS:

Maharaja Krishna Chandra Gajapati Medical College, Berhampur University, Ganjan District, Berhampur 760004, Orissa, India.
VSS Medical College, Sambalpur University, PO Sambalpur, Burla 768017, Orissa, India.
SCB Medical College, Utkal University, Cuttak 752001, Orissa, India.

Ladakh and Zaskar

If remote is what you want, this is it. The main town Leh (which is medium size with its own polo ground) is at 3505 metres and right at the tip of northern India. There are many festivals, approximately one a month, at the nearby Gompas. Acute mountain sickness is not uncommon. If you fly in you may well get it yourself.

THE MEDICAL SCHOOL:

Sonam Narbu Memorial Hospital, Leh, Ladakh, India. Tel: 01982 52014.

Private Hospitals in India

There are a number of private hospital groups, the largest is Apollo which has a number of centres. Some have previously taken elective students.

The Apollo Hospitals Group

www.apollohospitals.com

The Apollo Hospitals is a group of private hospitals throughout India, set up in 1983 by Dr P Reddy to try to bring international healthcare standards within the reach of every individual. They are major referral centres and centres of excellence providing high-tech specialities such as cardiac surgery. Although much of the medicine seen is Western, topical medicine is still common. From an educational point of view it can be argued that you learn more by seeing diseases and how to treat them here than you would seeing diseases and then not having the facilities or drugs to treat them in government hospitals. You may feel, however, that you didn't go to India to see the well-off in an air-conditioned hospital (although they do have schemes for the 'economically weaker'). The group has a number of hospitals in a number of states:

Apollo Speciality Hospitals, 320 Anna Salai, Nandanam, Chennai 600 035, Tamil Nadu, India Tel: (044) 4331741 Fax: (044) 4343996. This 200-bed hospital specializes in neuro and cancer.
Chennai (Madras): Apollo Hospitals, 121 Greams Lane, off Greams Road, Chennai 600 006, Tamil Nadu, India Tel: (044) 8293333 Fax: (044) 8234429. This is a super-speciality and the first Apollo hospital.
Hyderabad: A 400-bed high-tech speciality hospital (especially cardiac) and the Apollo Cancer Centre. Apollo Hospitals, Jubilee Hills, Hyderabad 500 034, Andhra Pradesh, India Tel: (040) 3607777 Fax: (040) 3608050
Madurai: Apollo Hospitals, Lake View Road, KK Nagar, Madurai 625 020. Tel: 0452 650892. Fax: 0452 650199. 135 beds.
Mumbai (Bombay): Apollo Cliniq, Bogilal Hargovind Das Building, 18/20, K. Dubash Marg, Mumbai 400 001, Maharashtra, India. Provides a clinic service to Bombay.
New Delhi: Indraprastha Apollo Hospitals Delhi, Mathura Road, New Dehli 110 044, Uttar Pradesh, India Tel: (011) 6830861 Fax: (011) 6823629. A 700-bed super-speciality hospital, the largest private hospital outside the USA. The ICU has an incredible 92 beds. Multi-organ transplants, non-invasive neuro-surgery, trauma … they do it all.
Ranchi: Abdur Razzaque Ansari Memorial Weavers Hospital, PO irba, Ranchi, Bihar, India Tel: (0651) 535717 Fax: (0651)535786. This is the first rural Apollo.

Japan

Population: 125 million
Language: Japanese
Capital: Tokyo
Currency: Yen
Int Code: +81

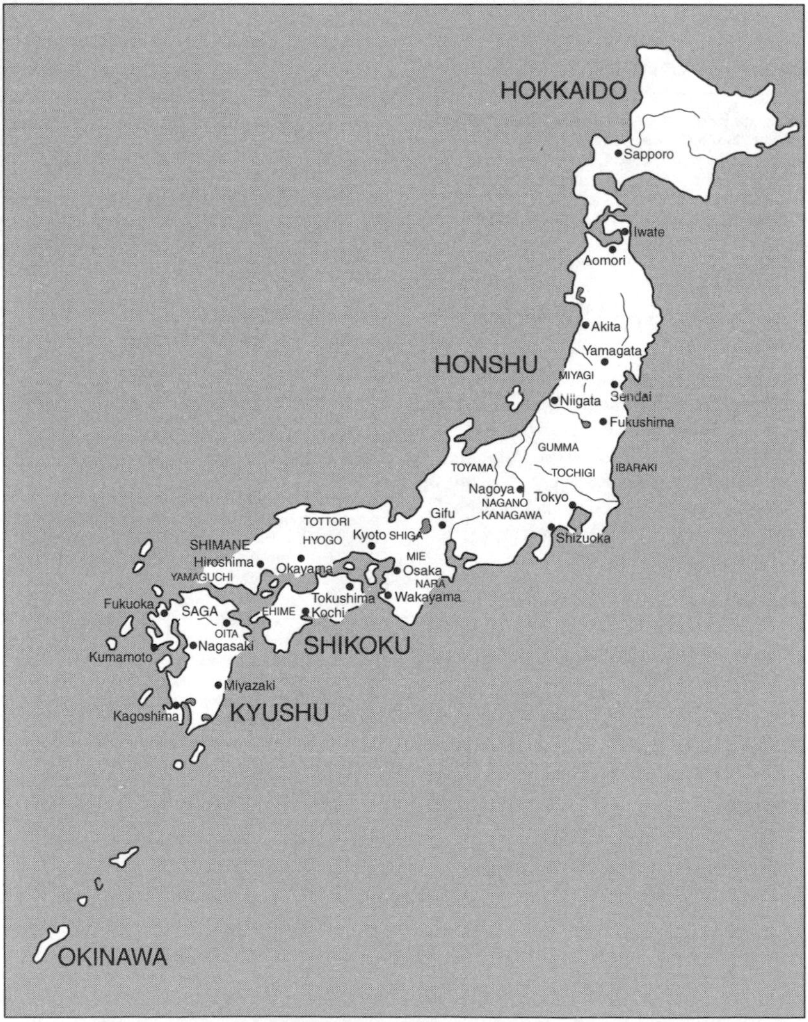

Japan, in the north Pacific, is made up of four islands and most cities are situated near the coast. It is well-known for its powerful economy and hardworking people. It is not a common elective or work destination, presumably due to language barriers. The schools are in general, however, very willing to offer exchanges. If you can understand Japanese, the world-wide web is a good place to start looking, although not that many schools have got on yet. For this reason, all the medical schools and their main teaching hospitals are listed below.

✪ Medicine:

Japan has a first class health system where most people pay into an insurance scheme related to their pay (see below). The poorest receive free treatment. Japan has some of the highest longevity and lowest infant mortality figures in the world. The common causes of death are heart and cardiovascular diseases, cancer (especially gastric) and tuberculosis. The ageing population will present a major problem to healthcare, but already intermediary healthcare services for the elderly are being set up.

Nearly all citizens in Japan participate in a medical care insurance programme. The current medical care insurance system consists of four different insurance groups depending on the size of the organization you work for and an elderly health-providing group. Although there are variations, under all schemes, patients may visit medical clinics and hospitals and be hospitalized when needed. They personally pay deductibles and co-payments. People of low income are eligible for medical assistance. They do not need to pay deductibles or co-payments.

✪ Working and advanced training in Japan:

Japan's Medical Practitioners Law strictly prohibits diagnosis and medical treatment by persons without the requisite medical licence. This therefore applies to foreign nationals. Technically, without a Japanese licence you are not allowed to do anything except observe. In 1987, 'The Law on Exceptions to the Medical Practitioners Law, Article 17' was passed which allows advanced clinical training. With a permit for advanced clinical training you are able to carry out all medical and surgical procedures (in a specified speciality) but only:

- Under guidance of a practitioner certified in advanced clinical training
- At a hospital permitted to give advanced clinical training (see below)
- Only if you can provide documents listed below

You are not allowed to write prescriptions and all notes must be countersigned by your supervisor. To apply for a permit you need:

- a medical practitioner's licence from your country
- A certificate of clinical experience (at least three years after qualification)
- Documents to prove you will return to your own country upon completion
- A certificate of language proficiency in Japanese or English
- Proof that you have not been 'struck off' in your country
- A certificate of your own medical health
- Insurance for any injury to patients
- Proof that you have no criminal record
- An application form (and 11,000 yen)
- Passport and photos

All this will give you a permit for up to two years in a specific field of surgery or medicine at a specific hospital. Write to: Office of National Examinations and Licences, Medical Professions Division, Health Policy Bureau, Ministry of Health and Welfare, 1-2-2 Kasumigaseki, Chiyoda-ku, Tokyo, Japan 100-45 Tel: 03-503-1711.

USEFUL ADDRESSES:

Japan International Educational Association, 4–5–29, Komaba, Meguro-ku, Tokyo 153, Japan Tel: 03 (467) 3521.
Ministry of Education, Kasumigaseki, Chiyoda-ku, Tokyo 100, Japan Tel: 03 (581) 4211.

Japan

Ministry of Foreign Affairs, 2–2–1, Kasumigaseki, Chiyoda-ku, Tokyo 100, Japan Tel: 03 (580) 3311.
Ministry of Health and Welfare, 1–2–2, Kasumigaseki, Chiyoda-ku, Tokyo 100, Japan Tel: 03 (503) 1711.

HOSPITALS OF UNIVERSITIES AND MEDICAL COLLEGES:

Aoto Hospital of the Jikei University, 6–41–2 Aoto, Katsushika-ku, Tokyo 125, Japan Tel: 03 (603) 2111.
Branch Hospital of Nagoya University, 1–1–20 Daiko-minami, Higashi-ku, Nagoya-shi, Aichi 461, Japan Tel: 052 (723) 1111.
Branch Hospital of Tokyo University, 3–28–6 Mejiro-dai, Bunkyo-ku, Tokyo 112, Japan Tel: 03 (942) 1151.
Fujigaoka Hospital of Showa University, 1–30 Fujigaoka, Midori-ku, Yokohama-shi, Kanagawa 227, Japan Tel: 045 (971) 1151.
General Medical Centre of Saitama Medical School, 1981 Aza-Tsujido-machi, Ooaza-Kamoda, Kawaboe-shi, Saitama 359, Japan Tel: 0492 (25) 7811.
Hachioji Medical Center of Tokyo Medical College, 1163 Tate-machi, Hachioji, Tokyo 193, Japan Tel: 0426 (65) 5611.
Higashi Hospital of Kitazato University, 863–1, Asamizo-da, Sagamihara-shi, Kanagawa 228, Japan Tel: 0427 (48) 9111.
Hospital of Aichi Medical Universtiy, 21 Aza-Karimata, Ooaza-Iwasaku, Nagakude-cho, Aichi-gun, Aichi 480–11, Japan Tel: 05616 (2) 3311 Fax: 0561 62 4866. www.aichi-med-u.ac.jp/index.html (Established in 1971, Aichi has 100 students a year and all major departments.)
Hospital of Akita University, 1–1–1, Hon-michi, Akita-shi, Akita 010, Japan Tel: 0188 (34) 1111.
Hospital of Asahikawa Medical College, 5–3–11, 4-sen, Nishi-Kagura, shikawa-shi, Hokkaido 078, Japan Tel: 0166 (65) 2111.
Hospital of Cancer Research Institute, Kanazawa University, 4–86 Yoneizumi-cho, Kanazawa-shi, Ishikawa 921, Japan Tel: 0762 (41) 8245.
Hospital of Chest Disease Research Institute, Kyoto University, 53 Kawahara-cho, Shougo-in, Sakyo-ku, Kyotot-in, Kyoto 606, Japan Tel: 075 (751) 3802.
Hospital of Chiba University, 1–8–1 Inohana, Chiba-shi, Chiba 280, Japan Tel: 0472 (22) 7171.
Hospital of Dokkyo University, 880 Ooaza-Kita-Kobayashi, Mibu-cho, Shimo-tsuga-gun, Tochigi 321-02, Japan Tel: 0282 (86) 1111.
Hospital of Ehime University, Ooaza-Shizugawa, Shienobu-cho, Onsen-gun Ehime 791–02, Japan Tel: 0899 (64) 5111.
Hospital of Fujita Gakuen Health University, 1–98 Dengakugakubo, Kutsukake-cho, Toyoake-shi, Aichi 470–1, Japan Tel: 0562 (93) 2000.
Hospital of Fukui Medical School, 23 Shmo-Aizuki, Matsuoka-cho, Yoshida-gun, Fukui 910–11, Japan Tel: 0776 (61) 3111.
Hospital of Fukuoka University, 7–45–1 Nanakuma, Jonan-ku, Fukuoka-shi, Fukuoka 814–01, Japan Tel: 092 (801) 1011.
Hospital of Fukushima Prefectural University, 1 Hikarigaoka, Fukushima-shi, Fukushima 960-21, Japan Tel: 0245 (48) 2111.
Hospital of Gifu University, 40 Tsukasa-machi, Gifu-shi, Gifu 500, Japan Tel: 0582 (65) 1241.
Hospital of Gunma University, 3–39–15 Showa-machi, Maebashi-shi, Gunma 371, Japan Tel: 0272 (31) 7221.
Hospital of Hamamatsu University, 3600 Handa-cho, Hamamatsu-shi, Shizuoka 431–31, Japan Tel: 0534 (35) 2111.
Hospital of Hirosaki University, 53 Hon-machi, Hirosaki-shi, Aomori 036, Japan Tel: 0172 (33) 5111.
Hospital of Hokkaido University, 5-chome, Nishi-Juushijo, Kita-ku, Sapporo-shi, Hokkaido 060, Japan Tel: 011 (716) 1161.
Hospital of Hyogo College of Medicine, 1–1 Mukogawa-cho, Nishinomiya-shi, Hyogo 663, Japan Tel: 0798 (45) 6111.
Hospital of Institute of Medical Science, Tokyo University, 4–6–1, Shiroganedai, Minato-ku, Tokyo 108, Japan Tel: 03 (443) 8111.
Hospital of Iwate Medical University, 19–1, Uchimaru, Morioka-shi, Iwate 020, Japan Tel: 0196 (51) 5111.
Hospital of Jichi Medical School, 3,311–1 Yakusiji, Minami-kawachi-cho, Kawachi-gun, Tochigi 329-04, Japan Tel: 0285 (44) 2111.
Hospital of the Jikei University, 3–19–18 Nishi-Shinbashi, Minato-ku, Tokyo 105, Japan Tel: 03 (433) 1111.
Hospital of Juntendo University, 3–1–3 Hongo, Bunkyo-ku, Tokyo 113, Japan Tel: 03 (813) 3111.
Hospital of Kagawa Medical School, 1750–1 Ooaza-Ikenobe, Miki-cho, Kida-gun, Kagawa 761–07, Japan Tel: 0878 (98) 5111.
Hospital of Kagoshima University, 1208–1 Ushiki-cho, Kagoshima-shi, Kagoshima 890, Japan Tel: 0992 (64) 2211.
Hospital of Kanazawa Medical University, 1–1 Daigaku, Uchinada-machi, Kawakita-gun, Ishikawa 920–02, Japan Tel: 0762 (86) 3511.
Hospital of Kanazawa University, 13–-1, Takara-machi, Kanazawa-shi, Ishikawa 920, Japan Tel: 0762 (62) 8151.
Hospital of Kansai Medical University, 1 Fumizono-cho, Moriguchi-shi, Osaka 570, Japan Tel: 06 (992) 1001.
Hospital of Keio University, 35 Shinano-machi, Shinjuku-ku, Tokyo 160, Japan Tel: 03 (353) 1211.
Hospital of Kitazato University, 1–15–1 Kitazato, Sagamihara-shi, Kanagawa 228, Japan Tel: 0427 (78) 8111.
Hospital of Kobe University, 7–5–2 Kusunoki-machi, Chuo-ku, Kobe-shi, Hyogo 650, Japan Tel: 078 (341) 7451.
Hospital of Kochi Medical School, Kohasu, Okatoyo-machi, Nangoku-shi, Koci 781–51, Japan Tel: 0888 (66) 5811.
Hospital of Kumamoto University, 1–1–1 Honjo, Kumamoto-shi, Kumamoto 860, Japan Tel: 096 (344) 2111.
Hospital of Kurume University, 67 Asahi-machi, Kurume-shi, Fukuoka 830, Japan Tel: 0942 (35) 3311.

Hospital of Kyorin University, 6–20–2 Shinkawa, Mitaka-shi, Tokyo 181, Japan Tel: 0422 (47) 5511.
Hospital of Kyoto Prefectural University of Medicine, 465 Kajii-cho, Noboru, Hirokoji, Kawarachodori, Kamigyo-ku, Kyoto-shi, Kyoto 602, Japan Tel: 075 (251) 5111.
Hospital of Kyoto University, 54 Kawahara-cho, Shougo-in, Sakyo-ku, Kyoto-shi, Kyoto 606, Japan Tel: 075 (751) 3111.
Hospital of Kyushu University, 3–1–1 Umaide, Higashi-ku, Fukuoka-shi, Fukuoka 812, Japan Tel: 092 (641) 1151.
Hospital of Medical Institute of Bioregulation, Kyushu University, 4546 Tsurumihara, Beppu-shi, Oita 874, Japan Tel: 0977 (24) 5301.
Hospital of Mie University, 2–174 Edobashi, Tsu-shi, Mie 514, Japan Tel: 0592 (2) 1111.
Hospital of Miyazaki Medical College, 5200 Kihara, Kiyoyake-cho, Miyazaki-gun, Miyazaki 889–16, Japan Tel: 0985 (85) 1510.
Hospital of Nagasaki University, Sakamoto-cho, Nagasaki-shi, Nagasaki 852, Japan Tel: 0958 (47) 2111.
Hospital of Nagoya University, 65 Maizuru-cho, Showa-ku, Nagoya-shi, Aichi 466-8550, Japan Tel: 052 (741) 2111 Fax: 052 744 2428 www.nagoya-u.ac.jp (Founded in 1871 the hospital is huge with 1035 beds and a new gene therapy centre.)
Hospital of Nihon Medical School, 1–1–5 Sendagi, Bunkyo-ku, Tokyo 113, Japan Tel: 03 (822) 2131.
Hospital of Niigata University, 754 Ichiban-cho, Asahi-machi-dori, Niigata-shi, Niigata 951, Japan Tel: 025 (223) 6161.
Hospital of Oita Medical College, 1–1506 Idaigaoka, Hazama-machi, Oita-gun, Iota 879–56, Japan Tel: 0975 (49) 4411.
Hospital of Okayama University, 2–5–1 Shikata-cho, Okayama-shi, Okayama 700, Japan Tel: 0862 (23) 7151.
Hospital of Osaka Medical College, 2–7 Daigaku-machi, Takatsuki-shi, Osaka 569, Japan Tel: 0726 (83) 1221.
Hospital of Osaka University, 1–1–50 Fukushima, Fukushima-ku, Osaka-shi, Osaka 553, Japan
Hospital of Research Institute for Microbial Diseases, Osaka University, 3–1 Yamadagaoka, Suita-shi, Osaka 565, Japan Tel: 06 (877) 5121.
Hospital of St Marianna University, 2–16–1 Sugao Miyamae-ku, Kawasaki-shi, Kanagawa 213, Japan Tel: 044 (977) 8111.
Hospital of Saga Medical School, Sanbonsugi, Ooaza-Nabeshiima, Nabeshima-cho, Saga-shi, Saga 840–01, Japan.
Hospital of Saitama Medical School, 38 Morohongo, Moroyama-machi, Iruma-gun, Saitama 350–04, Japan Tel: 0429 (95) 1111.
Hospital of Sapporo Medical College, 16-chome, Nishi-Minami-Ichijo, Chuo-ku, Sapporo-shi, Hokkaido 060, Japan Tel: 011 (611) 2111.
Hospital of Shiga University of Medical Science, Tukinowa-cho, Seta, Otsu-shi, Shiga 520–21, Japan Tel: 0775 (48) 2111.
Hospital of Shimane Medical University, 89–1 Shioji-cho, Izumo-shi, Shimane 693, Japan Tel: 0853 (23) 2111.
Hospital of Shinshu University, 3–1–1 Asahi, Matsumoto-shi, Nagano 390, Japan Tel: 0263 (35) 4600.
Hospital of Showa University, 1–5–8 Hatanodai, Shinagawa-ku, Tokyo 142, Japan Tel: 03 (784) 8000.
Hospital of Tokai University, 143 Shimokasuya, Isehara-shi, Kanagawa 259–11, Japan Tel: 0463 (93) 1121.
Hospital of Teikyo University, 2–11–1 Kaga, Itabashi-ku, Tokyo 173, Japan Tel: 03 (964) 1211.
Hospital of Tohoku University, 2-1, Seiryo-cho, Sendai-shi, Miyagi 980, Japan Tel: 022 (274)1111.
Hospital of Tokushima University, 2–50–1 Kuramoto-cho, Tokushima-shi, Tokushima 770, Japan Tel: 0886 (31) 3111.
Hospital of Tokyo Medical College, 6–7–1 Nishi-Shinjuku, Shinjku-ku, Tokyo 160, Japan Tel: 03 (342) 6111.
Hospital of Tokyo Medical and Dental University, 1–5–45 Yushima, Bunkyo-ku, Tokyo 113, Japan Tel: 03 (813) 6111.
Hospital of Tokyo Women's Medical College, 8–1 Kawada-cho, Shinjuku-ku, Tokyo 162, Japan Tel: 03 (353) 8111.
Hospital of Tokyo University, 7–3–1, Hongo, Bunkyo-ku, Tokyo 113, Japan Tel: 03 (815) 5411.
Hospital of Tottori University, 36–1 Nishi-machi, Yonago-shi, Tottori 683, Japan Tel: 0859 (33) 1111.
Hospital of Toyama Medical and Pharmaceutical University, 2630 Sugitani, Toyama-shi, Toyama 930–01, Japan Tel: 0764 (34) 2281.
Hospital of Tsukuba Univerity, 2–1–1 Amakubo, Sakura-mura, Shinji gun, Ibaragi 305, Japan Tel: 0298 (53) 3900.
Hospital of University of the Ryukyus, 207 Aza-Uehara, Nishihara-machi, Nakagami-gun, Okinawa 903–01, Japan Tel: 09889 (5) 3331.
Hospital of University of Occupational and Environmental Health, 1–1 Ibugaoka, Yahatanishi-ku, Kitakyushu-shi, Fukuoka 807, Japan Tel: 093 (603) 1611.
Hospital of Wakayama Medical College, 1 Nanaban-cho, Wakayama-shi, Wakayama 640, Japan Tel: 0734 (31) 2151.
Hospital of Yamagata University, Aza-Nishinomae, Iida, Zao, Yamagata-shi, Yamagata 990-23, Japan Tel: 0236 (33) 1122.
Hospital of Yamaguchi University, 1–2–3 Kasumi, Minami-ku, Hiroshima-shi, Hiroshima 734, Japan Tel: 082 (251) 1111.
Hospital of Yamanashi Medical College, 1110 Shimo-Kawahigashi, Tamaho-cho, Nakakoma-gun, Yamanashi 409–38, Japan Tel: 0552 (73) 1111.
Hospital of Yokohama City University, 3–46 Urabune-cho, Minami-ku, Yokohama-shi, Kanagawa 232, Japan Tel: 045 (261) 5656.
Ise Keio Hospital of Keio University, 2–7–28 Tokiwa, Ise-shi, Mie 516, Japan Tel: 0596 (22) 1155.
Itabashi Hospital of Nihon University, 30–1 Kami-machi, Ooyaguchi, Itabashi-ku, Tokyo 173, Japan Tel: 03 (972) 8111 www.med.nihon-u.ac.jp

Kashiwa Hospital of the Jikei University, 163–1, Kashiwa-shita, Kashiwa-shi, Chiba 277, Japan Tel: 0471 (64) 1111.
Kasumigaura Hospital of Tokyo Medical College, 3–20–1 Chuo, Amimachi, Inajiki-gun, Ibaragi 300–03, Japan Tel: 0298 (87) 1161.
Koshigaya Hospital of Dokkyo University, 2–1–500 Minami-Koshigaya, Koshigaya-shi, Saitama 343, Japan Tel: 0489 (65) 1111.
Misasa Branch Hospital of Okayama University, 827 Yamada, Misasa-cho, Tohaku-gun, Tottori 682–02, Japan Tel: 0858 (43) 1211.
Naruko Branch, Hospital of Tohoku University, 67–1, Aza-Shin-Yashiki, Naruko-machi, Tamatsukuri-gun, Miyagi 989–68, Japan Tel: 0229 (82) 2531.
Oohashi Hospital of Toho University, 2–17–6, Oohashi, Meguro-ku, Tokyo 153, Japan Tel: 03 (468) 1251.
Ooiso Hospital of Tokai University, 21–1 Tsukikyo, Oiso-machi, Naka-gun, Kanagawa 259–01, Japan Tel: 0463 (72) 3211.
Oomori Hospital of Toho University, 6–11–1 Oomori-nishi, Oota-ku, Tokyo 143, Japan Tel: 03 (762) 4151.
Rakusei New-Town Hospital of Kansai Medical University, 3–6, Ooeda-Higashi-shinrin-cho, Nishigyo-ku, Kyoto-shi, Kyoto 610–11, Japan Tel: 075 (332) 0123.
Surugadai Hospital of Nihon University, 1–8–13 Kandasuruga-dai, Chiyoda-ku, Tokyo 101, Japan Tel: 03 (293) 1711.
The First Hospital of Nihon Medical School, 3–5–5 Iidabashi, Chiyoda-ku, Tokyo 102, Japan Tel: 0 (261) 8331.
The Second Hospital of Nihon Medical School, 1–396 Kosugi-machi, Nbakahara-ku, Kawasaki-shi, Kanagawa 211, Japan Tel: 044 (733) 5181.
The Second Hospital of Tokyo Women's Medical College, 2–1–10 Nishi-Oku, Arakawa-ku, Tokyo 116, Japan Tel: 03 (810) 1111.
The Third Hospital of Jikei University, 4–11–1 Izumihon-machi, Komae-shi, Tokyo, 201, Japan Tel: 03 (480) 1151.
Tokyo Hospital of Tokai University, 1–2–5 Yoyogi, Shibuya-ku, Tokyo 151, Japan Tel: 03 (370) 2321.
Toyosu Hospital of Showa University, 4–1–18 Toyosu, Koto-ku, Tokyo 135, Japan Tel: 03 (534) 1151.
Tsukigase Rehabilitation Center of Keio University, 380–2 Tsukigase, Yugashima-machi, Amagi, Tagata-gun, Shizuoka 410–32, Japan Tel: 0588 (5) 1701.
Tsukushi Hospital of Fukuoka University, 377–1 Ooaza-Zokumyou-in, Chikushino-shi, Fukuoka 818, Japan Tel: 092 (921) 1011.

SPECIAL NATIONAL HOSPITALS WHICH ARE FUNCIONALLY EQUIVALENT/ SUPERIOR TO UNIVERSITY HOSPITALS:

Konodai Hospital, National Center of Neurology and Psychiatry, 1–7–1 Kono-dai, Ichikawa-shi, Chiba 272, Japan Tel: 0473 (72) 0141.
Musashi Hospital, National Center of Neurology and Psychiatry, 4–1–1 Ogawahigashi-machi, Kodaira-shi, Tokyo 187, Japan Tel: 0423 (41) 2711.
National Cancer Center, 5–1–1 Tsukiji, Chuo-ku, Tokyo 104, Japan Tel: 03 (542) 2511.
National Cardiovascular Center, 5–7–1 Fujishiro-dai, Suita-shi, Osaka 565, Japan Tel: 06 (833) 5012.
National Children's Hospital, 3–35–31 Taishido, Setagaya-ku, Tokyo 154, Japan Tel: 03 (414) 8121.

DESIGNATED HOSPITALS FOR CLINICAL TRAINING FOR MEDICAL PRACTITIONERS IN JAPAN:

Akita Red Cross Hospital, 1–4–36 Nakadori, Akita-shi, Akita 010, Japan Tel: 0188 (34) 3361.
Asahikawa Municipal Hospital, 1–1–65 Kanehoshi-cho, Asahikawa-shi, Hokkaido 070, Japan Tel: 0166 (24) 3181.
Chiba Rosai Hospital, 2–16 Tatsumidai-higashi, Ichihara-shi, Chiba 290, Japan Tel: 0436 (74) 1111.
Chugoku Rosai Hospital, 1–5–1 Hiro-Tagaya, Kure-shi, Hirochima 737-01, Japan Tel: 0823 (72) 7171.
Ehime Pefectural Central Hospital, 83 Kasuga-cho, Matsuyama-shi, Ehime 790, Japan Tel: 0899 (47) 1111.
Fukuoka-Chuo National Hospital, 2–2 Jiyo-nai, Chuo-ku, Fukuoka-shi, Fukuoka 810, Japan Tel: 092 (714) 01.
Gifu Prefectural Hospital, 4–6–1 Noitsushiki, Gifu-shi, Gifu 500, Japan Tel: 0582 (46) 1111.
Hiraga General Hospital, 64–2 Inukawara, Yathuhashi, Akita-shi, Akita 013, Japan Tel: 0182 (32) 5121.
Hirosaki National Hospital, 1 Ooaza-Tomino-cho, Hirosaki-shi, Aomori 036, Japan Tel: 0172 (32) 4311.
Hiroshima Prefectural Hiroshima Hospital, 1–5–54 Ujina-Kanda, Minami-ku, Hiroshima-shi, Hiroshima 734, Japan Tel: 0822 (54) 1818.
Hiroshima Railroad Hospital, 3–1–36 Futabanosato, Higashi-ku, Hiroshima-shi, Hiroshima 732, Japan Tel: 082 (262) 1170.
Hyogo Prefectural Amagasaki Hospital, 1–1–1 Higashi-Oumono-cho, Amagasaki-shi, Hyogo 660, Japan Tel: 06 (482) 1521.
Ishikawa Prefectural Central Hospital, Nu-153 Minami-Shinbo-cho, Kanazawa-shi, Ishikawa 920–02, Japan Tel: 0762 (37) 82.
Iwakuni National Hospital, 2–5–1 Kuroiso-machi, Iwakuni-shi, Yamaguchi 740, Japan Tel: 0827 (31) 7121.
Iwate Prefectural Central Hospital, 1–4–1 Ueda, Morioka-shi, Iwate 020, Japan Tel: 0196 (53) 1151.
Kagoshima Municipal Hospital, 20–17 Kajiyacho, Kagoshima-shi, Kagoshima 892, Japan Tel: 0992 (24) 2101.
Kameda General Hospital, 929 Higashi-machi, Kamogawa-shi, Chiba 296, Japan Tel: 04709 (2) 2211.
Kanazawa National Hospital, 3–1–1 Ishibiki, Kanazawa-shi, Ishikawa 920, Japan Tel: 0762 (62) 4161.
Kansai Denryoku Hospital, 2–1–7 Fukushima, Fukushima-ku, Osaka-shi, Osaka 553, Japan Tel: 06 (458) 5821.
Kawasaki Municipal Hospital, 12–1

Shinkawadori, Kawasaki-ku, Kawasaki-shi, Kanagawa 210, Japan Tel: 044 (233) 5521.

Kobe Municipal Central Hospital, 4–6 Minatoshima-nakamachi, Chuo-ku, Kobe-shi, Hyogo 650, Japan Tel: 078 (302) 4321.

Kochi Municipal Hospital, 1–7–45 Marunouchi, Kochi-shi, Kochi 780, Japan Tel: 0888 (22) 6111.

Kochi Prefectural Central Hospital, 2–7–33 Sakurai-cho, Kochi-shi, Kochi 780, Japan Tel: 0888 (82) 1211.

Kokuho Asahi Chuo Hospital, I–1326 Asahi-shi, Chiba 289-25, Japan Tel: 04796 (3) 8111.

Koritsu Showa Hospital, 2–450 Tenjin-cho, Kodaira-shi, Tokyo 187, Japan Tel: 0424 (61) 0052.

Kumamoto Municipal Hospital, 1–1–60 Koto, Kumamoto-shi, Kumamoto 862, Japan Tel: 096 (365) 1711.

Kumamoto National Hospital, 1–5, Ninomaru, Kumamoto-shi, Kumamoto 860, Japan Tel: 096 (353) 6501.

Kurashiki Central Hospital, 1–1–1 Miwa Kurashiki-shi, Okayama 710, Japan Tel: 0864 (22) 0210.

Kure Kyosai Hospital, 2–3–28 Nishi-Chuo, Naka-ku, Kure-shi, Hiroshima 737, Japan Tel: 0823 (22) 2111.

Kure National Hospital, 3–1 Aoyama-cho, Kure-shi, Hiroshima 737, Japan Tel: 0823 (22) 3111.

Kyushu Rosai Hospital, 1–3–1 Kuzuharatakamatsu, Kokuraminami-ku, Kita-Kyushu-shi, Fukuoka 800–02, Japan Tel: 093 (471) 1121.

Maebashi Red Cross Hospital, 3–21–36 Asahi-cho, Maebashi-shi, Gunma 371, Japan Tel: 0272 (24) 4585.

Matsudo Municipal Hospital, 4005 Kamihongo, Matsudo-shi, Chiba 271, Japan Tel: 0473 (63) 2171.

Mitsui Kinen Hospital, 1 Izumi-cho, Kanda, Chiyoda-ku, Tokyo 101, Japan Tel: 03 (862) 9111.

Miyazaki Prefectural Hospital, 5–30 Kita-Takamatsu-cho, Miyazaki 880, Japan Tel: 0985 (24) 4181.

Musashino Red Cross Hospital, 1–26–1 Kyonan-cho, Musashino-shi, Tokyo 180, Japan Tel: 0422 (32) 3111.

NTT Kanto Teishin Hospital, 5–9–22 Higashi-Gotanda, Shinagawa-ku, Tokyo 141, Japan Tel: 03 (448) 6651.

Nagasaki Chuo National Hospital, 2–1001–1 Hisahara, Omura-shi, Nagasaki 856, Japan Tel: 0957 (52) 3121.

Nagasaki Municipal Hospital, 6–39 Shinchi-macji, Nagasaki-shi, Nagasaki 850, Japan Tel: 0958 (22) 3251.

Nagoya Ekisaikai Hospital, 4–66 Shonen-cho, Nakagawa-ku, Nagoya-shi, Aichi 454, Japan Tel: 052 (652) 7711.

Nagoya National Hospital, 4–1–1 Sannomaru, Naka-ku, Nagoya-shi, Aichi 460, Japan Tel: 052 (951) 1111.

Nara Prefectural Nara Hospital, Hiramatsu-cho, Nara-shi, Nara 631, Japan Tel: 0742 (46) 6001.

National Medical Center Hospital, 1–21–1 Toyama-cho, Shinjuku-ku, Tokyo 162, Japan

Niigata Municipal Hospital, 2–6–1 Shichikuyama, Niigata-shi, Niigata 950, Japan Tel: 025 (241) 5151.

Oita Prefectural Hospital, 2–37 Takasago-cho, Oita-shi, Oita 870, Japan Tel: 0975 (32) 5141.

Okayama Red Cross Hospital, 65–1 Aoe, Okayama-shi, Okayama 700, Japan Tel: 0862 (22) 8811.

Okayama Saiseikai General Hospital, 1–17–18 Ifuku-cho, Okayama-shi, Okayama 700, Japan Tel: 0862 (52) 2211.

Okinawa Prefectural Central Hospital, 208–3 Miyazato, Gushikawa-shi, Okinawa 904–22, Japan Tel: 0997 (3) 4111.

Oomuta Municipal Hospital, 3–3, Shiranui-cho, Oomuta-shi, Fukuoka 836, Japan Tel: 0944 (53) 1061.

Osaka-Minami National Hospital, 677–2 Kido-machi, Kawachinagano-shi, Osaka 586, Japan Tel: 0721 (53) 5761.

Osaka Prefectural Hospital, 3–1–56 Mandai-higashi Sumiyoshi-ku, Osaka-shi, Osaka 558, Japan Tel: 06 (692) 1201.

Osaka Prefectural Nakamiya Hospital, 3–16–21 Miyanosaka, Hirakata-shi, Osaka 573, Japan Tel: 0720 (47) 3261.

Osaka Red Cross Hospital, 5–53 Fudegasaki-machi, Tennouji-ku, Osaka-shi, Osaka 543, Japan Tel: 06 (771) 5131.

Osaka Teishin Hospital, 2–6–40 Karasugatsuji, Tenouji-ku, Osaka-shi, Osaka 543, Japan Tel: 06 (771) 0545.

Rissho Koseikai Fuzoku Kosei Hospital, 5–25–15 Yayoi-cho, Chuo-ku, Tokyo 194, Japan Tel: 03 (383) 1281.

St Luke International Hospital, 10–1 Akashi-cho, Nakano-ku, Tokyo 104, Japan Tel: 03 (541) 5151.

Sakai Municipal Hospital, 2–1–1 Nishi, Shukuin-machi, Sakai-shi, Osaka 590, Japan Tel: 0722 (38) 5521.

Saku General Hospital, Ooaza-Usuda, Usuda-cho, Minami-Saku-gun, Nagano 384–03, Japan Tel: 0278 (82) 3131.

Sanraku Hospital, 2–5 Kanda-Surugadai, Chiyoda-ku, Tokyo 101, Japan Tel: 03 (292) 3981.

Sapporo National Hospital, 2 Kikusui, Shijo, Shiraishi-ku, Sapporo-shi, Hokkaido 003, Japan Tel: 011 (811) 9111.

Sasebo Municipal General Hospital, 10–3 Shimaji-cho, Sasebo-shi, Nagasaki 857, Japan Tel: 0956 (24) 1515.

Sendai Municipal Hospital, 3–1 Shimizu-koji, Sendai-shi, Miyagi 980, Japan Tel: 022 (266) 7111.

Shakai Hoken Hiroshima Municipal Hospital, 7-33, Moto-machi, Naka-ku, Hiroshima-shi, Hiroshima 730, Japan Tel: 082 (221) 2291.

Shakai Hoken Kokura Hospital, 1–1 Kibune-cho, Kokurakita-ku, Kitakyushu-shi, Fukuoka 802, Japan Tel: 093 (921) 2231.

Shizuoka Municipal Hospital, 10–93 Oute-machi, Shizuoka-shi, Shizuoka 420, Japan Tel: 0542 (53) 3125.

Shizuoka Prefectural General Hospital, 4–27–1, Kitayasu-Higashi, Shizuoka-shi, Shizuoka 420, Japan Tel: 0542 (47) 6111.

Shizuoka Red Cross Hospital, 8–2 Oute-machi, Shizuoka-shi, Shizuoka 420, Japan Tel: 0542 (54) 4311.

Shizuoka Saiseikai General Hospital, 1–1–1 Kojika, Shizuoka-shi, Shizuoka 422, Japan Tel: 0542 (85) 6171.

Sumitomo Hospital, 5–2–2 Nakanoshima, Kita-ku, Osaka-shi, Osaka 530, Japan Tel: 06 (443) 1261.
Tachikawa Hospital, 4–2–22 Nishiki-cho, Tachikaw-shi, Tokyo 190, Japan Tel: 0425 (23) 3131.
Takayama Red Cross Hospital, 3–11 Tenma-cho, Takayama-shi, Gifu 506, Japan Tel: 0577 (32) 1111.
Takeda General Hospital, 3–27 Yamashika-machi, Aizuwakamatsu-shi, Fukushima 965, Japan Tel: 0242 (27) 5511.
Tenri Yorozu Soudansho Hospital, 20 Mishima-cho, Tenri-shi, Nara 632, Japan Tel: 07436 (3) 5611.
The First Nagoya Red Cross Hospital, 3–35 Michishita-cho, Nakamura-ku, Nagoya-shi, Aichi 453, Japan.
The Second Nagoya Red Cross Hospital, 2–9 Myoken-cho, Showa-ku, Nagoya-shi, Aichi 466, Japan Tel: 052 (832) 1121.
The Second Tokyo National Hospital, 2–5–1 Higashigaoka, Meguro-ku, Tokyo 152, Japan Tel: 03 (411) 0111.
Tochigi National Hospital, 1–10–37 Nakatomatsuri, Utsunomiya-shi, Tochigi 320, Japan Tel: 0286 (22) 5242.
Tokyo Metropolitan Hiroo Hospital, 2–34–10 Ebisu, Shibuya-ku, Tokyo 150, Japan Tel: 03 (444) 1181.
Tokyo Metropolitan Komagome Hospital, 3–18–22 Honkomagome, Bunkyo-ku, Tokyo 113, Japan Tel: 03 (823) 2101.
Tokyo Teishin Hospital, 2–14–23 Fujimi, Chiyoda-ku, Tokyo 102, Japan Tel: 03 (238) 7144.
Tokyo-to Saiseikai Central Hospital, 1–4–17 Mita, Minato-ku, Tokyo 108, Japan Tel: 03 (451) 8211.
Tottori Prefectural Hospital, 730 Gotsu, Tottori-shi, Tottori 680, Japan Tel: 0857 (26) 2271.
Toyama Prefectural Central Hospital, 2–2–78 Nishi-Nagae, Toyama-shi, Toyama 930, Japan Tel: 0764 (24) 1531.
Tranomon Hospital, 2–2–2 Toranomon, Minato-ku, Tokyo 105, Japan Tel: 03 (588) 1111.
Tsu National Hospital, 1022 Shin-machi, Hisai-shi, Mie 514–11, Japan Tel: 05925 (5) 3120.
Wakayama Red Cross Hospital, 4–1 Komatsubaradori, Wakayama-shi, Wakayama 640, Japan Tel: 0734 (22) 4171.
Yamaguchi Prefectural Central Hospital, 77 Ooaza-Ozaki, Hofu-shi, Yamaguchi 747, Japan Tel: 0835 (22) 4411.

FORENSIC MEDICINE:
Tohoku University School of Medicine has a forensic medicine department, 2–1 Seiryo-machi Aoba-ku, Sendai 980–8575, Japan Tel: 81 22 717 8110 Fax: 81 22 717 8112 http://forensic.med.tohoku.ac.jp

Malaysia

Population: 20 million
Language: Malay
Capital: Kuala Lumpur
Currency: Ringgit
Int Code: +603

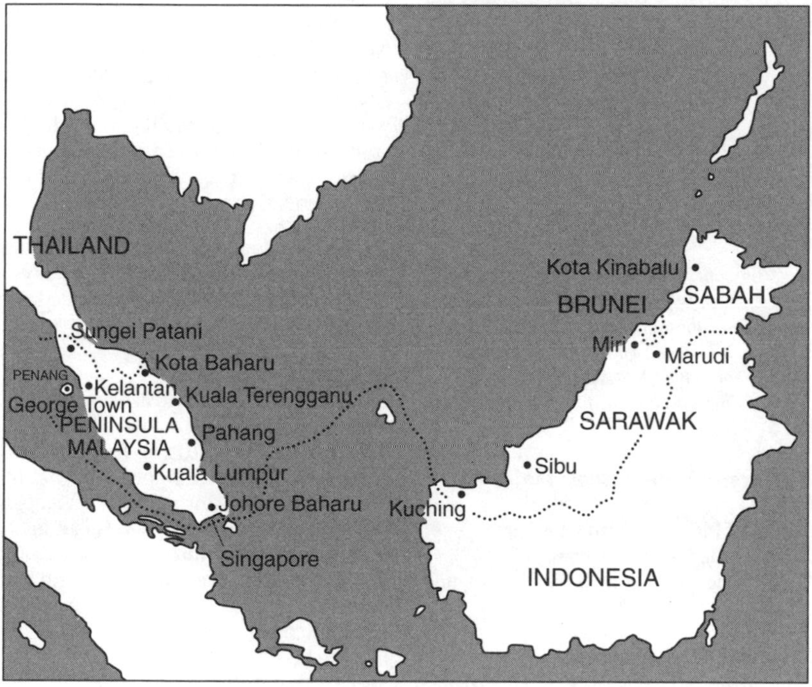

Malaysia consists of three territories: Malaya, Sarawak and Sabah. In recent years its economy has boomed and people in cities have become a lot richer, whereas those in rural areas have remained the same. It has some beautiful beaches and national parks to visit. There are three main races in Malaysia (Malay, Chinese and Indian), each with their own language and dialects. About 30% speak English although this obviously varies between rural and city areas. This can prove some barrier in history-taking, but don't let this put you off. Most doctors and nurses speak English.

✪ Medicine:

In the cities, Western medicine is the norm and a state-funded system exists. In rural areas, traditional medicine is still practised commonly. TB, HIV, malaria and dengue fever are relatively common.

➲ Visas and work permits: Commonwealth citizens do not require a visa for stays of up to 60 days. Some students, however, have found that their host institution has required them either to get a student visa, available on arrival or before you go. You need four passport-sized photos and an introduction letter from the hospital (cost is £30). Others have been told to get Professional Study Passes. The majority, however, have been told they don't need anything. Check with your host institution and the embassy as it obviously varies.

West Malaysia

Kuala Lumpar

KL is the capital of Malaysia and has recently undergone an economic boom. This is very evident from the abundance of huge new buildings. It is also a good base to explore the rest of peninsular Malaysia offering easy access to Taman Nagara (the National Park) and Singapore.

University Kebangsaan Malaysia (UKM)

Faculty of Medicine, Jalan Raja Muda
50300, Kuala Lumpar, Malaysia.
This is the central medical school and uses:

Hospital Kuala Lumpar

Jalan Pahang, 50586 Kuala Lumpur, Malaysia
Tel: 2921044 Fax: 03 2989845.

The hospital: A government-run tertiary referral centre and teaching hospital for the UKM right in the city centre. It is thought to be one of the biggest hospitals in Asia with 2585 beds on over 80 wards. The doctors (200 consultants) either work for the ministry of health or the university. The wards are divided into first, second and third class. A general medical ward has around 60 beds with three house officers. Ward rounds start at 7 am and last about four hours.

❍ Elective notes: The teaching is mainly bed-side during the round. Interesting cases include TB, tropical fevers (dengue and typhoid) and filariasis. AIDS and subsequent diseases are also common. There's lots of blood-taking, venflons, and ABGs to do, but not many other practical procedures. The third-class O&G department sees around 80 deliveries a day offering excellent experience. There is good teaching, although there is a question over whether it will remain a teaching hospital. Students have free rein of second and third class. Not all that many patients speak English.

Accommodation: Not provided, but is easily arranged and cheap. A hostel is typically £4–5 (30MYR)/night. If you apply through the university (see above address) they may be able to obtain accommodation with the residents.

Universiti Malaya, Faculti Perubatan, Lembah Pantai, Kuala Lumpar, Malaysia is the older medical school situated just outside the city. It uses:

University Hospital

Lembah Pantai 59100, Kuala Lumpur, Malaysia.

The hospital: Is 10 km from the city centre of Kuala Lumpur and is the teaching hospital for medical students at the University of Malaysia. It is a major tertiary referral centre. It has a friendly feel and more patients speak English than at Hospital KL. The A&E has a five-bed resus room and is one of the largest A&Es in the country.

❍ Elective notes: There is plenty to do with many procedures in A&E. The local medical students have tutorials that you are welcome to attend. The school has a very good teaching programme. Teaching is in English.

Accommodation: May be arranged on the university campus if you're persistent. Alternatively there is a YMCA.

The National Heart Institute

145 Jalan Tun Razak, 50400 Kuala Lumpar, Malaysia Tel: 298 1333 Fax: 2982824.

The hospital: Founded in 1992 due to

increasing cardiac disease. It is in the centre of KL with 300 beds and all the facilities of a modern hospital. It is a training centre for cardiothoracic surgeons and a tertiary referral centre for all of Malaysia. The cardiology department is the largest in the country with 10 consultants. There is a great deal of rheumatic as well as ischaemic heart disease.
Accommodation: Not provided but cheap places are available nearby.

OUTSIDE KUALA LUMPAR

Hospital Sultanah Aminah

Jalam Skudai, 80100 Johor Bahru, Johor, West Malaysia.
The hospital: Hospital Sultanah Aminah is a district general 1000-bed hospital in Johore Baharu, a busy, thriving town in the southern-most tip of the Malaysian peninsula. Facilities and investigations are limited. Due to the high incidence of rheumatic heart disease in Malaysia, cardiology is busy and a good place to go to practise hearing murmurs. Diseases to be seen include dengue fever, viral hepatitis, typhoid fever and TB. These often present late and advanced.
O Elective notes: Since it is not a teaching hospital, there are no local medical students so you have free reign throughout the departments.

Johore Specialist Hospital

39b Jln Abdul Samad, 80100 Johore Baharu, Johor, W. Malaysia.
A specialist private hospital. It's very friendly and there are usually no other students.

Hospital Sungei Patani

08000 Sungei Patani, Kedah Darulaman, Malaysia.
The hospital: About 3 km from the town centre and easily reached by regular buses. It is the largest district hospital in the south of Kedah and acts as a secondary referral centre for the surrounding smaller towns. It has three medical wards, each receiving about 200 admissions per month. There is also a six-bed ITU. There are four specialists (medical, surgical, O&G and radiology). There are also visiting physicians from Penang.
O Elective notes: There are no house officers so the presence of medical students is very much appreciated. The specialists and medical officers are very keen to teach. Diseases are like those in the rest of Malaysia ... TB, Hep B, HIV, snake bites and odd fevers. Sungei Patani (SP) is the second largest town in the state of Kedah (the 'rice-pot' of Malaysia). It is a fast developing town (in the golden triangle of the North) with a population of 30,000. There is very little to do in SP, but there is plenty to see in the surrounding areas.

Hospital Kuala Terengganu

Jalan Sultan Mohammed, Kuala Terengganu, Malaysia.
The hospital: A relatively modern busy DGH in the capital of Terengganu state on the east coast of peninsular Malaysia. It is a very Muslim area. The doctors and nurses speak English but the patients do not. Lots of TB, HIV, CVAs, MIs and dengue fever.
O Elective notes: Very friendly. Thursday afternoons and Fridays are the weekend but there is plenty of time off. Not much hands on. There is not actually that much to do in the vicinity but a nearby beach offers scuba diving. Maybe four weeks is enough.

Penang and Kelantan

Kelantan is a state on the north-east coast of peninsular Malaysia bordering Thailand. Islam is the main religion and it is the poorest state in Malaysia. Kota Baharu is the capital of Kelantan but is actually quite small. Penang is a tropical island, mainly wooded, off the west coast of Malaysia. The population totals 500,000 most of whom live in George Town where the state general hospital is situated.

For an elective in Penang write to the State Health Department for permission. The Director, Health Department, Pulau Pinang, Tingkat 37, Komtar 10590, Pulau Pinang. You will need to also get an immigration visa from the office in Penang during your first week. You need a letter from the hospital, and a letter from the Dept of Health.

Hospital Universiti Sains Malaysia (HUSM)

16150 Kubang Kerian, Kelantan Draul Naim, Malaysia Tel: 609 765 1700 Fax: 609 765 3370 http://kck4.usm.my/intro.html

Founded in 1979, the school of medical sciences does its preclinical years on the Penang campus and the clinical years in the Kelantan campus that houses USM Teaching Hospital. HUSM is the referral centre for the east coast states of peninsular Malaysia. It has 50 beds over 22 wards providing most major specialities. There is also an A&E. (Write to the Chairman of the Electives Committee, for application forms.)

Penang General Hospital (Hospital Pulau Pinang)

Jalan Residensi 10990, Pulau Pinang, Malaysia.

The hospital: The second-largest hospital in Malaysia with all specialities; for example it is one of only two centres performing invasive cardiology. It is just becoming a university hospital. Equipment is sparse but there is enough to get by. Dengue and other fevers are common as are malaria, TB and HIV.

O Elective notes: it is well set up for electives, write to the Deputy Director at the above address. Not much formal teaching, but plenty of bedside.

Accommodation: A wide variety is available in Penang from £2 (12 MYR)/night for a dorm to £12 (72 MYR) a night for an a/c room with shower. The YMCA is five minutes from the hospital (£8 (48 MYR)/night)

Hospital Lam Wah Ge

Jalan Tan Sri The Exe Him, 11600 Penang, Malaysia.

The hospital: About an hour out of the main tourist area of Penang. It is a charity hospital where patients are means tested as to the amount they can pay. Accordingly they are classed into first, second or third class patients.

O Elective notes: It is a very friendly hospital and, as it is not government-run, there are no local students. Everyone speaks immaculate English.

Accommodation: In the college of nursing in the hospital grounds and very cheap.

Hospital Tengky Ampuan Afzan

Jalan Tanah Puteh, 25100 Kuantan, Pahang, Malaysia.

The hospital: A DGH with departments including A&E, paeds, O&G.

O Elective notes: Lots of hands on experience can be gained here.

Accommodation: Can be arranged.

East Malaysia

Sarawak

Sarawak and Sabah are the Malaysian parts of Borneo. There is some beautiful countryside and it's excellent for mountaineers (Sabah has the highest mountains in south-east Asia). In Sarawak you can visit Bako National Park, Damai Beach and Wind Cave.

A useful address is: **State Health Department,** Tun Abang Haji Openg Rd, 93590 Kuching, Sarawak, Malaysia.

Sarawak General Hospital (Hospital Umum Sarawak)

Jalan Tun Abang Haji Openg Road, 93586 Kuching, Sarawak, East Malaysia Tel: 08 257555 Fax: 082 242751.

The hospital: A relatively large, modern, busy teaching hospital in Kuching, the beautiful capital of Sarawak, well-known for its rich history of culture and tradition. The A&E department admits an average of 160 patients per day and is one of the most advanced units in Malaysia.

O Elective notes: Elective students are allowed out on the ambulances where there is plenty of opportunity to practise resuscitation. In A&E there are histories to be taken (if you can understand them), patients to examine and minor procedures (e.g. stitching) to be done. General medical wards (four in total), like the rest of Malaysia, are divided into first, second and third class. Again, there are many opportunities for practical procedures. Cardiology outpatients is excellent for murmurs (high prevalence of rheumatic fever). There is a village healthcare team which goes out to visit different villages (e.g. Batu Nah 300 km north of Kuching or Marudi, five hours up river through dense rainforest) providing primary healthcare. You can travel with them either by boat or jeep, a must if you really want to sample Malay life, food and hospitality. It is often the elective highlight. It is becoming more difficult to organize these trips with the healthcare teams since some Aussie students overdid it with the rice wine in one of the villages in 1997. Officially the elective co-ordinator has stopped students going with them . . . just ask the healthcare team directly once you're there. More people tend to speak English here than in other parts of Malaysia.
Accommodation: Easy to organize as Kuching is popular with elective students and tourists. Many stay at St Thomas' Anglican Rest house (Jalan McDougall, Kuching Tel: 082 414027). There are many other elective students from Australia and Germany.

Sibu General Hospital

Batu 5½, Jalan OYA, Sibu, Sarawak, Malaysia Tel: 0884 34333.

The hospital: Has two consultants covering 40 beds and offers the opportunity to see many diseases rare to the West. Diseases seen include rheumatic and dengue fever, malaria, TB and amoebic abscesses.
O Elective notes: There's hands on experience in a number of procedures, including ECHO. Teaching is good and there are usually other elective students there so you can get yourself into groups. Food is great and the locals friendly (though few speak English). Sibu itself is 2½ hours by bus from the Niah caves and a five-hour ride from Miri.

Marudi Hospital

Miri Division, East Sarawak, Malaysia.

The hospital: A small rural hospital in a frontier town about five hours' express boat journey from Miri. It is deep in jungle. It serves not only Marudi but the local Kelabit, Kayan and Penan tribes that live along the river and in the deep interior. The hospital has four wards: male, female, paeds and maternity each with 8–10 beds. There is a basic operating theatre, a basic X-ray department and lab facilities. The three doctors tend to be very junior (few months to a couple of years out of school). The hospital also runs public health programmes. Lots of tropical diseases (malaria, Jap B encephalitis) here.

Sabah

Queen Elizabeth Hospital

Locked Bag No 2029, 886500 Kota Kinabalu, Sabah, East Malaysia Tel: 0 88 218166 Fax: 0 88 211999.

The hospital: The QEH is the main teaching hospital for Sabah with approximately 500 beds, but some have found it a bit grotty and overcrowded, although it is fairly well-equipped. It has most specialities (popular ones with elective students are dermatology, paeds, O&G, ophthalmology, medicine, TB, A&E, surgery, orthopaedics and radiology).
O Elective notes: You can decide when you get there or rotate around. It is very busy and it is a good place for seeing big livers, spleens, TB, malaria etc. Kota Kinabulu (KK) is a large city (population 200,000) and so there is a great deal to do. The local opthalmologist takes a special interest in medical students and organizes trips to the interior and smaller district general hospitals. You'll also go out with 'the Lion club' (a bit like Rotary) to take free medical services to

the villages in the jungle ... this has excellent reports. You get as much out as you put in. Good teaching but not much responsibility. Ward rounds are in English. Half the doctors are Indian and don't speak Malay and so it's not essential for you to learn it. However, like most places in Malaysia, the locals do not speak English. Repeatedly highly recommended. The are many islands a short boat trip from Kota Kinabulu. Sipadan Island is a tiny coal island near by advertised as the top scuba diving spot in the world ... it's well worth a visit, but can be pricey so be prepared to haggle. Also go to Sepilok Orangutan Sanctuary, Poring Volcanic Springs, Turtle Island and climb Mt Kinabulu (14,000 ft).

Note: To work here you have to pay RM 100 (£25) to the hospital library.

Accommodation: Try Jack's B&B (Jalan Karamunsing Karamungsing Warehouse Lot 17, KK, Sabah, Tel: 88 232367; see the Lonely Planet Guide; (£4.50 (25 MYR)/night). It's near the hospital (15 min), clean and serves fresh pancakes for breakfast.

The Maldives

Population: 300,000
Language: Dhivehi
Capital: Male
Currency: Rufiyaa
Int Code: +960

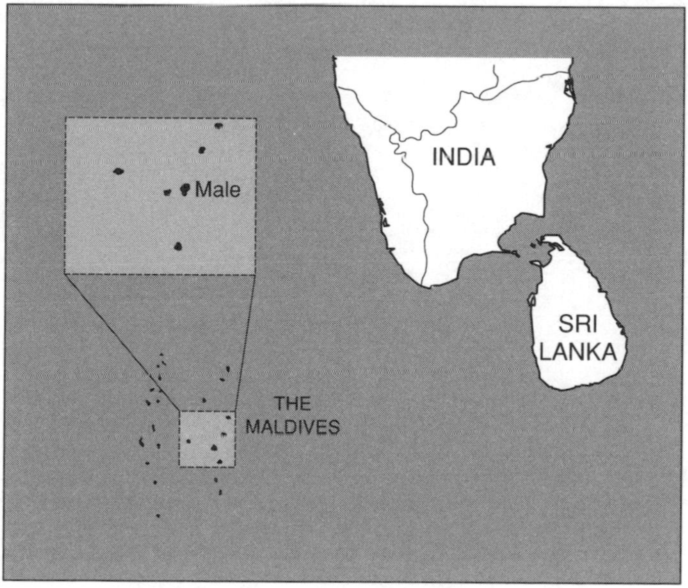

The Maldives are one of the world's poorest countries although it has become a well-known tourist destination for its beaches. It is an Islamic country and so alcohol is only allowed in expensive tourist resorts (not even in your own home). It is not a popular elective or voluntary work destination.

✪ Medicine:

The Maldives receives UN and WHO aid to provide a health service that is still vastly underfunded. There are no medical schools. The hospitals have to perform the function of GP units as well and hence everything from the trivial to the major is seen. Infectious diseases, such as typhoid, and hypertension and diabetes are fairly common. Some students have found universal precautions rather lacking so it may be worth taking your own gloves and goggles.

Male Hospital

Male, The Maldives.

The hospital: The main hospital, but some have found it more of a DGH. Currently they only accept UK and Australian students. Write to: The Ministry of Health, Male, Republic of the Maldives for elective details.

Seenu Regional Hospital

S. Hithadhoo, Addu Attoll, Republic of the Maldives.

The hospital: Founded in 1984 with 15 beds, it now has 50 and acts as a referral centre for the whole Attoll. It has one operating theatre, lab facilities and an X-ray machine. It is staffed by six doctors. Patients speak Divehi although the doctors speak English.

O **Elective notes:** As the hospital is so small you get to know everyone very quickly. The day usually finishes about 2 pm giving plenty of time for exploring, diving or sunbathing. There are some excellent dive spots, although the novelty of a tropical island does eventually wear off.

Accommodation: Usually provided free in a shared house a few minutes from the hospital.

Nepal

Population: 21.4 million
Language: Nepali
Capital: Kathmandu
Currency: Nepalese rupee
Int Code: +977

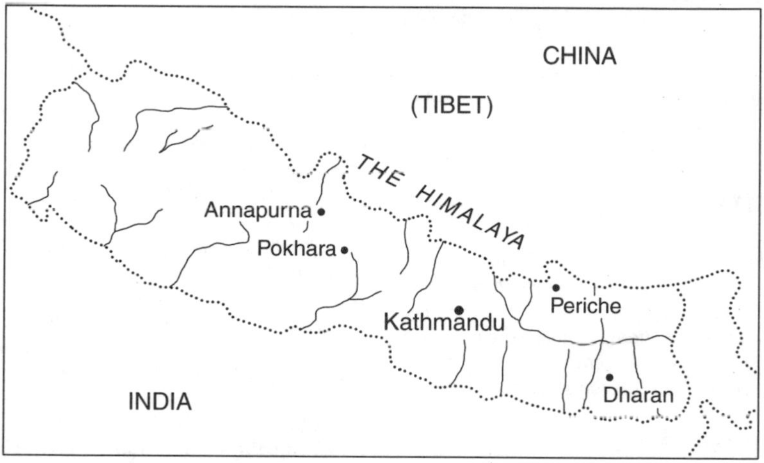

Nepal is one of the poorest countries in the world (average income US$150/year); however, the economy is improving rapidly. Eighty per cent of people rely on subsistence farming (and hence there is no shortage of food). Seventy-four per cent are illiterate. Working here not only gives the opportunity of practising basic medicine where it is very much needed, but also some spectacular scenery in the Himalayas.

✪ Medicine:

Until recently, medicine has been very primitive. There is only one doctor per 16,110 people, but 100 *dharmi-jhankri* (faith healers) for every doctor. Maternal and infant mortality are very high due to dangerous traditional birth practices. This is being tackled by a re-education programme for midwives. Patients have to pay for their healthcare. They seem small sums to us, but it often means they have to sell animals to get the money. Infectious diseases such as TB, malaria and Japanese encephalitis are common. HIV has become a problem mainly in the IVDU population. The incidence of leprosy is 6/1000 and average life expectancy is 54.

Most elective students go to the main hospitals in Kathmandu but there are plenty of opportunities in rural Nepal, the Himalayas and other towns. There are a great number of charities that also do work here. (*See* Section 3: The Appendix and the end of this chapter.)

➲ Visas and work permits:

Visitors' visas are easily obtained form the Royal Nepalese Embassy. A 60-day visa costs £30. These can be extended in

Kathmandu/Pokhara. Allow 2–3 weeks for the visa to be processed if posted (they can do it in 24 hours if by hand). They say that no special permit is required for elective students. Email: 101642.43@compuserve.com or visit http://www.south-asia.com/dotn. If holding a medical degree from a recognized institution you can register with the Nepal Medical Council, Ministry of Health, Ram Shah Path, Kathmandu.

◎ Climate:

Monsoon season is July to October causing many floods in the Terai plain. The rest of the year is fairly warm and sunny. It can get cold between December and February.

Kathmandu

Kathmandu is a big, bustling city, rapidly becoming a popular tourist destination. The people are extremely friendly. A trip in to the mountains from here is a must. The mountain villagers are very welcoming. There is jungle in the south where you can go elephant riding.

UNIVERSITIES:

The Institute of Medicine, Tribhuvan University

Maharajgung, PO Box 1524, Kathmandu, Nepal.

This is the main medical school; another has just been built in Pokhara.

HOSPITALS:

Bir Hospital

Tundikhel, Kathmandu, Nepal Tel: 01 221119/226963/221988 (A&E 223807).

The hospital: Bir Hospital is a large, busy general hospital receiving patients from all over Nepal. It is overcrowded and dirty. All the doctors are very friendly and speak good English, although few of the patients do.

O Elective notes: You are encouraged to do minor procedures and there are plenty of unusual conditions. The medical ward rounds last forever and are mostly conducted in Nepali ... however, interesting patients are translated for you. To work here for four weeks costs $100 and $50 for each week after that. It sounds like a lot, but the hospital really does need the funds (Registrars are paid £40/month) and you get great teaching and experience in A&E. You can visit other hospitals and there is time off to go trekking etc.

Accommodation: Not provided but there are plenty of cheap hostels and hotels in Thamel, which is close to the hospital and where most restaurants and bars are located. Food and drink is very cheap.

Kanti Children's Hospital

Maharajgunj, Kathmandu, PO Box 2664, Nepal Tel: 01 411550/414798.

The hospital: A large (170-bed), modern, busy government-run paediatric hospital on the north side of Kathmandu. It is the only paeds hospital in Nepal and provides all specialities bar orthopaedics and ENT. It has two medical, two surgical wards, four theatres, a NICU, a PICU, a burns unit and Casualty. Reasonable facilities are available, including ultrasound and ECHO. There are no doctors' fees but patients have to pay for medication (except at the doctor's discretion). Common conditions include malnutrition, congenital hip dysplasia, malaria, typhoid, Jap B encephalitis, meningitis, TB, childhood cancers and rheumatic fever. OPD is chaotic with doctors duty bound to see all patients who have paid their 6rpd (5p) and registered by 11 am.

O Elective notes: The teaching is excellent (the doctors speak English) and the cases interesting. A charge of $25 a week is made. When you see how desperate the patients are, you realize how much it is needed. The staff are incredibly friendly. Electives can be in medicine, surgery or A&E or you can rotate. There aren't many other students and the day finishes around 2 pm (the doctors have to do private work as they are only paid £50/month by the government). If you

are going here, RSPB comes highly recommended for superb teaching. Repeatedly highly recommended. Try to get out with the Social Action Volunteers who run clinics in villages.
Accommodation: Not provided but easy to find.

Prasuti Griha Government Maternity Hospital
Thapathali, PO Box 5307, Kathmandu, Nepal Tel: 01 211243/214205.
The hospital: Nepal's main maternity hospital with over 12,000 deliveries a year (i.e. 40 a day). There is also a small SCBU. It is well-run and clean though very lacking in resources.
O Elective notes: Lots of experience and the opportunity to do a research project.

Patan Hospital
United Mission to Nepal, PO Box 126, Patan, Kathmandu, Nepal. (Work and electives here can be arranged through Interserve.)
The hospital: A DGH run by the government and the United Mission to Nepal (UMN). It is in a rural area of south Kathmandu. It was built in 1982 and has 150 beds with medical, surgical, paeds and O&G wards. It has a busy OPD seeing 200,000 patients a year. COAD (± chest infections) due to the pollution in Kathmandu valley, smoking and smokey fires is very common. TB, meningitis, rheumatic heart disease and gastroenteritis are also common. Outreach clinics also take place.
Accommodation: Has previously been provided in a UMN guesthouse.

Pokhara

Pokhara is Nepal's second city 200 km west of Kathmandu. It's an excellent base for trekking the Annapurna circuit.

Manipal College of Medical Science
PO Box 155, Upallo Deep, Pokhara 16, Nepal.
The college is new having taken its first students in 1994. It is currently building its own 700-bed hospital which will be made into the local teaching hospital. They also run 'Eye camps' going out into the hills for a couple of weeks. All notes and medical discussions are in English.

Western Regional Hospital
Pokhara, Nepal Tel: 061 20066/20461.
The hospital: Run by the Nepali government and the INF. It has a good reputation. Surgical procedures are often due to leprosy and RTAs.

Green Pastures Hospital
Pokhara, Nepal.
The hospital: A tertiary leprosy referral hospital for the western region of Nepal. It is financed and staffed by the INF. It has 100 acute beds and 20 long stay beds. It has theatre facilities for reconstructive surgery. Due to the stigma, patients with leprosy are often thrown out of families. The hospital can arrange marriages between patients.
O Elective notes: After some teaching about leprosy, students are give jobs to do and patients to look after. There is quite a bit of responsibility. This elective is well-recommended. Apply through the INF VERY EARLY (see below).

Drug Education Programme
PO Box 5, Pokhara, Nepal.
The project: An 'outreach' project, going out and befriending drug addicts and alcoholics, giving needles and condoms and trying to prevent drug use. The language barrier can be a mild problem but don't let that put you off. People who have worked here have found in very rewarding.

RURAL HOSPITALS:

BP Koirala Institute of Health Sciences
Dharan, Nepal.
The hospital: Is on the site of a former British military hospital but is now under Government control and incorporates a

medical school and school of nursing. It has 150 beds. Rare diseases that are common include TB, malaria, kala-azar, rabies and tetanus.

Amda Hospital

Damak, Jhapa, Nepal.

The hospital: A welfare centre on the flatland of Nepal in Damak. It was set up by a Japanese-based charity for several thousand Bhutanese refugees. The UN now controls these camps.

United Mission to Nepal Hospital

Tansen, Nepal.

The hospital: A mission hospital on a hill overlooking a flood plain in south-west Nepal.

UMN Okhaldunga Hospital

c/o UMN Post Box 126, Kathmandu, Nepal.

The hospital: A 40-bed mission hospital built on a hillside in beautiful eastern Nepal. It is three hours' walk from the airstrip and three days' walk from the nearest road. The hospital community is a few Western doctors (GPs) and a few Nepali hospital workers. There are four wards, an OPD and a rudimentary outpatients clinic. Common conditions include TB, pneumonia, typhoid, diarrhoea, abscesses, trauma, burns and obstetric emergencies. Language is pretty much Nepalese, although the doctors speak English.

O Elective notes: This elective is very highly recommended, although you may feel isolated. There is a local bazaar 45 minutes' walk away. In the theatre there is plenty to be seen and assist in. It does have e-mail.

Accommodation: A guesthouse on site.

Kunde Hospital

Kunde, near Makhe Bazaar, Nepal (postal address: c/o Himalayan Trust, PO Box 224 Kathmandu).

The hospital: Kunde Hospital is run by a charitable organization (the Himalayan Trust) set up by Sir Edmund Hilary for the Sherpa people in the Everest region. It is more of a clinic with seven long-stay and two short-stay beds but is run very well. There is an operating table/examination couch and limited X-ray machine. Sherpa people are reluctant to stay in hospital as they believe that ghosts transmit illnesses and therefore hospitals are teaming with them. An impressive immunization scheme has been successful. They will not normally take elective students.

OTHER HOSPITALS:

ARGHAKHANCHI: Arghakhanchi Hospital, Arghakhanchi, Nepal Tel: 077 20188.
BANEPA: Scheer Memorial Mission Hospital, Banepa, PO Box 88, Nepal Tel: 011 61111/61112.
BHADRAPUR: Mechi Zonal Hospital, Bhadrapur Tel: 023 20024/20172/20011.
BHAIRAHAWA: Lumbini Eye Hospital, Siddhartha Nagar, Bhairahawa, Nepal Tel: 071 20265/20668.
BIRATNAGAR: Koshi Zonal Hospital, Biratnagar, Nepal Tel: 021 22900/21234/25619.
Rab Lal Golcha Eye Hospital, Biratnagar, Nepal. Tel: 021 23706/22022.
BIRGUNJ: Kedia Eye Hospital, Lipani, Birgunj, Nepal Tel: 051 21382.
Narayani Zonal Hospital, Birgunj, Nepal Tel: 051 21993/22153.
BUTWAL: Lumbini Zonal Hospital, Butwal, Nepal Tel: 073 20201/20200.
CHITWAN: Bharatpur Hospital, Bharatpur, Chitwan, Nepal Tel: 056 20022.
King Mahendra Memorial Eye Hospital, Bharatpur, Chitwan, Nepal Tel: 056 20333.
DAMAULI: Public Health Centre, Damauli, Tanahun, Nepal Tel: 065 60119.
DANG: Mahendra Hospital, Dang, Nepal Tel: 082 60119.
Rapti Eye Hospital, Tulsipur, Dang, Nepal Tel: 082 20165.
DHANGADHI: Far Western Regional Eye Hospital, Dhangadhi, Nepal Tel: 091 21112.
Seti Zonal Hospital, Dhangadhi, Nepal Tel: 091 21171/21111/21271.
DHARAN: Dharan Hospital, Dharan-4, Nepal Tel: 025 20134/20119.
Eastern Regional Hospital, Dharan, Nepal Tel: 025 20839/20845
GORKHA: Amppipal Mission Hospital, Amppipal, Gorkha, PO Box 126. KTM, Nepal.
Gorkha Hospital, Gorkha, Nepal Tel: 064 20288.
GULMI: Tamghas Hospital, Gulmi, Lumbini, Nepal Tel: 079 20188.
ILAM: Ilam Hospital, Ilam, Nepal Tel: 027 20044.
INARUWA: Inaruwa Hospital, Inaruwa, Nepal Tel: 025 20044.
JALESHWOR: Jaleshwor Hospital, Jaleshwor, Nepal Tel: 044 20170/20070.
JANAKPUR: Janakpur Zonal Hospital, Janakpurdham, Nepal Tel: 041 20133.

Shree Janaki Eye Care Centre, Janakpurdham, Nepal Tel: 041 20133/20397.
KAPILVASTU: Taulihawa Hospital, Kapilvastu, Nepal Tel: 076 60200.

KATHMANDU VALLEY:

Anand Ban Leprosy Hospital, Tika Bhairab, Lele, Lalitpur, GPO Box: 151, Nepal Tel: 01 290545/290538 Fax: 977 1 290538.
Ayurved Hospital, Naradevi, Kathmandu, Nepal Tel: 01 220764/228182.
Bankali Hospital, Gaushala, Kathmandu, Nepal Tel: 01 470302.
Bhaktapur Hospital, Dudhpati, Bhaktapur, Nepal Tel: 01 610676/610798.
Birendra Military Hospital, Chhauni, Kathmandu, Nepal Tel: 01 271940/271941/271965.
Birendra Police Hospital, Maharajgunj, Kathmandu, Nepal Tel: 01 412430/412530/412630.
Central Jail Hospital, Bagh Durbar, Tripureshwor, Kathmandu, Nepal Tel: 01 212442/212443.
Chest Hospital, Kalimati, Kathmandu, Nepal Tel: 270329.
Hospital for Disabled Children, Dhobighat, Jawalakhei, Lalitpur, GPO Box 2430, Nepal Tel: 01 525578.
Infectious Diseases Hospital, Teku, Kathmandu, Nepal Tel: 01 211344/211112/21294.
Maternity Hospital, Thapathali, Kathmandu, PO Box 5307, Nepal Tel: 01 211243/214205.
Mental Hospital, Lagankhel, Lalitpur, Nepal Tel: 01 521333.
Nepal Anti TB Hospital, Sanothimi, Bhaktapur, Nepal Tel: 01 610033/610706.
Nepal Eye Hospital, Tripureshwor, Kathmandu, Nepal Tel: 01 215466/213317/212102.
Patan Hospital, Lagankhel, Lalitpur, PO Box 252, Nepal Tel: 01 521048/521034/522266.
Shree Pashupati Homeopathic Hospital, Harihar Bhawan, Pulchowk, Lalitpur, Nepal Tel: 01 522092.
TU Teaching Hospital, Maharajgunj, Kathmandu PO Box 3578, Nepal Tel: 01 412303/412404/412505/412707.
Tokha Hospital, Tokha, Kathmandu, Nepal Tel: 01 213228.

MORE HOSPITALS:

LAHAN: Sagarmatha Chaudhari Eye Hospital, Lahan, Siraha, Nepal Tel: 033 20102.
MAHENDRANAGAR: Mahakali Zonal Hospital, Mahendranagar, Nepal Tel: 099 21111.
MALANGAWA: Sarlahi Hospital, Malangawa, Sarlahi, Nepal Tel: 046 20133/20183.
NAWALPARASI: Prithivi Chandra Hospital, Nawalparasi, Nepal Tel: 078 20188.
NEPALGUNJ: Bheri Zonal Hospital, Nepalgunj, Nepal Tel: 081 20158/20183/20193.
Fathe Bal Eye Hospital, Fultekra, Nepalgunj, Nepal Tel: 081 20598.
PALPA: Palpa Mission Hospital, Palpa, Nepal Tel: 075 20154.
POKHARA: Himalaya Eye Hospital, Dhari Patan, Pokhara PO Box 78, Nepal Tel: 061 20352 Fax: 977 061 20352.
Western Regional Hospital, Pokhara, Nepal Tel: 061 20066/20461.
RAJBIRAJ: Sagarmatha Zonal Hospital, Rajbiraj, Nepal Tel: 031 20196/20034.
SURKHET: Surkhet District Hospital, Surkhet, Nepal Tel: 083 20200.
TRISHULI: Trishuli Hospital, Nuwakot, Trishuli, Nepal Tel: 010 60188.

International Nepal Fellowship

69 Wentworth Road, Harborne, Birmingham B17 9SS Tel: 0121 427 8833 Fax: 0121 428 3110 ukoffice@inf.org.uk
In Nepal their address is: INF PO Box 1230, Kathmandu, Nepal (e-mail lp@nf.wlink.com.np).

They are involved in agricultural development and medical care throughout Nepal. It is not supposed to convert Nepales to Christianity and volunteers don't need to be Christian, just respect their beliefs. They run leprosy hospitals and rural clinics in Pokhara.

○ **Elective notes:** They offer some elective places but are often booked up over a year in advance. Doing a rural clinic elective with them comes highly recommended. It can involve trekking through to many villages with a couple of nurses to do a specific project.
Accommodation: Can be arranged for a minimal cost. The INF looks after elective students well. APPLY EARLY.

United Mission to Nepal

PO Box 126, Kathmandu, Nepal.
UMN run four hospitals in Nepal, for electives contact their UK Headquarters (*see* Section 3: The Appendix).

SOMETHING DIFFERENT:

Himalayan Rescue Association

PO Box 4944, Thamel, Kathmandu, Nepal
http://www.nepalonline.net/hra/
They have two posts in the Himalaya. One is in Periche (near the Everest Base Camp). This sees mainly Western trekkers with minor injuries and acute

mountain sickness. Visit the main website. They do not officially allow elective students, but qualified volunteers are required to work for periods of three months. The other post is **Himalayan Rescue Association Post**, Manang, Manag District, Nepal. (Write early as a porter has to carry this letter 90 miles from the nearest road up 3800 m.) This is on the Annapurna circuit and sees locals as well as trekkers. They have previously allowed elective students.

Pakistan

Population: 140.5 million
Language: Urdu
Capital: Islamabad
Currency: Pakistani rupee
Int code: + 92

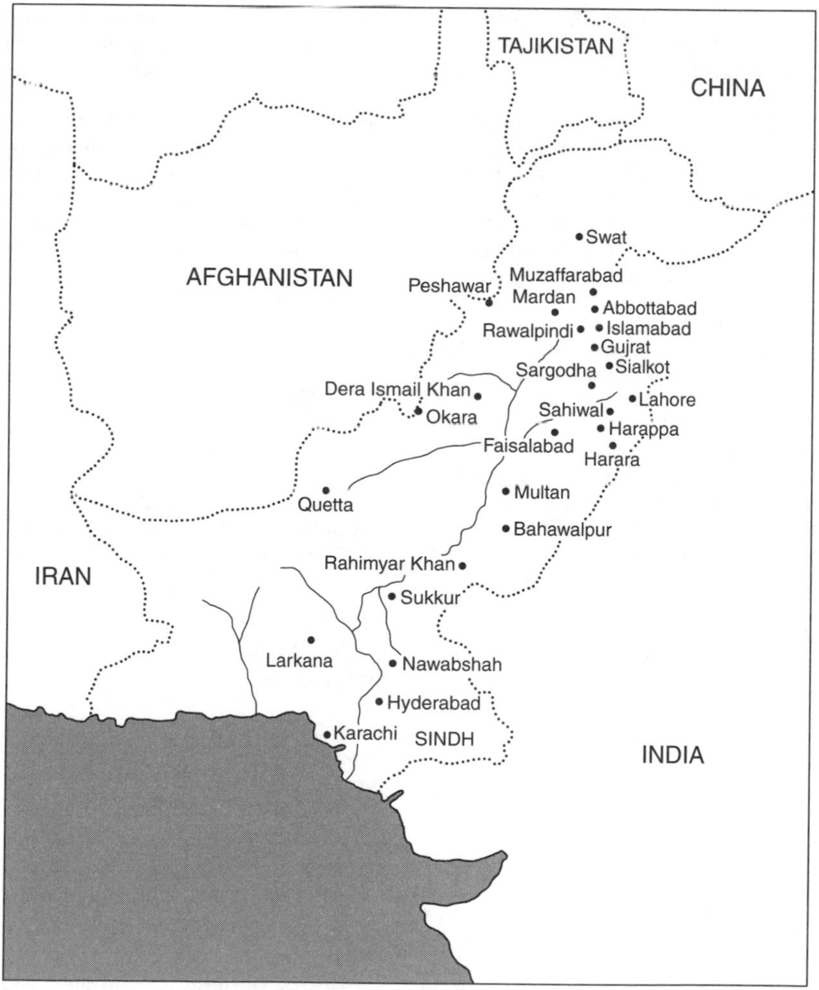

Pakistan has many political and domestic problems that unfortunately overshadow this beautiful country. Pakistan was originally created in 1947 as an independent Muslim Indian state. However, the disputes with India over Kashmir still exist and as Islamic militancy increases, discrimination against other religious minorities increases. There is a very large social gap between the rich and poor. The average annual income is $370, 1.7% of the average US income. Women's role in society is also very second-rate. There is a high male: female ratio implying that female neglect and infanticide still occurs. The religious make-up is 97% Muslim, 1.7% Christian and 1.5% Hindu.

WARNING: Think very seriously if you intend to go to Pakistan as a single white female. The cultural differences can cause many problems. Try to go in a pair or with a male colleague. At the time of writing there has recently been a military coup. You should probably enquire with the Foreign Office before going.

Medicine:
Pakistan is the ninth most populous country. Despite population growth falling, 50% of the population is under 15 years old. Official literacy rates are 40% but there is a wide variation. Healthcare is very poor with a shortage of staff, equipment and medicine. Infectious diseases (malaria, tuberculosis, diarrhoea and meningitis) are common causes of death. Infant mortality is amongst the highest in the world. The doctor:patient ratio is one per 1918. Because of high illiteracy and it being difficult to reach isolated women who do not leave their homes, family planning and education have been difficult. Government hospitals provide free treatment to the poor. However, no medicine is supplied and that has to be purchased by the family.

Pakistan vastly overproduces doctors, many of whom leave for greener pastures. In contrast there are very few nurses trained (approximately one for every 20 doctors). Doctors don't want to work in rural areas and there are very few female doctors.

Climate and crime:
Climate can vary considerably from the north (cold) to the south (hot, 30°C+). Rainfall peaks between July and August. Crime is frighteningly high compared to other Islamic countries. There is a high incidence of murder, rape, robbery and drugs crime. Abuse of women is also a major problem.

Visas and work permits:
Visas are needed for electives. You need an application form, letter from your clinical school and two passport photos. You need to register with police at your destination. Visas for study purposes are given after poof of acceptance at an organization in Pakistan is demonstrated. Short-term work offers are considered on the basis of qualifications, experience, eligibility and specific needs of the country. Doctors trained abroad usually have no problems, but check your degree is recognized by the Pakistan Medical and Dental Council, 30 Attaturk Avenue, Islamabad.

Lahore

Lahore has been described as the 'Paris of Asia', like no other city. It is an excellent place for sightseeing, the Lahore Fort, Badshahi Mosque and Iqbal Park as well as the city centre. There is a great deal of Mughal history.

MEDICAL SCHOOLS AND THEIR HOSPITALS:

King Edward Medical College
University of the Punjab, Nila Gumband, Anarkali, Lahore 54000, Pakistan Tel: 042 7354005 Fax: 042 7233796
www.kemc.edu

Founded in 1860, it is the oldest medical school in Pakistan. It uses a number of hospitals including the **Mayo Hospital**, **Lady Willingdon** and **Lahore General Hospitals**.

The Mayo Hospital: One of the largest in the country and founded in 1870. It was named after the then Viceroy of India. All specialities are available. There's an excellent range of pathologies in all subjects and a busy A&E. Friendly staff/students.

O Elective notes: Enthusiastic teachers but not much in the way of practical procedures as everyone is too busy.

Allama Iqbal Medical College

University of the Punjab, Allama Shabbir Ahmed Usmani Road, Lahore 54550, Pakistan Tel: 042 5160107 Fax: 042 5160771.

The medical school: Uses the **Jinnah Hospital** as its main teaching hospital. It is relatively new, clean and not overcrowded.

O Elective notes: There is a great deal of pathology and opportunity to investigate and manage people under supervision in A&E. There's also daily teaching with the local medical students.

Accommodation: Free, but very basic.

Fatima Junnah Medical College for Women

University of the Punjab, Shahrah-e-Fatima Jinnah, Lahore 54000, Pakistan Tel: 042 6369469 Fax: 042 6366058.

Founded in 1948 as more Muslim women doctors were desperately needed. Its teaching hospital is the near 1000-bed **Fatima Jinnah Hospital**. It's still women only.

OTHER HOSPITALS IN LAHORE:

Shaukhat Khanum Cancer Hospital

Lahore, Pakistan www.shaukatkhanum.org.pk

The hospital: Built in 1989 by Imran Khan in memory of his mother who died of cancer. It is a first class institution that diagnoses and treats those with cancer, irrespective of their ability to pay. It has a massive catchment area of 400 miles. Most of the Consultants are from the US and it has MRI and CT facilities.

O Elective notes: Their web site has an elective application form that can be downloaded. It's incredibly well-organized.

Accommodation: Very plush with a nominal charge of 6000 rupees (£80). Go with a friend if you can. There is a hospital car which previous students have used to go to the centre of town.

The Services Hospital

Lahore, Pakistan.

The hospital: A government hospital. Some reports describe the hospital as being understaffed and not all that clean.

Sheikh Zayed Hospital

Lahore, Pakistan.

The hospital: A postgraduate hospital with many specialities. Patients have to pay a small fee to be seen here.

O Elective notes: Recommended for the wide range of pathology but very little practical exposure.

Islamabad

Islamabad, the capital of Pakistan, is a beautiful, clean and pleasant city. It is surrounded by the Margalla Hills and Rawal Lake making it a very enjoyable place to work. Travel to Muree, a scenic hill station or Lahore. Hop across into India if you have a visa.

Margalla Institute of Health Sciences

Pitrus Bokhari Road, H-8/1, Islamabad, Pakistan Tel: 051 430260 Fax: 051 445966 www.margalla.com

The medical school: Has both clinical and academic activities on the same campus. Its teaching hospitals are:

- **Dar-ul-Shifa Hospital,** H–8/1, Islamabad with 150 beds expanding to 500 and having all major specialities. It is for the 'poor and needy'. A CT scanner is on the way.
- **Margalla Welfare Hospital,** Pirwadhai, Rawalpindi. Pirwadhai is a densly populated area with some very poor pockets.

- **Glora Welfare Hospital** (Ghosia-Mahria Trust), Gloria, Islamabad. The main campus is 15 minutes from the airport.

Quaid-I-Azam Postgraduate Medical College, Pakistan Institute of Medical Sciences

Islamabad, Pakistan.

The hospital: A government-run tertiary referral hospital and part of the postgraduate medical college. It is busy and overcrowded. Doctors here get paid £100/month.

Children's Hospital, Pakistan Institute of Medical Sciences

Sector G-8, Islamabad, Pakistan.

The hospital: A tertiary referral hospital taking children from most of north Pakistan and Azad Kashmir. There is a wide range of illness in this multi-racial society. There are many Afghanistani and Sudanese refugees. Encephalomyelitis and malnutrition are common causes for admission.

Elective notes: If pushy, you can get to do procedures such as lumbar punctures, or liver biopsies. Clinics also throw up a whole range of petty to life-threatening conditions. The hospital is a postgraduate teaching centre so there is plenty of teaching if you want it.

Accommodation: Provided and excellent by Pakistani standards, but the food is a bit monotonous.

Karachi

Karachi is the largest city in Pakistan.

Aga Khan University Medical College

PO Box 3500, Stadium Road, Karachi 74800, Pakistan Tel: 21 493-0051 Fax: 21 4946623

www.akuweb.com/medical_college.html

The medical school: Founded in 1983 it has a strong commitment to community medicine. Forty per cent of Karachi's population live in 'Katchi abadis' (slums) and hence this, and medicine in rural Pakistan, are important areas of learning.

Elective notes: There are many other students. Lots of 'group seminars and tutorials' if you're into that kind of thing. Work can be quite intense. Once a week there is community medicine. A&E is busy with quite a few gunshots and punishment beatings.

Dow Medical College

University of Karachi, Baba-e-Urdu Road, Karachi, Pakistan www.dmc.edu

This is a large medical school (founded in 1945) with a 1400-bed hospital.

Sindh Medical College and Jinnah Postgraduate Medical Centre

University of Karachi, Rafiqui HI Shaheed Road, Karachi 75510, Pakistan Tel: (9221) 519006 09.

The medical school: Is one of the biggest teaching hospitals in Pakistan and is under the University of Karachi. Hospitals used include: JPMC, the National Institute of Cardiovascular Diseases and the National Institute of Child Health.

Liaquat National Hospital

Stadium Road, Karachi 5, Pakistan Tel: 419612 13 14

The hospital: Started as an outdoor hospital in 1958. It is a non-profit making privately managed public hospital. It has 475 beds and the OPD sees 550 patients a day. It has nine operating theatres and a CT scanner. All surgical specialities, including chest and neuro, are carried out.

Imam Clinic and General Hospital

ST-5 Block-I North Nazimabad, Karachi SD 74700, Pakistan Tel: (21) 6625111.

Rawalpindi

Rawalpindi Medical College

University of the Punjab, Tipu Road, Rawalpindi, Pakistan.

The medical school and its hospitals serve Islamabad and Rawalpindi and act as a referral centre for Northern Punjab and Azad Kashmir. It's teaching hospitals are:

- **Rawalpindi General Hospital,** Murree Road, Rawalpindi, a major teaching hospital offering the basic specialities as well as psychiatry, orthopaedics, urology and cardiology. It has Rawalpindi's only CT.
- **Holy Family Hospital** which has 400 beds (soon to increase to 800) and is all air-conditioned. It is advanced with MRI scanner.
- **District Headquarters Hospital**, is in the inner city and has a trauma centre, neurosurgery and chest department.

Al Shifa Eye Hospital

Jhelum Road, Rawalpindi, Pakistan
www.alshifa-eye.org.pk

The hospital: Next to the Pakistani Institute of Ophthalmology. It is near the city centre and Islamabad is about 30 min in the car. It receives from all of north Pakistan.

Accommodation: Cheap.

OTHER MEDICAL SCHOOLS IN PAKISTAN:

Ayub Medical College, University of Peshawar, Abbottabad, Pakistan.
Bolan Medical College, University of Baluchistan, Quetta, Pakistan.
Chandka Medical College, University of Sind, Jamshoro, Larkana, Pakistan.
Khyber Medical College, University of Peshawar, Peshawar, Pakistan
Liaquat Medical College, University of Sind, Jamshoro, Larkana, Pakistan.
Nawabshah Medical College for Girls, University of Sind, Nawabshah, Pakistan.
Nishtar Medical College, Bahuddin Zakaria University, Nishtar Road, Multan, Pakistan Tel: 061 72979 Fax: 061 571648. (Founded in 1951 it uses the Nishtar Hospital.)
Punjab Medical College, Sargodha Road, Faisalabad, Pakistan Tel: 041 72970 Fax: 041 762846. (Founded in 1970, the school uses the Allied Hospital (1150 beds) and the DHQ Hospital (500 beds) to serve Faisalabad, Pakistan's third-largest city.)
Quaid-e-Azam Medical College, Islamia University, Circular Road, Bahawalpur, Pakistan Tel: 0621 884289 Fax: 0621 7189. (Founded in 1970, the school uses the Bahawalpur Victoria Hospital with 1300 beds, CT, cardiac, hand and limb transplant surgery.)

RURAL HOSPITALS:

Kunri Christian Hospital

Kunri, Umarkot, Sindh 69160, Pakistan.

The hospital: In Kunri, a small 'desert town' in south-east Pakistan. It is very hot (up to 40 °C). It has 60 inpatient beds plus wards for ophthalmology and TB. The hospital tends to concentrate on women and children (75% of admissions are female). Malaria, malnutrition, TB, tetanus and rickets are common. There is a busy theatre and OPD. There's a large O&G workload. It is a friendly place. All the doctors operate and it is a good place to see a wide variety of surgery. It's all done under ketamine. There is a huge TB programme at present. It is a Christian hospital (Church of Pakistan) in a very Muslim area. This is very restrictive, especially if you are female (do not go into town alone and you will need to wear Pakistani dress). Males can't eat with female staff. Most of the staff are Pakistani with a couple of Westerners.

❍ **Elective notes:** A hard elective but a good experience.

Accommodation: Provided with bed, bathroom and kitchen for 50R (80p) per night. Food is chapattis and curry for 15R.

Bach Christian Hospital

PO Qulandarabad, Abbotabad District, Harara, Pakistan. (Contact 'Interserve')

The hospital: A mission hospital in the foothills of the Himalayas. Plenty of unusual pathology.

❍ **Elective notes:** Staff very friendly and welcoming. Lots to explore and you can visit local clinics.

Accommodation: Excellent apartment available.

Tank Christian Hospital

Tank, near Dera Ismail Khan, NWFP, Pakistan (arrange though 'Interserve').

The hospital: A well-staffed mission hospital and very friendly. Tetanus, TB, malaria and gunshots are relatively common. It is in a very remote area, next to the tribal homeland of the Pathans.

❍ **Elective notes:** It's a mission hospital so you should at least be sympathetic to the Christian faith. It's well-staffed so not many procedures but students have

had good teaching in past. There's not much responsibility. Excellent exploring to be done nearby.
Accommodation: Excellent flat available.

Memorial Christian Hospital

Paris Road, Sialkot 51310, Pakistan Tel: 432 265868 Fax: 432 265869.
The hospital: Sialkot is a busy industrial town in north-east Pakistan, 10 km from the volatile Kashmir/India border. It can get VERY hot (45 °C) in June and cool in winter (5–10 °C). The hospital was established by the Presbyterian Church of the USA in 1886 and moved to its current site in 1932. It is run by 20 Pakistani doctors and a couple of Westerners. It has 300 beds (but 400 patients including those in the corridors). It has basic lab and radiology facilities. The hospital provides care to 120 villages in a rural outreach programme. There is also a school of nursing and midwifery. Although it is charity-run, a small charge of 20p for a consultation and £2 for an admission is asked. Relatives cook meals on stoves provided by the hospital. The 'Intensive Care Unit' has one pulse oximeter. Plenty in OPD to see and do.
O Elective notes: Students are supposed to be 'committed Protestant Christians in sympathy with the hospital's aims'.

Shilokh Mission Hospital

Jalapur Jattan, Gujrat District, Pakistan
Tel: 04 331 592113.
The hospital: A 150-bed rural mission hospital run by the Sialkot Diocese Church of Pakistan. It has medical, surgical, O&G and ophthalmological services.

HOSPITALS IN PAKISTAN APPROVED BY THE PAKISTAN MEDICAL AND DENTAL COUNCIL FOR HOUSE JOB/INTERNSHIP IN ADDITION TO TEACHING HOSPITALS:

ABBOTTABAD: Civil Hospital
CMH
DERA ISMAIL KHAN: District Headquarters Hospital
GUJRANWALA: CMH
Faisal Shaheed Memorial Hospital Trust
ISLAMABAD: Federal Government Services Hospital
Pakistan Institute of Medical Sciences
JHELUM: CMH
District Headquarters Hospital
KARACHI: Abbasi Shaheed Hospital
Akhter's Eye Hospital
Baqai Hospital
KV Site Hospital
Lady Dufferin Hospital
Liaquat National Hospital
LRBT Hospital
Mary Adelaide Leprosy Centre
Masoomeen Hospital
National Institute of Child Health
Naval Surgery
PAF Hospital, Mauripur
PNS Shifa
Sind Government Hospital, Liaquatabad
Skin and Hygiene Centre
Social Security Hospital, Landhi
Sobraj Maternity Home
Spencer Eye Hospital
SRS Hospital
KHARIAN: CMH
LAHORE: Cairns Hospital, PWR
CMH
Data Darbar Hospital
Fatima Memorial Hospital
Gulab Devi Hospital for Chest Diseases
Ittefaque Hospital
OPD Society of Rehabilitation of Disabled
Shaikh Zayed Hospital
Shalamar Hospital Trust
United Christian Hospital
LARKANA: District Headquarters Hospital
MARDAN: District Headquarters Hospital
MULTAN: CMH
MUZAFFARABAD: CMH
OKARA: CMH
PESHAWAR: CMH
Health Care Medical Centre
Marhaba Hospital
QUETTA: CMH
Sardar Bahadur Khan TB Sanatorium, PWR
RAHIMYARKHAN: District Headquarters Hospital
RAWALPINDI: Cantonment General Hospital
SAHIWAL: District Headquarters Hospital
SARGODHA: District Headquarters Hospital
PAF Base Hospital
SIALKOT: CMH
District Headquarters Hospital
SUKKUR: District Headquarters Hospital
SWAT: Saidu Group Hospitals
WAH CANTT: POF Hospital

Papua New Guinea

Population: 4.5 million
Languages: English and Motu
Capital: Port Moresby
Currency: Kina
Int Code +675

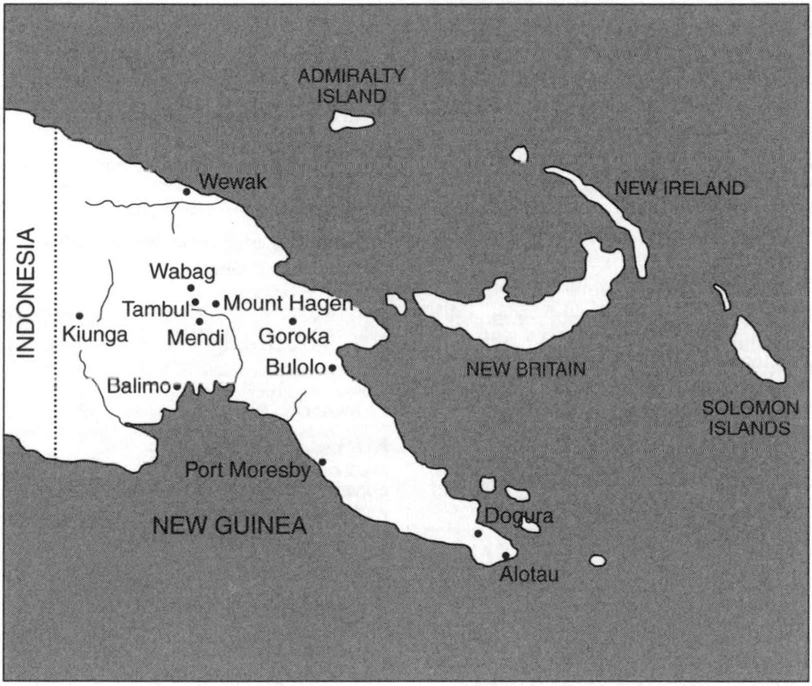

Papua New Guinea is a fascinating place, the eastern half of an island north of Australia. It has great diversity from volcanic highlands to tropical beaches and swamps. It has more languages (over 700) than any other country in the world. Most people, however, can speak Pidgin. Since it gained independence from Australia in 1975, not a lot has changed. Many areas are still extremely remote and don't have easy access to medical care.

✚ Medicine:

In each province there is a government-run hospital, but this doesn't amount to much. A number of missionary hospitals provide care in deep jungle. Very few Westerners go to the government-run ones and hence the latter will be concentrated on here. The health system makes best use of the few doctors, and nurses often treat patients alone, only asking the doctor if unsure. Infectious diseases are extremely common e.g. TB (of every part of the body), malaria, leprosy and elephantiasis, especially in the Western Province. In paeds it's malnutrition and pneumonia. In some areas, hypertension and NIDDM are increasing as diet is becoming Westernized. Orthopaedics is busy with the country's outdoor work, houses on stilts and passion for rugby. However, there are very few orthopaedic operations for risk of infection. They are all treated with traction. Trauma and violence are very common for a number of reasons:

- Alcohol (since it was legalized with independence) has created major problems. There is a culture of going out and getting completely trashed. Marijuana use is also increasing. Violence stems directly from the alcohol, but also the need for money to fund it.
- Women get a rough time as shown by the fact the government has had to produce a leaflet entitled 'Wife Beating is Illegal'. In many parts of the country women are not allowed to initiate a conversation with a man, they don't eat at the same table or even sleep in the same house with males (including their husband). A wife has to be bought by the husband, but with high unemployment and low pay many can't afford 20 pigs etc. and hence rape has become a major problem. It isn't reported, not that the authorities would do anything anyway.
- 'Payback' is an inherent part of PNG culture. If your clan has a grievance with the member of another clan then you all get together and knife him (or anyone in his clan) sparking a vicious circle. Sixty per cent of the population is under 24 and many of these young men are unemployed with no social role and hence have nothing else to do.

➲ Visas and work permits:
A visa is required to enter or do an elective in PNG. Contact the embassy for this and work permits.

Note: Girls, beware … most of the smaller communities are fine (although it is advisable to wear a long skirt); however the capital (Port Moresby) is not that safe for single white females. Try to observe local customs. Use common sense, Friday (pay-day) is not a good day to go to town as all the locals will be getting pissed and rowdy.

Port Moresby

The capital has PNG's only medical school.

University of Papua New Guinea
Faculty of Medicine, PO Box 5623,
Boroko, PNG.
This has a busy teaching hospital with 600–700 deliveries a month. It's the only tertiary referral centre in PNG.

RURAL HOSPITALS:

Sopas Adventist Hospital
PO Box 112, Wabag, Enga Province, PNG,
Fax: 54 71231.
The hospital: Busy with around 100 beds and floor space. Outpatients is also very busy. There are usually only one or two doctors and so students are very much appreciated and will find they are running clinics fairly quickly. There are many bush knife and gunshot wounds as the locals here still believe in payback and tribal fighting despite their conversion the Christianity. Two full days a week are devoted to surgery.
❍ Elective notes: The hospital is pretty isolated and it is only really safe to go out with hospital staff. Try to go with someone else. It is all friendly but everyone is very busy. Overall, people

have thoroughly enjoyed it. You don't need to be an Adventist or a Christian to go here. There are also nursing students. Enga Province is remote and in the beautiful cool tropical rainforest highlands. It was one of the last areas to be 'discovered'. Most of the locals are subsistence farmers. It is a 'dry' province so leave the duty free at home (cars are searched occasionally).

Wewak General Hospital

PO Box 395, Wewak, East Sepik Province, PNG.

The hospital: Wewak is one of the main hospitals (365 beds) on the north coast of Papua New Guinea and receives referrals from smaller hospitals in the region. Specialities include medicine, surgery, O&G and paeds. There is a severe lack of facilities. Mobile clinics are also run from here. The only way to get to the villages along the Sepik River is by canoe. Conditions seen include: malaria (+++), TB, broken limbs (wife and daughter beating), asthma, meningitis and pneumonia. The staff are incredibly welcoming and friendly.

O Elective notes: There are plenty of practical procedures in A&E and loads of deliveries and ops in O&G. It's excellent for surgery too. The hospital is on a beautiful coastline with golden sand and blue sea.

Accommodation: A backpackers' lodge is in town, but something usually becomes available in the hospital.

St Barnabus Health Centre

PO Box 21, Dogura, Milne Bay Province, PNG.

The hospital: Dogura is a very small rural village with one basic store, a school and the health centre. The health centre consists of an outpatients, a theatre and four wards. Facilities are very poor. There are beds but few mattresses. There is a very old X-ray and ultrasound machine. Currently, the centre is run by one VSO doctor (who also does surgery), one VSO midwife and six PNG nurses. The 'patrol' goes out into the mountains (for days) to do rural clinics and immunization. The hospital has electricity for three hours a day. The phone is (intermittently) run from a car battery. Malaria is the major problem here with 30% being chloroquine-resistant.

O Elective notes: This elective comes extremely highly recommended if you want a bit of responsibility with the chance to practise clinical skills in a friendly developing world setting. Excellent beaches, snorkelling and walking. This is a beautiful part of the country. Dogura is a 10-minute flight from Alotau, i.e. very isolated. Alotau itself is a small town with one hotel (expensive £40/night). Get anything you may need here before going to Dogura.

Accommodation: Has previously been provided.

Nazarene Hospital

PO Box 456, Mount Hagen, WHP, PNG.

The hospital: A 100-bed general mission hospital consisting of medical, surgical, paeds and O&G wards. There is one operating theatre, an outpatients, A&E and pharmacy. It's run by 3–4 doctors (mainly American missionaries).

O Elective notes: There are excellent opportunities for students both in outpatients and theatre. Plenty of responsibility on call without the feeling of being left alone or dumped on. Learn Pidgin before you go as it means you can converse with patients directly. Note this is a Christian mission run by an American missionary. You probably should be Christian if applying. No smoking/drinking on site. Also, the surrounding areas are not safe and so you shouldn't go out alone. Girls need to wear a skirt. Highly recommended though.

Accommodation: Provided.

OTHER HOSPITALS:

- **Goroka Base Hospital**, Goroka is another hospital that's recommended.
- **Kainantu Hospital**, Kainantu is in the highlands. It has 125 beds.
- **Mendi Hospital,** Mendi in the highlands has a good student programme and comes recommended.

- **Veiferi'a Hospital,** Veiferi'a. This is a Catholic mission hospital.

UFM-RUN HOSPITALS:

Contact **UFM Worldwide**, 47a Fleet Street, Swindon, Wiltshire SN1 1RE Tel: 01793 432255.

A Christian faith is a prerequisite to work here. They usually will want to meet you. They can provide accommodation at their hospitals.

Rumginae Health Centre

PO Box 41, Kiunga, Western Province, PNG Fax: 583416.

The hospital: Rumginae is in a tropical jungle near the source of the Fly River. It has 60 beds with three doctors serving 20,000 people. Resources are limited but it provides a good service. It has medical, TB, antenatal and postnatal wards. There is a minor op theatre but major stuff goes to Tabubil (100 km away). There is a busy OPD run entirely by nurses and community healthcare workers. X-rays and u/s can be done.

Balimo Health Centre

PO Box 4, Balimo, Western Province, PNG Fax: 661492.

The hospital: Set in the flood plain of the Aramia River (with crocodiles). Balimo is a health centre rather than a government-run hospital. However, it has a surgeon (unlike the government-run hospital) and a school of nursing (nurses are trained to diagnose and refer). Balimo has 100 beds with wards for surgery, general medicine, acute admissions, nutrition, leprosy and TB. It has a well-equipped operating theatre. It serves 30,000 but receives referrals from all over the Western Province. There is a busy OPD. Medical patrols extend the work to villages upstream. Some of these are up to nine hours away in dugout canoe. TB, malaria and leprosy are common.

O Elective notes: In addition to ward rounds and clinics radio 'sked' is a lunchtime affair in which doctors in Balimo give advice to surrounding health workers in other villages via short-wave radio. Students can also do a few minor procedures.

Philippines

Population: 70 million
Languages: Pilipino and English
Capital: Manila
Currency: Philippine peso
Int Code: +632

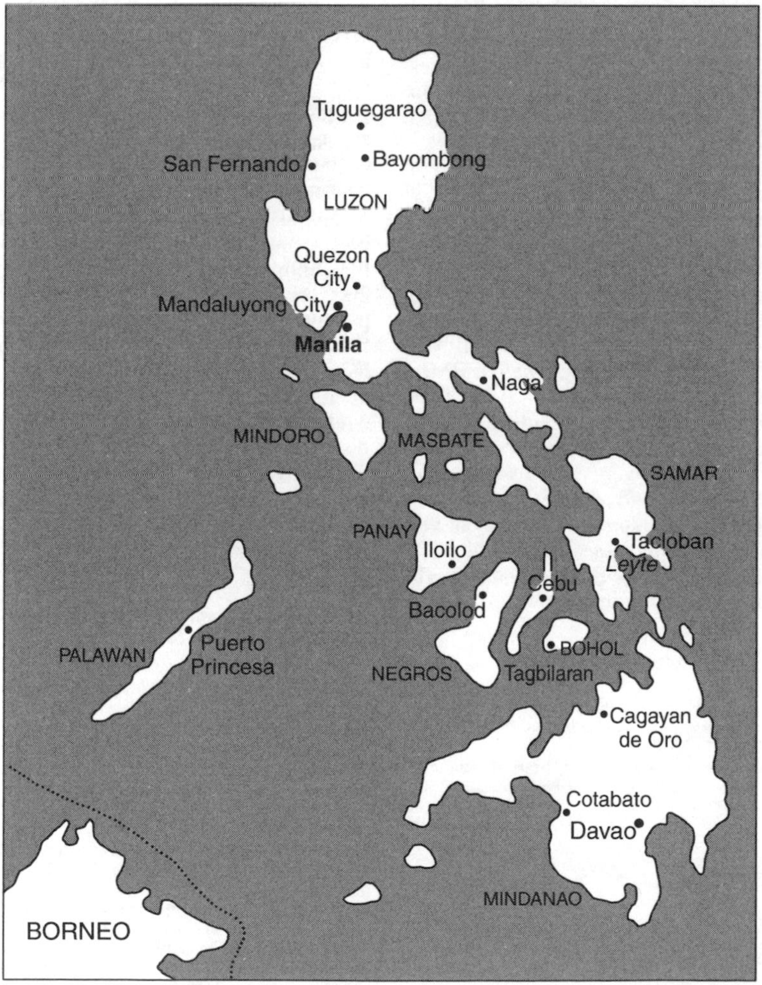

The Philippines lie in the west of the Pacific Ocean and comprise over 7000 separate islands in three main groups (the Luzon, Visayan and Mindanao/Sulu islands). It is a land where earthquakes and volcanoes tend to keep the people poor. Most in the country are Catholic, though Islamic in the south. Very few of the local population can speak English and the lack of translators doesn't make it a popular elective destination.

⊕ Medicine:
Most people have to pay for healthcare which even then is pretty poor. Most hospitals are private and there are few Government ones. Infectious diseases, including TB and typhoid, are common. Malaria has been successfully reduced, however.

➲ Visa and work permits:
A temporary non-immigrant visitor's visa should be applied for in person at the embassy. You'll need a passport, one photo, proof you can fund yourself and, ideally, a letter from the hospital where you're going. Visas can usually be picked up the next day. They will deal with postal applications if a registered SAE is enclosed. A student visa is required if enrolling on a course. Tell the embassy that you are only shadowing for a few weeks and ensure that they are happy that you don't need a student visa (which is a lot more hassle and cost). Work permits require a petition from the institution employing you.

USEFUL ADDRESSES:

Philippine Medical Association, PMA Building, North Avenue, Quezon City, Manila, Philippines Tel: 929 4974/3514.
Department of Health, San Lazaro Compound, Rizal Avenue, Sta. Cruz, Manila, Philippines Tel: 711 9502/9503 Fax: 743 1829.

Manila

Manila is a huge city with a major traffic problem. There are plenty of cinemas, restaurants and shops. There are some nice beaches nearby and inland are rainforests and volcanoes. The people are friendly with a great sense of humour.

There are 27 medical schools in the Philippines, five in Manila. To arrange an elective it is usually best to do it directly through the hospital and therefore the main hospitals throughout regions are listed below. The oldest medical school in Manila is:

University Santo Tomás
The Catholic University of the Philippines, Faculty of Medicine and Surgery, España Street, Manila 2801, Philippines.
It uses:

Philippines General Hospital
Taft Avenue, Manila, Philippines Tel: 521 8450 Fax: 524 2221.
The hospital: A tertiary referral centre receiving patients from all over the country and acts as a teaching hospital for a number of universities. It has nearly 2000 beds crammed into wards of 50 patients and sees 700,000 patients a year. It is a government hospital but patients have to pay for medications or doctors/charities pay. It is very poorly equipped. TB, rheumatic fever and heart diseases are fairly common.
O Elective notes: Write to the Clinical Director. Patients don't speak English but the doctors do (with an American accent).

SPECIALITY AND MAJOR HOSPITALS:

Dr Jose Fabella Memorial Hospital, Lope de Vega, Sta. Cruz, 1003 Manila, Philippines Tel: 734 5561.
Lung Center of the Philippines, Quezon Avenue, Quezon, Metro Manila, Philippines Tel: 924 6101 Fax: 924 0696.
National Center for Mental Health, Nueve de Febrero Street, Mandaluyong City, Metro Manila, Philippines Tel: 531 8682.
National Kidney Institute, East Avenue, Quezon City, Metro Manila, Philippines Tel: 924 3601 Fax: 924 0701.
Philippine Children's Medical Center, Quezon Avenue, Quezon City, Metro Manila, Philippines Tel: 924 6601 Fax: 924 0840.
Philippine Heart Center, East Avenue, Quezon City, Metro Manila 1100, Philippines Tel: 923 1301 Fax: 922 0551.

Philippine Orthopaedic Center, Banawe Avenue, Quezon City, Metro Manila, Philippines Tel: 712 4569 Fax: 712 4746.
San Lazaro Hospital, Quiricada Street, Sta. Cruz 1003, Manila, Philippines Tel: 732 3776 Fax: 711 6966.

RESEARCH HOSPITALS:

Institute for Tropical Medicine, Alabang, Muntinlupa, Philippines Tel: 842 2828 Fax: 842 2245.
Schistosomiasis Control and Research Hospital, Palo, North Leyte, Philippines Tel: (053) 323 3083.

OTHER HOSPITALS IN MANILA:

Capitol Medical Center, Scout Magbanua St, Quezon City, Philippines Tel: 99 15 71 Fax: 928 1571.
Cardinal Santos Medical Center, Wilson St, San Juan, Philippines Tel: 721 3361 Fax: 78 5 60.
Children's Medical Center, Phils, Inc, 11 Banawe St, Quezon City, Philippines Tel: 712 0845 Fax: 712 0801.
Chinese General Hospital, 286 Blumentritt, Manila, Philippines Tel: 711 4141 Fax: 711 3967.
De Los Santos Medical Center, 201E Rodriguez Sr. Blvd, Quezon City, Philippines Tel: 78 70 11.
Dr Jesus C Delgado Memorial Hospital, 7 Kamuning Road, Quezon City, Philippines Tel: 96 53 63 Fax: 926 53 63.
Makati Medical Center, 2 Amorsolo St, Makati, Philippines Tel: 815 99 11.
Medical Center Manila, 1122 Gen Luna St, Ermita, Manila, Philippines Tel: 59 16 61 Fax: 59 00 21.
Medical City General Hospital, Lourdes Drive, Ortigas Business Complex, Mandaluyong, Philippines Tel: 631 8626.
Olivarez General Hospital, Sucat Road, Paranaque, Philippines Tel: 828 79 66 Fax: 827 87 47.
St Luke's Medical Center, 279 E Rodriguez Sr Blvd, Quezon City, Philippines Tel: 722 6161.

MEDICAL CENTRES:

Baguio General Hospital and Medical Center, Baguio City 2600, Philippines Tel: (074) 442 3738.
Davao Medical Center, Davao City, Davao del Sur, Philippines Tel: (082) 73974.
Dr P Garcia Memorial Research and Medical Center, Cabanatuan City, 3100 Nueva Ecija, Philippines Tel: (044) 463 1607.
East Avenue Medical Center, East Avenue, Diliman, Quezon City, Metro Manila, Philippines Tel: 98 0611.
Jose R. Reyes Memorial Medical Center, Rizal Avenue, Sta Cruz, 1003 Manila, Philippines Tel: 711 9491 Fax: 732 1077.
Mariano Marcos Memorial Hospital and Medical Center, Batac, Ilocos Norte, Philippines Tel: (077) 792 3144.
Rizal Medical Center, Pasig, Rozal, Metro Manila, Philippines Tel: 671 4216 Fax: 671 4216.
Vicente Sotto Sr Memorial Medical Center, Cebu City, Philippines Tel: 72801.
Western Visayas Medical Center, Mandurriao, Iloilo City, Philippines Tel: (033) 77742.
Zamboanga Medical Center, Zamboanga City, Philippines Tel: (062) 991 0573.

Palawan

Palawan is a small island on the west of the Philippines. It has been largely unspoilt by Western influence. Travel around the island can be slow with many roads closed. The alternative method of transport is by sea.

Palawan Provincial Hospital

Puerto Princesa, Palawan, Philippines.
The hospital: The people in the hospital (100 beds) are very friendly and keen to practise their English. There's also a fair bit of malaria, TB and gastroenteritis. In A&E you'll need an interpreter as the locals do not speak enough English. Most of the illnesses are fairly basic (e.g. dehydration), but in the extreme.
O Elective notes: The clinical director is a top chap from Ipswich.

OTHER REGIONAL HOSPITALS:

Batangas Regional Hospital, Batangas City, Philippines Tel: (043) 725 2011.
Bicol Regional Hospital, Naga City, Camarines Sur, Philippines Tel: (5421) 332 775.
Cagayan Valley Regional Hospital, Tuguegarao, Cagayan, Philippines. Tel: (078) 446 1410.
Cotabato Regional Hospital, Cotabato City 9600, Philippines Tel: (64) 212 373.
Davao Regional Hospital, Tagum, Davao Del Norte, Philippines Tel: (082) 701 0747.
Eastern Visayas Regional Medical Center, Tacloban City, Leyte, Philippines Tel: (38) 321 3129.
Governor G Galleres Memorial Hospital, Tagbiliran City, Bohol, Philippines Tel: (038) 3165.
Ilocos Regional Hospital, San Fernando, La Union, Philippines Tel: (072) 412 691.
Jose B Lingad Memorial General Hospital, San Fernando, La Union, Philipines Tel: (44) 961 3921.

Mariano Marcos Veterans Memorial Hospital, Bayombong, 3700 Nueva Vizcya, Philippines Tel: 321 2090.
Northern Mindanao Regional Training Hospital, Cagayan de Oro City, Philippines Tel: (8822) 3646.
Quirino Memorial Medical Center, Quirino Compound, Project 4, Quezon City, Philippines Telefax: 721 3089.
Tondo Medical Center, Balut, Tondo, Philippines Tel: 251 8420.
Western Visayas Regional Hospital, Bacolod City, Philippines Tel: (034) 74131.

Singapore

Population: 2.8 million
Official Languages: Malay, Chinese, Tamil and English
Capital: Singapore City
Currency: Singapore dollar
Int Code: +65

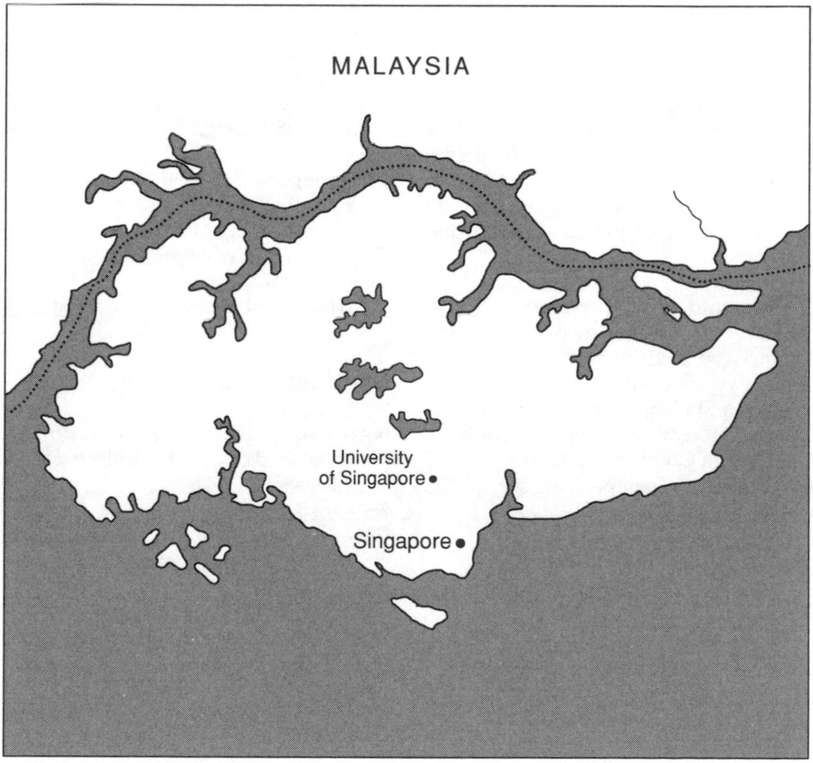

Singapore is a lovely island country in south-east Asia with nearly three million inhabitants in a space less than the distance from Edinburgh to Glasgow. Despite this there are many green areas and the environment is very clean.

Medicine:
Singapore has an advanced efficient health system. This is partly due to its wealth, but also the fact that families are encouraged to preserve the extended family and therefore care for elderly

relatives at home. There are one medical school and three major government subsidized general hospitals: Singapore General, Tan Tock Seng and the National University Hospital. The Eastern General Hospital is just being completed. Primary care consists of private GPs and government polyclinics. Private practice is very much on the rise in Singapore. The government has introduced a scheme of mandatory saving so that a proportion of salary goes into a fund that can be used for a pension or healthcare. The proportion of the bill to be paid by patients is set at different levels depending on their 'class'. Class A patient also get better rooms. Class C gets the same treatments, but not the frilly bits (typically 30 beds to a ward). Older patents speak only their Chinese dialect or Malay or Tamil. Communication between staff is usually in English. The leading causes of mortality are heart and cerebrovascular diseases and cancers.

➲ Visas and work permits:

Any foreigner wishing to study in Singapore needs a Student Pass. To obtain one of these you need to:

- Fill in a Student Pass application form (Form 16, available from the Singapore High Commission (below))
- And send two passport-sized photographs
- Two copies of your passport two copies of the acceptance letter from the College/University in Singapore

Note: It can take up to six weeks to process your application. They may then ask you to pay a security deposit. The cost of a student pass is S$15/year.

Recently, the dispensing of employment passes has changed from the Ministry of Home Affairs to the Ministry of Manpower (contact the Work Permit Department at 5383033 or the Singapore Immigration and Registration at 3916100). As a doctor, you will probably need a P pass; as a paramedical professional you may need a Q pass. Full details are available from the High Commission or MOM's Employment Pass Department, Fifth Floor, SIR Building, 10 Kallang Road, Singapore 208718.

USEFUL ADDRESSES:

For employment opportunities contact: Centre Director in London, Contact Singapore, Charles House, Lower Ground Floor, 5–11 Regent Street, London SW1Y 4LR Tel: 020 7976 2090 Fax: 020 7976 2091 e-mail cslondon@sings.demon.co.uk

A licence to practise medicine is available after completing one year as a houseman at an approved hospital from: The Singapore Medical Council, Ministry of Health, 55 Cuppage Road, Singapore 0922.

Singapore Medical Association, 2 College Road, Level 2, Alumni Medical Centre, Singapore 169850 Tel: 223 1264 Fax: 224 7827 www.sma.org.sg e-mail: sma_org@pacific.net.sg

Ministry of Health www.gov.sg/moh

UNIVERSITIES:

National University of Singapore

Faculty of Medicine, 10 Kent Ridge Crescent, Singapore 119260
www.med.nus.edu.sg

This was founded in 1905 and has access to over 5000 beds. Language of instruction is English. They have a very well-organized elective programme and will send you a list of hospitals (including the three big ones) and departments you can choose from. They can arrange accommodation at minimal cost (the National is nearest to the halls). Some students have previously arranged electives directly with the hospital.

Note: Singapore students have a summer holiday between March and June. This means that some departments won't take students. For those that do there will be little structured teaching. Between November and February is a good time to go as the students have finals and there are therefore many revision sessions. By March (when they have finals) everyone is too stressed to care!

Another useful address is: **The Graduate School of Medical Studies**, National University of Singapore, Blk MD5, Level 3, 12 Medical Drive, Singapore 117598 Tel: (65) 874 3353 Fax: (65) 773 1462.

National University Hospital

Singapore.

The hospital: A large 957-bed tertiary hospital (opened 1985) that also has the National University Children's Medical Centre on its grounds. Both have every speciality imaginable right down to hand and reconstructive microsurgery.

Singapore General Hospital

Outram Road, Singapore 169608.

The hospital: The country's largest (1600-bed) teaching hospital catering for a huge proportion of the Singapore population. It is divided into seven blocks, eight floors each. It is very busy and there is a wide range of pathology. All specialities including A&E and a department of forensic medicine are here. The doctors have heavy workloads.

O Elective notes: Try to go in term time. It's highly recommended.

Accommodation: Previously been available in houseman's quarters for £300 (818 SGD)/7weeks.

Tan Tock Seng Hospital

11 Jalan Tan Tock Seng, Singapore 308433 Tel: (65) 256 6011 Fax: (65) 252 7282.

The hospital: One of the hospitals affiliated to the National University of Singapore. It was established in 1844 as the first and only local hospital for the sick and poor. It is in fairly old buildings but a new modern 14-storey block (giving 1211 beds) has just been built. It is well known for its stroke centre (neurology, neurosurgery and rehab) and respiratory medicine. It is the second-largest general hospital in Singapore. It is not far from the city centre and next to an MRT station. Most conditions are similar to other developed countries, although NIDDM is more prevalent. There is usually excellent teaching with the local students. The surgery department is reputed to be the best in Singapore. The head of the department is extremely amiable, approachable and an excellent teacher. This elective is great revision for surgical finals although most time is in outpatients, not theatre.

Singapore National Eye Centre

11 Third Hospital Avenue, Singapore 168751 Tel: (065) 2277 255 Fax: (065) 2277 290.

This is the principal specialist eye facility in Singapore and in the compound of Singapore General Hospital.

Alexandra Hospital, Alexandra Road, Singapore 159964 Tel: 473 5222 Fax: 479 3183.
Woodbridge Hospital, Institute of Mental Health, 10 Buangkok Green, Singapore 539747.

HOSPICE CARE:

Hospice Care Association. 6 Dunearn Road, Singapore 1130.

SOMETHING DIFFERENT:

Institute of Science and Forensic Medicine

11 Outram Road, Singapore 169078
Fax: 65 2290749
www.gov.sg/moh/isfm/overview.html

The institute has seven forensic pathologists and deals with the gruesome and not-so-gruesome aspects of forensic pathology.

Sri Lanka

Population: 19 million
Language: Sinhalese
Capital: Colombo
Currency: Sri Lanka rupee
Int Code: +94

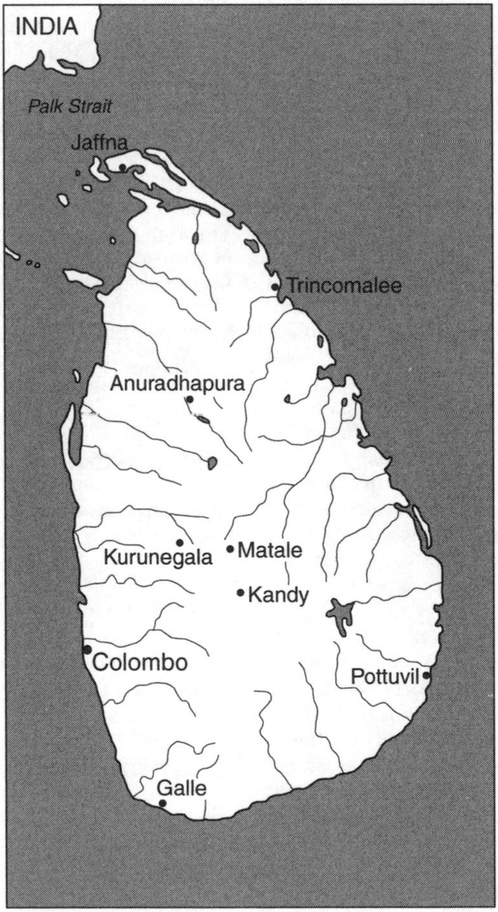

Sri Lanka is definitely worth a visit. It's small enough to explore thoroughly in a relatively short time but there is plenty to do. The capital, Colombo, is dirty and typically Third World, but further south the beaches are astonishingly beautiful. To the north there are many tourist attractions. Kandy is a very pretty city set up high in the hills and

therefore relatively cool. It's an ideal base for seeing the rest of the island. The bus and train services are very good and cheap. With 1000 miles of beaches Sri Lanka offers superb snorkelling and diving. There is also a very rich history. Visit Anuradhapura, the ancient capital from 380 BC and Polonnaruwa from 1100 AD. The rugged central uplands offer a number of mountains with shrines and fortresses on the summit. Go on safari in Yalla and Wilpattu. In Nuwala Eliya, if you're smart enough (jacket and tie) you can visit the Hill Club. The cost of living is generally much higher than you might have expected ....beware of touts and con merchants. The civil war in which the Tamils are fighting for an independent state is in the north-east area of the island. DO NOT GO THERE.

Medicine:
Medical training follows the British system since it is a former colony. Therefore notes are written in English and all the doctors speak it. Many people in large towns can also speak it; if they can't there is usually someone around to translate. There are two systems of medicine:

- Western medicine practised by fully qualified doctors who have done five years of training at one of the five medical schools. They are aided by Assistant Medical Practitioners (AMPs or Apothecaries) who have done two years of Western training and practice mainly in rural areas.
- Many rural people practise Auyrvedic medicine (indigenous medicine).

The primary care service is provided by Western-style GPs and small surgeries run by AMPs in rural areas. These provide good maternity and paediatric care. Secondary healthcare consists of remote 'one man stations' with a doctor or AMP and 'base' hospitals in towns. These provide general medical, surgical, obs and paeds facilities. Tertiary care is provided by one of the big town hospitals. They are often poorly equipped and overcrowded. A few people pay for private care. Infectious diseases including malaria and TB are pretty common.

Visas and work permits:
A visitors' visa is required for an elective. Contact the embassy.

USEFUL ADDRESS:

The Sri Lankan Medical Association, Wijerama House, No 7 Wijerama Avenue, Columbo 7, Sri Lanka.

MEDICAL SCHOOLS AND THEIR TEACHING HOSPITALS:

Colombo

University of Colombo
Faculty of Medicine, PO Box 271 Kynsey Road, Colombo 8, Sri Lanka.
This is the oldest (1870) and largest medical school in Sri Lanka.

National Hospital/Columbo General Hospital
Ward Place, Colombo, Sri Lanka.
The hospital: Is the largest teaching hospital (3000 beds) and the quality of care and teaching is high. The hospital is government-run, very busy and has limited resources. Common problems are diabetes, malaria, dengue fever, TB, valve disease and leprosy.
Elective notes: In the mornings there are ward rounds, tutorials and case presentations. The teaching is excellent; however, the 'hands on' experience is somewhat limited unless you speak Sinhalese. The students are very happy to translate. Surgery has also come highly recommended. It is possible to go on a variety of outpatient clinics e.g. leprosy clinics, paeds visits and to TB hospitals. Electives here are well-organized and you can do what you want when you arrive. Medical student hours are about 8 am–2 pm.
Accommodation: Mrs Peiris, 62/2 Park Street comes recommended.

The Lady Ridgeway Hospital for Children
Borella Colombo 10, Sri Lanka.
The hospital: The paediatric hospital for the medical school. Much of the

pathology is tropical disease. Congenital problems are also common. Community clinics to shanty towns are run from here.

O Elective notes: A number of other students are often around though not normally elective students. Everyone is friendly and welcoming. The hospital has limited facilities but it is a good learning experience.

The De Soysa Maternity Hospital
Colombo 8, Sri Lanka.
This is the specialist maternity hospital for Sri Lanka.

Peradeniya

University of Peradeniya
Faculty of Medicine, Peradeniya, Kandy, Sri Lanka.

Peradeniya General Hospital, University of Peradeniya
Peradeniya, Kandy, Sri Lanka.

The hospital: Perandeniya Teaching Hospital is the largest hospital outside the capital, Colombo. It consists of a medical unit comprising two wards and a compliment of 150–200 patients. There are usually upwards of 60 admissions per day. Mornings consist of consultant ward rounds (huge) and teaching (all in English).

O Elective notes: Very few locals speak English so liase closely with the 'home' students of which there are around 40. There are plenty of heart murmurs to hear and spleens to feel. Due to the pressures of numbers, practical procedures are not plentiful.

Galle

University of Ruhuna
Faculty of Medicine, PO Box 70, Galle, Sri Lanka Tel: (09) 32321 Fax: (09) 22316. (The School uses Karapitiya Hospital at the same address.)

The hospital: A major, 1200-bed teaching hospital (third-biggest in Sri Lanka). It is four miles from old town Galle. It is a tertiary referral centre for southern Sri Lanka. An excellent range of pathologies from many congenital/ rheumatic heart disorders through to tropical diseases (malaria, filariasis, leprosy, tropical splenomegaly).

O Elective notes: Few patients speak English but are more than happy for you to examine them. No formal teaching, but bedside teaching is all in English. There are plenty of students about (30 in a clinic!) so there isn't much hands on but teaching is good. Go to Unawatuna beach in the afternoons. The university charges US$40/week to do an elective here.

Accommodation: Cheap family houses can be arranged through the university, but a tourist place (such as Seaview Guesthouse) on the beach may be better.

OTHER MEDICAL SCHOOLS:

North Colombo Private Medical College, PO Box 6, Talagolla Road, Ragama, Colombo, Sri Lanka.
University of Jaffna, Faculty of Medicine, Thirunelvely, Jaffna, Sri Lanka.

SOME RURAL HOSPITALS:

Kurunegala Hospital
Kurunegala, Sri Lanka.

The hospital: Is in the hill country and has a great deal of tropical medicine (malaria, typhoid, dengue fever).

O Elective notes: Although interesting, students have complained of endless ward rounds.

Matale Base Hospital
Matale, Sri Lanka.

The hospital: Excellent for surgery, although facilities are extremely poor. There are two operating tables in one theatre.

Thailand

Population: 60 million
Language: Thai
Capital: Bangkok
Currency: Baht
Int Code: +66

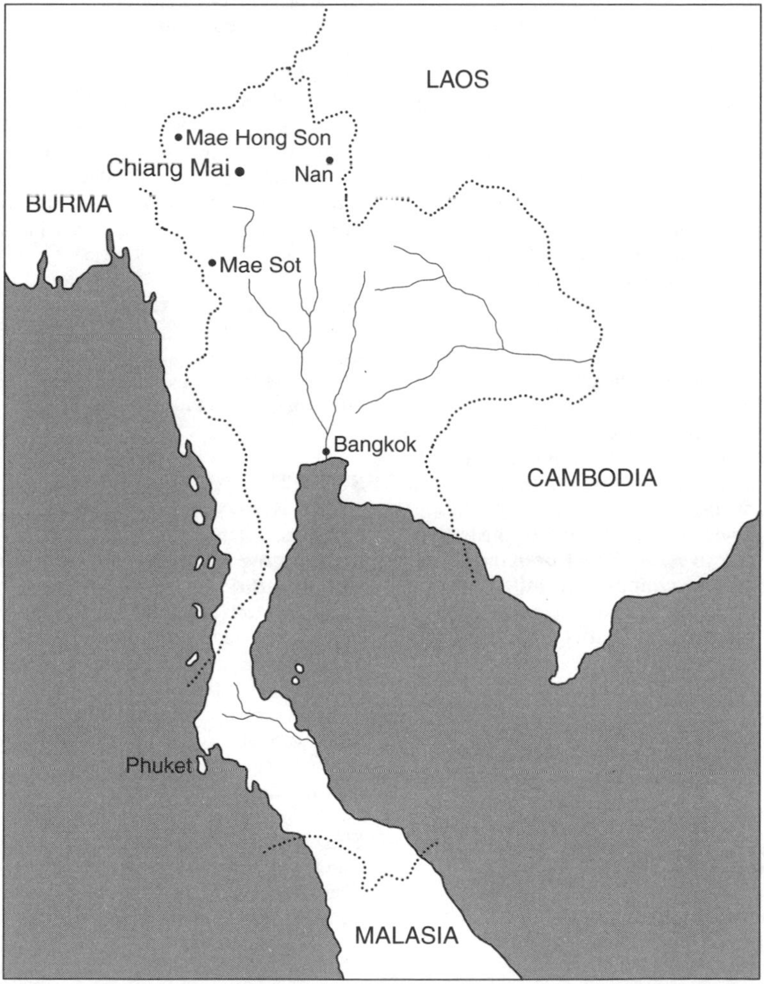

Thailand lies between the Indian and Pacific Oceans and has Burma, Laos, Cambodia and Malaysia as neighbours. In recent years, business in Bangkok has been booming; however, the north still remains very poor. Although Thailand is not a very popular destination, most medics and students head for these northern parts. Because of the problems in Burma a number of refugee camps are set up just over the border in Thailand. This area has provided some very interesting electives.

Medicine:
Specialist medical care can really only be found in Bangkok. Improvements though have occurred in rural areas. This has been achieved by training more primary healthcare workers rather than more doctors. A system runs by which the poor can obtain a certificate so that they do not have to pay for healthcare. HIV is a major problem in Bangkok, especially among the many prostitutes (over 80% prevalence in this group).

Visas and work permits:
A visa is required to enter Thailand for more than 15 days. Enquire with the embassy for more details. Most students do not require special permits, but check with the embassy. Work permits are required for anything more than voluntary work.

A very helpful source of information for electives is **The Foreign Medical Student Exchange Committee**, Faculty of Medicine, Siriraj Hospital, Mahidol University, 2 Prannock Road, Bangkoknoi, Bangkok 10700, Thailand.

SOME MEDICAL SCHOOLS AND TEACHING HOSPITALS:

Bangkok

Chulalongkorn University
Faculty of Medicine, Rajdamri Road, Bangkok 10500, Thailand
http://md2.md.chula.ac.th/
Founded in 1947 the school uses Chulalongkorn and Siriraj hospitals (over 1000 beds).

Mahidol University
Faculty of Medicine, Siriraj Hospital, 2, Pharnnok Road, Bangkok 10700, Thailand.
This is the oldest medical school in Thailand and also uses the Siriraj Hospital.

Chiang Mai

Chiang Mai University
110 Intawaroros Road, Muang District, Chiang Mai 50200, Thailand Tel: 053 221122 Fax: 053 217144
www.medicine.cmu.ac.th
Founded in 1959 this is the only medical university in the north and uses the largest hospital, the Maharaj Nakorn Chiang Mai Hospital. This has 1800 beds and all major specialities in three buildings. The school was originally designed to produce more doctors for rural Thailand and there is a close co-operation with rural health centres. The campus (including hospital) is in west Chiang Mai at the base of Doi Suthep (1000 m). It is 5 km from the airport.

SOME RURAL HOSPITALS:

Fang Hospital
Amphur Fang, Chiang Mai 50110, Thailand.
The hospital: A 150-bed hospital in a relatively rural area close to Chiang Mai. The doctors are all extremely friendly. Many problems are HIV, TB, typhoid, malaria and gunshots. Road traffic accidents are also common. Visits to local hill tribes are carried out. The hospital only has very basic equipment (X-ray is the only imaging).

Srisungwan Hospital
Mae Hong Son, Thailand.
The hospital: 140 beds and seven doctors. Wards include O&G, male and female medical and surgical, paeds, an ITU and a monk's ward. There are two operating theatres, ultrasound and X-ray

facilities. It is a highly respected hospital in Thailand despite its small size. It has public and private wards. The public have malaria, TB, meningitis, heroin addictions, gunshot wounds. The private wards have the diseases of the West: NIDDM, MIs, cancers. Malaria is a huge problem in the region accounting for 50% of hospital admissions.

O Elective notes: You will need to attempt to learn some Thai. This is not a holiday elective but very educational. You can get out to trek and also to visit Burmese refugee camps.

Nan Hospital

Nan, Thailand.

The hospital: Nan is a provincial, secondary referral hospital for surrounding rural hospitals. Nan itself is remote in the north of Thailand close to the Thai–Laos border. All the doctors are incredibly friendly and good at teaching. Trauma (from motorbike accidents), dengue fever, malaria, snakebites, TB, hepatocellular cancer and HIV are all common.

O Elective notes: Beautiful surroundings and excellent opportunities for practical procedures and in theatre but beware of the HIV rate.

Phya Thai Phuket International Hospital

28/36–37 Sri Sena Road, Tambol Taladyai,
Amphur Muang, Phuket 83000, Thailand
Tel: (076) 252603–06 Fax: (076) 252646–7
e-mail phyathai@phuket.ksc.co.th
website: www.phyathai.com

The hospital: First class facilities and equipment as a significant percentage of patients are overseas tourists. It has all major specialities. The hospital is 15 minutes walk from town. However, sometimes there are not so many patients. Local patients often don't speak English. All the doctors do and are very friendly.

O Elective notes: Phuket is a lovely island but if you don't have transport the actual area around the hospital can get a bit dull. There's plenty of time to explore.

Accommodation: Furnished rooms adjacent to the hospital are provided (2000baht/month (£33)). It has fridge, freezer, a/c but NO HOT WATER.

NORTHERN THAI HEALTH STATIONS:

The Thai German Highland Development Project is a German organization that donates money towards the development of hill tribes. The Thai government contributes 20%. There are a number of Health Stations usually run by around three paramedics providing basic health needs, treatment of malaria, TB etc. Contact the foreign medical student exchange for more details.

A SPECIAL NOTE ON THE SITUATION WITH BURMA:

Due to the poverty (despite it being the top heroin exporter in the world) and civil war, Burma's health care is almost non-existent and hospitals tend to only cater for military personnel. There are no hospitals in rural areas. There is high infant mortality and many people have TB, malaria and HIV. The intense fighting has resulted in many people fleeing to the jungle (not without its dangers). Others have crossed the border as refugees into Thailand. In total there are over 100,000 such refugees in many camps along the border. They are not recognized as refugees by the Thai Government or the UN and so are dependent on NGOs such as Medicins sans Frontières, the Red Cross and the Burmese Border Consortium. The camps are often attacked by Burmese soldiers who cross the border. If you are thinking of working here up-to-date information is vital. Contact one of these groups. The foreign medical student exchange can also give advice. An example of one of the camp health centres is the tremendously successful Dr Cynthia's clinic in Mae Sot.

Mae Sot

An area in north-west Thailand 7 km from the Burmese border. It has 50,000 people in it including Thai and Burmese refugees. Mae Sot has a huge gem trade and is a lively border town with day and night markets, restaurants and bars. Medicins sans Frontières (MSF) and Shoklo Malaria Research Unit (SMRU) crowds hang out here in the evenings.

Dr Cynthia's Clinic

PO Box 67, Mae Sot, Tak 63110, Thailand
Tel: 55 533 644 Fax: 55 544 655
e-mail win7@loxinfo.co.th

This was set up by Dr Cynthia Maung, originally from Karen, who had to flee during the student uprising in 1988. Many of her colleagues with her in the jungle died from malaria. She has now set up a clinic for the refugees in Mae Sot. It relies on money from the NGOs to function. Many volunteer doctors, medical students and teachers come to help. Dr Cynthia, her brother (also a doctor) and 50 medical assistants (refugees) who are trained at the clinic, run it. It works as an outpatients but also has 15 beds (no nurses, the relatives have to do that), a basic lab, maternity and child health clinics and a computer (with Internet access). All services are free. It trains 50 medics a year who go to other camps and across into the Burmese jungle to give treatment to those with no access to healthcare. There is a great deal of malaria and drug resistance is a major problem. TB, peptic ulcers and worm infestations are also common. There is basic education into personal hygiene. To organize an elective or to work here write or e-mail to the above.

Note: Dr Cynthia is (obviously) incredibly busy so don't expect a quick reply. It is also expensive for them to e-mail back so you may only get one reply. Ring before you go to ensure all is OK.

O Elective notes: Medical students run clinics with medics trained in the clinic. They act as translators. When there are no students the medics run the clinics themselves so they are very experienced. Students are also involved in teaching the local medics. There is a great deal of responsibility in going here and it is exhausting work. Mae Sot itself is a pleasant town, safe and the people are very warm-hearted but venturing into the jungle is dangerous. Gunfire can be heard at night and tourists have been kidnapped. There are many languages. Make attempts to learn a bit of each.

Accommodation: Has previously been in the clinic. As there is the possibility it may be attacked and it is now crowded with refugees you are best to stay in a guesthouse in town (see the Lonely Planet Guide). No. 4 Guest House comes recommended.

Shoklo Malaria Research Unit

PO Box 46, Mae Sot, Tak Province, 63110, Thailand Tel: 55 531531 Fax: 55 544442. (It has close links with Prof White, Centre for Tropical Medicine, University of Oxford, John Radcliffe Hospital, Headington, Oxford OX3 9DU, UK.) Alternatively get in touch with the faculty of Tropical Medicine, Wellcome–Mahidol University, 420/6 Rajvithi Road, Bangkok 10400, Thailand Tel: 2460832 Fax: 00 2 2467795.

SMRU is made up of an international group of scientists and physicians and researches into resistant strains of malaria. Most of its work is done in the Maela refugee camp on the Thai–Burmese border (the MSF has a hospital in the camp).

Accommodation: Provided by the SMRU in their base camp. It is now too dangerous to stay in the border camps for fear of raids. Cost is about 2000baht (£33).

PRIVATE HOSPITALS IN BANGKOK:

Kluaynamthai Hospital 1, 80 Soi Rongpayaban 2, Rama 4 Rd, Prakanong, Bangkok, 10110, Thailand Tel: (02) 381 2006 Fax: (02) 391 3582.

The Thonburi Hospital Public Co, Ltd 34/1 Issaraphap Road, Soi 44, Bangkok-Noi Bangkok 10700, Thailand Tel: (02) 412 0022 Fax: (02) 412 6005 www.thonburi-hosp.com

AUSTRALIA and NEW ZEALAND

Australia

Population: 17.8 million
Language: English
Capital: Canberra
Currency: Australian dollar
Int Code: +61

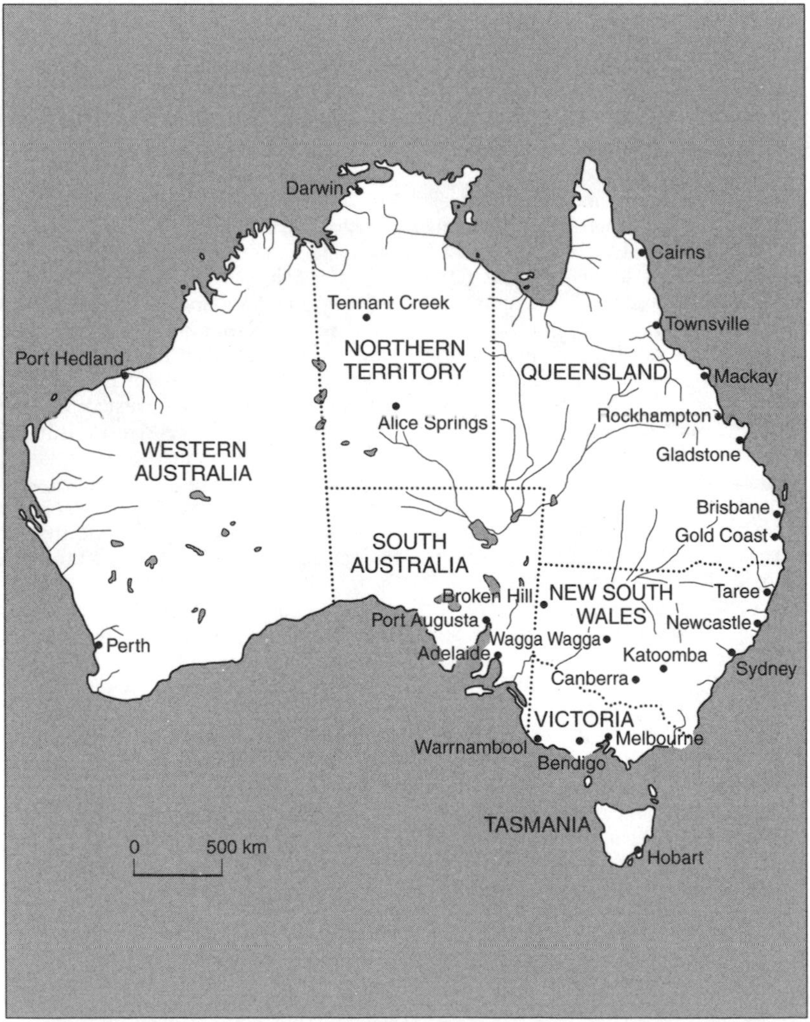

The world's sixth-largest country comprises six states and the Northern Territory. Its variety of landscapes range from snowy mountains to magnificent beaches, arid deserts to tropical rainforests. Most Australians live on the coast; indeed, all cities bar Canberra are on the coast. Working in Australia can therefore almost guarantee some sun, sand and surf as well as spectacular diving and a multitude of water sports.

✪ Medicine:

Australia has an impressive public health system with high standards and short waiting lists. There are many world-renowned city hospitals as well as the well-known Royal Flying Doctor Service serving the outback communities. There is a great deal of disparity however. The Aboriginal community is still grossly under represented in society with higher rates of alcoholism, trauma and medical conditions compared to their white counterparts. The average life expectancy of an Aboriginal male is still only 47 years. Australia's main health priorities at present include Aboriginal health, cancer prevention (especially skin, lung, cervical and breast), heart disease and injury prevention.

There is less distinction between private and public healthcare with many people having some form of health insurance. The National Insurance scheme is called Medicare. A normal consultation with a GP costs about $30 (£15) for which Medicare give a rebate of $24 (£12). The patient therefore has to pay about $6 (£3) to see a GP. Accident and Emergency is free and therefore some people go to A&E with what should really be GP conditions. There's one doctor per 434 people and the leading causes of death are heart and cerebrovascular diseases and cancer. Whilst on the subject of health, it is worth mentioning something about the demography of HIV in the Asia–Pacific region. The rapid increase in countries such as Thailand is of great concern to its neighbours. By the mid-1990s in Australia there were approaching 3000 reported cases of AIDS, 96% of which were male. There are two main populations. Most is known about the city group especially prevalent in inner Sydney. The Aboriginal community is the other group. They are experiencing a massive increase especially in areas such as Palm Island. Hepatitis C is also a major problem among intravenous drug users in Sydney, in some areas reaching 60% prevalence in this group.

Working in Australia either as a doctor, nurse, physiotherapist or medical student provides the opportunity to practice a wide range of medicine – from advanced First World medicine in the cities, to almost Third World medicine in the Aboriginal communities.

➲ Visas and work permits

To do an elective in Oz you require a visitor's visa ('tourist' class (Class 676)) available free of charge from the High Commission (*see* Section 3: The Appendix). If staying for more than an elective and enrolling on a full time course you will need a student visa. If reading this, you are probably from a gazetted country (i.e. trusted by the Aussie's not to be a baddy; a full list is available from the embassy). For this you need to fill in forms, get letters, send money etc. They will also require a medical examination and CXR from a recognized physician. More details can be found by calling 0891 699 333. This is a 'cost-a-packet' automated information line. Fortunately there is a 'poor hard up students' line 020 7887 5637 open from 2 pm to 4 pm. There is an emergency line: 020 7887 5314 open at all times. Alternatively, visit their web site: www.ida.com.au/backpackers/visas.html

✪ Working in Australia:

This can require a great deal of planning. There are two options: temporary work (up to a year), and permanent work.

TEMPORARY WORK: Six months or a year in a speciality in Australia either as an SHO or Registrar is very attractive and commonly done. It is also relatively easy to get jobs, especially in

'Areas of Need' in the rural outback. It is far more difficult to get a pre-registration job, however. You are better to wait and register at home. To obtain a visa for temporary work as a medical practitioner you need to have a medical and a chest X-ray. You do not have to have sat the Australian Medical Exams. Most contracts however will require that:

- You will return to home at the end of your contract
- You will not apply to sit the AMC exams

They really don't want you to stay. Breaking these rules will make it extremely difficult for you to apply for more/permanent work out there at a later date. If under 25 you can apply for a working holiday visa (about £60). This allows you to stay in Australia for a year and work for up to three months for a single employer. Although you can practise medicine with this visa, a number of hospitals require you to have a full medical practitioner visa so ring and check first of all. The best way to find these temporary jobs is either to look in the *BMJ*, apply through agencies (such as Slade) or contact the hospital in which you would like to work directly. Most jobs are for a minimum of three months.

PERMANENT WORK: This has become extremely difficult to obtain over the last few years. Australia has been flooded with overseas doctors and hence they are making it as difficult as possible. Again, PRHO jobs are virtually impossible to get. Once registered, you can either migrate immediately and join a postgraduate training scheme or alternatively, complete SHO training and membership and then leave. Either way there are many obstacles.

The first obstacle is getting in. You need to obtain residency status in Oz from the Department of Immigration and Multicultural Affairs before you can apply to sit the AMC exams. Allow up to a year (or even longer) for a migration application to be accepted. You need proof of identity (birth certificate), education (school and degree certificates), health (medical and CXR) and character (no convictions (you may get away with the odd one, after all, they used to be compulsory!)). It's all done on a points system and as a doctor you score minus 25 for skills (they really don't want you!). It can be made a bit easier if you marry an Australian.

Secondly you will need to sit the AMC exams. These are the Australian 'finals' and hence test undergraduate as well as graduate knowledge. They also cover the specialities and therefore you are best to sit these as soon as possible after qualifying while it's all still fresh (you can't sit it before qualifying like the American exams). The exam is in two parts, a written and a clinical. Passing the written allows limited registration with the AMC. This enables a year's work (like pre-registration house year), although the year is at your UK level. The clinical exam has to be taken within three years, allowing full registration. To work as an independent doctor (e.g. a GP) you will either need specialist exams that are recognized, to work in an 'unmet area of need' (which can change) or to work in a hospital setting for 10 years. For more details write to the **Australian Medical Council**, PO Box 293, Woden ACT, Australia 2606 Tel: 02 6285 1633 Fax: 02 6285 2943.

You will also need to register with the appropriate State Medical Board:

Medical Board, PO Box 4221, Darwin, Northern Territory 0801 Tel: 08 8999 2944 Fax: 08 899 2426.
Medical Board of the ACT, PO Box 1309, Tuggeranong, ACT 2901, Australia Tel: 02 6205 1600 Fax: 02 6205 1602.
Medical Board of Queensland, 19th Floor, Forestry House, 160 Mary Street, Brisbane, Queensland 4000, Australia Tel: 07 3227 5777 Fax: 07 3225 2527.
Medical Board of South Australia, 91 Payneham Road, St Peters, South Australia 5069 Tel: 08 8362 7811 Fax: 08 8362 7906.
Medical Board of Western Australia, 34 Colin Street (PO Box 1182) West Perth, Western Australia 6005 Tel: 08 9481 6599 Fax: 08 9321 2119.
Medical Council of Tasmania, 2 Gore Street, South Hobart, Tasmania 7004 Tel: 03 6223 8466 Fax: 03 6223 4579.
Medical Practitioners Board of Victoria, 3rd Floor, 1 Palmerston Crescent, South Melbourne. Victoria 3205, Australia Tel: 03 9695 9500 Fax: 03 9682 8060.

New South Wales Medical Board, PO Box 104, Gladesville, NSW 2111, Australia Tel: 02 9879 6799 Fax: 02 9816 5307.

See p. 196 for a list of rural workforce agencies.

OTHER ADDRESSES:

Royal Australian College of Surgeons, Surgeons Gardens, Spring Street, Melbourne, Victoria 3000, Australia Tel: 03 9249 1200 Fax: 03 9249 1219.
Red Cross National Office 206 Clarendon Street, East Melbourne, Victoria 3002, Australia.

Climate & crime:

The north of Australia is warm all year round and particularly humid during the summer monsoon. The east and sout-east are fairly temperate. The warmest months are December to February (25–30°C), the coolest are June to August. Although not a violent country, crime is increasing in some inner city and Aboriginal areas.

Elective notes:

Australia is a very popular destination. Early planning is vital as most hospitals work on a 'first come, first served' basis. It's also worth noting that Australian students have a massive summer holiday between November and February. This can mean the hospitals get a bit quiet; brilliant if you want individual attention and the chance to do procedures, not so good if you want formal teaching and to make friends. If you have to go at this time of year, think about going with a friend.

If you want to do Aboriginal work, aim for the northern territories and Darwin. If you're planning to travel around Oz, book flights before you go as they can work out half the price of booking them once you're there. Aussies are proud of their country and will want you to go and see it.

AUSTRALIAN UNIVERSITIES AFFILIATED TO MEDICAL SCHOOLS:

SOUTH AUSTRALIA:
Flinders University The School of Medicine, The Flinders University of South Australia, Bedford Park, SA 5042, Australia.
The Medical School, University of Adelaide, Frome Road, Adelaide, SA 5000.

VICTORIA:
Monash University The Faculty of Medicine, Monash University, Wellington Road, Clayton, VIC 3168, Australia www.med.monash.edu.au
University of Melbourne Faculty of Medicine, University of Melbourne, Gratton Street, Parkville, VIC 3052, Australia www.unimelb.edu.au

QUEENSLAND:
The University of Queensland Medical School, Herston Road, Herston, QLD 4006, Australia www.uq.edu.au

TASMANIA:
University of Tasmania The Faculty of Medicine, University of Tasmania, 43 Collins Street, Hobart, TAS 7000.

NEW SOUTH WALES:
University of Newcastle The Faculty of Medicine, University of Newcastle, Newcastle, NSW 2308, Australia www.newcastle.edu.au
University of New South Wales The Faculty of Medicine, University of New South Wales, PO Box 1, Kensington, NSW 2033, Australia www.unsw.edu.au
University of Sydney The Faculty of Medicine, University of Sydney, Sydney, NSW 2006, Australia www.usyd.edu.au

WESTERN AUSTRALIA:
University of Western Australia The School of Medicine, University of Western Australia, Perth, WA 6000, Australia.

SOME INTERNET SITES:
Australia Medical Services Directory: www.midcoast.com.au/cms
Health Care of Australia: www.hcoa.com.au/

NEW SOUTH WALES

Sydney

Sydney is Australia's largest city with the largest suburban area of any city in the world (twice the size of Beijing, six times the size of Rome). It has the famous Opera House, harbour and plenty of beaches. Nightlife is superb with many shows on Oxford Street (student tickets available 30 minutes before the performance). There is a fantastic beach culture in the summer (shuts down between

May and September) and the temperature can reach 40°C with high humidity. Outside Sydney there are some excellent national parks, blue marines and skiing. A trip to the Blue Mountains is a must. Coaches to Brisbane (12 hours) and Melbourne (10 hours) overnight are much cheaper than flights (about £25 one way).

UNIVERSITIES IN NEW SOUTH WALES:

There are two universities based in Sydney: the University of New South Wales and the University of Sydney. Each has specific hospitals affiliated to them.

University of New South Wales:

Faculty of Medicine, Anzac Parade, Sydney 2052, Australia www.unsw.edu.au (Elective Co-ordinator, Faculty of Medicine UNSW Tel: 02 9385 2452)

- St Vincent's
- St George's
- Prince of Wales/Prince Henry
- Sydney Children's Hospital
- Liverpool Hospital

The Prince Henry, Prince of Wales and Sydney Children's Hospital form a group in themselves. They make up a 1000-bed teaching hospital and medical school located in Sydney's eastern suburbs (15 min drive from the city centre). They are spread over two campuses (the Randwick campus, incorporating the Prince of Wales and Sydney's Children's Hospitals, and The Prince Henry Hospital at Little Bay, 8 km south).

University of Sydney

The Secretary, Faculty of Medicine, Edward Ford Building (A27), University of Sydney, NSW 2006, Australia
Tel: 02 9351 3132 Fax: 02 9351 6645
www.usyd.edu.au

- Royal Prince Alfred Hospital
- Royal North Shore Hospital
- Concord Hospital
- Westmead Hospital
- Nepean Hospital
- New Children's Hospital
- Canberra Hospital (*see* Australian Capital Territory)

To do elective work in any of the above hospitals you have to write to the affiliated University. They will then process your application as outlined below. You may state a preference as to where and in what department you wish to work. To give yourself a head start it may be worth writing to your chosen destination directly first of all and then writing to the University saying they have offered you an elective placement. Whatever you do apply EARLY.

The University of Sydney will ask you to provide the following in your next letter:

- Areas of work which are of special interest
- The precise dates you require an attachment
- Letter from your Dean
- A recent passport photo
- Curriculum vitae
- A bank cheque drawn on an Australian bank for $A100

The earlier you apply the more likely you are to get what you want. Once a place is found a further fee of $A100 is required for enrolment. The clinical schools also have an administrative fee (e.g. Canberra charges A$300 for four weeks, A$500 for 4–8 weeks). It's all very expensive, but well-organized. Some electives can be time-limited to a maximum of eight weeks.

With the University of New South Wales you often pay nothing.

UNIVERSITY OF NSW HOSPITALS:

St Vincent's Hospital

Victoria Street, Darlinghurst, Sydney, NSW 2010, Australia Tel: (02) 9339 1111 Fax: (02) 9332 4142.

The hospital: A medium-sized teaching hospital of NSW university (approximately 400 beds) right in the city centre (20 min walk to the Opera House and Harbour Bridge). It's between Sydney's red light district (King's Cross) and the gay district (Oxford Street). Not surprisingly, the area is therefore always buzzing, day and night. Also, not surprisingly there is a high incidence of HIV among patients (one in 20) and Darlinghurst has the highest concentration of homeless people in Sydney. The A&E department treats 100+ patients a day. The hospital covers internal medicine, surgery, trauma and psychiatry.

WARNING: this is a dangerous area at night (mainly muggings); however it is perfectly safe during the day.

❍ Elective notes: The consultants are pretty relaxed and it's not too difficult to get the afternoons off to get down the beach (they'll encourage you to see Australia). The casualty teams are happy for you to see patients first and do minor procedures such as suturing. Most major trauma goes to other hospitals; however there are no Australian students here so you have free rein. GI surgery also has good reports. From previous reports some supervisors in the psychiatry department are not very well-organized. It is one of the few hospitals in Sydney that doesn't charge tuition fees.

Accommodation: There is no private accommodation in the hospital and they recommend you stay in a local hostel ($100–$150 a week). However, most elective students stay in a place called Lavinus Nolan House, 433 Bourke Street, Darlinghurst, NSW 2030 (contact Sister Mary Clooney) approximately 10 min walk from the hospital, just off Taylor square. It's a residence in the grounds of St Margaret's Womens' Hospital (a private hospital) and costs about A$120 (£60)/week for your own room and good facilities. It's well-situated for buses to Circular Quay and the beaches (Bondi beach = 30 min bus ride). The nun who runs the residence is pretty strict (especially on the no visitors rule!), but it is thoroughly recommended as you'll be hard pushed to find a place so central so cheaply. Some elective students stay at a youth hostel in Coogee Beach (about 30 min bus ride away). They also report this as a good option. The YHA by the coach station is good for short-term accommodation.

St George's Hospital

Belgrave Street, Kogarah, NSW 2217, Australia Tel: (02) 9350 1111 Fax: (02) 9350 3960.
www.unsw.edu.au/stgh/stghome.html The web site lists all staff.

The hospital: A large, high-tech hospital in the south-eastern suburbs of Sydney (five minutes to the station then 15 min on the train).

❍ Elective notes: The A&E is busy and in other specialities (e.g. GI) it's all advanced stuff. You are welcome to attend the Sydney students' tutorials, but in some specialities (e.g. orthopaedics) reports suggest that consultants have been very keen that students explore Oz.

Accommodation: Has been provided in a flat a couple of minutes from the hospital at a rather expensive rate. They can supply a list of local guesthouses. The more central hospitals in Sydney (Royal Prince Alfred or St Vincent's) may be more sociable. Bondi beach is a short train and bus ride away.

Prince of Wales Hospital

High Street, Randwick, Sydney NSW 2031, Australia Tel: (02) 9282 2222 Fax: (02) 9382 2033 http://yorrick.pow.unsw.edu.au/
www.powh.edu.au/
http://clinical.web.unsw.edu.au/powh/

The hospital: A tertiary referral centre next to Sydney's Children's Hospital and fairly friendly. Originally a destitute children's asylum, it was converted into a military hospital during the world wars. It was converted back to civilian use in 1953. There are 313,000 people in its catchment population, although nearly half of its patients are from outside this area. The Randwick campus is currently under redevelopment to include facilities such as a new acute service, a helipad, the new Royal Hospital for Women and a Hyperbaric Unit. It's fairly central (20 min bus ride from the centre).

❍ Elective notes: The A&E is typical of any Western hospital and you can do as much as you want.

Note: If you're doing orthopaedics and want to see sporting injuries, most

go to private clinics; however, the professor is very keen that you explore Oz. Highly recommended if you're wanting more of a laid back elective.
Accommodation: At the Prince Henry Hospital (*see below*). They may be able to arrange accommodation on-site, but not until you arrive.

Sydney Children's Hospital

(Used to be Prince of Wales Children's Hospital), High Street, Randwick 2031/2, Sydney, NSW, Australia www.powh.edu.au/
The hospital: A modern hospital (next to the adult Prince of Wales (*see above*)) in the suburbs of Sydney, but not too far from the centre (6 km). It is also undergoing major changes to provide an even better service.
O Elective notes: Very easy going and you can choose to do as much or as little as you wish.
Accommodation: At the Prince Henry Hospital (some have not been impressed by it, *see below*).

The Prince Henry Hospital

Anzac Parade, Little Bay 2036, Sydney, NSW, Australia Tel: (02) 9382 5555 Fax: (02)9382 5029 www.powh.edu.au/
The hospital: Was founded in 1881 during an outbreak of smallpox in Sydney. The Coastal Hospital was erected at 'sufficient distance from Sydney to ensure safety and confidence'. It was renamed Prince Henry in 1934 and since 1959 has been affiliated with the Prince of Wales as part of the University of NSW teaching hospitals. Currently, the acute services of this hospital are being relocated to the Randwick campus (*see* Prince of Wales) while the Prince Henry becomes a centre of excellence for rehabilitation and aged care.
Accommodation: The Prince of Wales and Sydney Children's Hospital both have their accommodation on the Prince Henry site. The plus points are that it is cheap and next to a lovely golf course and beach. The major problem is that it is six kilometres from these other hospitals and in the opposite direction to the city (making it about an hour's bus ride from the centre). You may be better organizing your own accommodation.

The Liverpool Hospital

Elizabeth Street, Liverpool 2173, Sydney, NSW, Australia Tel: (02) 9828 3000 Fax: (02) 9828 3307
www.med.unsw.edu.au/livtrauma (trauma dept)
The hospital: Has a good trauma unit as well as the regional perinatal centre (The Caroline Chishom Centre).

UNIVERSITY OF SYDNEY HOSPITALS:

Royal Prince Alfred Hospital

Missenden Road, Camperdown, Sydney NSW 2050, Australia Tel: (02) 9515 6111 Fax: (02) 9515 6133. (Contact: The Electives Co-ordinator, Central Clinical School, RPA at this address.)
The hospital: Being linked to Sydney University, this is one of the Bohemian student areas of Sydney, 10–20 min bus ride from the city centre. It's a friendly hospital with specialities in breast cancer and liver transplantation. There is a very busy A&E department.
O Elective notes: With the busy A&E there's plenty of opportunity for practical procedures and doing early investigations. Reports show that the cardiology firm is intense work (cardiology ward rounds start at 7 am). There is a specialist breast cancer unit (The Sydney Breast Cancer Institute) based within the hospital. If this is your specialist interest it is well worth writing to them. There is a specialist liver transplant unit. They'll give you a radio-pager and expect you to be ready within two hours notice to go on an organ retrieval. Great if this involves helicopters or fast jets to New Zealand … not so good if you wanted to go for a night out in Sydney.
Accommodation: For elective students is in the nurses' home (Queen Mary's) with other students, so there is the oppor-

tunity to meet many new people. However, there are only two rooms available for medical students ($35 (£18)/week). If you don't get a room, ask one of the local students . . . many go away and are happy to rent out their room for a month or so. Failing that, Billerbong Gardens Hostel ($100 (£50)/week) is the next nearest. There's also a superb gym with aerobics classes and pool (outdoor). Lots of cafés and bars are close by.

The Royal North Shore Hospital

Pacific Highway St Leonard's, North Sydney, NSW, Australia 2065 Tel: (02) 9226 7111 Fax: (02) 9926 7779.

The hospital: The RNSH is a large (950-bed), modern teaching hospital in north Sydney (St Leonard's), 15 min by train (four stops across Harbour Bridge) from the city centre and 40 min from Manly Beach. There are many students present. This area is very safe.

O Elective notes: The busy A&E (with helicopter service) and oncology departments come particularly recommended. The intensive care department can provide a well-organized elective. Like the rest of Australia, it seems that the staff are very keen for you to go out and see Oz while you're there (vascular surgery may be the exception to this)! Oncology (it would appear) is very relaxed! There's no formal teaching for elective students, but you can attend the Sydney medical students tutorials which are very good and also the weekly medical Grand Round (free lunch provided). The Elective Co-ordinator introduces you to your ward. The staff and other medical students are very friendly and you can do something different every night.

Note: Apply early here as it fills up quickly. Repeatedly highly recommended.

Accommodation: The nurses' home costing $70 (£35) per week (the price has actually come down over the years) is between grotty and reasonable (many have noted cockroaches in the kitchen). You meet many other students. There is a canteen close by and a couple of cheap restaurants. Another place you can stay is Billy Blue Palace (expensive, but the accommodation is good and food is provided) or the rather extravagantly named St Leonard's Mansions ($100 (£50)/week, 7 Park Road, St Leonard's Tel: 9439 6999 Fax: 9437 5890) which may well have the largest population of funnel web spiders in Sydney (ALWAYS wear shoes!) There is a good gym and heated outdoor swimming pool on the hospital site and the hospital is conveniently on a bus route to the beach.

Advice for electives: Some have found it beneficial to write directly to the department you want to work in (A&E is the most popular) and *then* to the Clinical School Electives Co-ordinator. If you write direct to the clinical school they will give you four choices and allocate you where available. Either way you won't be exempt from the $100 (£50) registration fee to the University of Sydney, nor the $250 (£125) administration fee of the Northern Clinical School.

Concord Hospital

Hospital Road Concord, Sydney, NSW 2005, Australia.

The hospital: A large teaching hospital in one of Sydney's western suburbs, founded to repatriate soldiers after the war, but was later handed over to the local authority. Although not far, it can take a little while to get into Sydney. There are very friendly staff in a lovely hospital.

O Elective notes: It can get very quiet and dull, especially when the students are not there. The Upper GI team is good, keen to give informal teaching and get you assisting in theatre. The formal teaching for the Aussie students is on a Friday afternoon and well worth attending.

Accommodation: In the hospital and cheap (about $60 (£30)/week), but remember it can be difficult to get in and out of Sydney, especially at night. Some have stayed in the Queen Mary Building at Royal Prince Alfred Hospital (20 min from Sydney, 45 from Concord).

Westmead Hospital

Hawksbury Road, Westmead, Sydney 2145, NSW, Australia Tel: (02) 9845 5555
www.westmead.nsw.gov.au/
www.usyd.edu.au/su/radiology/westmead.htm

The hospital: A large (900-bed) teaching hospital in a suburb of Sydney (45 min train ride from the city). It claims to be the largest teaching hospital in the Southern Hemisphere (covering 95 acres). It has both state and private divisions. The hospital covers many specialities, but is especially known for its neonatal and paediatric medicine (there is a 30-bed unit for emotionally disturbed children). There is a busy A&E.

O Elective notes: There is excellent teaching and many clinics to attend. The cardiologists are keen to teach, but expect you to turn up to the catheter lab which can get a bit repetitive. Some units (such as Oncology) may expect a small project. A&E is well-organized. With the neonatal and paediatric group they also run something called ISAM (Intravenous Substance Abusing Mothers) clinics. There is an affiliated dental school.

Accommodation: Pretty basic ($20 (£10)/week), so plan to spend your weekends in Sydney. Having said that, it's cheap and there's nowhere else to stay in Westmead. Cooking facilities are good and it's convenient for the train station. There is a pool and some tennis courts. It's one hour to Bondi Beach.

Nepean Hospital

PO Box 63, Penrith 2751, Sydney, NSW, Australia.

The hospital: About a one-hour train ride from Sydney at the foot of the Blue Mountains. It provides most general specialities to the local area.

O Elective notes: The consultants are fairly relaxed … put in what you want. It's good, but if it's Sydney you want, remember the distance. The train can get dodgy late at night.

Accommodation: Provided in the nurses' home at about $20 (£10)/week. It's fine, but a bit quiet.

The New Children's Hospital

(Previously the Royal Alexandra Hospital for Children) Hawkesbury Road, Westmead 2145, Australia Tel: (02) 9845 0000 Fax: (02) 9845 3489 www.nch.edu.au (an amazing web site).

The hospital: NCH is the major paediatric hospital (350 beds) for NSW and the South Pacific. It is the home of the University of Sydney's Department of Paediatrics and was purpose-built in 1996. It has superb facilities for staff, patients and relatives. It has a special paeds A&E. This hospital is also superb for other medical professionals, for example speech therapists (Tel: 9845 2076), physiotherapists (Tel: 9845 3369), nurses (Tel: 9845 3023) and teachers (Tel: 9845 2813). Briefly, some of the departments include: Gene Therapy Research Unit, The Children's Hospital Insitute of Sports Medicine (CHISM) (8% of children in A&E have sports injuries), cardiology/cardiac surgery, clinical genetics, cochlear implant centre, emergency, endocrinology, immunology and infectious diseases, intensive care, psychological medicine, respiratory medicine, rheumatology, spina bifida, surgery and trauma. It is also associated with the Neonatal and Paediatric Emergency Transport Service (NETS), a flying doctor service especially for kids transporting 1500 children a year by helicopter.

The hospital is 28 km west of Sydney, accessible by the Sydney metro (get off at Parramatta). A direct shuttle bus goes from the airport. Full details are available on their incredible web site. This also displays current job opportunities.

O Elective notes: The opportunities in an elective here are vast and can be decided upon arrival. NETS is worth a special mention. They are happy for elective students to go on retrieval, but it takes a couple of days to train up before you can go on the helicopter. The views of Sydney, however, make it well worth it. Elective places here are hard to come by … you really should apply 12 months in advance. Write to the Electives Co-ordinator at the above address.

Note: It is a long way out of Sydney (45 min on the tube). The hospital has close links with the King George V Hospital in central Sydney. This is a tertiary referral maternity hospital delivering 4700 babies a year.

Accommodation: Available at about $35 (£17)/week and has air-conditioning and a swimming pool. However, there are no cooking facilities. Tel: 98452958 e-mail: hostel@nch.edu.au.

Sydney Hospital and Sydney Eye Hospital

Macquaire Street, Sydney 2000, NSW, Australia Tel: (02) 9382 7111 Fax: (02) 9382 7320 www.ozemail.com.au/~sydhosp

The hospitals: Are the oldest in Australia, dating back to 1788. Currently there are 113 inpatient beds and there are three academic departments affiliated with Sydney University and/or the University of NSW. Services include general medicine, surgery, orthopaedics, ENT, hand surgery, ophthalmology and drug, alcohol and sexual health. It has an A&E and specialist eye A&E.

O **Elective notes:** Nice hospital, very central (10 min walk to the Opera House). The general part of the hospital is pretty small. Excellent if you're interested in eyes.

OTHER HOSPITALS IN NEW SOUTH WALES:

The only University outside Sydney in NSW is the **University of Newcastle** – The Faculty of Medicine, University of Newcastle, Newcastle, NSW 2308, Australia www.newcastle.edu.au

Royal Newcastle Hospital

Pacific Street, Newcastle 2300, NSW, Australia Tel: (02) 4923 6000 Fax: (02) 4923 6204.

The hospital: The main teaching hospital for the University and accordingly has most specialities.

Newcastle Mater Misericordiae Hospital

Edith Street, Waratah 2290, Newcastle, NSW, Australia Tel: (02) 4291 1211 Fax: (02) 4960 1197 www.newcastle.edu.au/department/md/htas

The hospital: The Newcastle Mater is a 192-bed public teaching hospital owned by the Sisters of Mercy (Singleton) and managed by Catholic Health Care. Operating under agreement with the Department of Health NSW through the Hunter Area Health Service, the Mater provides services to people of the Hunter Area and referring regions. Newcastle is a coastal city 160 km north of Sydney. There is easy access to beaches, lakes and vineyards. The surrounding economy is based on industry, mining and tourism.

Manly Hospital

Darley Road, Manley, NSW 2095, Australia Tel: (02) 9977 9611 Fax: (02) 9977 8907.

The hospital: A small district general hospital serving the northern beach towns and coastal commuter belt of north-east Sydney. It is three-quarters of a mile north of the town Ventremup. It's on a steep slope and has a magnificent view of Sydney Harbour. It was founded late last century and has been built up since. However, serious cases are referred to the Royal North Shore Hospital five miles away.

O **Elective notes:** By applying here you can do a number of specialities. They can also arrange general practice for you.

Broken Hill Base Hospital

PO Box 457, 174 Thomas Street, Broken Hill 2880, NSW, Australia Tel: (08) 8088 0333 Fax: (08) 8088 1715.

The hospital: In the outback of NSW, over 1000 km from Sydney with a half-hour time difference from the rest of the state. The nearest large town is Adelaide (five hours' drive away). Broken Hill ('Silver City') allegedly has a population of 27,000, but you may feel that most of them have gone away. The hospital has 100 beds. The town's claim to fame is that it appears in the film 'Priscilla, Queen of the Desert' – the hotel with the gaudy paintings actually exists. The hospital serves the Far West Health Region covering a vast area of desert and countryside (1½ times the size of the UK). It has one consultant surgeon and one consultant physician with the rest of the specialities being covered by visiting specialists from all over the state.

O Elective notes: You can do whatever you want, rotating from one week to the next. There is the opportunity to fly with the flying docs (if you're persistent) (this is where the Royal Flying Doctors are based). It's also worth going out into one of the outlying Aboriginal communities for a day or longer.

Accommodation: Approximately $70 (£35)/week and is in the nurse's home, where most people who work in the hospital live. Food is also provided cheaply from the canteen. It's very friendly and there's always something going on. Someone will have a car or if you talk to the right people you might be able to borrow a hospital car. There's lots of beer to drink. Sydney is 16–18 hours away by coach, two and a half-hours by plane. Things to do in the vicinity include: camel riding, go down a disused mine, visit Silverton (and go down active silver mines), visit Menindee caves, bush-camping . . . or do the local's favourite . . . sunset watching. You can go on the postal round with the postman for $230 (£115) – he flies to the different houses making 50–70 landings on his route.

Wagga Base Hospital

20 Docker Street, Wagga Wagga, NSW 2650, Australia.

The hospital: Wagga is actually the largest inland town in NSW and so is fairly busy. It's friendly but FREEZING COLD in the winter. The hospital is a fairly typical DGH.

O Elective notes: The medical students extradited there from Sydney consider it some sort of Siberia. The staff are friendly and the consultants keen to teach. It's great if you like skiing.

Overall advice: it's good, but if you're only visiting one place in Oz . . . try somewhere else.

Accommodation: Free and the town is nice, if unexciting.

Blue Mountains District Anzac Memorial Hospital

Locked Bag No 2, Katoomba, NSW 2780, Australia.

The hospital: Katoomba is a quiet town in the Blue Mountains, surrounded by stunning scenery and only two hours (109 km) by train ($10 (£5)) from Sydney. The hospital has 95 beds covering general surgery and medicine, paeds, O&G, care of the elderly and A&E. A&E receives from several towns and a very large area of National Park. It's mainly outdoor activity injuries (fractures etc.) that are seen. This is, however, a great place to go if you're the outdoors type with rock-climbing, caving, pot-holing and horse riding easily accessible.

Note: While the rest of Oz is in sunshine, this place is usually in mist. It is also home to many funnel web and red back spiders.

Accommodation: Free for students in the nurse's home, but is a bit run-down. It may be a bit lonely if you're on your own.

Manning Base Hospital

PO Box 35, Taree, NSW 2430, Australia.

The hospital: Manning Base Hospital is located in Taree, a 3 and a half hour drive north of Sydney just off the highway to Brisbane. The area is popular with tourists and the retired. Taree itself has a high unemployment rate and considerable social problems amongst the local Aboriginal cluster. The hospital has approximately 180 beds providing A&E, surgical, medical, paediatric, obstetric and gynaecological as well as psychiatric services.

O Elective notes: It does have a few medical students from Newcastle (Australia) present on their rural attachment. The staff are friendly, but there may be some lack of supervision for elective students and you may well find yourself out on a limb. There may be little opportunity to practise practical procedures. Transport here is limited, but the staff are friendly and will offer lifts. **Accommodation:** Available in the nurses' quarters for $60 (£30) per week.

OTHER HOSPITALS:

Auburn Hospital, Norval Street, Auburn 2144, NSW, Australia Tel: (02) 9563 9500 Fax: (02) 9563 9510.
Balmain Hospital, Booth Street, Balmain 2041, NSW, Australia Tel: (02) 9395 2111 Fax: (02) 9395 2119.
Bankstown Hospital, Eldridge Road, Bankstown 2200, NSW, Australia Tel: (02) 9722 8000 Fax: (02) 9722 8316.
Blacktown Hospital, Blacktown Road, Blacktown 2148, NSW, Australia Tel: (02) 9830 8000. Fax: (02) 9830 8020.
Canterbury Hospital, Canterbury Road, Campsie 2194, NSW, Australia Tel: (02) 9789 9111 Fax: (02) 9789 3450.
Cessnock District Hospital, View Street, Cessnock 2325, NSW, Australia Tel: (02) 4990 1166 Fax: (02) 4990 6113.
Gladesville Hospital, Victoria Road, Gladesville 2111, NSW, Australia Tel: (02) 9477 9123 Fax: (02) 9477 2005.
Hornsby Ku-Ring-Gai Hospital, Palmerston Road, Hornsby 2077, NSW, Australia Tel: (02) 9477 9123 Fax: (02) 9477 2005.
Lismore Base Hospital, 60 Uralba Street, Lismore 2480, NSW, Australia Tel: (02) 6621 8000 (02) 6621 708.
Orange Base Hospital, Sale Street, Orange 2800, NSW, Australia Tel: (02) 6362 1411 Fax: (02) 6362 0306.
Royal Womens Hospital, 188 Oxford Street, Paddington 2021, NSW, Australia Tel: (02) 9382 6111 Fax: (02) 9382 6513.
Rozelle Hospital, Cnr Church and Glover Streets, Leichardt 2040, NSW, Australia Tel: (02) 9556 9100 Fax: (02) 9818 5712.
Sutherland Hospital, 430 Kingsway Street, Caringbah 2299, NSW, Australia Tel: (02) 9540 7111 Fax: (02) 9540 7197.
Tamworth Base Hospital, Dean Street, Tamworth 2340, NSW, Australia Tel: (02) 6766 1722 Fax: (02) 6766 6638.

PRIVATE HOSPITALS:

Cape Hawke Community Private Hospital, Breckenridge Street, Forster 2428, NSW, Australia Tel: 61 65 546077 Fax: 61 65 558750 www.midcoast.com.au/prof/medical/hosp/chcph.html
Mayo Private Hospital, Potoroo Drive, Taree 2430, NSW, Australia Tel: 6165 521466 Fax: 6165 626759 www.midcoast.com.au/prof/medical/hosp/mayo/mayo.html
Sydney Adventist Hospital, 185 Fox Yalley Road, Wahroonga, NSW 2076, Australia Tel: 61 2 9487 91 Fax: 61 2 9487 92 www.sah.org.au/sahwelc.htm (The South Pacific flagship of the Seventh-day Adventist healthcare system. This operates a 324 bed unit.)
The Hills Private Hospital, 499 Windsor Road, Baulkham Hills 2153, NSW, Australia Tel: 639 3333 Fax: 639 5950 www.midcoast.com.au/prof/medical/hosp/hills.html

SOMETHING DIFFERENT:

The NSW Institute of Forensic Medicine

42–50 Parramatta Road, PO Box 90, Glebe, NSW 2037 Australia.

For some gruesome murders, appalling suicides (and the odd natural death) this can at least be described as an interesting elective. Not great for communication skills with patients. The chappy to contact is the Associate Professor, director of the NSW Institute of Forensic Medicine at the above address. Alternatively, write to the Electives Co-ordinator Dept of Clinical Education, Royal Prince Alfred Hospital, Missenden Road, Camperdown, NSW 2050, Australia.

VICTORIA

Melbourne

Melbourne is the 'culture capital' of Oz with great shops, restaurants and theatres. It is also the sports capital, being home to Aussie Rules football, Grand Prix and the tennis open. Travel around the city is easy and cheap. Beaches are a 45-minute tram ride from the centre (excellent transport system). Weather is hottest in January and February, but it can be unpredictable. Out of the city, things to do consist of: Coreal Ocean Road, Grampians National Park, Philip Island (see the penguins) and Yarra and Clare Valleys. There is also excellent skiing.

There are two universities in Victoria, one in Melbourne, the other in Clayton (20 km outside Melbourne).

University of Melbourne, Faculty of Medicine, University of Melbourne, Gratton Street, Parkville, VIC 3052, Australia www.unimelb.edu.au (This has three teaching hospitals.)
Monash University, The Faculty of Medicine, Monash University, Wellington Road, Clayton, VIC 3168, Australia (4145 beds) www.med.monash.edu.au

HOSPITALS IN MELBOURNE:

Royal Melbourne Hospital

132 Grattan Street, Parkville 3050, Melbourne, Australia Tel: (03) 9342 7031 Fax: (03) 9342 7802
www.medrmh.unimelb.edu.au/

The hospital: A large, busy inner-city hospital with several hundred beds and all specialities affiliated with the University of Melbourne.

O Elective notes: It's a very friendly place, at least for nephrology and vascular surgery, gastroenterology, endocrinology (mainly outpatients), neurology and cardiology and you can do as much or as little as you want. You won't be able to do general medicine, surgery, paeds or O&G as these are full with Aussie students. The staff are very keen for you to explore Australia. Not so good for practical skills as there are loads of other students around, but on the other hand, this makes the social life good. There are many lectures and tutorials for you to attend if you want. It's a 15-minute walk into the centre of Melbourne. Psychiatry has had some very good reports. You must apply to the Dean of the Clinical School, Royal Melbourne Hospital.

Accommodation: There is excellent accommodation for elective students at only A$ 11.50/week (contact the clinical school Charles Cornibere Residence). Swimming pool and sauna are in the residence; the University Gym is just a short walk away ($29 (£15)/month membership).

St Vincent's Hospital

41 Victoria Parade, Fitzroy 3065, Victoria, Australia Tel: (03) 8288 2211 Fax: (03) 9288 3399 www.medstu.unimelb.edu.au/

The hospital: Was founded in 1883 and is one of the three teaching hospitals in Melbourne. It is, however, modern and right in the city centre.

O Elective notes: The clinical school takes in 80 students per year who tend to be hard-working, but good fun. There is a high doctor to patient ratio and therefore the staff have plenty of time for teaching. In dermatology, like the rest of Oz, malignant melanomas are the hot topic. This hospital has often been thoroughly recommended.

Accommodation: The clinical school has its own building with 14 bedrooms and excellent facilities. It's $25 (£10)/week with free washing machine, drier, tea, coffee, cleaning lady, free local calls etc.

Royal Children's Hospital

(Affiliated with the Royal Women's Hospital) (University of Melbourne)
Flemington Road, Parkville, Melbourne, Victoria 3052, Australia Tel: (03) 9345 5522 (Switch) Fax: (03) 9345 5789
www.rch.unimelb.edu.au/

The hospital: A very busy tertiary referral centre (330 beds) and great if you're into paediatrics. It has all the rarities of a tertiary referral centre as well as the usually illnesses as it is the local children's hospital. Melbourne city centre (2 km away) is 30 minutes on foot, 10 minutes by tram.

O Elective notes: There are loads of students so it's good on social life but poor on practical skills. The teaching programme is excellent. You get into small tutorial groups ('tutes') and get regular lectures, quiz sessions and case presentations.

Accommodation: A flat for elective students just a short walk from the hospital. There are two bedrooms, each sleeping two plus a bathroom, kitchen and living room. Rent = $60 (£30). It's clean, but appliances have a habit of breaking. The hospital is famous for it's McDonalds in the foyer, but don't worry, there are plenty of good pubs and restaurants close by.

The accommodation only takes four and so it is important to apply early (a year in advance is advisable); however,

Australia

if it is full you can try Brookes Gillespie House (part of the University: Brookes Gillespie House, 740 Swanson Street, Carlton, Melbourne).

To apply here you can either contact the Elective Student Co-ordinator (and risk being charged an administration fee of $250 (£125)) or apply directly to one of the consultants.

Royal Women's Hospital

132 Grattan Street, Carlton, Victoria 3053, Australia Tel: (03) 9344 2000 Fax: (03) 9348 1840 www.rch.unimelb.edu.au

The hospital: A 400-bed obstetric, gynaecological and neonatal paediatric hospital. It is the largest Australian hospital specializing in women's and infant's health and is a major teaching hospital.

Monash University

The Faculty of Medicine, Monash University, Wellington Road, Clayton, VIC 3168, Australia www.med.monash.edu.au

Monash University is situated approximately 20 km outside Melbourne. It incorporates the Alfred and Box Hill Hospitals as well as the Monash Medical centre in Clayton.

The Alfred Hospital

PO Box 315, Commercial Road, Prahran, Victoria 3181, Australia Tel: (03) 9510 2000/2513 Fax: (03) 9276 2222.

The hospital: A 10-minute bus ride from the city centre. It's one of the big teaching hospitals in Melbourne. The Alfred has big research interests in trauma, intensive care, diving medicine and chest medicine. This wide range of interests means that there are many interesting patients to see. The main beach (St Kilda) is a 15-minute walk away.

O Elective notes: The consultants and registrars are friendly and keen to teach. They are also as keen for you to see Australia as you are.

Accommodation: Not always provided; however, some units will try there best to find you some cheaply.

Monash Medical Centre

246 Clayton Road, Clayton, Melbourne, Victoria 3168, Australia
www.mmcc.monash.edu.au/

The hospital: Is about 20 km outside Melbourne and accepts patients from the southern suburbs.

O Elective notes: For paediatrics at least it is very friendly, but can be quiet in the summer.

HOSPITALS IN COUNTRY VICTORIA:

The Austin Hospital

Studley Road, Heidelberg 3081 Victoria, Australia Tel: (03) 9496 5000 Fax: (03) 9458 4779 www.austin.unimeb.edu.au

The hospital: This is a well-advanced centre of excellence having a PET scanner, a liver transplant unit, cardiac surgery, neurosurgery, cardiology, neurology, endocrinology, oncology, GI and spinal injuries unit. There is a very good physiotherapy department. The psychiatry department sees a number of patients with PTSD from Vietnam. It is 10 km north-east of Melbourne.

O Elective notes: Very busy but the staff are keen to teach.

Accommodation: Provided on-site for around $20 (£10)/week with gym and pool.

The Bendigo Hospital

Lucan Street, PO Box 126, Bendigo, Victoria 3550, Australia

The hospital: Bendigo is an old gold mining town two hours north of Melbourne and a tourist destination in its own right. The hospital is a medium-sized DGH serving a large surrounding area. Bendigo itself is a lovely place. From here you can travel to Melbourne, the Great Ocean Road, Philip Island, Healesville, the Yarra Valley, the Dandenong Mountain range and Sydney for a long weekend.

O Elective notes: You can do A&E, medicine, surgery, orthopaedics, obstetrics and gynaecology or oncology. There are Aussie students there in term time. They and the other staff are all friendly.

The interns and registrars rotate from Melbourne, so there's always a bit of a party atmosphere as people come and go and its easy to get lifts to Melbourne. You can do as much/little as you wish. There is no fee to the hospital.
Accommodation: Cheap, $25 (£12)/ week in the nurses' home in the hospital.

Warrnambool and District Base Hospital

Ryot Street, Warrnambool, Victoria 3280, Australia Tel: (03) 5564 1666 Fax: (03) 5564 9660.
The hospital: Warrnambool is a small city on the south coast of Victoria towards the end of the Great Ocean Road (population 28,000). It's a relatively quiet, medium-sized hospital.
O Elective notes: There are few Aussie medical students so you can quickly become a member of the team and get doing practical skills. You can choose any speciality and the consultants are willing to teach, but there is no formal teaching. As you may expect, nightlife is fairly quiet, but there are plenty of good, cheap places to eat and drink. The local bay is good for swimming and surfing, but can get cold and windy in the winter.
Accommodation: In the nurses home opposite the hospital costing $50 (£25)/week. There's a decent canteen. Warrnambool is pretty remote, especially if you don't have a car. It's three hours from Melbourne, but it's easy to get to Great Ocean Road and the Grampians.

Mornington Peninsula Hospital/ Frankston Community Hospital

8–10 Hastings Road, Frankston, Victoria 3199, Australia Tel: (03) 9783 6077.
The hospital: A modestly sized acute general hospital with 344 beds of which 140 are surgical. There are four general surgeons in the professorial unit.

Geelong Hospital

Geelong, Victoria, Australia.
The hospital: A fairly small DGH one hour from Melbourne.
O Elective notes: There are no students there so you have free rein. It is very close to some famous surf beaches.

OTHER HOSPITALS IN VICTORIA:

Ballarat Base Hospital, Drummond Street, Ballarat 3350, Victoria, Australia Tel (03) 5320 4000 Fax: (03) 5333 1562.
Box Hill and District Hospital, Nelson Road, Box Hill 3128, Victoria, Australia Tel: (03) 9895 3333 Fax: (03) 9895 3176 www.boxhill.org.au/boxhill
Caufield Hospital, 260 Kooyong Road, Caufield 3162, Victoria, Australia Tel (03) 9276 6000.
Dandenong and District Hospital, David Street, Dandenong 3175. Victoria, Australia Tel: (03) 9791 6000 Fax: (03) 979 5709.
Fairfield Hospital, Yarra Bend Road, Fairfield 3078, Victoria, Australia Tel (03) 9345 5522. Fax: (03) 9482 6572.
Frankston Community Hospital, 8–10 Hastings Road, Frankston, Victoria 3199, Australia Tel: (03) 9783 6077.
Goulburn Valley Base Hospital, Shepparton, Victoria 3630, Australia.
Mildura Base Hospital, Thirteenth Street, Mildura 3500, Victoria, Australia Tel: (03) 5022 3333 Fax: (03) 5023 3470.
Peter MacCallum Cancer Clinic, 481 Little Lonsdale Street, Melbourne, Victoria 3000, Australia Tel: (03) 9641 5555.
Preston and Northcote Community Hospital, 205 Bell Street, Preston 3072, Australia Tel (03) 9285 2222 Fax: (03) 9487 2524.
Repatriation General Hospital, Heidelberg, Banksia St West, Heidelberg 3081, Victoria, Australia Tel (03) 9496 2111 Fax: (03) 9862 3658.
St George's Hospital, 283 Cotham Road, Kew, Victoria 3101, Australia Tel: (03) 9272 0444.
Tallangatta Hospital, Tallangatta, Victoria 3700, Australia.
The Melbourne Clinic, 130 Church Street, Richmond, Victoria 3121, Australia Tel: (03) 9429 4688.
Wangaratta District Base Hospital, Green Street, Wangaratta 3677, Victoria, Australia Tel: (03) 5722 0111 Fax: (03) 5722 0105.
Western Hospital, Gordon Street, Footscray 3011, Victoria, Australia Tel (03) 9319 6666 Fax: (03) 9317 7815.
Wimmera Base Hospital, Baillie Street, Horsham 3400, Victoria, Australia Tel (03) 5381 911 Fax: (03) 5382 0829).

SOMETHING DIFFERENT:

Victorian Institute of Forensic Medicine

Kavanagh Street, Southbank, Melbourne, Victoria, Australia Tel: 613 9684 4444.
For those wishing to study forensic/coronial services, contact the Professor at the above address. They expect a small project to be done while you're there.
Accommodation: Sometimes provided, if not there are plenty of youth hostels in central Melbourne.

SOUTH AUSTRALIA

Adelaide

Although considered by many to be more of a 'country town' than a city, Adelaide has wonderful beaches, wines and a good music scene. It's not usually on the tourist route and hence is not so often visited on electives. This is a good place to go however if you've 'done' Australia before and want to work in a very friendly major teaching hospital.

There are two universities in South Australia, both in Adelaide.

Adelaide

The Medical School, University of Adelaide, Frome Road, Adelaide, South Australia 5000 (2179 beds).

Flinders University

The School of Medicine, The Flinders University of South Australia, Bedford Park, South Australia 5042 (775 beds).

The Royal Adelaide Hospital

North Terrace, Adelaide 5000, South Australia Tel: (08) 8222 4000 Fax: (08) 8223 4761.

The hospital: A very friendly major hospital. You can walk to the city centre in two minutes and it's surrounded by Botanical Gardens and parks. It is a centre for diving medicine and a world centre for training in baromedicine. The hospital itself came from humble backgrounds. It started as the Colonial Infirmary in 1837. Three of its four patients died. It is now one of Australia's largest teaching hospitals.

O Elective notes: There is high-quality teaching in both medicine and surgery. Great if you're a bit of a diver. As an elective student you are given a great deal of responsibility.

Accommodation: A$22 (£11)/ week in the nurses' home.

Adelaide Women and Children's Hospital

72 King William Road, North Adelaide 5006, South Australia Tel: (08) 8204 7000 Fax: (08) 8239 0417 www.wch.sa.gov.au/

The hospital: A major hospital providing extensive services both within the hospital and on rural outreach clinics. Departments include cardiology, child development, endocrine and diabetes, gastroenterology, neurology, oncology, orthopaedic, paediatric intensive care and renal. They are currently developing Telehealth services to facilitate videoconferencing to the rural and remote areas.

Flinders Medical Centre

Bedford Park, Adelaide, South Australia 5042 Tel: 00618 204 5511 Fax: 00618 204 5450 www.flinders.sa.gov.au

The hospital: Being a teaching hospital for the Flinders University nearly all specialities are catered for. This 430-bed hospital is superb for Accident and Emergency. It has a very modern A&E department with a CT scanner next door. The hospital itself is outside the city centre, but buses are cheap. It allegedly has a better working atmosphere than the Royal Adelaide.

O Elective notes: There's lots of teaching and responsibility. Many opportunities to do practical procedures such as suturing. Aussie medical students actually go here to do their electives. There are many things to do: Kangaroo Island, many wineries (Coonawwarra, Clare, McLaren, Barossa Valleys . . . one-hour drive).

Accommodation: Can be arranged within the hospital.

HOSPITALS OUTSIDE ADELAIDE:

Pika Wiya Health Service

PO Box 2021 Port Augusta 5700, South Australia.

The hospital: In the outback of South Australia 200–300 km north of Adelaide. Its population is about 17,000 with a large Aboriginal community. Pika Wiya is a health service specifically for Aboriginal people and is run in general practice style. There is an 80-bed hospital, however, but no resident doctors, so the Pika Wiya doctors have to cover that too. Clinics are in Port Augusta and Davenport, both giving lots of hands on medicine.

O Elective notes: Spend time with the child health service and paediatrician as both go out into the local communities giving real experience of Aboriginal life. The flying doctors in Port Augusta are willing to take students up, so there's even more opportunity to get to meet real Australians.

Accommodation: In Port Augusta. The social life is not as bad as you may think. People are often happy to lend you a car or give you a lift and there is often the odd student from Adelaide. You must visit the nearby Flinders Mountain Range. Warning: You may get lonely.

OTHER HOSPITALS IN SOUTH AUSTRALIA:

Mount Gambier Hospital Inc, Lake Terrace West, Mount Gambier 5290, South Australia Tel (08) 8724 2211 Fax: (08) 8723 0008.
Queen Elizabeth Hospital, Woodville Road, Woodville 5011, South Australia Tel: (08) 8222 6000 Fax: (08) 8222 6010.
Queen Victoria Hospital, 160 Fullerton Road, Rose Park 5067, South Australia Tel (08) 8332 4888 Fax: (08) 8333 9171.
Whyalla Hospital, Wood Terrace, Whyalla 5600, South Australia Tel (08) 8645 8300 Fax: (08) 8645 3007.

QUEENSLAND

Brisbane

(Population: 1.4 million, Australia's third-largest city) Brisbane is a relaxed city, 25 km upstream from the mouth of the Brisbane River with many places to eat, drink and watch sport. It has good weather and there are loads of things to do on the 1240 miles of Queensland coast: Fraser Island, Byron Bay, Surfer's Paradise, Whitsunday Islands, the sunshine coast and the Great Barrier Reef. Magnetic Island is a good place to try jet-skiing at a reasonable price and for white water rafting try the Tully River at Mission Beach. If you're in Cairns for a day and have a sense of humour try 'Uncle Brian's Fun, Falls and Forest' Day Trip. Around Brisbane itself are the beautiful Hinterlands, superb for those interested in bush walking or mountaineering (but remember Australia has eight of the world's ten most poisonous snakes!). September to October is a good time to visit as the weather is starting to get hot but box jellyfish are not yet out so it's safe to swim in the sea. Despite Australia's 'Slip, Slap, Slop' policy, malignant melanomas and other skin conditions are still highly prevalent. Brisbane has become the skin capital of the world. Therefore dermatology and skin surgery are good specialities here. Expect loads of hassle if you turn up in the melanoma clinic with a tan.

To do your elective anywhere in Queensland you **must** apply to The Postgraduate Medical Education Foundation of Queensland Ltd, Medical School, Herston Road, Herston Q4006 Australia Tel: 61 7 3365 5047 Fax: 61 7 3365 5036 www.medicine.uq.edu.au/elective.htm

Apply **at least six months in advance** and pay £75 ($150) administration fee. They can then place you somewhere in Queensland (the earlier you apply, the more chance you will get your first choice). Also request accommodation at this time. The University of Queensland can then levy further charges (which can be pretty steep, up to $700 (£350) for four weeks).

Again, as in the case for Sydney, you can put yourself at an advantage by writing to your desired destination before writing to the Postgraduate Medical Education Foundation. It's much better to say that 'Dr "X" from "Y" hospital has said he would be delighted to have me do an elective in his department.'

The Royal Brisbane Hospital

Herston Road, Herston 4006, Brisbane, Queensland, Australia Tel: (07) 3253 8111 Fax: (07) 3857 4462
www.medicine.uq.edu.au/RBH/hospital.htm

The hospital: A large (800-bed, 500,000 admissions/year) hospital 15-minute bus ride (two miles) from the city centre. It is right next to the Queensland Medical School on the northern side of Brisbane and shares its campus with the Royal Children's Hospital, Royal Women's Hospital and the Queensland Institute of Medical Research. All specialities are covered bar cardiology and transplant surgery, which are covered at the Prince Charles hospital.

O Elective notes: There is a laid back, welcoming attitude but also excellent teaching with a library and computer lab onsite which you are free to use. Units such as gastroenterology may be a bit too specialized and you learn nothing. It's a 25-min walk to the city centre, 20-min bus ride to the airport. If you want to travel Oz, this is a good start as the Greyhound bus stops at the front gates and the staff are keen that you explore.

Note: This is a popular place, so make enquires early.

Accommodation: Lady Lamington Home Nurses Quarter is quaint ($70 (£35)/week = $11.50 (£5.75)/night; prices may well be going up, however) and there's a swimming pool and gym for residents. The canteen's not great, but it's only five minutes' walk to the food store in Fortitude Valley.

The Royal Children's Hospital Brisbane

Herston Road, Herston 4006, Brisbane, Queensland, Australia Tel: (07) 3253 8111 Fax: (07) 3857 4462

The hospital: Part of a site of three hospitals situated in the Herston area of Brisbane (the other two being the Royal Brisbane and the Royal Women's Hospital). Each year the RCH admits 16,000 children to its wards, sees 18,000 children in A&E, sees 99,800 outpatients and has 3600 admissions for cancer. The 168 beds comprise 12 for transplants, 24 for neurosurgery and 20 neonatal beds.

Accommodation: In the nurses' home. It's comfortable and cheap ($10 (£5)/night). It's friendly as all elective students stay here (note, think about the Mater if you're staying some time as that's free).

The Mater Misericordiae Hospital

Raymond Terrace, South Brisbane 4101, Queensland, Australia Tel: (07) 3840 8111/8518 Fax: (07) 3840 3846/1548
www.medicine.uq.edu.au/Mater/default.htm

The hospital: The Mater Hospital is one of Brisbane's teaching hospitals. Located on the South Bank of Brisbane, it's within walking distance of the city centre (20 minutes).

O Elective notes: As an elective student you are attached to a group of finalists and therefore you get some excellent teaching and opportunities to do minor procedures. There are also X-ray and pathology meetings, but not much ward-based activity.

Accommodation: Provided free to students by the hospital, although kitchen facilities are poor. You can buy meal tickets for the canteen.

Mater Children's Hospital

Department of Paediatrics and Child Health, South Brisbane, Queensland 4101, Australia (part of the Mater Misericordiae Hospitals).

The hospital: Fairly large and good for developing skills in examining and assessing children. Neonatology, Accident and Emergency, general paediatrics and child psychiatry (mainly emotional and behavioural disorders) departments have all been praised. The paediatrics is very similar to that in any Western hospital. It's close to the city centre, so there's plenty to do in your time off.

Accommodation: Free to students and has a pool. There's a manmade beach nearby.

Princess Alexandra Hospital

Ipswich Road, Woolloongabba 4102, Brisbane, Australia Tel: (07) 3240 2111/5346 Fax: (07) 3240 2420/5399
www.uq.edu.au/~mddricha/index.html,
www.medicine.uq.edu.au/PA/default.htm

The hospital: A large (900-bed), modern general hospital (tertiary referral) on the south side of the Brisbane river. It covers all major adult specialities with the exception of cardiac surgery. It is nationally recognized for spinal injuries and solid organ transplant. It is affiliated with the University of Queensland and sees 60,000 inpatients a year. The hospital is a couple of miles from the city centre, a 10–20-minute train ride from the nearby station (500 yards). There are many job opportunities for doctors, radiographers and nurses. Check their web site for the latest.

O Elective notes: The doctors are friendly and enthusiastic, with a realistic attitude to the amount of work that you should do! Ward rounds on the general surgery side start at 7.30 am, but the accommodation is only two minutes from the ward. There is a large hepatobiliary department and there's the opportunity to assist in liver and kidney transplants. For orthopaedics there are ten consultants, each with their own special interest. There are many motorcyclists in Queensland, so this tends to be a busy department. This elective comes well-recommended.

Accommodation: $11 (£5.50)/night in the nurses' home (Diamantina House) with good facilities, including a 25-metre outdoor swimming pool. Other sports facilities are available at the St Lucia campus of Queensland University a 10-minute walk and five-minute ferry ride across the Brisbane River. There are regular 'kegs' (free beer nights) for doctors and medical students.

HOSPITALS OUTSIDE BRISBANE:

Townsville General Hospital

Eyre Street Townsville 4810, Queensland, Australia Tel: 61 77 819 368 or (07) 4781 9211 Fax: 61 77 819 649 or (07) 4772 1373
www.medicine.uq.edu.au/TownsV/default.htm

The hospital: A large modern(ish) hospital with many specialist departments. It's even more relaxed than many other Aussie hospitals allowing you to do what you want at a slightly slower pace. Not that much to do in Townsville, but Magnetic Island is only 15 minutes away by ferry. This is a lovely island and offers some of the best diving in Australia ... the courses are pretty cheap here as well.

Accommodation: Basic, but in the hospital grounds and not expensive.

Gladstone Hospital

PO Box 299, Gladstone, Queensland 4680, Australia.

The hospital: A small hospital in a rather bleak looking industrial town. There are only nine doctors, but many visiting consultants. It is busy and the doctors are keen for you to do practical procedures, minor ops and suturing. The staff are friendly.

Accommodation: Free in the (condemned!) but quaint nurses' home. The canteen varies in standard.

Mackay Base Hospital

Bridge Road, Mackay, Queensland Q4740, Australia

The hospital: Mackay is a small town in north Queensland. The MBH is a 220-bed, very busy, sociable hospital. There are usually about 12 students present (mostly Australian). This is a popular hospital for British doctors on a 'working holiday' and so the social life is very good.

O Elective notes: A&E has a quite a reasonable turnover and they are keen for you to do minor surgery and suturing. General medicine, ICU and CCU have also been very popular with previous visitors. They are a bit more serious about attendance than other Australian hospitals, but are keen to teach. The town has a number of pubs and clubs and is very pretty. However, note that public transport is very limited so you have to rely on (expensive) taxis to get about. If you can borrow a car you're only two hours from Airlie Beach opening the gateway to the Whitsunday Islands and Barrier Reef. The Eungella National Park is fairly close to town.

Accommodation: Free and in the newly renovated nurses' home. There is a swimming pool outside the quarters with palm trees and BBQ. The food in the canteen is expensive and not great, so most people cook in the quarters. The Aussie students live there too, so social life is good.

Gold Coast Hospital

108 Nerang Street, Southport QLD 4215, Australia

The hospital: Gold Coast Hospital is a teaching hospital about 70 km south of Brisbane in a very popular holiday strip of Queensland. It has recently undergone some major improvement. It provides all major specialities except cardiothoracic surgery, radiotherapy and burns. There are a number of UK doctors working throughout the hospital. A&E is busy and an excellent experience if you get stuck in. There are many surfing injuries as the Gold Coast is otherwise known as surfer's paradise.

O Elective notes: If there when Queensland students are on holiday (e.g. September/October) you'll get more experience (but less lectures); however, make sure you spend some time in A&E or it can get a bit boring. If the students are around, you are welcome to go to their teaching. The respiratory department has been popular with time off to explore the local areas. The Gold Coast is well suited for exploring the eastern coastline of Oz. There's loads to do and plenty of night-life. The beach is a 20-minute walk away.

Accommodation: In the nurses' quarters costs $19.50 (£12)/week and there's a swimming pool.

Bundaberg Base Hospital

Bourbong Street, Bundaberg 4670, Queensland, Australia Tel: (07) 4152 0222 Fax: (07) 4173 1779.

The hospital: Bundaberg is a coastal town of 32,000. Its main industry is sugar cane farming, mainly for the production of Bundaberg rum. The hospital is friendly and laid back, many of the doctors being British. If doing A&E, quite a few of the injuries are work-related.

Accommodation: In the hospital with the other doctors. Bundaberg is the cheapest place in Queensland to do a scuba diving course and there is easy access to the coral Whitsunday Islands and Fraser Island.

Rockhampton Base Hospital

Canning Street, Rockhampton 4700, Queensland, Australia Tel: (07)4931 6211.

The hospital: Rockhampton is a mining community and the beef capital of Australia, just inland of the south Queensland coast. The hospital is friendly and the medics are keen to teach. There are many lunch time tutorials (and free lunch). Many of the docs are Brits. There's little to do in Rockhampton itself so you have to rely on the interns for social life.

Accommodation: Basic but only $60 (£30)/week. There is a swimming pool and tennis court on-site.

Cairns Base Hospital

The Esplanade, Cairns, North Queensland, Australia.

The hospital: Currently undergoing renovation. A&E has four major trauma beds, eight minor cubicles and a four-bed obs ward. The usual trauma, ODs etc. are common, but there are also box jellyfish stings, snake bites and barotrauma in local divers. Not wildly busy though. There is the occasional bit of tropical medicine to see and quite a bit of diabetes. Outreach clincs are run (by plane) into the bush.

O Elective notes: It's a good place for the Barrier Reef but the weather is unpredictable and there's no beach nearby (10 mins by car). It is organized through the University of Queensland and there is a $150 (£75) fee.

Accommodation: Not at present, but may change.

Toowoomba Base Hospital

Private Mailbag No 2, Toowoomba, Queensland 4350, Australia Tel: (076) 316 310 Fax: (076) 391 098.

The hospital: 100 km west of Brisbane in Toowoomba (80,000). It is on a plateau that defines the Darling Downs.

The Hospital has 485 beds serving the 500,000 people between Queensland's border and the eastern Darling Downs. It has general medicine and surgery, orthopaedics, O&G, paeds, anaesthetics, psychiatry and A&E services.

❍ **Elective notes:** They are very keen to have students.

OTHER HOSPITALS IN QUEENSLAND:

Ipswich Hospital, East Street, Ipswich 4305, Queensland, Australia Tel (07) 3810 1111 Fax: (07) 3812 1419.
Maryborough General Hospital, 185 Walker Street, Maryborough 4650, Queensland, Australia Tel: (07) 4123 8222 Fax: (07) 4123 1606.
Repatriation General Hospital, Newdegate Street, Greenslopes 4120, Queensland, Australia Tel (07) 3394 7111 Fax: (07) 3394 7745.
Royal Women's Hospital, Bowen Bridge Road, Herston 4006, Queensland, Australia Tel (07) 3253 8111 Fax: (07) 3857 4462.

PRIVATE HOSPITALS:

Greenslopes Private Hospital, Newdegate Street, Greenslopes, Queensland, Australia Tel: 61 7 3394 7284 Fax: 61 7 3394 7789.
Park Haven Private Hospital, 9–13 Bayswater Road, Hyde Park, Queensland 4812, Locked Bag 913, TMC Townsville, Queensland 4810, Australia Tel: 61 7 422 8822 Fax: 61 7 4721 3365.
www.parkhaven.com.au

WESTERN AUSTRALIA

Larger than western Europe, Western Australia exports 60% of Australia's gold, 11% of the world's iron ore and has Perth as its capital.

Perth

(Population just over one million). Perth is Australia's fourth-largest and most isolated city. It is clean with plenty to do: try sandsurfing, take a day trip to Rottnest Island, taste wine in Swan Valley and camel ride through the Bush. There are heaps of good pubs and clubs in Perth and the weather is extremely pleasant even in the winter. South of Perth you have the Margaret River area, home to some of Oz's finest wines, limestone caves and surf. The town of Augusta has whale-watching cruises during the season and at Pemberton you can climb one of the tallest trees in the world (the Gloucester Tree at 61 m high).

There is one University in Western Australia.

University of Western Australia

The School of Medicine, University of Western Australia, Perth, WA 6000. Another address is University of WA, QEII Medical Centre, Nedlands WA 6907 Tel: (08) 9346 2316. Currently the elective fee is around A$250 (£125).

Royal Perth Hospital

Wellington Street/Box 2213, Perth 6000, WA Tel: (08) 9224 2244 Fax: (08) 92243511
www.rph.wa.gov.au/

The hospital: Claims to be Western Australia's premier teaching hospital located at the city centre. Its history traces back to the first colonial hospital in a tent on Garden Island in June 1829. Today, the 955-bed hospital seeing 67,000 admissions a year is on two separate sites, in Wellington Street in the City of Perth and at Shenton Park 8 km away (Royal Perth Hospital, Selby Street, Shenton Park 6008 Tel: (08) 9224 2244 Fax (08) 9224 3511). It is also associated with the Royal Perth Rehabilitation Hospital (address below). Services include: emergency services, coronary angioplasy, cardiothoracic surgery, stroke treatment, bone marrow transplantation, immundeficiency diseases, interventional neuro-radiology, burns treatment, plastics and max-fax, rehab and a spinal unit.

❍ **Elective notes:** General medicine is a friendly department and you are encouraged to attend ward rounds and outpatient clinics. All in all … fairly laid back. Good teaching and the grand round has a free lunch. An elective here is arranged through the University of Western Australia. Beaches and night-life are nearby.

There are some wonderful nursing opportunities here.

Accommodation: Provided at the hospital ($50 (£25)/week) for a room (a/c), lounge and kitchen.

Sir Charles Gardiner Hospital (Queen Elizabeth II Medical Centre)

Verdun Street, Nedlands 6009, Perth, Western Australia Tel: (08) 9346 3333 Fax: (08) 9389 2534.

The hospital: A large, modern teaching hospital in the suburbs of Perth. Both general medicine and surgery are reported to be very friendly and well-organized and there is a newly refurbished A&E. The hospital is a short bus ride (about an hour's walk) from the city centre.

O **Elective notes:** The department of respiratory medicine offers good opportunities to specialize and do projects if you wish. In A&E you'll get one red back spider/scorpion bite a day. It's a good place to get procedures under your belt. The staff are keen for you to go off and explore Oz.

Accommodation: Pretty basic (in Anstey House) and only $60 (£30)/week with overseas doctors, nurses and other students. The hospital is very close to King's Park which has walks through natural bushland and great barbecuing facilities. The University of Western Australia (very picturesque) is about 10 minutes' walk away and has an excellent gym. At night during the summer months an open-air cinema is also put on here. The beaches are accessible by bus. Some students have found they can't use the computers and there aren't many pubs nearby.

Princess Margaret Children's Hospital

Roberts Road, Subiaco 6009, Perth, Western Australia Tel: (08) 9340 8222 Fax: (08) 940 8111.

The hospital: The Princess Margaret is a pleasant, friendly place, reasonably busy and the only specialized paediatric hospital in Western Australia The paediatrics is fairly similar to that of the UK, with the exception of aboriginal children who are often flown in from the communities. The hospital is in one of the nicest areas of Perth and is not far from the city centre.

O **Elective notes:** There are fifth- and sixty-year students on attachment and elective students are free to join any of their teaching.

Accommodation: None at the PMH, but it is provided at the Charles Gardiner Hospital a short bus journey away. The PMH have a good doctor's room with a pool table and free muffins every day.

Freemantle General Hospital

Alma Street, Freemantle 6160, Perth, Western Australia. Tel: (08) 9431 3333.

The hospital: A modern hospital, relaxed and friendly in a suburb of Perth. The Professorial unit is great if you're after intensive medicine followed by intensive relaxation.

OTHER HOSPITALS IN WESTERN AUSTRALIA:

Armadale–Kelmscott Memorial Hospital, Albany Highway, Armadale 6112 WA Tel: 08 9391 2000.
Bentley Health Service, Bentley Hospital, Mills Street, Bentley 6102, WA Tel: 08 9334 3666.
Graylands Hospital, Brockway Road, Mt Claremount 6010, WA Tel: 08 9347 6600.
Hawthorn Hospital, 100 Flinders Street, Mt Hawthorn 6016, WA Tel: 08 9444 8166.
Joondalup Health Campus, Shenton Avenue, Joondalup 6027, WA. Tel: 08 9405 2211.
Kalamunda District Community Hospital, Elizabeth Street, Kalamunda 6076, WA Tel: 08 9293 2122.
King Edward Memorial Hospital for Women, Bagot Road, Subiaco 6008, WA Tel: 08 9340 2222.
La Salle Hospital, Eveline Road, Middle Swan 6056, WA Tel: 08 9347 5500.
Lemnos Hospital, Selby Street, Shenton Park 6008, WA Tel: 08 9382 0760.
Mt Henry Hospital, Cloister Avenue, Como 6152, WA Tel: 08 9313 1555 Fax: 00618 9450 1036.
Osbourne Park Hospital, Osbourne Place, Stirling 6021, WA Tel: 08 9346 8000.
Perth Dental Hospital, 196 Goderich, Perth 6000, WA Tel: 08 9220 5777.

Repatriation General Hospital, Hollywood, Monash Avenue, Nedlands 6009, WA Tel (08) 9346 6000 Fax: (08) 9386 3153.
Rockingham–Kwinana District Hospital, Elanora Drive, Rockingham 6168, WA Tel: 08 9527 2777
Royal Perth Rehabilitation Hospital, Selby Street, Shenton Park 6008, WA Tel: 08 9382 7171.
Swan District Hospital, Eveline Road, Middle Swan 6056, WA Tel: 08 9347 244.
Woodside Maternity Hospital, 18 Dalgety, Fremantle 6160, WA Tel: 08 9339 1788.
Wooroloo Hospital, Linley Valley Road, Wooroloo 6558, WA Tel: 08 9573 1228.

PRIVATE HOSPITALS IN WESTERN AUSTRALIA:
Attadale Hospital, 21 Hislop Road, Attadale 6156, WA Tel: 08 9330 1000.
Bethesda Hospital Inc, 25 Queenslea Drive, Claremont 6010, WA Tel: 00618 9340 6300.
Bicton Hospital, 220 Preston Point Road, Bicton 6157, WA Tel: 08 9339 1133.
Colin Street Day Surgery, 51 Colin Street, West Perth 6005, WA Tel: 08 9321 4256.
Freemantle Kaleeya Hospital, Staton Road, East Fremantle 6158, WA Tel: 08 9339 1655.
Glengarry Hospital, 53 Arnisdale Road, Duncraig 6023, WA Tel: 08 9447 0111.
Gosnells Family Hospital, 2 Hamilton Court, Gosnells 6110, WA Tel: 08 9490 1333.
Hollywood Private Hospital, Monash Avenue, WA 6009, Perth, WA Tel: 00618 9346 6000.
Mercy Hospital, Thirlmere Road, Mt Lawley 6050, WA.
Mount Hospital, 150 Mounts Bay Road, Perth 6000, WA Tel: 08 9480 1822.
Mount Lawley Private Hospital, 14 Alvan, Mount Lawley 6050, WA Tel: 08 9370 2500.
Niola Private Hospital, 61–69 Cambridge, Leederville 6007, WA Tel: 08 9380 1833.
Perth Surgicentre, 38 Ranelagh Cresent, South Perth 6151, WA. Tel: 08 9367 4322.
South Perth Community Hospital Inc, South Terrace, Como 6152, WA Tel: 08 9367 7966.
St John of God Hospital Murdoch, 100 Murdoch Drive, Murdoch 6150, WA.
St John of God Hospital Subiaco, 175 Cambridge, Subiaco 6008, WA Tel: 08 9382 6111 Fax: 08 9381 7180.
Stirling Community Hospital, 32 Spencer Avenue, Yokine 6060, WA Tel: 08 9276 5244.
Undercliffe Hospital Complex, 20 Coogan Avenue, Greenmount 6056, WA Tel: 08 9294 1211.

Australia

USEFUL ADDRESSES:

Avon Health Service combining Northam Regional Hospital (a 40-bed unit) Robinson Street, Northam, WA 6401 Tel: (08) 96901300 Fax: (08) 96901319; York District Hospital (a 12-bed unit), Trews Road, York, WA 6302 Tel: (08)96411200 Fax: (08)96411706; Avon Community Heath, 222 Fitzgerald Street, Northam, WA 6401 Tel: (08) 96225080 Fax: (08) 96222734 www.avon.net.au/~health/

Health Department of Western Australia, 189 Royal Street, East Perth, WA 6004.
The Government of Western Australia, European Office, 5th Floor, Australia Centre, Corner of Strand and Melbourne Place, London WC2B 4LG, UK Tel: 020 7240 2881 Fax: 020 7240 6637 e-mail agent_general@wago.co.uk

NORTHERN TERRITORY

Royal Darwin Hospital

Rocklands Drive, Casuarina 0810, NT, Australia Tel (08) 8922 8888 Fax: (08) 8920 8286.

The hospital: The hospital has 300 beds and is a teaching hospital of Flinders University. Twenty-five per cent of the population is Aboriginal. It is close (300 km) to Kakadu National Park World Heritage Area. There are many Aboriginal settlements.

○ Elective notes: It's a very relaxed and friendly lifestyle. Darwin's population is about 60,000 so there is plenty to do.

Alice Springs Hospital

Gap Road/ PO Box 2234, Alice Springs 0870, NT, Australia Tel: (08) 8951 7777 Fax: (08) 8952 2712.

The hospital: Has just under 200 beds and departments, including paediatrics, obstetrics and gynaecology, surgery, medicine, A&E, psychiatry and anaesthetics. Half the patients are Aboriginal. On the paediatrics wards you'll see lots of gastroenteritis, pneumonia and failure to thrive. There is also a flying doctors base. The A&E is very busy especially on a Friday night.

○ Elective notes: Doctors are friendly and encourage you to do practical procedures (especially in A&E) and take long weekends to explore Ayers Rock, Kings Canyon and Western MacDonnells. They are good teachers. The town has shops, banks restaurants etc. but is by no means big.

Note: Apply well in advance if you want to go.

Accommodation: Previously a problem, now it is free and very good.

Tennant Creek Hospital
PO Box 346, Tennant Creek, NT 0861, Australia Tel: (08) 89 62 3132 Fax: (08) 89 62 4399.

Tenant Creek is 12-hour bus ride from Darwin and many would ask why the hell go there. Tennant Creek has the dubious claim to fame of being one of the few towns in the world with a population of 3500 to appear on most world maps. This is because it's the only real settlement between Darwin and Alice Springs. It's half way between the two and (according to unreliable Australian legend) was founded when a beer wagon bound for one of the local telegraph stations broke down. This attracted others, but as the golden liquid began to dry up they had to explore the area around. One lucky chap discovered a different type of golden stuff and even more people came in. It became a gold mining town and to this day there are still two gold mines which provide most of the employment. The town also provides the administration centre for the Barkley region (about the size of England), and a supply centre for many of the cattle stations and Aboriginal settlements in this region.

The hospital: Serves an area about the size of England and has just over 20 beds (12 general medical, four paeds and four obs and gynae) and they are always full. There are usually four doctors: the medical superintendent, two district medical officers (running bush clinics and most of the patient management in the hospital) and a resident medical officer on eight weeks' rotation from Alice Springs (running A&E and some bush clinics). There's a one-man path lab, a radiographer and a community care team (doing immunizations, screening and health awareness programmes (HIV, DM and skin cancer) in the Bush. There is a six-seater air ambulance that can transport patients from the settlements in the Barkley region to either Tennant Creek or Alice Springs. There's one GP in the town.

❍ **Elective notes:** There are many great experiences to be had, A&E, ward work and frequent clinics, either reached by many days 4WD cross-country driving or flying. These clinics give excellent insight into Aboriginal life and health as well as being amazingly sociable and relaxing. Contact the superintendent to organize this. Don't give up (fax), it's a great elective.

OTHER HOSPITALS IN NORTHERN TERRITORY:

Katherine Hospital
Gorge Road, Katherine 0850, NT, Australia Tel: (08) 8973 9211 Fax: (08) 8973 9375.

Australia

AUSTRALIAN CAPITAL TERRITORY (ACT)

Canberra

The Canberra Clinical School
Canberra, ACT Tel: (02) 6244 3649
Fax: (02) 6281 5616.
http://xray.anu.edu.au/hospital/clinsch

The Canberra Clinical School is affiliated with the University of Sydney and is a popular destination for elective students from Europe, Japan, Canada, New Zealand and Australia itself.

Elective students can attend a maximum limit of eight weeks (contact the University of Sydney). There is the University enrolment fee of $100 (£50) (covering insurance and other costs) and an administration fee of $300 (£150) for elective periods of up to four weeks, and $500 (£250) for elective periods of 4–8 weeks. These fees are payable to the Canberra Clinical School before arrival.

To apply, write stating which discipline you prefer to The Elective Officer at the clinical school.

The Canberra Hospital (The Woden Valley Hospital)
Yamba Drive, Garran 2605, Canberra ACT
Tel: (02) 6244 2930 Fax: (02) 6281 3935
http://xry.anu.edu.au/fhospital.html

The hospital: A large teaching hospital with 500 beds in the centre of Canberra (population 300,000). It's three hours to snowfields, beaches and outback Australia. It's a friendly, cosmopolitan, political city (and the National Capital). The hospital itself is a little isolated, 20 minutes' walk to the shopping centre.

O Elective notes: An elective with the cardiothoracic or neurosurgery unit comes thoroughly recommended. Plenty of time for sightseeing. The staff and other students are friendly and welcoming. The electives officer is very efficient.

Accommodation: On-site in the Canberra Hospital at a cost of $4.70 (£2.50) per night (student rate), with a redeemable bond of $50 (£25) to be paid on arrival together with two weeks' rent payable in advance. There's a pool for residents.

Australia

OTHER HOSPITALS IN ACT:

Calvary Public Hospital, Haydon Drive, Bruce, 2617, ACT Tel (02) 6201 6111 Fax (02) 6252 9201.
Jindalee Nursing Home, Goyder Street, Narrabundah 2604, ACT Tel (02) 6295 5511 Fax. (02) 6239 6686.

TASMANIA

Tasmania is a large island off the south coast of Australia. It offers some spectacular scenery and diving.

University of Tasmania

The Faculty of Medicine, University of Tasmania, 43 Collins Street, Hobart, TAS 7000.

HOSPITALS IN TASMANIA:

Douglas Parker Rehabilitation Centre, 31 Tower Road, Newtown, Hobart 7008, TAS Tel: (03) 6228 1801 Fax: (03) 6278 1373.
Launceston General Hospital, Charles Street, Launceston 7250, TAS Tel: (03) 6332 7111 Fax: (03) 6332 7018.
Queen Victoria Hospital (Maternity), Charles Street, Launceston 7250, TAS Tel : (03) 6337 2777 Fax (03) 6337 2729.
The Royal Hobart Hospital (General) 48 Liverpool Street, Hobart 7000, TAS Tel: (03) 6222 8308 Fax: (03) 6231 2043.

The Flying Doctors

Think of Australia and think of medicine, and this is what get. Because of this, an elective with one of the 14 stations operating a Flying Doctor service is extremely hard to come by. Do not let that put you off. If you apply early (very early ... apply two years+ in advance) and to as many places as possible you are in with a chance. It is certainly worth it.

The Royal Flying Doctor Service (RFDS) is legendary around the world and is still providing to the needs of thousands. Eighty per cent of Australia is RFDS territory. Reverend John Flynn started it all. In 1912 he wanted to be able to provide a medical service to those terribly isolated in Australia's interior. Many people had died horrible, lonesome deaths in these very isolated parts. There were two major problems: first, how could the patient alert the doctor and, second, how could the doctor get there? Two very new inventions solved these, the radio and the aeroplane. Most people laughed off the idea, but Flynn persisted and in 1933 the Australian Aerial Medical Service was born. Today the RFDS flies four million miles a year, makes 169,000 patient contacts a year (3000 a week), 17,000 emergency evacuations and conducts 5000 clinics (95/week) in places that would otherwise be entirely isolated. All this is done with just 350 staff. They also conduct radio clinics, provide 2500 medical packs to isolated areas and have provided the communication network for the 'School of the Air'.

Administration of the 14 bases is divided between seven sections, each of which is completely autonomous, meeting the particular needs of their area. Generally speaking, the sections follow a state pattern. There are, however, exceptions: The Victorian section's field of operations is in the Kimberley region in the north-west of Western Australia with radio bases at Derby and Wyndham. Two other sections operate in Western Australia. These are the Western Australian Section (Port Hedland, Jandakot, Carnarvon and Meekatharra) and the Eastern Goldfields Section (Kalgoorlie). The South Australia Section is responsible for both South Australia (Port Augusta) and the Northern Territory (Alice Springs). The other three sections are New South Wales (Broken Hill), Queensland (Charleville, Mt Isa and Cairns) and Tasmania.

RFDS ADDRESSES:

www.rfds.org.au
Stuart Terrace, The Superintendent, Alice Springs RFDS, Alice Springs, NT 0870.
Captain Clyde Thomson, Director of the New South Wales, RFDS Section and Base, PO Box 463, Broken Hill Airport, Broken Hill, NSW 2880.
The Superintendent, Cairns Royal Flying Doctor Service, 1 Junction Street, Cairns, QLD 4870.
The General Manager, The Royal Flying Doctor Service, 29 Douglas Street, Carnarvon, WA 6071.
The General Manager, The Central Section of the Royal Flying Doctor Service, 2 Beulah Road, Kent Town, SA 5067.
The Superintendent, Charleville Royal Flying Doctor Service, Old Cauuamulla Road, Charleville, QLD 4470.
The General Manager, The Eastern Goldfields Royal Flying Doctor Service Section and Base, 56 Piccadilly Street, Kalgoorlie, WA 6430.
The General Manager, The Royal Flying Doctor Service, The Main Street, Meekatharra, WA 6642.
The Superintendent, Mount Isa Royal Flying Doctor Service, Barkly Highway, Mount Isa, QLD 4825.
The General Manager, Port Augusta RFDS, 4 Vincent Terrace, Port Augusta, SA 5700.
The General Manager, The Royal Flying Doctor Service, The Esplanade, Port Hedland, WA 6721.
The General Manager, RFDS Queensland Section GPO Box 550, QLD 4001.
The General Manager, The Royal Flying Doctor Service, Tasmanian Section, PO Box 199, Launceston, TAS 7250.
The General Manager, The Victoria RFDS Base, Clarendon Street, Derby, WA 6728.
The General Manager, The Victoria RFDS, 2a River Street, South Yarra, VIC 3141.
The General Manager, The Western Australia Royal Flying Doctor Service Section, 3 Eagle Drive, Jandakot Airport, WA 6164.

Flying Obs and Gynae Service

124 McDowall Street, PO Box 264, Roma, Queensland 4455, Australia Tel: (076) 22 2966 Fax: (076) 223520.

The service: Based in Roma, about eight hours west of Brisbane. Every day the eight-seater plane flies out with a Consultant and Reg in O&G and an anaesthetist. In the remote hospitals in the outback one of the seniors runs a clinic while the other runs the surgery. Surgery includes D&Cs, laparoscopies, hysterectomies and the odd C-section. It is a very friendly group that runs the service.

O Elective notes: This is an excellent elective (if you don't get air-sick). You are often really needed in theatre and get made to feel part of the team. With supervision they let you do a number of procedures. You must apply at least a year in advance as this is very popular.

Accommodation: Provided in the nurses' quarters of the hospital in Roma.

FURTHER READING:

Working in Australia by Steve Kisely and Judy Jones, BMJ Classified, pp 2–3, 2 January 1999.

Rural Workforce Agencies:

New South Wales Rural Doctors Network, Suite 19 Level 3, 133 Kings Street, Newcastle, NSW 2300 Tel: 02 4929 1811 Fax: 02 4929 1911 e-mail icameron@nswrdn.aust.com
Northern Territory Remote Health Workforce Agency, PO Box 1195, Alice Springs NT 0871 Tel: 08 8952 3881 Fax: 08 8952 3536 ntrhwa@oct4.net.au
Queensland Rural Medical Support Agency, PO Box 167, Kelvin Grove DC QLD 4059 Tel: 07 3356 1880 Fax: 07 3352 7557 e-mail nlawrence@gpnetwork.net.au
Rural Workforce Agency of Victoria, Suite 8, Level 4, 456 Swanson Street, Carlton VIC 3053 Tel: 03 9349 4899 Fax: 03 9349 4211 e-mail rwav@rwav.com.au
South Australian Rural and Remote Medical Support Agency, Calvary Hospital, 89 Strangeways Terrace, North Adelaide SA 5006 Tel: 08 8239 1222 Fax: 08 8239 1777 e-mail sarrmsa@sarrmsa.com.au
Tasmanian General Practice Divisions Limited, PO Box 104, Newstead TAS 7250 Tel: 03 6334 3255 Fax: 03 6334 3651 e-mail tasgpdiv@gpnetwork.net.au
Western Australia Centre for Rural and Remote Medicine, 328 Stirling Highway, Claremont WA 6010 Tel: 08 9384 2611 Fax: 08 9385 2938 e-mail gregdown@cyllene.uwa.edu.au
A couple of locum agencies: **Australian Medical Placements,** PO Box 74, Torrensville, South Australia 5031 Tel: 08 8443 4455 Fax: 08 8443 4466 e-mail medplace@webmedia.com.au
Rivers Medical Group, Unit 5A, 163 Canning Highway, East Freemantle, Western Australia 6158 Tel: 08 9319 8288 Fax: 08 9319 8299.

New Zealand

Population: 3.6 million
Language: English
Capital: Wellington
Currency: New Zealand dollar
Int Code: +64

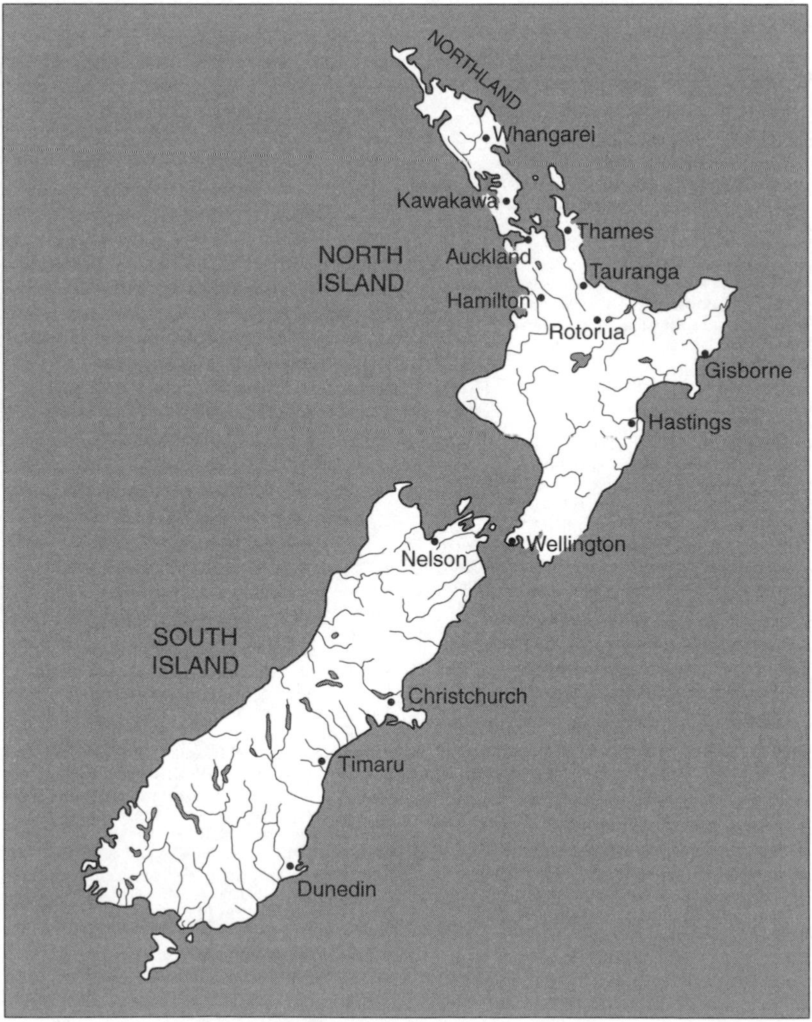

New Zealand, 1000 miles off the coast of Australia, comprises the North and South Island as well as a number of smaller islands. The North has a larger population and has hot springs and geysers, whereas the (adrenaline) South is more mountainous and is the place to be based if you're an outdoors type. Nearly half the population lives in one of the three big cities (Auckland, Wellington or Christchurch).

Medicine:

New Zealand is a world leader in public health services being the first to introduce a welfare state. They did try to charge for hospital beds, but it was so unpopular it was scrapped. The vast majority of conditions are as for any developed country (cardiovascular diseases and cancers); however, the big exception is in the Maori population. A number of hospitals, mainly in Northland on North Island, serve areas rich in Maori people. They tend to suffer more with infectious diseases, such as rheumatic fever, and diseases resulting from their Westernization, such as diabetes and hypertension. Trauma, both deliberate and accidental, is also more common.

New Zealand medical practice, at least in peripheral hospitals, can be very relaxed ... T-shirts and definitely no white coat. New Zealand medical students spend their final (sixth) year as trainee interns. They have done all their finals and they spend a year rotating through medicine, surgery, O&G, paeds and psychiatry. It's similar to being a House Officer without the on-call or prescribing. They are paid half a house surgeon's salary, but since they are still paying school fees, the gain is negligible. Most elective students are given a similar role (without pay!).

Visas and work permits:

British students are not required to obtain visas and British citizens can stay up to six months if not taking paid work. A few students have previously paid £45 for a visa. For up-to-date information on visas and work permits either ring the embassy on their rip-off line (*see* Section 3: The Appendix) or look on www.immigration.gopt.nz Australian citizens are free to travel between Oz and NZ.

Climate and crime:

The climate varies greatly from an almost subtropical north to a cold windy south. The best weather is after Christmas. Crime rates are incredibly low making 'Crimewatch' more of a 'lost and found' service.

Elective notes:

There are two universities in New Zealand, the University of Auckland and the University of Otago (based in Dunedin). There are, however, four clinical schools, Auckland, Wellington, Christchurch and Dunedin. The last three are the clinical schools of the University of Otago. There are big summer holidays in the run up to Christmas. Therefore there aren't many students around. You lose on the social life but do get a bit more attention.

Work:

New Zealand (like Australia) is oversupplied with foreign doctors. Four thousand have entered since 1992 and NZ as a whole only requires 6000. They got in because a loose immigration policy did not check whether a person's overseas qualification was recognized locally. Many of these are now sitting exams to register or are unemployed. Legislation is tightening quickly. Within the next year it is thought that the ONLY foreign doctors who will be able to practise in NZ without sitting registration exams will be Australian. You should therefore have a job offer before leaving for NZ and should get your contract checked by the **Association of Salaried Medical Specialists (ASMS)**, PO Box 5251, Wellington, NZ Tel: 4 499 1271 Fax: 4 499 4500.

For a list of health and hospital services (but not hospital addresses) visit www.hospitals.co.nz/public.html

For lists of job vacancies and advice on obtaining medical work in New Zealand visit New Zealand Health Jobs www.nzhealth.co.nz

NORTH ISLAND

Auckland

Auckland (NZ's biggest city) is about the size of LA, but has only 800,000 people. Transport can therefore be tricky without a car. There is plenty to do in the city which also has a pretty good nightlife. It does have some outdoor activities (white and black water rafting, swimming with dolphins, volcano walking, skydiving) … but if that is specifically what you're after, Christchurch or somewhere else in the South Island is probably better.

University of Auckland

School of Medicine, Private Bag 92019, Auckland, New Zealand Tel: 9 373 7599 Fax: 9 373 7481.

The medical school's principal hospital is Auckland Hospital and electives here should be arranged through the Elective Co-ordinator at the above address. There is an administration fee of NZ$350. They are very helpful but NZ is a popular place … apply very early. Some people have avoided going through the University and gone direct to hospitals to save the $350. The University says you must go through them to make it official. The four main hospitals in Auckland are: North Shore, Middlemore, Green Lane and Auckland.

Auckland Hospital

Park Road/Grafton Road, Auckland, New Zealand.

The hospital: Auckland Hospital is the main tertiary referral centre for the North Island (and some Pacific islands) and is therefore very busy. It's right in the middle of the city. A&E receives a great deal of trauma. On-site there is also the Starship Hospital (almost a theme park), an impressive busy specialist paediatric hospital that serves the whole of NZ and the South Pacific Islands.

O Elective notes: In A&E you'll get to do many minor procedures. There are eight-hour shifts and students can come in for any shift. Formal teaching occurs twice a week in the form of X-ray meetings and journal clubs. Elective students are very much encouraged to take the weekends off for exploring. In January and February there are no local students and you are probably made to feel more part of the team because of this. Neurology rarely has students.

Accommodation: Provided in the on-site residency with other students and staff. It is good (NZ$110/week).

Green Lane Hospital

Green Lane, Auckland 1005, New Zealand.

The hospital: Green Lane is a small hospital to the south of the city centre (15–20 minutes by bus). This is the place to go for cardiology (especially paediatric cardiology as it's more specialized than Auckland Hospital).

O Elective notes: It's well-equipped with friendly doctors and helpful staff; however, it can get a bit quiet. There are Auckland students, so there is consistent teaching and exploring is encouraged.

Accommodation: On-site in a hostel which is also open to the general public ($80/week). This means you meet a wide variety of people, though many are not young and the nightlife can be pretty poor.

North Shore Hospital

Shakespeare Road, Milford, Auckland, New Zealand.

The hospital: North Shore lies north across the Waitemata Harbour from the main city (approximately 35 mins by bus). It has acute medical, surgical, obstetric and psychiatric services. There are no paeds or acute orthopaedics departments. An ITU has just been built. The A&E department offers a wide variety of experience, although most major trauma goes to the main Auckland Hospital.

O Elective notes: There's plenty of opportunity to suture wounds, set fractures and attend resuscitations. It has all its own local facilities and a beach.

Accommodation: In the nurses' home with OTs and physios. All facilities are available and it's very relaxed and friendly. Book early as some have left it too late to get accommodation (in which case stay in Central City Backpackers, 26 Lorne St, £30/wk).

Middlemore Hospital

Private Bag 93311, Auckland, New Zealand.

The hospital: A trauma centre and situated in the rough end of town.

Wellington

For the capital city, Wellington is fairly small, but it is friendly and there is a lot going on. It has a beautiful harbour and many tourist attractions, including the 'Bee-hive' parliament complex, museums, gardens and cable car.

Wellington School of Medicine

Mein St, Newtown, Wellington, PO Box 7343, Wellington South, NZ Tel: 64 4 385 5456 Fax: 64 4 385 5566.

To do an elective in Wellington contact The Overseas Elective Co-ordinator at the above address. You have to fill in a form stating what you have already done, stick a photo on it, get malpractice insurance, tick subjects you would like to do (from paediatric surgery to neurology; research, GP, public health and psychiatry are also available) and send it back.

Wellington Hospital

Mein Street, Newtown, Wellington, PO Box 7343, New Zealand.

The hospital: In Newtown, about a 30-minute walk (five-minute bus ride) from the city centre. It is a tertiary referral centre and teaching hospital and hence has most specialities.

Elective notes: You tend to follow one of the interns and gradually take on their work! Lots of tutorials and lectures if you wish. Good experience and Wellington is a good base in the centre of NZ. The students are very friendly and invite you out to parties etc. You partially act as a trainee intern, but you get to sit in on clinics (which the real ones don't). Paeds is highly recommended. It is in Wellington Children Hospital which is two wards off the main hospital.

Accommodation: Sometimes arranged in the residency. Other times it is in the Riddleford Hostel next to the hospital ($90/week). Free tea and coffee for medical students!

Wakefield Sports Med

Wakefield Specialist Centre, Rintoul Street, Newtown, Wellington, New Zealand Tel: 389 7460 Fax: 389 7461 (A private sports specialist clinic a few minutes from Wellington General Hospital.)

Northland

Northland has some beautiful beaches and is excellent for diving (with dolphins), fishing and sailing. It has some amazing countryside and is great if you're an outdoors type. The Bay of Islands is particularly impressive. There are many Maori people here making interesting folk-law and medicine.

Whangarei Area Hospital

Northland Health Limited, PO Box 742, Whangarei, New Zealand Tel: 0 9 430 4100 Fax: 0 9 430 4110.

The hospital: Whangarei Area Hospital is a modern hospital with a relatively busy A&E department containing 12 beds. Whangarei (a two-hour drive from Auckland) is Northland's largest city. It is the major referral centre for Northland with surgical, medical, intensive care, coronary care, paeds, psych, oncology, renal, O&G and emergency services. Opened in 1901, it now has 250 beds. There is a helicopter service to bring in referrals. It is also a training centre for Auckland Medical School so TIs (not students) get sent here. There is quite a lot of trauma from RTAs. There is a large Maori population who often practise 'home kills' of animals and sustain lacerations in the process ... lots of nerve blocks and suturing practice. There is a busy paeds ward (18 beds) and a paeds emergency department. There's also a great deal of orthopaedics.

O Elective notes: They have previously tried to arrange a helicopter ride in the air ambulance for visiting students. Only elective students are here so its not overcrowded. There are quite a few British doctors and nurses. It's a good elective. Write to the Medical Staff Co-ordinator at the above address. A fee of $75 is charged. Whangarei isn't very picturesque, although the harbour is quite nice. It is a great base from which to explore the Northland and the Bay of Islands. There is a good bus service.
Accommodation: Provided at $70/week (£30) and is good, although cooking facilities leave a lot to be desired. There are a good canteen and a swimming pool for residents.

Bay of Islands Hospital

PO Box 290, Kawakawa, New Zealand.
The hospital: Bay of Islands is a small (approx 30-bed) rural hospital with a day surgical ward and a general medical ward with some paediatric beds. It is run by four doctors. There is also a small maternity unit and A&E. Kawakawa itself is a pretty small, mainly Maori village, 15 km from the coast. The population is around half Maori/Polynesian and half white with many from poor social circumstances. Specialists (from Whangarei) visit and run clinics.
O Elective notes: You can also get to do some minor procedures. The staff (including the four doctors) are friendly and offer lifts to local areas to see the sites. Recommended for 4–5 weeks. GP work can be arranged on arrival. Transport is tricky, though easy enough if you want to get to Auckland (four hours, south). It has a few shops, a pub and a vintage railway. Borrow a bike to get to the lovely beach at Paitia (famous for dolphin and whale watching, watersports and boogy boarding down giant sand dunes). (Write to the medical secretary to organize a trip here.)
Accommodation: Free. It can either be in the nurses' home or in a cottage with other medical staff. The canteen food isn't great, but again is free (make sure you book it with the kitchen). There's a good sports centre 15 minutes from the hospital.

Whakatane Hospital

Stewart Street, Whakatane, Bay of Plenty, North Island, New Zealand.
The hospital: A 200-bed general hospital with 40% of its population being Maori. All the major specialities are here and the staff are helpful both in and out of the hospital.
O Elective notes: You'll probably be the only student and you can do as much or as little as you want. There are tutorials and the opportunity to visit community clinics. The area has quite a lot of thermal activity (volcanoes and hot springs). Organize this elective early.
Accommodation: Provided free of charge in the old nurses' home.

Rotorua

Rotorua is a brilliant place for an elective or work. It's central North Island, so a good base to explore from and has a lot of geothermal activity. Things to do include hot spa pools, naturally warm rivers to swim in, bush walks and mountain biking. This also makes for some pretty novel therapies (see Queen Elizabeth Hospital below). Nearby there is white water rafting, black water rafting, caving and skydiving. The ski fields are two hours away (but can be closed if the local volcanoes are covering them in ash). There are lots of fast food places, cafés and a five-screen cinema. Nightlife is quiet, but if you like rugby, this is paradise.

Rotorua Hospital

Lakeland Health, Private Bag 3023, Rotorua, New Zealand Tel: (07) 348 199.
The hospital: A small friendly district hospital with 120 beds. It has two medical, a surgical, orthopaedics, paediatrics, O&G, psychiatry and geriatrics wards. Most of the patients are Maori so you see lots of diabetes and its complications. Other common conditions in Maori paeds are malnutrition and rheumatic fever. Amoebic meningitis is

also a problem because of the thermal baths (two cases a year). Don't put your head under water. The luge and mountain bike trail provide a descent bit of trauma.
O Elective notes: There are no NZ medical students, only trainee interns who are willing to teach. It's all pretty laid back … the hospital day starts at 8 am, but yours starts whenever you get out of bed! Ward rounds are in Polo Shirts. Apply very early (up to 18 months in advance).
Accommodation: And food (not great) are provided at the hospital for NZ$100/week (about £50). You share accommodation with trainee interns from Auckland Medical School.

Queen Elizabeth Hospital for Rheumatology and Rehabilitation

PO Box 1342, Whakaue Street, Rotorua, New Zealand.
The hospital: Situated on the edge of Lake Rotorua, it has 50 patients and is run by three consultants. It has two rheumatology and one orthopaedic ward. Common conditions include, RA, OA, gout, scleroderma, psoriasis, fibromyalga and SLE. There is also an OPD. Treatments include (given for three weeks): exercise, physio, OT, balneotherapy (the use of hot mud, mud baths, hot springs, massage, steam treatment or wax therapy), counselling, relaxation and drugs.

Gisbourne

Gisborne Hospital

Tairawhiti Healthcare Ltd, Private Bag 7001, Gisborne, New Zealand.
The hospital: On the outskirts of the town (population 30,000) on the east coast of North Island. There are two medical, two surgical wards, an ICU, a paeds dept and A&E. There is a large Maori population in the East Cape and this is reflected in the medicine with a high percentage of rheumatic fever, diabetes and renal dysfunction. The general medical wards are covered by three consultant physicians and students tend to be allocated to one. There are no middle-grade staff, but there are numerous house officers.
O Elective notes: There's plenty of teaching on the rounds, in lunchtime sessions and in practical procedures. The consultants also go on outreach clinics offering a great opportunity to see the countryside and GP-run hospitals north of Gisborne. This is a good elective, but you may feel a bit out of the way and it has a slower pace of life than others. There is a lot to explore around Gisbourne (which has a cinema).

Note: The hospital is about an hour's walk from anywhere; therefore, get a bike!
Accommodation: Free. The house officers all live in and the social life is actually quite good.

Thames

Thames Hospital

Waikato Area Health Board, Thames, PO Box 707, New Zealand.
The hospital: Thames is a small district general hospital with both medical and surgical wards.
O Elective notes: You can choose to spend your time in one area or rotate. The busiest time is their summer (i.e. over Christmas). Most action is in the emergency department where all admissions are seen first. This is a relaxed, friendly elective with good teaching, but the staff are also keen for you to go explore the surrounding countryside. There are some lovely walks and beaches nearby. Thames itself (1½ hours by bus from Auckland) is a small, quiet town, but the people are genuine and there is plenty to do. Try to go with someone or visit somewhere else as well.
Accommodation: The nurses' hostel costs around $50 (£20)/week and is usually pretty full so there's plenty of life.

Tauranga Hospital

Western Bay Health, Cameron Road, Tauranga, New Zealand.
The hospital: Tauranga Hospital is a

large modern hospital with enthusiastic and friendly staff.

O Elective notes: Tauranga is a reasonable-sized town with quite a few things to do. There is an airport for flights to the South Island. The beaches are excellent for swimming, surfing and fishing. Described as an excellent elective.

Hastings Memorial Hospital

c/o Health Care, Hawkes Bay, Hastings, New Zealand.

The hospital: A very friendly small hospital with a good range of services (surgery, orthopaedics, O&G, paeds, medicine).

O Elective notes: An immensely friendly hospital well worth visiting. Responsibility if you want it, time off if you don't.

Accommodation: Provided.

Waikato Hospital

Private Bag 3200, Hamilton, New Zealand
Tel: 0 839 8880 Fax: 07 839 8897.

SOUTH ISLAND

Christchurch

Christchurch (population 300,000) is a top base from which to start exploring New Zealand. If you go in winter, the skiing is supposed to be excellent in the Southern Alps. Since it is in the South Island it is also very convenient if you're after the silly sports (bungee, ski-diving etc.). Christchurch itself is very 'British' and, although there is a great deal outside, it's not so great for wild nights out.

Christchurch School of Medicine

Christchurch School of Medicine, Christchurch Hospital, PO Box 4345, Christchurch, New Zealand
Tel: 03 364 0824 Fax: 03 364 0935.

The school is in and uses Christchurch Hospital for its clinical training. It is the major teaching hospital of the University of Otago (based further down the coast). They can arrange electives in all specialities although some students have found they can't do general medicine or surgery as they are full with their own students. This is an extremely popular destination. Write incredibly early to the above address.

Christchurch Hospital

PO Box 4345, Christchurch, South Island, New Zealand.

The hospital: Christchurch Public Hospital is the major acute hospital for the city and surrounding area. It has many large and well-organized departments. Quite a few British doctors work here. There are many local as well as elective medical students.

O Elective notes: Elective students tend to be treated as trainee interns. Some departments include:

- *Cardiology:* comprising a 30-bed long-stay ward, a day ward, CCU, intensive care, catheter lab and outpatients all of which you can rotate through.
- *Emergency:* a busy friendly unit seeing 60,000 patients a year with a 40% admission rate. Arguably one of the best attachments. Not much planned teaching but plenty by the bedside.
- *Bone Marrow Transplant:* The team look after those with an underlying haematological problem. Students have previously been able to do lumbar punctures, bone marrow biopsies and give intrathecal medication. Warning: young people die, be prepared for this.
- *Oncology:* Highly recommended, but less practical experience.
- *Neurosurgery, Endocrinology, Dermatology.*
- *Orthopaedics* (only acute and trauma here) Offers some excellent teaching and the opportunity to visit the Burwood Spinal Injuries Unit, world-renowned for treating tetraplegics and reconstruction surgery (*see below*); the department is also pretty relaxed allowing plenty of time to go exploring.

Accommodation: Not provided. There is a local YMCA right opposite the hospital, $90 (£40)/week for a shared room and another $70 (£30)/week for cafeteria food as there are no self-catering facilities. Apparently, if you're there for more than a couple of weeks you can haggle and get it cheaper. Sports facilities in the YMCA are good. Book well in advance.

Spinal Injuries Unit

Burwood Hospital, Private Bag 4708, Christchurch, New Zealand.

The hospital: One of two in New Zealand dealing with a whole spectrum of spinal injuries. Acute spinal patients are rapidly transported here for their acute management and then extensive rehabilitation lasting two to four months.

O Elective notes: The consultants are very knowledgeable and keen to teach; however, for obvious reasons clinical experience can be slow. The patients are the ones who teach you the most. The unit itself is 11 km outside the city centre with an excellent bus service.

Accommodation: Provided in a nurses' hostel on-site or can be arranged in the city. Sports facilities are available in the hospital.

Princess Margaret Hospital

Private bag, Christchurch, New Zealand.

The hospital: A smaller hospital in Christchurch. A number of British doctors work here.

Burwood Hospital

Burwood Road, Christchurch, New Zealand.

The hospital: The only child psychiatric inpatient unit in the South Island.

Dunedin

Dunedin is a relatively isolated town, not a city, in South Island. The total population is 115,000 of whom 15–20,000 are students. The people often have Scottish relatives and there are many Scottish street names. All the student nightlife is pub-based and a good laugh. Queenstown and Janaka (skiing) are close (snowboarding is booming) and there's lots of glaciers and beautiful countryside.

Otago Medical School

PO Box 913, Gt King Street, Dunedin, New Zealand Tel: 03 479 7416 Fax: 03 479 0401.

Otago can arrange electives in its main teaching hospital, Dunedin, or a number of others in the vicinity. Write to the Overseas Electives Co-ordinator at the Administration Office at the above address.

Note: There is a charge of NZ$250 (£110).

Dunedin Hospital

Dunedin, New Zealand.

The hospital: A teaching hospital with all specialities (neurosurgery, cardiothoracics, a good anaesthetics dept (with pain team), ortho, ENT etc.). It is similar to any other First World hospital.

O Elective notes: Elective students often get given positions as trainee interns. In anaesthetics, students have previously done quite a lot of procedures.

Accommodation: No hospital accommodation is available but they help you arrange some.

Southland Hospital

Invercargill, Dunedin, South Island, New Zealand.

The hospital: Is also part of the medical school on the south side of town and acts as a DGH and has 200 beds. It has a good neurology department. It is a very friendly hospital.

O Elective notes: You can either act as a trainee intern or go to clinics. Very hands on in A&E with respect to minor injuries. Highly recommended; however, the hospital is about one hour's walk from the town centre. Apply through Otago Medical School.

Accommodation: In the doctors' residence.

Nelson

Nelson is a small coastal town (population 45,000) located in the extreme north of South Island. There's plenty to do ... walks, kayaking, skydiving, skiing, river surfing, bungee jumping, jet boating, and horse riding. Marlborough Sounds and Abel Tasman National Parks are not too far away. It's New Zealand's sunniest city and weather is hottest around Jan/Feb ... take a raincoat in Nov/Dec. Nightlife isn't great, but the locals are friendly. Surrounding Nelson there are fantastic golden beaches.

Nelson Hospital

Private Bag, Nelson, South Island, New Zealand Tel: (03)546 1800 Fax: (03)546 1680.

The hospital: Nelson Hospital is medium-sized (100 beds) with friendly (but no middle-grade) staff. It is the largest hospital for over 500 km.

O Elective notes: Students are treated as trainee interns and there are plenty of practical procedures to do. There's lots of teaching as there are no local students (although there can be quite a few elective students). You can do as much or as little as you want. A&E doesn't get much major trauma but lots of minor injuries. This is a more relaxed elective than in the cities. You also get to do more. Very highly recommended (repeatedly).

Accommodation: Has been provided at $140 (£60)/week sharing with other elective medical students. However, it has occasionally been closed. There are youth hostels in town (Dave's Palace does special medical student discounts, around $60 (£25)/week) There are a small gym and swimming pool in the hospital grounds.

Timaru

Timaru Public Hospital

Health South Canterbury, High Street, Private Bag 911, Timaru, New Zealand.

The hospital: The only medical centre between Dunedin and Christchurch and has a wide catchment area extending up into the Southern Alps, including Mount Cook and Mount Aspiring National Park. It covers all basic specialities, has 250 beds and three theatres. There is a maternity hospital with a further 50 beds.

O Elective notes: It is a very friendly hospital and a few procedures and assisting in theatre can usually be done.

Accommodation: Up to three students can stay in hospital flats that are not expensive.

THE CARIBBEAN

The Caribbean

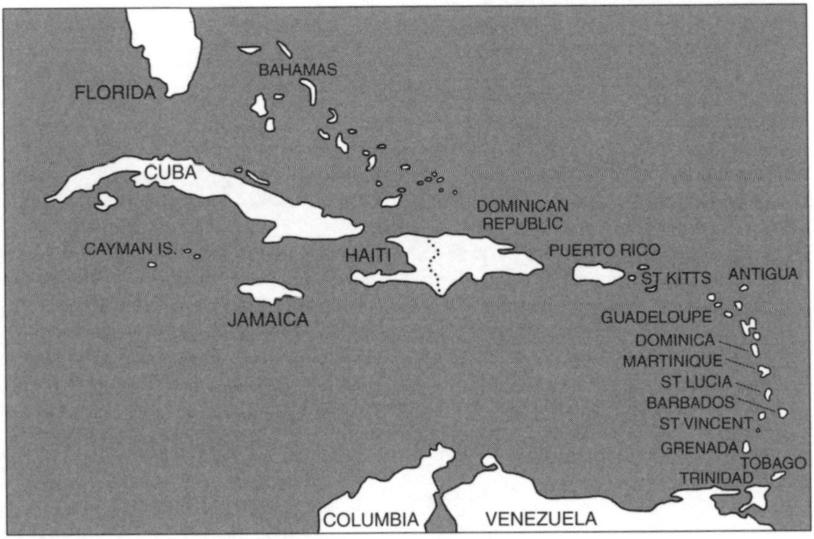

The Caribbean is an idyllic place to work if you like the sun and beautiful beaches. Beware, however, the islands are very different. Some have wonderful health facilities and others can be classed as Third World. Even within an island itself (for example, Jamaica) the wide disparity can mean superb private care for a minority and very poor conditions for others. This chapter goes through the islands from west to east. Some are independent. Some still have ties with America or Europe. Look at the map above to find out their relations. You may well be able to offer your services to various boats travelling between islands in return for free transport (look out for notices at the dockyards). It should be noted that HIV is an increasing problem, especially in some of the Islands of the West Indies, with a few of the islands having the world's highest rates for heterosexual transmission.

◎ Climate:

The Caribbean as a whole has a subtropical climate with very mild winters. It's hottest between June and September (30 °C), but this is also when rainfall tends to peak. Hurricanes seem to be an increasing threat between July and December.

To do an elective at one of the hospitals that are affiliated with the University of the West Indies (Antigua, Dominica, St Vincent, St Lucia, Grenada, Martinique, Jamaica, Guadalope, St Joseph, St Martin and Barbados) you can write directly to the University. However, to give yourself a head start, write to where you want to go first and then (if they require it) write to the University stating that you have been offered an elective placement. The University address is under Jamaica.

The eastern Caribbean states (St Lucia, St Vincent and the Grenadines, and St Christopher and Nevis) are part of the Commonwealth. Most information is below but if you need more details contact the High Commission for Eastern Caribbean States, 10 Kensington Court, London W8 5DL (Tel: 020 7937 9522 Fax: 020 7937 5514) or the Ministry of Health: Chausee Road, Castries, St Lucia.

The Bahamas

Population: 300,000
Official Language: English
Capital: Nassau
Currency: Bahamian dollar
Int Code: +1 242

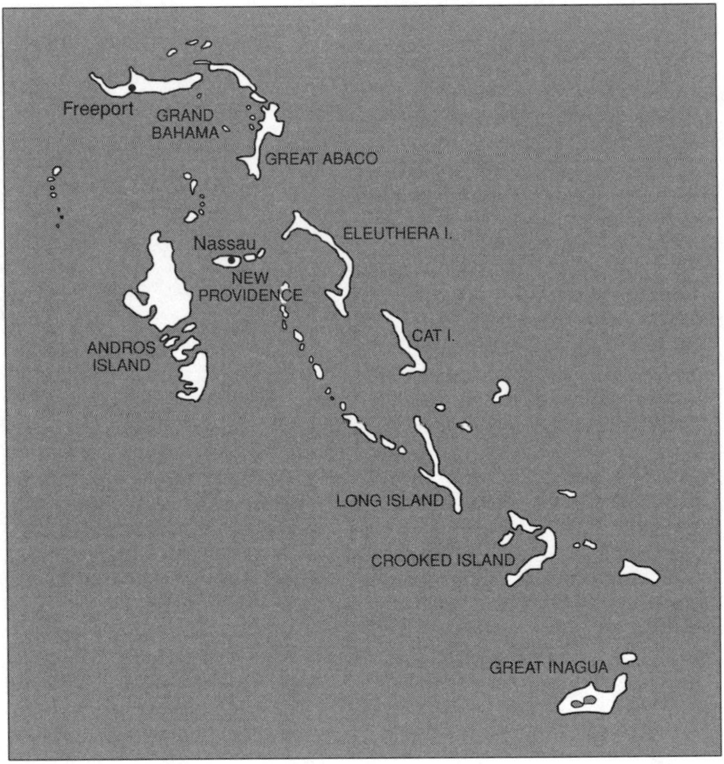

The Bahamas are a group of 700 islands and 2400 cays of the south Florida coast. Only 30 islands, however, are inhabited. As well as a large tourist industry, the Bahamas have more recently become a major offshore financial centre.

✪ Medicine:

The Ministry of Health and the Environment is responsible for the provision of general healthcare in the Bahamas. There are both private and Government-maintained hospitals providing a modern and comprehensive healthcare system. The system is not free, but curative treatment is generally available to all residents in the Government-maintained hospitals notwithstanding the ability to pay. The Government health care system is funded by a National Insurance scheme paid by employers and employees on the Bahamas. It covers those employed and those previously employed on the islands. Hospitals are only maintained on the two most populated islands: Nassau and Grand Bahama (over 83% of the population resides on these two islands, with over 67% living in Nassau alone), but general clinics are available on all the major islands with resident physicians. A rapid response emergency Air Sea Rescue programme is available throughout the islands, provided with the assistance of the American Coast Guard. Private boats can also transport patients. Doctor:population ratio = 1:692, but for every inhabitant there are six tourists per year. Leading causes of mortality are heart disease, cancers, crime, accidents and obstetric.

➲ Visas and work permits:

Contact The High Commission of the Commonwealth of the Bahamas, Bahamas House, 10 Chesterfield Street, London W1X 8AH Tel: 020 7408 4488 Fax: 020 7499 9937.

No clear information is available regarding the need for students to obtain a study visa. UK and American citizens can land as visitors with just a passport and stay up to eight months, although anyone staying longer than an 'average holiday' has to apply for an extension.

In most lines of work, the Government of the Bahamas has to offer the job to a suitably qualified Bahamian before an outsider and then, if given to an expatriate, a costly work visa is obtained. However, for nurses, doctors and kindred services, no work permit is required. Write to:

The Ministry of Health
PO Box N-3730, Nassau, The Bahamas Tel: (242) 322 7425 Fax: (242) 322 7788.

USEFUL ADDRESS:

The Bahamas Medical Council
PO Box N-9802, Nassau, NP. Bahamas
Tel: (242) 328 2260 Fax: (242) 328 1211.

◎ Crime:

Illegal weapons are easily obtainable and hence gunshot injuries and murders do occasionally occur.

HOSPITALS IN NASSAU:

The Princess Margaret Hospital

Naussau, The Bahamas.

The hospital: A Government-maintained hospital providing 484 beds. Its departments include: A&E, medical, surgical, maternity, paediatrics, intensive care, eye and chest medicine, speciality clinics and dialysis. There is also a GP service.

O Elective notes: There are plenty of patients and things to see. Although it's in English it can be difficult to understand. There are quite a few friendly local students.

Accommodation: Not provided. Sunshine guesthouse is recommended.

The Doctors Hospital

PO Box N-3018, Nassau, Bahamas
Tel: 322 8411.

The hospital: An acute care privately operated hospital with 72 beds. Medical specialities include: emergency medicine, ENT, general surgery, orthopaedics, obstetrics and gynaecology, ophthalmology, internal medicine, gastroenteology, urology, cardiology and paediatrics. It has recently been renovated.

Sandilands Rehabilitation Centre

Nassau, The Bahamas.

The hospital: A Government-maintained geriatric and psychiatric hospital with 477 beds. The facility includes a security unit, a family guidance centre and a combined substance abuse centre for drug and alcohol abuse.

The Lyford Cay Hospital/Bahamas Heart Institute

Naussau, The Bahamas.

The hospital: A private hospital specializing in plastic and reconstructive surgery. There is a cardiac diagnostic centre providing doppler echocardiography, 24-hour ECGs, exercise ECGs, and pacemaker implants.

HOSPITALS IN FREEPORT, GRAND BAHAMA:

There's one general hospital and two specialist medical centres:

Rand Memorial Hospital

Freeport, Grand Bahama.

The hospital: A Government-owned community-type hospital providing general medical care broadly similar to that offered by the Princess Margaret Hospital. It has 92 beds and a full medical staff.

The Sunrise Medical Centre

Freeport, Grand Bahama

The hospital: A private medical facility providing specialist services in general medicine, dental, obstetrics and gynaecology, oral and max-fax surgery, orthodontics and optometry.

Lucayan Medical Centre

Freeport, Grand Bahama.

The hospital: A private medical facility offering specialist services in family medicine, internal medicine, obstetrics, gastroenterology, kidney diseases, ophthalmology, paediatrics, psychiatry, surgery, urology and anaesthetics.

Cuba

Population: 10.8 million
Language: Spanish
Capital: Havana
Currency: Cuban peso
Int Code: +53

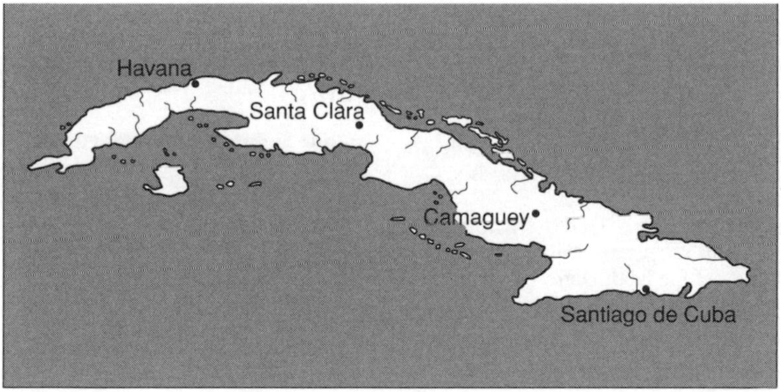

The Caribbean's largest island is also the only Communist one. It is a former Spanish colony and the culture, language and traditions have persisted. The USA put sanctions on Cuba in 1962 in response to the presence of Soviet nuclear weapons on the island. Despite the collapse of Communism in the Soviet Union the restrictions remain making life pretty tough financially. The social life is, however, excellent with street and beach parties, beer and rum. There is a lot to see around the island.

✪ Medicine:

Although it has limited resources, Cuba has a very impressive healthcare system. Life expectancy (76 years) is the highest in Latin America. Basic drugs and materials (such as X-ray films) are in very short supply due to the US blockade. Havana's large pharmaceutical industry manages to supply what is needed. Cuba's ophthalmalogical services are world-renowned as being very advanced. The doctor:patient ratio is one per 333. Despite the stretched resources the doctors tend to be very friendly and keen to teach. Leading causes of death include heart disease, cancers and malnutrition.

Medical students here train for a particular speciality, e.g. to become a paediatrician and hence don't need to study other subjects.

O Elective notes:

Ask the hospital if there is anything they want you to bring. Also take a bike with you as there isn't much in the way of public transport. Most elective students have had to stay in hotels which has proved expensive.

HAVANA:

Medical School

Instituto Superior de Ciencias Médicas de la Habana, Calle 146 y Avenida 31, Playa, La Habana.

This is the oldest and largest Cuban medical school using many hospitals in the area.

Hospital Nacional Ameiseiras

Havana, Cuba.

The hospital: This is one of the main hospitals. It has most major specialities, however, as for most of Cuba, facilities and drugs are limited.

Hospital Clinico Quirlurgico

'Dr Gustavo Aldereguia Lima', Ave 5 de Septiembre y Calle 51 A, Cienfuegos, Cuba.

The hospital: Is a DGH, friendly and offers a full range of services. Resources are poor but the health care still manages to be very good.

O Elective notes: Medical students especially from South American countries come here and there is plenty of teaching.

Hospital Fajardo

Zapata Y D, Vedado, Havana CR: 10400, Cuba.

Polyclinico Plaza de la Revolucion

Havana, Cuba.

This is like a GP surgery, i.e. primary healthcare.

OTHER MEDICAL SCHOOLS ON CUBA:

Instituto Superior de Ciencias Médicas 'Carlos J Finlay', Carretera Central Oeste y Madame Curie, Camagüey.
Instituto Superior de Ciencias Médicas de Santiago de Cuba, Avenida de las Américas y Calle E, Reparto Sueño, Santiago de Cuba.
Instituto Superior de Ciencias Médicas de Villa Clara, Carretera Acueducto y Circunvalación, Santa Clara, Cuba.

The Cayman Islands

Population: 33,000
Language: English
Capital: George Town
Currency: Dollar
Int Code: +1 345

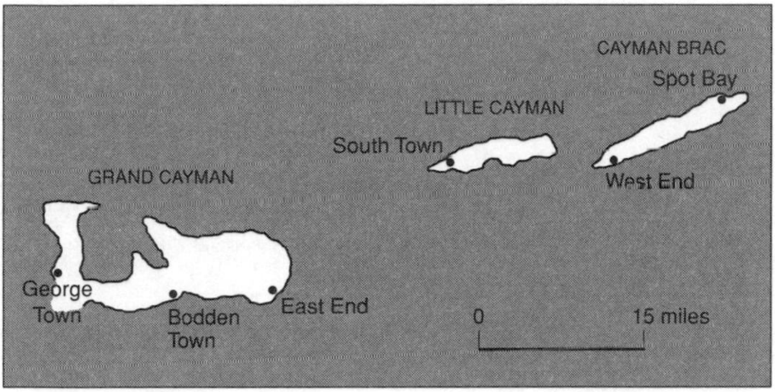

The three islands that make up the Caymans are situated 190 miles north-west of Jamaica. Tourism is the major economy here; however, the Caymans are also a major financial centre because of the absence of tax and foreign exchange controls. The two largest islands have hospitals. Grand Cayman has a modern well-equipped 120-bed hospital. Cayman Brac (the second largest island) has a small cottage hospital.

➲ Visas and work permits:
Very few medical students have done electives in the Cayman Islands. Approach the hospital directly to find out more about visa requirements and accommodation.

Persons holding British, Commonwealth or US qualifications are able to practise in the Cayman Islands once they have been locally licensed through the Health Practitioners Board (the Chief Medical Officer is the Chairman of the Board). Persons employed at the George Town hospital are on a Government contract – this is equivalent to a work permit. It is worth mentioning that the Government has a policy of having to try to give the job to a Caymanian before an outsider. However, with such a small population it shouldn't be a problem for medics.

George Town Hospital
PO Box 915, Grand Cayman, Cayman Islands Tel: 345 949 8600 Fax: 345 945 1754.
The hospital: A modern well-equipped 120-bed hospital. It has a wide range of services and a number of specialists on

the staff. In cases where specialist treatment is not available locally, patients are airlifted to Miami where the Government has an arrangement with certain hospitals.

OTHER MEDICAL ORGANIZATIONS ON THE ISLANDS:

Cayman Islands Red Cross, Cayman Island Medical and Dental Association, Cayman Against Substance Abuse (CASA), Alcoholics Anonymous, Cayman Island Cancer Society.

There are also many private practitioners. A few are listed below. When writing address them as follows: Name, PO Box, Grand Cayman, Cayman Islands BWI.

Dr Abraham (Paediatrician) Box 30675sMB Cayman Medical and Surgical Centre, Rankin's Plaza Eastern Avenue Tel 945 7050 Fax 945 7855.
Dr Addleson (GP) Box 30073MB Pasadora Place Smith Road Tel 945 2881 Fax 949 6826.
Dr Bhargava (Plastics) Box 30950SMB Plasadora Place, Smith Road, George Town Tel: 945 1565 Fax 945 6826.
Dr Carlsen (Plastics) Box 30719SMB Cosmetic Surgery Hospital, Crewe Road Tel: 949 5968 Fax 949-6571.
Dr Caudeiron (Obstetrics) Box 30722SMB Professional Medical Centre, Walkers Road, George Town Tel 949 9090 Fax 949 9633.
Dr Fiona Foster (GP) Box 286GT Island Centre, Smith Road, George Town Tel 949 8086 Fax 949 9228.
Cayman Medical and Surgical Centre Box 30618SMB, Rankin's Plaza Tel 949 8150 Fax 949 7855.
Cayman Orthopaedic Group Box 11698APO Smith Road Plaza, Smith Road Tel 945 8380 Fax 945 8405 (Dr Perez Ali, Ted English, Steve Richie, Vir Sennik, Frank Smith and Bill Vivani).
Dr Shirley Cridland (Paediatrician) Box 1332GT, Smith Road, Geroge Town Tel: 9949 5225 Fax 945 1066.
Dr De Alwis (Obstetrics) Box 10826APO, Professiobnal Medical Centre, Walkers Road Tel: 945 6066 Fax 945 1695.
Dr Michael Hetley (Dive Medicine/GP) Cayman Clinic Box 2309GT Crewe Road, George Town Tel: 949 9400 Fax 945 5828.
Dr Patricia Hill (Paediatrician) Box 10790APO, 247 Smith Road, George Town Tel 945 8527 Fax 945 8528.
Dr John Madden (GP/Dive Medicine) Box 30618SMB, Cayman Medical and Surgical Centre, Rankin's Plaza, Eastern Avenue Tel 949 0923 Fax 945 7040.
Dr Meggs (Obsterics and Gynaecology) Island Medical Centre, Box 229SAV Tel 949 8969 Fax 949 8920.
Professional Medical Centre Box 273GT Walkers Road Tel 949 6066 Fax 945 2695. (Drs S Tomlinson (GP/Surgeon), R Crichlow (Ophthalmologist), L Cona (GP) and a number of visiting specialists.)
Dr Richmond-Peck (Obstetrics) Box 31600SMB Cayman Medical and Surgical Centre Tel 945 7044 Fax 949 7855.
Dr Gordon Smith (Paediatrican/Dive Specialist/GP) Box 2777GT Professional Medical Centre Tel 949 2970 Fax 949 7543.
Dr Sandra Voice (Plastics) Box 30719SMB Cosmetic Surgery Hospital, Crewe Road Tel 949 2080 Fax 949 2805.

Jamaica

Population: 2.4 million
Language: English
Capital: Kingston
Currency: Jamaican dollar
Int Code: +1 876

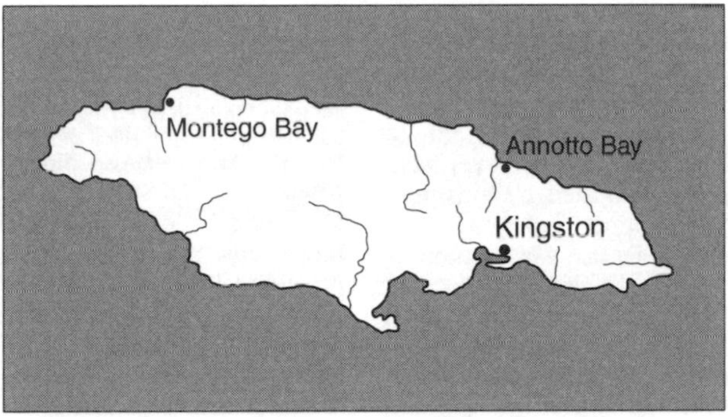

Jamaica is one of the larger islands in the Caribbean, separated from the southern coast of Florida by Cuba. It is the peak of one of the great volcanic mountains that form the seabed, and so consists of central mountainous jungle surrounded by a strip of flat land around the coast. The idyllic beaches and exclusive holiday resorts that are associated with Jamaica are mainly on the north coast. The capital, Kingston, is a city of about one million people and is on the much poorer south coast. The University of the West Indies and the associated teaching hospital, University Hospital West Indies, sit on two adjacent sites in the northern outskirts of the city.

After gaining independence in 1962, Jamaica underwent great political changes resulting in massive inflation and a large disparity between rich and poor. In the early 1990s 50% of households did not have a WC and 29% did not have electricity. These disparities are reflected in Jamaica's health problems.

Kingston has a well-earned reputation for violence with a murder rate of 15 per 100,000 a year (two murders/day), one of the highest in the world. The violence tends to be in certain areas. Most of this is confined to gangland feuds, but foreigners are occasionally targeted, usually for money. Jamaicans equate white with rich, so if white, expect to be plagued by beggars and drug pushers. Women get even more hassle with proposals of marriage as well. Despite all this, the University, hospital and surrounding areas are relatively safe, especially during daylight hours.

There is much to see and do outside Kingston. The best way to travel around the island is by car. However, this can be expensive, so you may have to cram into the minibuses that make the five-hour trip across the mountains to the north coast. You may think that Jamaica is an English-speaking country: it is, but you may well have difficulty understanding the history in 'Patois', and local dialect.

Medicine:
Both tropical and Western diseases are common. Trauma, both from violence and from RTAs (50% each), is seen regularly. Cancers, heart and cerebrovascular disease are the most common causes of death. Diabetes mellitus has increased by 300% since the 1960s, presumably through Western influence. The complications of this are putting a major strain on the health service. Child malnourishment is common and 90 clinics around the island try to deal with it. Approximately 15,000 children live on the streets of Kingston. Gastroenteritis is the most common cause of hospital admission. Other infectious diseases are common.

A few diseases are important to Jamaica. Malaria and Yellow Fever have now both been eradicated by mosquito eradication. Vomiting sickness is a disease common in the winter months unique to Jamaica. Vomiting occurs approximately three hours after a meal and can be fatal in a few days. It has been found to be due to eating undercooked ackee (a fruit introduced by Captain Bligh in 1793). Ingestion of Barracuda fish sometimes also causes poisoning. Jamaican neuropathy (tropical spastic paraparesis) is now known to be due to HTLV-1, present in 5% of the population and 28% of Jamaican prostitutes. Veno-occlusive disease of the liver due to drinking *Crotalaria retusa* bush tea is also seen. One in ten Jamaicans carry the sickle cell gene reflecting their African descent and the previous prevalence of malaria in Jamaica.

The Jamaican psychiatrist also has a different job to most. There are a number of reasons for this: the social backdrop, cultural differences and the financial constraints under which they work. Although Christianity is very strong in Jamaica, many children are born without commitment between their parents. It is common for a young woman to have children and leave them with the grandmother while she goes out to work. The father has no responsibilities. Single parenting is therefore part of the norm with one woman having several children by two or three 'babyfathers'. Another cultural difference is the widespread use of cannabis and to a lesser extent, cocaine. Therefore, drug-induced psychoses are more common. Also, due to the poor funding in the healthcare system, physical treatments are used very early on to expedite discharge. This means higher doses of antipsychotics and early ECT.

The **University Hospital**, **Kingston Public Hospital** and the **Cornwall Regional Hospital** in Montego Bay are class A secondary and tertiary referral centres. Class B hospitals (providing in- and outpatient services in general surgery, internal medicine, obstetrics and gynaecology and paediatrics) are located in St Ann's Bay, Savannah-la-Mar, Mandeville and Spanish Town. There are also about a dozen smaller class C hospitals that are parish-based with two or three doctors providing general medicine, child and community care. Specialist hospitals include: The **Victoria Jubilee** (maternity), the **Bustamante Children's Hospital**, the **Mona Rehabilitation Centre** (physiotherapy and OT for sufferers from polio, spasticity, amputation and paraplegia), the **Bellevue** (psychiatry), the **National Chest Hospital** and the **Hope Institute** (palliative care). About 450 doctors work in the public hospital and health centres. Elsewhere there are 750 doctors working within the private healthcare system.

University of the West Indies

Faculty of Medical Sciences, The Registry, Kingston, Jamaica, WI Tel: 1 876 9271297 Fax: 9272556.

The University of the West Indies was initially a University College associated with the University of London. The faculty of medicine was the first faculty to be established due to the lack of medics on the island. It proved impossible to adapt Kingston Public Hospital into a teaching hospital and so a new University hospital was specially designed.

The University has a well-organized elective programme both in Jamaica and on other islands. It can send an application form on which you request a speciality. They can also help with accommodation by recommending private residences. One address that comes recommended is: Mrs Soares, 16, Beverly Drive, Beverly Hills, Kingston 6, Jamaica, WI Tel: 809 978 3806. She is an elderly Jamaican lady living in an affluent part of Kingston. A number of local students live there. Usual cost is around £10/day. Another is Mrs S Grant, 43, University Crescent, Kingston 6, Jamaica, WI.

The University Hospital of the West Indies

Mona, St Andrew, Kingston 7, Jamaica WI.

The hospital: Is the major teaching hospital and is situated on the Mona campus. It has just over 400 beds making it larger than Kingston Public Hospital. It has pretty good facilities and caters for most specialities, although there are specialist hospitals. The department of psychiatry has a 20-bed ward which, due to different approaches to psychiatric management in Jamaica, is rarely much more than half full. There is also a day ward. There are connections with the large long-stay psychiatric hospital (Belleview Hospital, *see* below). There is an MRC sickle cell laboratory on the Mona Campus.

O Elective notes: It's a busy hospital with plenty to see and do in A&E. There's a high standard of well-organized teaching.

Accommodation: Can be difficult. The Dean's Office can put you in touch with people who run boarding houses for students (*see above*).

Cornwall Regional Hospital

Mt Salem, Montego Bay, St James, Jamaica, WI.

The hospital: The main public hospital in Montego Bay. It is busy especially for O&G, casualty and surgery. Casualty sees quite a lot of penetrating injuries. There are less shootings than in Kingston and it is a nicer area.

O Elective notes: Good experience, but not loads of responsibility.

Accommodation: They try to provide it, but no guarantees.

Annotto Bay Public Hospital

Annotto Bay, St Mary, Jamaica, WI Tel: +1 876 996 2222.

The hospital: A very busy rural hospital. It is pretty isolated but has all main specialities (surgery, medicine, O&G, paeds). It is poorly funded.

O Elective notes: Plenty of chances to practise clinical skills. You can visit St Ann's Bay Public Hospital or Port Antonio Public Hospital which are nearby. Good teaching on wards. The hospital is fairly isolated.

Bellevue Hospital

Kingston, Jamaica, WI.

The hospital: The largest psychiatric hospital in the Caribbean. It is a state-funded hospital in deepest Downtown. It is part of Jamican folklore and is like something out of a horror film. It has 23 wards spread out over extensive grounds containing 1500 patients; Yardies from the neighbouring ganglands; drugs-runners; pimps and prostitutes. All bar seven of the wards are long-stay wards and Bellevue also acts as a dumping ground for old Jamaicans whose relatives have emigrated. This is a place of institutionalization – schizophrenics lying in bed all day, mentally retarded patients not even getting sanitary care. Some patients can be very violent. The hospital, however, has guards that carry assault rifles.

There are only 4–5 doctors and one nurse per ward. The doctor sees about 60 outpatients in the morning and 90 in the afternoon. Most patients are probably incorrectly diagnosed. WARNING: this is a dangerous place … think seriously before going here if you are white.

Haiti and the Dominican Republic

Haiti

Population: 7.2 million
Language: French and French Creole
Capital: Port-au-Prince
Currency: Gourde
Int Code: +509

Due to the political unrest in Haiti (the western third of Hispaniola) it is difficult to find out information. It is an incredibly poor country and most people can't afford healthcare, instead getting help from voodoo priests. This is reflected in a life expectancy of only 57. Malnutrition, infectious diseases, such as malaria and TB. and political killings are the big killers. There is only one doctor for 7040 people.

The Dominican Republic, however, (that occupies the other two-thirds of Hispaniola) is a popular tourist destination with Italians and Germans. It has a number of medical schools:

Iberoamerican University (UNIBE)
School of Medicine, Av Francia 129, Santo Domingo, Dominican Republic Tel: (809) 689 4111 Fax: (809) 686 5821.

Dominican Republic

Population: 7.8 million
Language: Spanish
Capital: Santo Domingo
Currency: Dominican Republic peso
Int Code: +1 809

This is a new medical school (founded 1982) also in the nation's capital. It trains a number of foreign students.

Universidad Autónoma de Santo Domingo (USAD)
Departmento de Medicina, Facultad de Ciencias de la Sald, Ciudad Universitaria, Santo Domingo, Dominican Republic.
This is the oldest medical school and situated in the nation's capital.

Universidad Nordestana (UNNE)
Facultad de Ciencias Médicas, Apartado 239, San Francisco de Marcorís, Duarte, Dominican Republic.
A much smaller teaching hospital to the north of the island. Its teaching hospital has 350 beds.

St Kitts

Population: 41,000
Language: English
Capital: Basseterre
Currency East Caribbean dollar
Int code: +1 869

St Kitt's is a small beautiful island and a popular tourist destination. It is a former British colony and lies at the top of the Leeward Islands chain. The government provides a basic health service. To find out more write to: The Chief Medical Officer, Church Street, PO Box 186, Basseterre, St Kitts, WI.

JNF Hospital

St Kitts, West Indies.

The hospital: A small hospital. TB, HIV, diabetes, thyroid disorders and hypertension are very common. The hospital is very friendly.

Antigua

Population: 65,000
Official Language: English
Capital: St John's
Currency: East Caribbean dollar
Int Code: +1 283/268

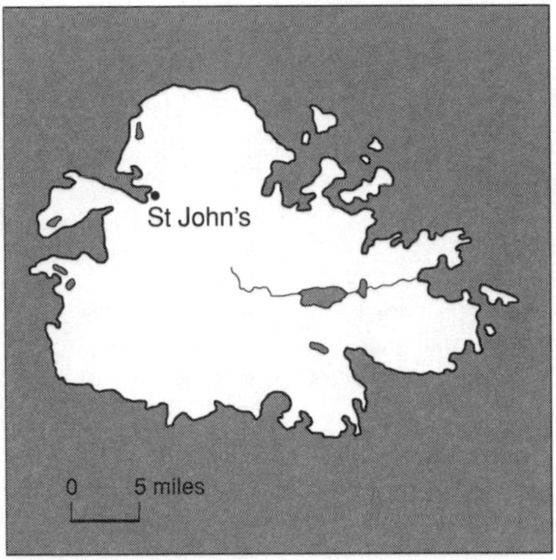

The island is a Third World Country and has been a colony of the Spanish, French and British. Tourism is the island's main industry and accounts for about half the workforce. Approximately 65,000 people live on Antigua, of whom 90% are of African descent but the British influence is clear with their passion for cricket. There are beautiful beaches that are all open to the public. Prime beaches to visit are located on the east coast, Dickenson and Runaway beaches, Deep Bay and Hawksbill Beach to the west of St John's and Darkwood beach to the south. Antigua has some excellent diving with coral canyons, the most popular diving site being at Cades Reef. The going rate is about £20 for a single tank and £175 for a certification course. Snorkelling from shore is readily available with wrecks and many shoals of fish that can be easily visualized. Windsurfing schools are located at Dickenson Bay. The main places to visit on the island are Nelson's Dockyard, Jolly Harbour and Shirley Heights. Nelson's Dockyard is the island's main port of entry for yachts; it has many restaurants, a small market, a museum and various other historical buildings with a colonial atmosphere. Jolly Harbour is a new marina with various shops and boutiques located on the quay. At night there are many bars and discos. Shirley Heights is an eighteenth-century fort ruins with a wonderful hilltop view. Within the ruins is a bar that offers a public barbecue on Sundays with a live steel band. Other places of interest include: Devil's Bridge, a coastal sea arch and Fig Tree Drive, a road that passes by pineapple patches and tall plants.

To get around you can hire a bike or car or use the bus services. The roads, however, are very poor with many potholes. In order to drive on Antigua, you will need a temporary 90-day driving licence which cost about £8. Car rental is about £20/day. Taxis are government-run, but always confirm with the driver the price before the journey. When you've done all that head to Barbuda, Antigua's dependency 30 miles north-east with even more beautiful beaches.

O Medicine:
Pretty good for the Caribbean. There are state-run hospitals providing treatment free. GPs are not free and therefore everything comes to hospital.

Holberton Hospital
PO Box 2797, St Johns, Antigua, West Indies Fax: +1 283 462 6073.
The hospital: Located in St John's which is the capital of the island. From the outside it looks like a small rundown warehouse. It has 60 beds comprising four wards and an 'intensive care unit'. Although poorly sanitized, it does have a good X-ray department, including a CT scanner. The beds are huddled close to each other on crumbling wards often without curtains around them. There are ants and insects everywhere, including the theatres.
O Elective notes: There is a ward round in the morning, after which there are few doctors on-site. The hospital is run by three casualty officers and the on-call teams who work from home. By 7 am the casualty department waiting room is full. There is quite a bit of trauma due to the state of the roads and lack of road law. Local anaesthetic is reserved for children. Consultants conduct one clinic a week from a shed at the bottom of the main hospital drive. To arrange this elective contact the hospital administrator MONTHS before you intend to go. It works out cheapest and quickest to fax.
Accommodation: Hospital accommodation is basic. The are many insects and the shower consists of a high-up tap. No mosquito nets are provided. Try Mrs E. Murphy, Murphy's Apartments, All Saint's Road, St Johns, Antigua, but this can be expensive.

Dominica

Population: 71,000
Language: English
Capital: Roseau
Currency: East Caribbean dollar
Int Code: +1 767

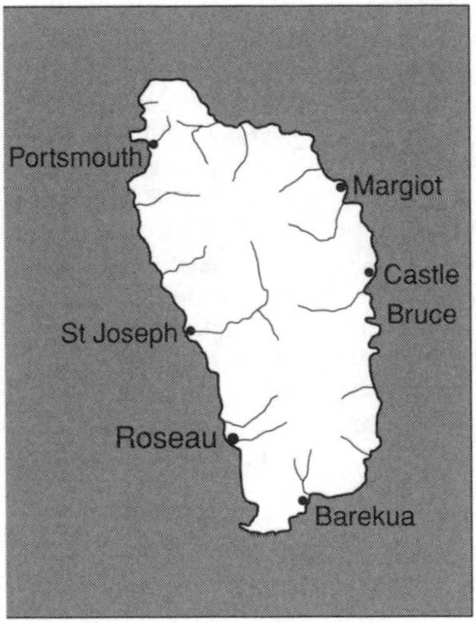

Dominica is a small island in the eastern Caribbean measuring only 46 km by 25 km. The volcanic mountains rise spectacularly out of the sea and are richly forested. The highest peak is Morne Diablotin, 1447 m high and is within the Northern Forest reserve. There is an abundance of rivers, lakes and impressive waterfalls which make excellent swimming. The east coast is very dramatic being washed by the fierce Atlantic waves much in contrast to the west which faces on to the Caribbean sea and is more typically sandy beaches and palm trees.

A third of the population lives in Roseau. Most of the islanders are of African descent with about 3000 native Caribs who reside in a large reserve on the eastern side of the island. The Caribs settled in the fourteenth century and called the island 'Waitikubuli'. It was rediscovered by Christopher Columbus and pronounced a British colony until its independence in 1978. There is still a strong Carib and Creole tradition found in the art and basketwork, music and clothes. This is combined with the Rastafarians and Catholic religions that have superseded. The local language is Patois, but English is mostly spoken. There is high unemployment and most women are involved in the upbringing of at least five children. Agriculture is the main income and there is an effort to export bananas, chillies and bay leaves, although the annual hurricanes destroy many of the crops. Subsistence farming and local produce provides enough food for most people and despite a low standard of living compared with other Caribbean islands, none seems to suffer from malnutrition. Tourism is increasing rapidly and this island is sure to change.

✪ Medicine:

Medical care is provided from 44 health centres and the main hospital in the capital. There is private healthcare, but most have to make do with the Government's cover.

Princess Margaret Hospital

Roseau, Commonwealth of Dominica.

The hospital: The main hospital on the island with 800 beds. It's mostly an old building, but the French have constructed a new wing (foyer, radiology and A&E). The staff are very friendly, most of whom trained in the University of the West Indies in Jamaica or Cuba. There are also VSO workers. Despite the lack of facilities, lab tests, imaging and drugs, the standard of care is very impressive. Common disorders include diabetes, hypertension, TB, intestinal parasites and yaws.

Accommodation: Available in a local B&B ($12/night).

Martinique

Population: 371,000
Language: French and Creole
Capital: Fort-de-France
Currency: French franc
Int Code: +596

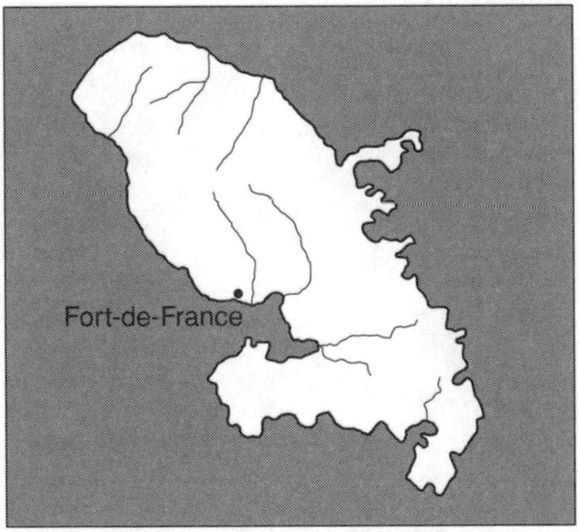

Martinique is a beautiful small French island next to St Lucia. There are plenty of white sandy beaches and clear blue sea ... perfect if you want to learn to dive or windsurf. The people are mostly black Caribbeans although there are many French settlers. So if you want to hit the beach, enjoy Creole food, get a tan and practise your French, this is the place to go. You will need good French to converse with patients.

Service de Médecine Interne (4B)
Chu De Fort-De-France, 97261 Fort-De-France, Martinique, French West Indies.

The hospital: Relatively large: the A&E department has a helicopter service and the hospital covers all the main specialities.

O Elective notes: The medical wards are extremely laid back. Turn up in the mornings, do a ward round and a few procedures (e.g. bone marrow aspirates, pleural drains, ECGs, blood gases etc.) and then go explore. One of the consultants has a haematology interest so you can see advanced cases of leukaemia, Hodgkin's and AIDS.

St Lucia

Population: 145,000
Language: English
Capital: Castries
Currency: East Caribbean dollar
Int Code: +1 758

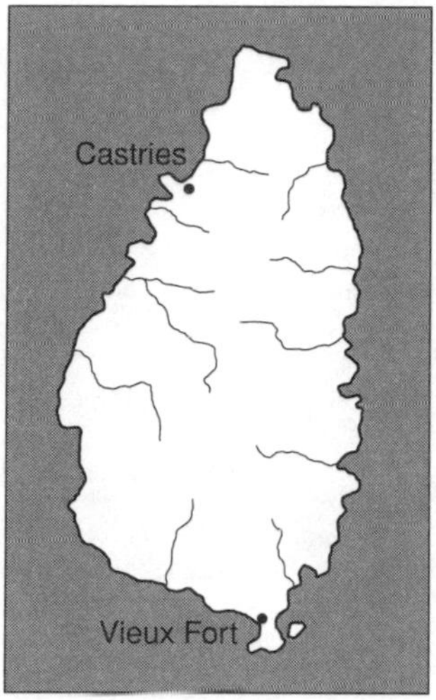

St Lucia is a beautiful island (possibly the most beautiful in the Caribbean) with good beaches and amazing rainforests. It has been both a French and British colony and retains the character of both. Today it relies on tourism, mainly from cruise ships, and banana growing.

St Jude Hospital
Vieux Fort, St Lucia, West Indies.

The hospital: St Jude's is St Lucia's largest hospital and is situated by the town Vieux Fort. It is charity-run by the Sisters of Mercy and is staffed almost exclusively by volunteers. As a result students are much more involved, appreciated and given far more responsibility than at home. Every morning there is a huge general outpatients clinic at which all students are expected to attend and see patients. There is a wide variety of conditions and they tend to be advanced as patients have to pay to attend.

❍ **Elective notes:** This is an invaluable experience and you'll learn at a terrific rate. There'll be five or six doctors (often American) around to ask if you need help. There's good teaching and plenty of practical procedures. Outpatients finishes at 2 pm at which point you are free to go if not on-call. On-call is on a 1:4 rota and involves staying in the OPC until 4 pm and then working in the emergency room. There is plenty of trauma and acute medicine to be seen here. Rheumatic fever, TB and sickle cell disease are pretty common. The volunteers are all very friendly and welcoming and organize frequent trips and beach parties. This elective comes extremely highly recommended.

Accommodation: And meals are provided. There are plenty of people around and usually one or two American students so going on your own is fine.

St Vincent

Population: 111,000
Language: English
Capital: Kingstown
Currency: East Caribbean dollar
Int Code: +1 784

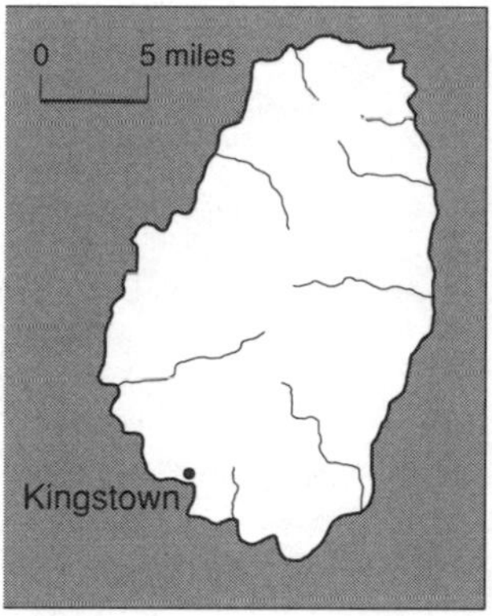

St Vincent is a beautiful volcanic island manly relying on banana production and élite tourism. Associated with it arc a group of mainly coral islands, the Grenadines. Kingstown itself is a little run down and the people can be a bit rude if you're a single white female, but this is not true of the other Grenadine islands. There's a lot to do around St Vincent – botanical gardens, volcanoes, rainforests, waterfalls etc. However, the best places to go for deserted paradise are the smaller Grenadine islands with their white sands, palm trees and clear blue water ideal for diving and snorkelling.

Kingstown General Hospital

Kingstown, St Vincent, West Indies.

The hospital: Kingstown General Hospital has 210 beds and serves the whole of St Vincent and the Grenadines. Specialities include A&E, general medicine and surgery, paediatrics, O&G, ophthalmology, ENT and radiology. The hospital has most of the necessary equipment although much is old and in short supply. They also lack simple things such as tourniquets and make do with gloves and catheters. X-ray and ultrasound are the only imaging techniques.

❍ Elective notes: Most of the doctors are friendly and helpful. They are of many nationalities, mainly Indian. They don't give much formal teaching, but are keen to answer questions. The hospital is always busy, but especially so in the afternoons when medical students from the nearby American offshore medical school descend in huge numbers. This is your cue to escape as nothing much happens once they arrive. This elective is thoroughly recommended if you want a stress-free, relaxing time.

Accommodation: Provided in the nurses' hostel, a five-minute walk from the hospital. It's cheap and convenient and meals can be provided very cheaply if you like rice.

Barbados

Population: 260,000
Language: English
Capital: Bridgetown
Currency: Barbados dollar
Int Code: +1 246

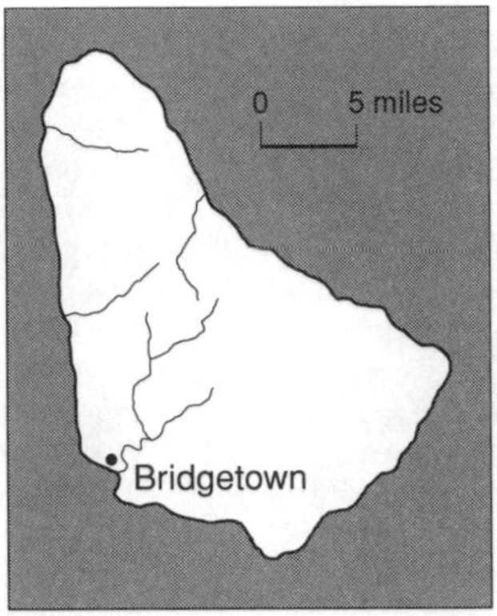

Barbados is one of the larger islands that comprise the West Indies. It is made of coral unlike the other Caribbean islands which are volcanic. Measuring 22 miles by 14 it has a resident population of about 260,000 which, during peak season, reaches roughly 400,000. As part of the Commonwealth (independence granted in 1966), the Queen is still the Monarch, but a separate Parliament operates here. The island is divided into 'parishes', like counties in the UK. The majority of Barbadians (colloquially Bajans) are black of African descent, with the other 5% being white of Scottish/English descent. The island's economy consists of tourism, sugar and rum. Bridgetown is the capital and is not the typical capital you would expect from a Third World country. Crime is not really a problem here although in recent years people have had to start locking doors and there is the occasional mugging. Occasionally you will be bothered by a VERY friendly Bajan offering to 'walk you home safely'. He will ask for money at some point. It's best just to say that you're a doctor at the hospital and fed up with being asked. Tourist attractions include: Welchman Hall gully, Harrison's cave, the picturesque coastline at Bathsheba, Farley Hill National Park and Barbados wildlife reserve. There is an abundance of water sports available. Barbados is the place to learn to scuba dive (five-day PADI courses). Tell them you work in the hospital as this can give you up to 50% off courses. There is also water-skiing, jetskiing, windsurfing, sailing and fishing on many beaches. The cricket is also a MUST see. Other events include the races at Garrison Savannah, Oistins Easter fish festival, Congaline Carnival, Open air opera, the Jolly Roger cruise and the Mount Gay rum tour. As you might expect, the nightlife is also pretty active with a number of clubs along the coastline (drink as much as you

can for about £6). Transport is provided cheaply by government taxis or private ZR vans (50p a ride). WARNING ... there is no law against drink-driving.

⊕ Medicine:

Provided by both Government-subsidized hospitals/clinics and private hospitals. It is Western diseases that are the killers although NIDDM (prevalence = 20% in the general population) and HIV are increasing.

Queen Elizabeth Hospital

Bridgetown, Barbados, WI Tel: 1 246 429 5112 Fax: 1 246 429 6738.

The hospital: The QEH is the main hospital on the island situated near Bridgetown (10 minutes' walk from the centre). There are other smaller hospitals on the island, although there are no other surgical theatres except at the private hospital 'Bayview'. The wards are all male or female. The décor can also leave a bit to desire. The lattice brickwork on one of the wards allows a pleasant draft but doesn't keep the birds out! There is also a lack of comforts for the visiting doctor although the place is very relaxed (7.30 am clinics may not start until 10.30). Medications are flown in from Florida. The hospital does have a (temperamental) CT scanner, but this contrasts with the fact that they regularly run out of steroids, saline, blood and aspirin. Orthopaedics is very busy with trauma due to the lack of seatbelts. There is a lack of hip prostheses for the ageing population and amputation is becoming more common. If you can't afford to go privately you can order your new hip by mail from Miami and bring it with you on the day of your operation.

O Elective notes: There is difficulty for the visiting student to do much in theatre (chances are, you won't get to scrub up), but the teaching makes up for this (there are 20 West Indian students in each of the two final years). There is no pressure to go, but you will learn a lot. You are invited to clinic where your help is very much appreciated. You're treated as a doctor. Some of the common diseases consist of diabetes (NIDDM) and its complications. HIV is quite a major problem here. HTLV-1 is also endemic.

Dress: No jeans, no bared shoulders (therefore be careful with sundresses), dresses to the knees and shirt and tie for the boys. No white coats.

Electives can be done in: general medicine, general surgery, orthopaedics, ophthalmology, A&E, pathology, radiology, ENT, child health, psychiatry, family medicine, community health and anaesthesiology. They are all done at the QEH except family medicine (conducted in a GP unit) and community health (conducted at the Randel Phillips Polyclinic). You can organize this through: The Faculty of Medical Sciences, Queen Elizabeth Hospital, Bridgetown, Barbados, WI. A US$50 admin fee is requested. Write VERY EARLY to the administrative assistant (or fax/call on the above number). There is then a further fee of US$150 on commencement of the elective. Electives longer than 8–10 weeks may have a further charge.

Accommodation: Not actually provided. The Electives Co-ordinator can arrange it for you (it tends to be a cosy cartel of ex-secretaries' houses, some of which charge a lot and aren't in great areas of town). There can be 20–30 elective students there at any one time so the Co-ordinator may get confused as to where you are sent. Try to get confirmation before you go. The best is reported to be Mrs Carter (Mrs Carter, Interlaken, Worthing, Christchurch, Barbados). BDS$500 gets you a nice double room or you can share for BDS$375 each. WARNING: Insects are very common. Malaria is not a problem although dengue fever outbreaks do occur. Most will provide a net, but take some insect repellent. Food is not cheap in supermarkets, but eating out is.

Language: English, but you may need a translator to decipher the accent!

Note: If you apply to Bayview (private hospital on Barbados) they give lovely accommodation in a plantation house for free.

Grenada

Population: 92,000
Language: English
Capital: St George's
Currency: Eastern Caribbean dollar
Int Code: +1 473

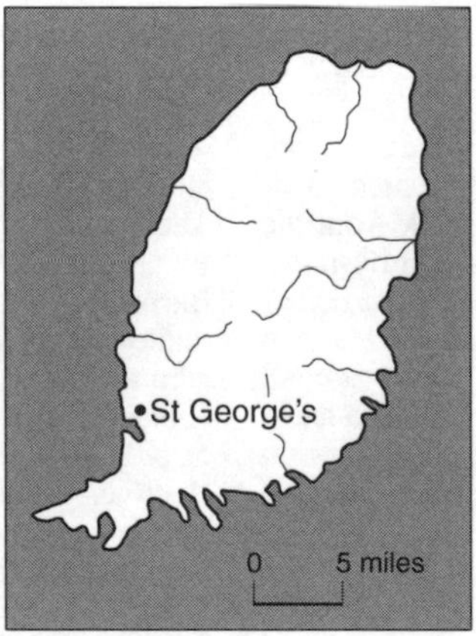

Grenada is one of the most southern islands and has close ties with Cuba. Previously many Cubans have worked in Grenada's hospitals. The country has an offshore American pre-clinical medical school.

Grenada General Hospital

St George's, Grenada, West Indies.

The hospital: A friendly medium-sized hospital overlooking the harbour entrance to St George's. Departments include general medicine and surgery, orthopaedics, O&G, anaesthetic and paeds. Hypertension, diabetes and pre-eclampsia are relatively common with TB, dengue fever, rheumatic fever and leptospirosis also being seen. It is pretty overcrowded with limited facilities. There is a busy psychiatry department that has close links with Mount Gay Psychiatric Hospital and many parishes. Not surprisingly the unit is very stretched with only relatively basic treatments. The preclinical medical school and library are here.

O Elective notes: The junior doctors do a 1:2 and therefore are grateful for any help, although there isn't pressure to. There's good teaching with formal lectures. It's popular with Australian students. Lots of sunbathing and beer drinking. If you're female you may find the local men show a lot of interest. It's a safe place and shouldn't worry you. TIP: Hang around the yacht club as there are often rich people looking for extra hands. Dive the 'Bianca C' wreck.

Mount Gay Hospital

St George's, Grenada, West Indies.

The hospital: Built for 80, this psychiatric hospital has 120 beds/mattresses. It's busy, cramped and has poor facilities.

Trinidad and Tobago

Population: 1.3 million
Language: English
Capital: Port of Spain
Currency: Trinidad and Tobago dollar
Int Code: + 1 868

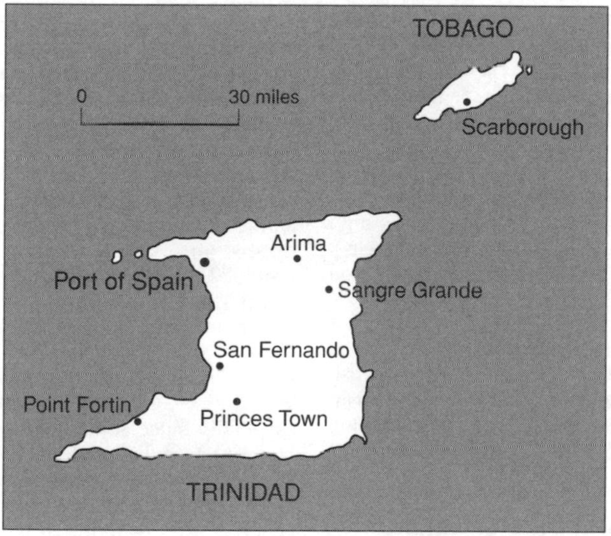

Trinidad, seven miles off the coast of Venezuela is one of the least-visited Caribbean Islands. The language is English (hence if you want Third World medicine without language barriers, this is a good choice). Its sister island, Tobago, gets all the tourism, whereas Trinidad is more industrial with sugar being a major income. It is, however, still a beautiful island and the people are probably more genuine due to the lack of tourism. January–February are good times to go as they build up towards carnival time (which takes place on the days before Ash Wednesday), but book accommodation well in advance. There are big parties every night, steel bands fill the evenings with their practice and everyone has a smile on their face (not surprisingly, this is also a busy trauma time in A&E). The people are friendly and fun-loving and from a diverse cultural descent (African, Indian and more recently Chinese). Crime is increasing and be wary of wandering streets at night, especially if you're a lone female. There is an idyllic beach on

Trinidad (Marcus Bay) and mountain ranges covered in forests. However, for the real beauty visit Tobago (approx £30 flight, £10 ferry). You can go on a scuba course (£180) or just lie on the beach.

Medicine:

The healthcare system consists of both a public and a smaller private sector. The public uses a three-tier system. Primary care is provided by 102 health centres with doctors, nurses and midwives across the country. Delivery units are attached to a number of these. There is secondary care through three county and four district hospitals. Tertiary care is from two general hospitals, one in the south and one in the north. These have specialists in all fields. Primary care in the private sector is via 600 GPs. The two teaching hospitals (for the University of the West Indies) on Trinidad are the Port of Spain and Mount Hope.

NIDDM is very common as are its complications. HIV on both islands is also very prevalent (reports say as high as 70% in young people in some areas). Leptospirosis is also common on Trinidad due to the number of rats.

Visas and work permits:

No visa is required for EU, British Commonwealth or US citizens to visit. Work permits are not required if working for less than 30 days, otherwise you must apply to the Embassy.

Port of Spain General Hospital

Charlotte Street, Port of Spain, Trinidad, West Indies Tel: 1 809 623 2951.

The hospital: Port of Spain General Hospital is a very large (900-bed), busy hospital admitting for the whole of the Port of Spain, the capital of Trinidad. It is a public hospital and only those Trinidadians not rich enough to afford private healthcare come here (about 95% of the population). Conditions on the wards are pretty basic and there are few advanced facilities (no CT/MRI for example). Each team on the medical unit admits on a 1:6; normally about 40–50 patients come in.

Elective notes: A&E is either fairly or very busy but the hours are very flexible (important around carnival time). There's plenty of practical experience (stitching, putting on plasters, basic medical management). All drugs prescribed are in trade names . . . so take a *BNF*. The doctors and staff are very friendly and helpful. There's plenty of advanced pathology, tropical diseases and trauma. HIV and drug abuse are common. This, with poverty, makes psychiatry an interesting speciality. The local students are a pretty keen bunch, but they get plenty of teaching that you are more than welcome to attend.

Note: State on application whether you want the Port of Spain or Mount Hope hospitals as some people have arrived and been attached to students at Mount Hope. You can either arrange this through the UWI or the hospital. The latter is recommended.

Accommodation: Make sure you confirm your accommodation and price before you go as some people have been ripped off. A list of guesthouses is provided. La Maison Rustique, 16 Rust Street, St Clair is in a safe area and recommended. Another is Miss May Cherrie, 22 Stone St, Port of Spain. Note: There are usually many elective students . . . this is socially very good, especially since some areas of Trinidad are not particularly safe and you tend to stick together. Also think about getting a Hilton Pool pass as Port of Spain has no beach within walking distance. (Beer prices 37p (supermarket), 70p (bar).) Accommodation is also available at Mount Hope.

Mount Hope Hospital

The Eric Williams Medical Sciences Complex, Uriah Butler Highway, Champs Fleurs, Trinidad, West Indies Tel: 1 809 645 2640.

The hospital: Built in the early 1980s to solve Trinidad's health problems. It has equipment and facilities similar to most Western hospitals; however, people have to pay for their care. So few people can afford it that only 10% of beds may be

occupied. People don't turn up for out-patients and even for operations as they can't pay. Therefore it is not a busy place. The staff are friendly and keen to teach; however, not much is seen. Students have in the past felt they saw more at the Port of Spain General, although there are plenty of lumps and bumps if doing surgery (good for short case practice). It is about 10 miles out of the city centre (although it can take up to an hour to get there).
Accommodation: A list of guesthouses is provided. Occasionally accommodation has been available in the hospital.

San Fernando General Hospital

Harris Promenade, San Fernando, Trinidad, West Indies Tel: 1 809 652 3581.
The hospital: Has the major specialities. There's a wide range of diseases and 'hands on' experience is encouraged.

Tobago Regional Hospital

Fort Street, Scarborough, Tobago, West Indies Tel: 868 639 2551.
The hospital: The small hospital (30 medical beds) for Tobago. It is friendly but has relatively poor facilities. There's medicine, surgery, O&G department. Diabetes, hypertension and HIV are all common. There's a busy A&E.
❍ Elective notes: There's good teaching and Tobago is more beautiful than Trinidad. You must learn to dive.
Accommodation: Stay at the Hope Cottage Guest House, Calde Hall Road, The Fort, Scarborough, Tobago.

OTHER HOSPITALS IN TRINIDAD AND TOBAGO:

Arima District Hospital, Queen Mary Avenue, Arima, Trinidad, WI Tel: 1 809 667 3503.
Caura Chest Hospital, Couva, Central Trinidad WI Tel: 1 809 662 2211.
Couva District Hospital, Couva, Central Trinidad, WI Tel: 1 809 636 2411.
Eric Williams Medical Sciences Complex Authority (including the women's hospital) Mt Hopem, Trinidad, WI Tel: 1 809 645 2640.
Mayaro District Hospital, Mayaro, East Trinidad, WI Tel: 1 809 630 4346.
Point Fortin District Hospital, Point Fortin, South Trinidad, WI Tel: 1 809 48 3281.
Port of Spain General Hospital, Charlotte Street, Port of Spain, Trinidad, WI Tel: 1 809 623 2951.
Princes Town District Hospital, Princes Town, Trinidad, WI Tel: 1 809 655 2255.
St Ann's Hospital, St Ann's Road, Port of Spain, Trinidad, WI Tel: 1 809 624 1151.
St James Medical Complex, St James, Port of Spain, Trinidad, WI Tel: 1 809 622 4173.
San Fernando General Hospital, Harris Promenade, San Fernando, Trinidad, WI Tel: 1 809 652 3581.
Sangre Grande County Hospital, Sangre Grande, East Trinidad, WI Tel: 01 809 668 2273.
Tobago County Hospital, The Fort, Scarborough, Tobago, WI Tel: 01 809 639 2551.

PRIVATE HOSPITALS:

Adventist Hospital, Western Main Road, Cocorite, Port of Spain, Trinidad, WI Tel: 01 809 622 1191.
Langmore Health Foundation, Palmyra Village, San Fernando, Trinidad, WI Tel: 01 809 652 2244.
Nicoll Nursing Home, 44 Coblentz Avenue, Port of Spain, Trinidad, WI Tel: 01 809 624 7566.
Southern Medical Clinic, 26–24 Quenca and St Vincent Streets, San Fernando, Trinidad, WI Tel: 01 809 652 2078.

EUROPE

Austria

Population: 8 million
Language: German
Capital: Vienna
Currency: Schilling
Int Code: +43

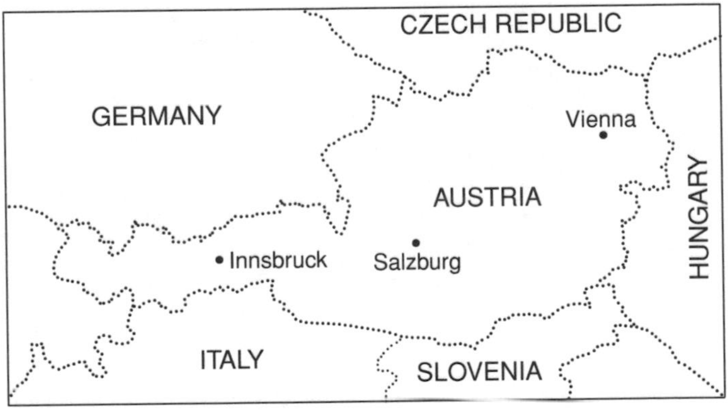

Austria is a landlocked country in central Europe that has a great deal to offer the visiting medic. You can ski in the Alps or sample some of the culture in one of its cities. Despite this, probably because of language difficulties, Austria is not by any means a popular destination with students or doctors.

✪ Medicine:

A healthcare system exists that provides a pretty good service to the population. Western diseases are the norm.

➲ Visas and work permits:

No visa is required to visit or do an elective in Austria if from the EU. Contact the embassy for information on work permits.

Notes for elective students: There is an **Exchange programme for medical students** within the **International Federation of Medical Students (IFMSA)**. The programme offers to medical students the possibility to work in a medical institution (e.g. hospital). In Austria the exchange programme is organized by the **Austrian Medical Students Association (AMSA)** (The National Exchange Office, AMSA, c/o Liechtensteinstrasse 13, A–1090 Vienna, Austria). Students coming to Austria are assigned to a University hospital in Graz, Innsbruck or Vienna. Free board and lodging are provided. Working languages are German and English, though obviously German is needed to communicate with patients. July to September are AMSA's preferred times of exchange as this is when most elective students are present.

The IFMSA exchange is operated on a bilateral basis . . . for each student they accept they send one out to the applicant country. This can be a problem in the UK since, as there is no medical students association, there is no one to organize this. For this reason, direct exchanges between hospitals in the UK and Austria are therefore proposed. A useful place to start looking for hospitals in Austria is from the main University in Vienna **Allgemeines Krankenhaus**, Wien Universitätskliniken A-1090 Wien, Währinger Gürtel 18–20 Tel: 0222 40400 0 www.akn-wien.ac.uk

Belarus

Population: 10.1 million
Language: Belorussian
Capital: Minsk
Currency: Belorussian rouble
Int Code: +375

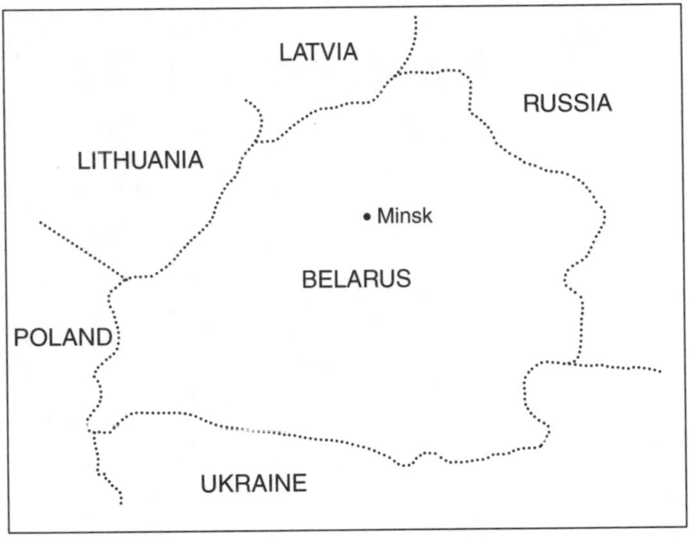

Belarus is a landlocked country bordered by Latvia, Lithuania, Poland, Russia and the Ukraine. Since its split from Moscow in 1991, Belarus has only had agriculture as a viable resource. Since the Chernobyl disaster in 1986 in next-door Ukraine, many Belorussians have suffered severe ill health.

Medicine:

Belarus had a relatively good healthcare system but has been under increasing strain since the Chernobyl nuclear disaster. Cancer and leukaemia rates have risen dramatically resulting in the need for many new specialist wards. Belorussian doctors, via the 'Know-How' Fund, are being trained in specialist techniques such as bone marrow transplantation to try to cure these conditions. (There is one doctor per 246 people.) The big killers include heart disease and cancer.

Climate and crime:

Varies from warm (20 °C) in the summer to very cold (–10 °C) in the winter. Crime has increased greatly since independence due to poverty.

➲ **Visas and work permits:**
Application for a visa can be made in person or by post. Fill in an application form from the Embassy and send/take it with: a valid passport, a passport photo, formal invitation from the individual or corporate (government body, company or organization) on their letter-headed notepaper or alternatively a letter of support, and finally, the appropriate fee payable only in the local currency, to the Embassy of the Republic of Belarus. (Fees are currently: Visitor visa £40, Business £40, Student £10).

You may need a short interview but it's the consular officer's assessment of your intentions that carries weight in the end. The visas take 5–10 working days to process.

Once in you should register your passport with the Ministry of Foreign Affairs of the Republic Belarus or the Ministry of Internal Affairs. If staying in a hotel, they'll register you at the reception. (Register within three days of arrival). (*See* Section 3: The Appendix for Embassy address.)

For information on hospitals contact:

The Ministry of Foreign Affairs of the Republic of Belarus
222 030 Minsk, ul.Lenina, 19. Consular Department, Belarus Tel: 00375 172 22 26 40 Fax: 00375 172 22 26 63.

Belgium

Population: 10.1 million
Languages: Dutch, French and German
Capital: Brussels
Currency: Belgium franc
Int Code: +32

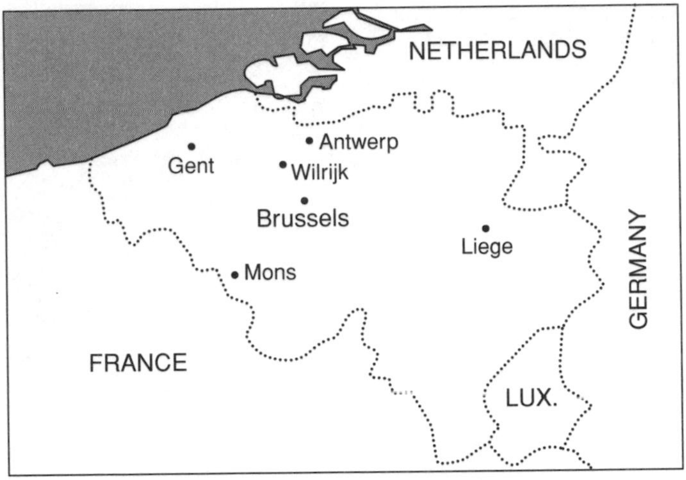

Belgium (bordered by France, Germany, the Netherlands and Luxembourg) has become almost the capital of Europe. It is not commonly visited by UK students. Since it is also on the Socrates/Erasmus programme, only a brief list of medical schools is given below.

Medicine:

Belgium has some of the best healthcare in the world. However, it is not free. Most Belgians belong to an insurance scheme entitling them to a 75% rebate on costs. Belgium is particularly renowned for fertility treatments and organ transplants.

Visas and work permits:

Neither are required for entry by EU members. Contact your local embassy if outside this region.

Climate and crime:

A typical maritime climate, warmest between June and August. Crime is pretty low.

UNIVERSITIES:

Rijksuniversitair Centrum Antwerpen, Faculteit voor Geneeskunde en Farmacie, Groenenborgerlaan 171, B-2020 Antwerpen, Belgium.
Université Catholique de Louvain, UCL 5020, Avenue Emmanuel Mounier 5010 or 10 avenue Hippocrate (for the hospital), B-1200 Bruxelles, Belgium. http://www.md.ucl.ac.be/luc/luc_eng.htm (This is one of the oldest and largest medical schools in Belgium with around 800 beds.)
Université Libre de Bruxelles, Faculté de Médecine et de Pharmacie, Boulevard de Waterloo 115, B-1000 Bruxelles, Belgium.
Vrije Universiteit Brussel, Faculteit van de Geneeskunde en de Farmacie, Laarbeeklaan 103, B-1090 Brussels, Belgium.
Limburgs Universitair Centrum, Universitarie Campus, Faculteit voor Geneeskunde, B-3610 Dipenbeek, Belgium.
Rijksuniversiteit Gent, Caculteit der Geneeskunde, Akademisch Ziekenhuis, De Pintelaan 185, B-9000 Gent, Belgium.
Katholieke Universiteit Leuven, Faculteit der Geneeskunde, Minderbroedersstraat 17, B-3999 Leuven, Belgium.
Université de l'Etat á Liége, Faculté de Médecine, Place du 20 août 7, B-4000 Liege, Belgium.
Université de l'Etat á Mons, 24 avenue du Champ de Mars, B-7000 Mons, Belgium.
Facultés universitares Notre-Dame de la Paix, Faculté de Médecine, Rue de Bruxelles 61, B-5000 Namur, Belgium. (Preclinical only) Clinical students are transferred to
Universitair Instelling Antwerpen, Faculteit voor Geneeskunde en Farmacie, Universiteitsplein 1, B-2610 Wilruk (CLINICAL ONLY)

Languages: Dutch at: Antwerp, Vrije Universiteit Brussel, Diepenbeek, Ghent, Katholieke Universiteit Leuven and Wilrijk; French at Université Catholique de Louvain, Université libre de Bruxelles, Brussels, Mons, Liége and Namur.

Croatia

Population: 4.5 million
Language: Croatian
Capital: Zagreb
Currency: Kuna
Int Code: +385

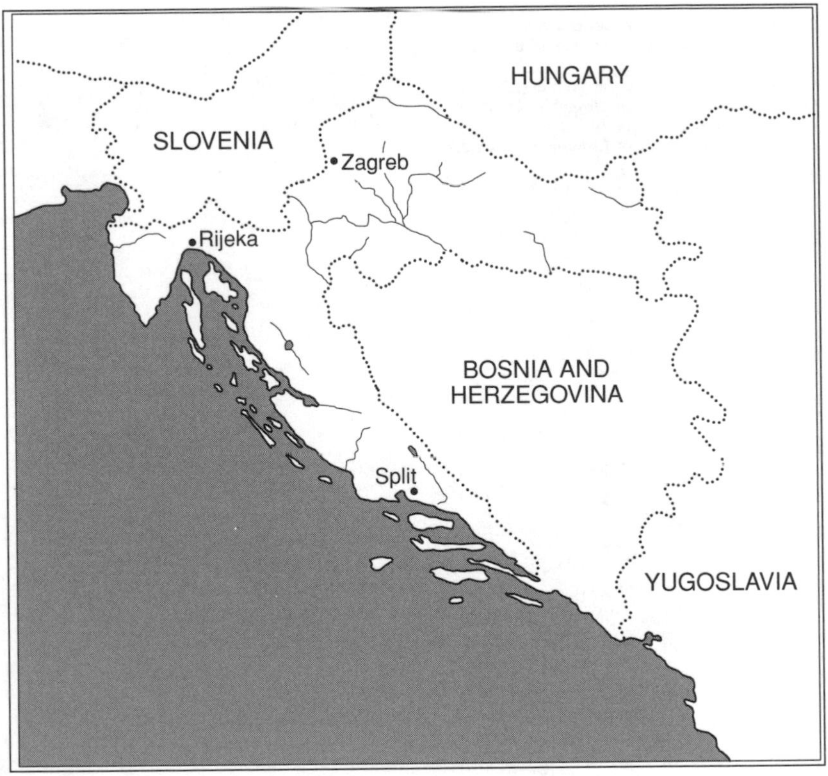

Croatia has been involved in heavy conflicts recently with the break-up of Yugoslavia and the war with Bosnia. Although tourism in some areas is picking up, confirm safety with the Foreign Office before organizing work or an elective.

✚ Medicine:
Although most people are covered by a health insurance scheme, the war has put a great deal of pressure on resources. Western diseases are still the big killers.

➲ **Visas and work permits:**
Due to the small numbers of students that go here, no accurate information can be gained regarding the need for student visas. Contact the embassy for up-to-date details.

University of Zagreb Medical School

10 000 Zagreb p.p. 1026, Croatia
Tel: 385 1 4566 777 Fax: 385 1 272 050
http://mamef.mef.hr

Founded in 1917, Croatia's first medical school now uses many clinics and institutes. These include, the **Clinical Hospital Center Zagreb** (providing all major medical and surgical specialities as well as O&G and paeds, **'Sestre Milodsrdnice' Clinical Hospital, 'Merkur' Clinical Hospital, 'Sveti Duh' General Hospital, 'Fran Mihaljevic' Clinical Hospital for Infectious Diseases, 'Vuk Vrhovac' University Clinic for Diabetes, Endocrinology and Metabolic Diseases, 'Jordanovac' Clinical Hospital for Pulmonary Diseases and Thoracic Surgery, University Clinic for Traumatology, Paediatric Clinic, University Clinic for Tumors, Rehab and Orthopaedic Institute** and **'Vapee' Psychiatric Hospital**.

Sveti Duh General Hospital

Sveti Duh 64, 10000 Zagreb, Croatia.

The hospital: Has 800 beds and offers most specialities except paediatrics and dermatology. There is a six-bed coronary care unit and a specialized cardiology ward. It is an incredibly busy, understaffed hospital where the juniors have few responsibilities (the consultants do all the prescribing). The teaching, however, is excellent. There are very few other students.

Accommodation: Not provided.

University of Rijeka School of Medicine

Bracé Branchetta 20, 51000 Rijeka, Croatia
Tel: 051 651 111 Fax: 051 675 806
http://mamed.medri.hr/eng/index.html
e-mail dekanat@medri.hr

University of Split Medical School

Soltanska 2, 21000 Split, Croatia Tel: 385 21 565 073 Fax: 385 21 365 389
www.mefst.hr/mefst/medsch.htm
e-mail: office@mefst.hr

Cyprus

Population: 700,000
Language: Greek
Capital: Nicosia
Currency: Cyprus pound
Int Code: +30

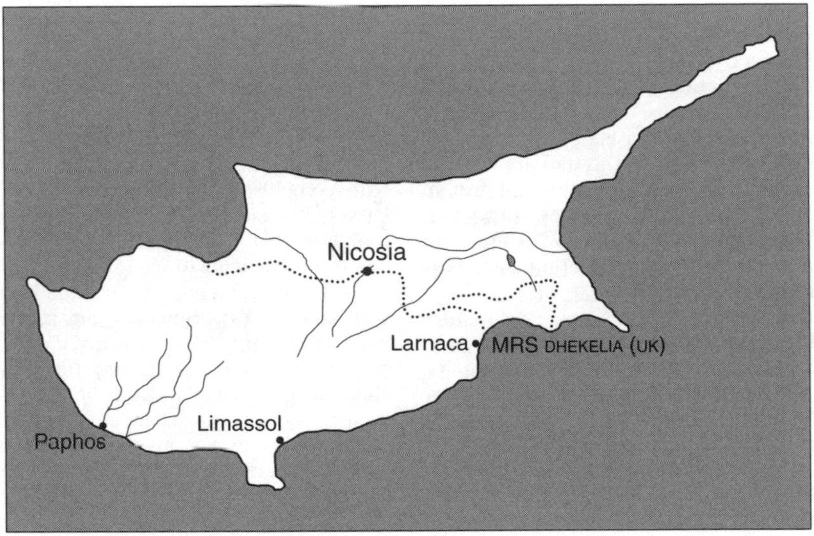

Lying in the eastern Mediterranean, Cyprus became divided in 1974 following an invasion by the Turkish military. This has left the Greek Cypriot Republic of Cyprus in the south and the Republic of Northern Cyprus which is only recognized by the Turks. There's plenty of history and things to do: Aphrodite's birthplace and many beaches. Egypt is not too far. People do know some English but fluent Greek is ideal.

✪ Medicine:

Healthcare is advanced, more so in the south. Western diseases (heart diseases, cancers, accidents) are the common causes of mortality. If you're wanting medicine half-way between European and middle-eastern this is the place! There is no GP service so everything just turns straight up in hospital.

◎ Climate and crime:

It can get very hot in the summer (up to 35 °C) and winters are mild. Crime is not a major problem. Lone girls get a great deal of male attention but not threatening.

Nicosia General Hospital

Nicosia, Cyprus.

The hospital: The tertiary referral centre for Cyprus. It carries out some sophisticated surgery.

Archbishop Makarios III Hospital

Acropolis, Nicosia, Cyprus Tel: Cyprus 02 305090.

The hospital: Built ten years ago principally as a specialist paeds hospital with departments in thalassaemia, cardiology, oncology, endocrinology, metabolic disorders, surgery and NICU. It also has some O&G and ENT.

❍ **Elective notes:** There are many clinics to attend and interesting pathologies to see. Not much hands on though.

Accommodation: Not provided.

Paphos General Hospital

Paphos, Cyprus.

The hospital: Serves a population of 25,000 Cypriots and in the holiday season 50,000 tourists.

❍ **Elective notes:** The staff are friendly and tend to speak very good English so do not worry if your Greek isn't great. The working day is 8 am to 2 pm so there is plenty of time for exploring. Surgery is recommended.

Limassol General hospital

Limassol, Cyprus.

The hospital: Is in a well-set out new building just north-west of Limassol. It is a very busy hospital made busier by the fact there is no GP service. Quite a lot of thalassemia and other things to see, including, kala-azar, scarlet fever and metabolic diseases.

❍ **Elective notes:** It's busy but has very friendly staff who go out of their way to teach.

Accommodation: Not provided, Castle Hotel Apartments (2 Prophitis Elias Street, Potamos Yernasoyias) is recommended.

Larnaca General Hospital 'Archbishop Makarios III'

Larnaca, Cyprus Tel: 04 630300 Fax: 04 630222.

The hospital: Built in 1986 and offers all basic specialities. It serves the local population, of which half are true inhabitants and half are refugees who have fled the Turkish invasion of the north. The population doubles in the summer with tourists.

MRS Dhekelia

Dhekelia Garrison, BFPO 58, Cyprus (only if British and best to be involved in the army).

Army general practice: This is an excellent opportunity to see general practice in an army setting. The typical day consists of an early start (5.30 am) with compulsory physical training e.g. basketball, circuits or running. Ward rounds start at 7.30 am with usually only one or two patients to see (children with asthma, post-epileptic fit or squaddies with sore backs. Clinic at 8 am sees a wide range of problems (the GPs see families as well as soldiers) finishing about 1 pm. There's ALS or trauma training most weeks. There are plenty of opportunities to get involved in other aspects of general practice such as nursing, midwifery, physiotherapy, speech therapy, social work etc. You can also take part in the military exercises. There's plenty of spare time ... learn to water-ski, kneeboard and there are opportunities for helicopter and gliding lessons. The weather, even in December, is excellent.

Accommodation: And food is excellent in the Garrison Officers' Mess.

Czech Republic

Population: 10.3 million
Official Language: Czech
Capital: Prague
Currency: Czech koruna
Int Code: +42

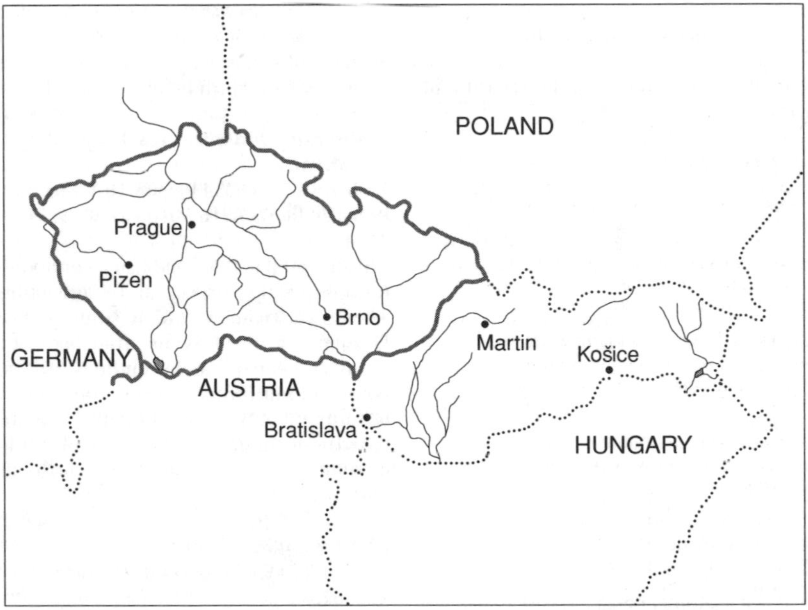

The Czech Republic comprises Bohemia and Moravia and was formally part of Czechoslovakia. Czechoslovakia separated from the former Soviet Union in 1989, since then free elections have taken places and in 1993 a peaceful split of the country into the Czech Republic and Slovakia was agreed. Working here gives a unique opportunity to witness medicine changing as the area rapidly becomes Westernized. It's a great country if you're interested in music, architecture, history or the arts as all can be found in abundance in Prague. Book as many concerts as you can at the Rudolfinum as they are popular and very cheap. Although a few people speak English, knowing some Czech is a huge advantage to coming here. It is not a popular destination for electives or work.

✪ Medicine:

Medicine is improving, however, rich Czechs still travel to Germany to have complex operations. Infant mortality has been high and cancers, heart, cerebrovascular diseases are common causes of mortality. Doctor:population ratio = 1:270.

➲ Visas and work permits:
As a foreign student studying in the Czech Republic, you may be required to obtain a Long Term Residence Permit (contact the Embassy). This is obtained by filling out the appropriate form and sending a letter (in Czech) from the institution offering you a place. You should do this at least 8–10 weeks before departure. A small charge (about £4) is made.

For working you will require a Work Permit from the District Labour Office in the area of your work in the Czech Republic. Ask you employer to get in touch with them. They have to prove that the job cannot be given to a Czech national. You will then need a Long Term Residence permit as well.

USEFUL ADDRESSES:

Health Care Educational Institute in Brno, (Institut pro dalsí vzdêlávání pracovníku ve zdravotnictví) Vinarská 6, 656 02 Brno, Czech Republic Tel: 05/4332130, 43210451 Fax: 05/43211177.
Institute for Clinical and Experimental Medicine (Institut klinické a experimentální medicíny) Vídeñská 800, 140 00 Prague 4, Czech Republic Tel: 02/4721464 Fax: 02/4721324.
Institute of Haematology and Blood Transfusion (Ústav hematologie a krevní transfúze) U nemocnice 1, 128 20 Prague 2, Czech Republic Tel: 02/298741–5 Fax: 02/292911.
Institute of Health Information and Statistics, (Ústav zdravotnických informaci a statistiky) Information Dept, Palackécho nám 4, 120 00 Prague 2, Czech Republic Tel: 02/2497 2712 or 2497 2243 Fax: 02/2491 5882.
Ministry of Health, Palackého nám 4, 128 01, Prague 2, Czech Republic Tel: 024971111 Fax: 02/290092, 24972111.
National Institute of Public Health (Státní zdravotní ústav) Šrobárova 48, 100 42, Prague 10, Czech Republic Tel: 02/67310578, 67310191 Fax: 02/67311188 e-mail PROVAZ2@SCEARN
Postgraduate Medical School, (Institut postgraduálního vzdêlávání ve zdravotnictví) Budêjoviká 15, 141 00 Prague 4, Czech Republic Tel: 02/749529, 61211332 Fax: 02/423692.
Research Institute for Pharmacy and Biochemistry (Výzkummy ústav pro farmacii a biochemii) Kourimská 17, 130 60 Prague 3, Czech Republic Tel: 02/67310936 Fax: 02/67310261.
Union of Health Care Institutions (Sdruzení zdravotnicých zarizení) Lidická 86, 797 36 Prostêjov, Czech Republic Tel: 0508/521254.

UNIVERSITIES AND HOSPITALS:

The Charles University has three faculties in Prague and two outside.

Inside:

- Lékarská Fakulta Univerzity Karlovy, Katerinská 32, 121 08 Praha 2
- Lékarská Fakulta Univerzity Karlovy, V úvalu 84, 150 18 Praha 5
- Lékarská Fakulta Univerzity Karlovy, Ruská 87, 100 00 Praha 10

Outside:

- Lékarská Fakulta Univerzity Karlovy v Hradci Králové, Šimkova 870, 500 38 Hradec Králové
- Lékarská Fakulta Univerzity Karlovy v Plzni, Husov 13, 306 05 Plzeñ

The Charles University was founded in the thirteenth century in Prague and each faculty has its own speciality. An example is the third faculty hospital:

University Hospital Karlovy Vinohrady

Srobarova 50, 10034 Prague 10, Czech Republic Tel: 02 6716 3010 Fax: 02 6731 2664.

This hospital is large and has a very prestigious plastic surgery and burns unit. There is also a new cardiac surgery unit. Despite this there is an atmosphere of decay and general underfunding.

Accommodation: Depends on which department and at which faculty you are based. For the third medical faculty it is in a nurses' flat opposite the hospital costing £1/day.

III Chirurgick Klinika

Londynska 15, 12808, Praha 2, Czech Republic.

The third surgical clinic is in a converted apartment block away from the main medical faculties in the upmarket area of Prague known as Vinohrady. The ground floor accepts emergencies and has an outpatients department. The next three floors comprise 76 beds and two intensive care units as well as the three theatres. The surgery department covers general surgery for Postal Area 3 in Prague, but also thoracic surgery for the whole of the Czech Republic.

❍ Elective notes: There are ward rounds to attend (other doctors will whisper translations to you) and plenty of investigations and surgery to see

(e.g. cardiac catheterization, ECHOs, bypasses etc.)
Accommodation: Has been free previously.

OTHER MEDICAL SCHOOLS:

Universita JE Purkyne
Lékarská Fakulta, Komenského nám.2, 662 43 Brno, Czech Republic.

Universita Palackeho
Lékarská Fakulta, Leninova 8, 770 00 Olomouc, Czech Republic.

Foreigners also visit the following hospitals in Prague.

First Medical Clinic of Prague Ltd, Vyšehradská Str, 120 00 Prague 2, Czech Republic Tel/Fax: 02/292286 Tel: 02/298978, 90000686. (The largest medical clinic catering to foreigners in Prague.)
Hospital HOMOLKA, Roentgenova 2, 150 00 Prague 5, Czech Republic Tel: 02/52922144 (dpt. for foreigners), 02/5293048 (public relations) Fax: 02/57210689.
Hospital MOTOL, Vúvalu 84, 150 00 Prague 5, Czech Republic Tel: 02/24433690 (dpt. for foreigners) Fax: 004202/24431020.

HOSPITALS IN PRAGUE AND NEARBY AREA:

Note: *Nemocnice* = Hospital
Chirurgická nemocnice u Šv Klementa, Nábr L Svobody 2, 110 00 Praha 1, Czech Republic Tel: 02/2481 0226.
Fakultní nemocnice Bulovka, Budínova 2, 18000 Praha 8, Czech Republic, Tel: 02/6608 2963.
Fakultní nemocnice Královské Vihohrady, Srobárova 50, 100 00 Praha 10, Czech Republic Tel: 02/6716 2200.
Fakultní nemocnice v Motole, Vúvalu 84, 150 00 Praha 5, Czech Republic Tel: 02/2443 1010.
Fakultní Thomayerova nemocnice, Videnlská 800, 140 00 Praha 4, Czech Republic Tel: 02/472 1634.
Interní nemocnice v Bubenci, Chittussiho 1, 160 00 Praha 6, Czech Republic Tel: +4202/2431 0194.
Mestská nemocnice v Roztokách, Tiché údolí 376, 252 63 Roztoky U Prahy, Czech Republic Tel: 02/39 77 38.
Nemocnice Beroun, Profesora Veselého 490, 266 01 Beroun, Czech Republic Tel: 0311/230 06.
Nemocnice Kolín, Zizkova 146, 280 02 Kolín, Czech Republic Tel: 0321/284 14.
Nemocnice Mestec Kráhlové, E Benese 343, 289 03 Mèstec Králové, Czech Republic Tel: 0324/932 71.
Nemocnice milosrdných sester Sv K Boromejského v Praze Vlasská 36, 110 00 Praha 1, Czech Republic Tel: 02/2451 0904.
Nemocnice Mladá Boleslav, V Klementa 147/II, 293 01 Mladá Boleslav, Czech Republic Tel: 0326/227 23.
Nemocnice na Františku, Na Františku 8, 110 00 Praha 1, Czech Republic Tel: 02/2481 0502.
Nemocnice na Homolce, Roentgenova 2, 150 00 Praha 5, Czech Republic Tel: 02/5292 2531.
Nemocnice na Zizkové, Kubelíkova 16, 130 00 Praha 3, Czech Republic Tel: 02/627 2002.
Nemocnice Nymburk, Boleslavská 425, 288 00 Nymburk, Czech Republic Tel: 0325/2601.
Nemocnice s poliklinikou, Brázdinská 1000, 250 01 Brandys nad Labem/Stará Boleslav, Czech Republic Tel: 0202/34 00.
Nemocnice s poliklinikou Kladno, Vancurova 1548, 272 01 Kladno, Czech Republic Tel: 0312/22 77.
Nemocnice s polildinikou Mêlník, Prazská 528, 276 01 Mêlník, Czech Republic Tel: 0206/62 31 46.
Nemocnice s poliklinikou Sedlcany, Tyršova 160, 264 01 Sedlcany, Czech Republic Tel: 0304/220 55.
Nemocnice s poliklinikou Slany, Polit veznu 576, 274 01 Slany, Czech Republic Tel: 0314/25 54.
Nemocnice **Rakovník**, Dukelskych hrdinu 200, 269 00 Rakovník, Czech Republic Tel: 0313/2245.
Nemocnice svaté Alzbety, Na slupi 6, 12000 Praha 2, Czech Republic Tel: 02/2491 5694.
Nemocnice ve Vysocanech, Sokolovská 304, 190 00 Praha 9, Czech Republic Tel: 02/6631 2011.
Ústrední vojenská nemocnice, U Vojenské nemocnice 1200, 160 00 Praha 6, Czech Republic Tel: 02/3800 2203.
Všeobecná fakultní nemocnice v Praze, U nemocnice 2, 120 00 Praha 2, Czech Republic Tel: 02/2491 0377.
Zeleznicní nemocnice Praha, Italská 37, 120 00 Praha 2, Czech Republic Tel: 02/2421 1534.

Denmark

Population: 5.4 million
Language: Danish
Capital: Copenhagen
Currency: Danish krone
Int Code: +45

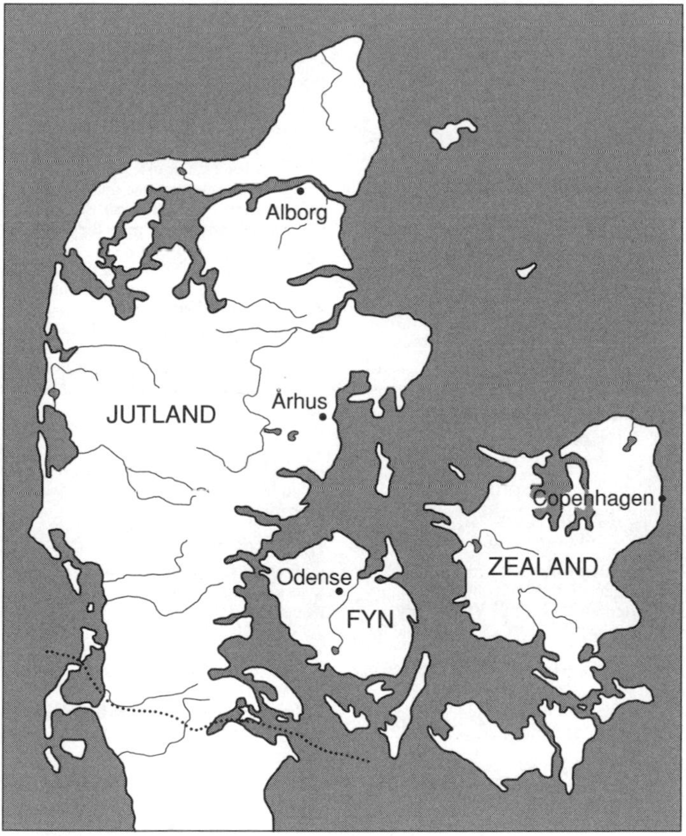

Denmark is made up of 500 islands of which only 100 are inhabited. The largest are Zealand (on which Copenhagen lies), Funen and Jutland. This fragmented nature of Denmark means that nowhere is more than 51 km from the sea. Denmark has a population of just over five million of whom 70% is concentrated in the cities. The capital, Copenhagen, has 1.4 million inhabitants. Most Danes speak English.

Medicine:

Denmark was one of the first countries to establish a national health service and it is still in place today providing free healthcare to all, paid for by taxes. It is well-run and the range of conditions seen is typical of a developed country.

There are three medical schools. Training is a total of 6.5 years (three years pre-clinical and three and a half clinical). Most of the clinical teaching of students from the University of Copenhagen takes place at a number of teaching hospitals in the Greater Copenhagen area. The teaching hospitals are all publicly funded and controlled. For clinical rotations, students are assigned to one of three 'Klinikudvalg', comprising one or more teaching hospitals.

Visas and work permits:

US, EU, NZ and Australian citizens do not need a visa to visit Denmark. Under the EU-scheme, EU citizens can stay up to three months without a visa to search for work.

COPENHAGEN MEDICAL SCHOOL AND HOSPITALS:

Bispebjerg Hospital, Bispebjerg Bakke 23, 2400 København NV, Denmark Tel: 35 31 35 31 Fax: 35 31 39 99.
Frederiksberg Hospital, Norde Fasanvej 59, 200 Frederiksberg, Denmark Tel: 38 34 77 11 Fax: 39 34 77 55.
Københavns Amts Sygehus, Sct Elisabeth, Hans Bgbinders Alle 3, 2300 København S, Denmark Tel: 31 55 45 00 Fax: 32 84 56 54.
Københavns Amts Sygehus, I Glostrup, Ndr. Ringvej, 2600 Glostrup, Denmark Tel: 43 96 43 33 Fax: 43 96 06 16 (*see below*).
Københavns Amts Sygehus I Herlev, Herlev Ringvej, 2730 Herlev, Denmark Tel: 44 53 53 00 Fax: 44 53 53 32.
Københavns Amts Sygehus I Gentofte Niels Andersensvej 65, 2900 Hellerup, Denmark Tel: 31 65 12 00 Fax: 39 77 76 7710.
Københavns Universitet, Det Laegevidenskabelige Fakultet, Panum Instituttet, Blegdamsvej 36, DK-2200, København, Denmark.
Kommunehospitalet, Øster Farimgsgade 5, 1399 København, Denmark Tel: 33 38 33 38 Fax: 33 38 39 99.
Rigshospitalet (incl Finsen) Administrationen, afsnit 522, Blegdamsvej 9 2100 København Ø, Denmark Tel: 35 45 35 45.
Sundby Hospital, Italiensvej 1, 2300 København S, Denmark Tel: 32 34 32 34 Fax: 32 34 39 99.

Copenhagen County Hospital (Glostrup Hospital)

Sdr Ringvej, Glostrup 2600, Denmark.

The hospital: Glostrup hospital is owned and run by the county of greater Copenhagen, along with Herlev and Gentotfe Hospitals. The Copenhagen county hospital at Glostrup was built in 1953. It has all major specialities. There are 25 bed units of 23 beds each – 575 beds in total. Each ward has 10 bedrooms, interviewing rooms, living room, toilets and bathrooms as well as offices for staff. It employs around 400 doctors.

ÅRHUS MEDICAL SCHOOL AND HOSPITALS:

Åarhus Universitet

Det Laegevidenskeabelige Fakultet, Vennelyst Boulevard 9, DK-8000 Aarhus C, Denmark Tel: 8942 1166 Fax: 8942 1109 www.health.au.dk

Århus Amtssygehus, Tage Hansens Gade 2, 8000 Århus C, Denmark Tel: 89 49 75 75 Fax: 89 49 72 49.
Århus Kommunehospital, Norrebrogade 44, 8000 Århus C, Denmark Tel: 89 49 33 33 Fax: 86 18 52 39.
Marselisborg Hospital, PP Ørumsgade 11, 8000 Århus C, Denmark Tel: 89 49 33 33.
Skejby Sygehus, Brendstrupgårdsvej, 8200 Århus N, Denmark Tel: 89 49 55 66 Fax: 89 49 60 00.

ODENSE MEDICAL SCHOOL AND HOSPITAL:

Odense Universitet, Det Laegevidenskabelige Hovedområde, Campusvej 55, DK 5230, Odense, Denmark (The Odense Universitetshospital address is: Sdr Boulevard 29, DK-5000, Odense C. Tel: 6611 3333 Fax: 6613 285. www.ouh.dk)
Odense Universitetshospital, Sdr Boulevard 29, 5000 Odense C, Denmark Tel: 66 11 33 33 Fax: 66 13 28 54.

Finland

Population: 5 million
Languages: Finnish and Swedish
Capital: Helsinki
Currency: Markka
Int Code: +358

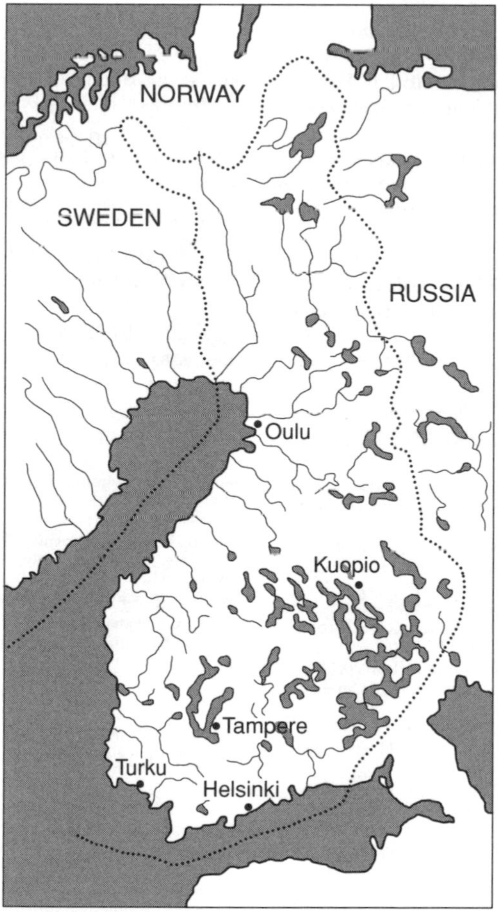

Situated right in the north of Europe, Finland reaches up into the Arctic Circle. It has some beautiful countryside, great if you like walking.

Medicine:
Finland has a sound healthcare policy aiming to improve both the standard and distribution of healthcare even further.

Despite this, cardio and cerebrovascular diseases are the big causes of mortality and male life expectancy is low for European standards. Women, however, are above average. Violent deaths (suicides, traffic accidents etc.) are very common compared to the rest of Europe while cancers are below expected. The healthcare system is run by health authorities through 21 hospital districts. They can either provide aspects of healthcare or purchase it from the private sector. Although the state provides sickness insurance (through local and employers taxes), patients are still expected to contribute to the cost of their healthcare. To belong to a health centre can cost up to FIM100/year. One day in hospital costs FIM125 (including examinations, procedures and medication) and an outpatients appointment sets you back FIM100.

➲ Visas and work permits:

For EU nationals no visa is required for a three-month stay. Technically, students should obtain a residence permit although some elective students have not found this necessary. Residence permits are easy to obtain if you have a contract for work. Visit: http://virtual.finland.fi

MEDICAL SCHOOLS IN FINLAND:

There are five universities with medical schools that tend to deal with the more specialized treatments:

University of Helsinki, PO Box 33 (Yliopistonkatu 4), FIN-00014 University of Helsinki, Finland Tel: 9 1912 2177 Fax: 9 1912 2176 www.helsinki.fi/

University of Kuopio, PO Box 1627, FIN-70211 Kuopio, Finland Tel: 17 16 2042 Fax: 17 16 3496 www.uku.fi (The Kuopio University Hospital PO Box 1777, FIN-70211, Kuopio, Finland Tel: 17173 311 Fax: 17172 116) is one of the largest providers of healthcare in Finland having 1000 beds. It has specialist burns, heart and hand surgery units.

University of Oulu, PO Box 191 (Kirkkokatu 11A), FIN-90101 Oulu, Finland Tel: 8 553 1011 Fax: 8 553 4040 www.oulu.fi/

University of Tampere, PO Box 607. FIN-33101 Tampere, Finland Tel: 3 215 6549 Fax; 3 215 6503 www.uta.fi/index-be.html

University of Turku, FIN-20014 Turku, Finland Tel: 2 333 6582 Fax: 2 333 6370 www.utu.fi

France

Population: 58 million
Language: French
Capital: Paris
Currency: French franc
Int Code: +33

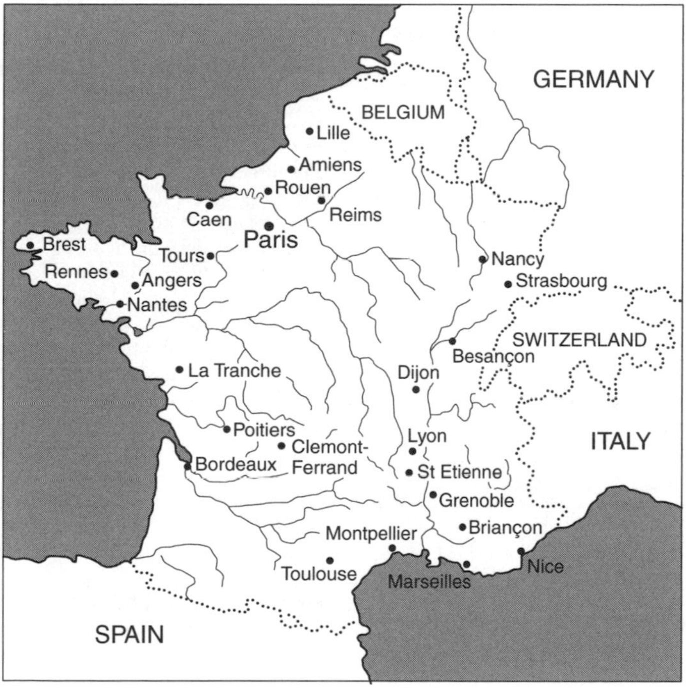

Famed for its fine food, wine and fashion, France offers a great deal for the visiting medic. Paris has its well-known attractions, but the south has other attractions such as skiing and beaches. That said, France is not a popular elective destination for English-speaking students, possibly because of its close proximity to the UK. It is also very easy to arrange exchange programmes through the Socrates/Erasmus programme. For these reasons, only a brief list of a few medical schools is given below. The 'Yahoo' France home page is a useful resource for finding more hospitals. If you are interested in the skiing more than the medical aspect, try approaching one of the many ski patrols. Pretty fluent French is obviously needed to get the most out of an elective/working here.

✪ Medicine:

Medical care is run on both a state and private healthcare system. As you would expect, disease prevalence is as for any developed country.

➲ Visas and work permits:
Like most of the EU, no visa is required for visiting medical students. Contact the Embassy for details regarding length of work for more details on the need for a permit.

◎ Climate and crime:
Climate varies from mild to almost Mediterranean in the south. The Pyrenees and Alps can obviously get very cold, but usually have clear blue skies.

MEDICAL SCHOOLS IN PARIS:

Université de Paris Sud, UFR de Médecine Fremlin-Bicêtre, 63 rue Gabriel Péri, F-75006 Paris, France.
Université de Paris, UFR de Médecine Necker-Enfants malades, 156 rue de Vaugirard, F-75015 Paris, France.
Université de Paris, UFR de Médecine Saint-Antoine, 184 rue Faubourg-Saint-Antoine, F-75012 Paris, France.
Université de Paris VII, UFR de Médecine Lariboisière-Saint-Louis, 10 Avenue de Verdun, F-75010 Paris, France.
Université de Paris VII, UFR de Médecine Xavier Bichat, 16 Rue Henri Huchard, F-75018 Paris, France.
Université de Pierre et Marie Curie (Paris VI), UFR Broussais-Hôtel-Dieu, 15 rue de l'Ecole de Médecine, F-75006 Paris, France.
Université Pierre et Marie Curie (Paris VI), UFR de Médecine Pitié-Salpêtrière, 91 Boulevard de l'Hôpital, F-75634 Paris Cedex 13, France.
Université René Descartes (Paris V), UFR de Médecine Cochin-Port Royal, 24 Rue du Faubourg Saint-Kacques F-75014 Paris Cedex 14, France.

HOSPITALS OCCASIONALLY USED FOR ELECTIVES:

Hôpital Cochin
Rue du Fallbourg St Jacques, 75014 Paris, France.
The hospital: A large hospital in the south of the city and has wards covering all of the medical and surgical specialities.

Centre Medico-Chirurical Foch
40 rue Worth, 92151 Suresnes, France Tel: 1 46 25 20 00 Fax: 1 42 04 59 23.
The hospital: A medium-sized hospital in Suresnes on the outskirts of Paris. It has a good reputation for general medicine.

Hôpital de Cimez
4 Avenue Reine Victoria, Cimiez, Nice, France.
The hospital: Serves a large population from Monaco to Fréjus (about 1.5 million) it has most specialist field and is a teaching hospital affiliated with the University of Nice. There are a number of subdivisions, however, with some services (e.g. maternity) being at a different site.

L'Archet II Centre Hospitalier Universitaire de Nice
151 Route de St Antoine de Ginestiere, BP79 06202, Nice Cedex 03, France.
The hospital: The new section of one of the major hospitals serving Nice and most of the Cote d'Azur. It has superb facilities and is on a hilltop with beautiful views of Nice below.
❍ Elective notes: Medical students are treated as house officers and do on-calls. For electives, the timetable is free so you can go to theatre, A&E or OPD. There aren't many procedures as senior staff do them and blood taking is done by nurses. Florence is a mere three-hour drive away.
Accommodation: You have to find yourself but the government organization, le Crous, can help.

Hôpital Charles Nicolle
Rue de Germont, Rouen 76 00, France.
The hospital: A very large regional teaching hospital. Rouen is a large industrial city in Normandy on the Seine. The hospital is on the right bank on the edge of the old red light district. Paris is one hour by train.

Centre Hospitalier
05105 Briançon, Alps, France.
The hospital: A friendly district hospital in the French Alps. Lots of skiing pathology and its own helicopter rescue service. You need good French to make this worthwhile. There are many Italian tourists so Italian is a plus.

Grenoble

Is surrounded by ski resorts and hence a place to consider going to if you're really after a skiing holiday.

Faculté du Médicine de Grenoble
Domaine de la Merci 38706 La Tronche, France.
There are two hospitals in Grenoble (population 400,000), one (in the south near the Olympic village) deals with acute trauma. The larger, hospital Albert Michallon (near the University Campus) is huge and has most fields of medicine. Write to Le Chef de Service Scolarité at the Bureau Relations Internationales at the above address.

OTHER MEDICAL SCHOOLS IN FRANCE:

École Libre de Médicine, 56 Rue du Port, F-59046 Lille Cedex, France.
Université d'Aix-Marseille, UFR de Médecine, 27 Boulevard Jean Moulin, F-13005 Marseille, France.
Université d'Angers, UFR des Science médicales et pharmaceutiques, Rue Haute de Reculée, F-49045 Angers Cedex, France.
Université de Besançon, UFR de Médecine, 4 place Saint Jacques, F-25030 Besançon Cedex, France. (Founded 1806.)
Université de Bordeaux, UFR de Médecine, 146 Rue Léo Saignat, F-33076 Bordeaux, France.
Université de Brest, UFR de Médecine, 22 Avenue Camille Desmoulins, F-29279 Brest Cedex, France.
Université de Caen, UFR de Médecine, Avenue de la Côte de Nacre, F-10432 Caen Cedex, France.
Université Claude Bernard, UFR de Médecine Grange Blanche, 8 Avenue Rockefeller, F-69373 Lyon Cedex 08, France.
Université de Clermont-Ferrand, UFR de Médecine, Boulevard Churchill, F-63000 Clermont-Ferrand, France.
Université de Dijon, UFR de Médecine, 7 Boulevard Jeanne d'Arc, F-21033 Dijon, France.
Université François-Rabelais, UFR de Médecine de Tours, 2 bis Boulevard Tonnellé, F-37032 Tours Cedex, France.
Université de Lille II, UFR de Médecine, 1 place de Verdun, F-59045 Lille, France.
Université de Louis Pasteur, UFR de Sciences médicales, 4 Rue Kirschleger, F-67085 Strasbourg Cedex, France.
Université de Montpellier, UFR de Médecine, 2 Rue Ecole de Médecine, F-34060 Montpellier Cedex, France.
Université de Nancy I, UFR A et B de Médecine, 9 avenue de la Forêt de Haye, BP 184, F-54506 Vandoeuvre-les-Nancy Cedex, France.
Université de Nantes, UFR de Médecine et Techniques médicales, 1 Rue Gaston Veil, F-44000 Nantes, France.
Université de Nice, UFR de Médecine, Chemin de Valombrose, F-06034 Nice, France.
Université de Paris, UFR de Médecine et de Biologie humaine, 74 rue Marcel Cachin, F-93000 Bobigny, France.
Université Paris Val-de-Marne, UFR de Créyeil, 51 Avenue de Lattre de Tassigny, F-94000 Créteil, France.
Université Paul Sabatier, UFR de Médecine Toulouse-Rangeuil, 133 route de Narbonne, F-31062 Toulouse Cedex, France.
Université de Picardie, UFR de Médicine, 12 Rue Frédéric Petit, F-80000 Amiens, France.
Université de Poitiers, UFR Mixte de Médecine et de Pharmacie, 34 Rue de jardin des Plantes, F-86034 Poitiers Cedex, France.
Université de Reims, UFR de Médecine, 57 Rue Cognacq-Jay, F-51097 Reims, France.
Université René Descartes, UFR de Médecine Paris-Ouest, 104 Boulevard Raymond-Poincaré, F-92380 Garches, France.
Université de Rennes, UFR 'Clinique et Thérapeutique médicales', Avenue Professeur Léon-Bernard, F-35043 Rennes, France.
Université de Rouen, UFR de Médecine et de Pharmacie, Avenue de l'Université, BP 97, F-76800 Saint-Etienne-Du-Rouvray, France.
Université de Saint-Etienne, UFR de Médecine, F-42100 Saint-Etienne, France.
Université scientifique et médicale de Grenoble, UFR de Médecine, Domaine de 'La merci', F-8700 La Tranche, France.

Germany

Population 81.6 million
Capital: Berlin
Language: German
Currency: Deutsche Mark
Int Code: +49

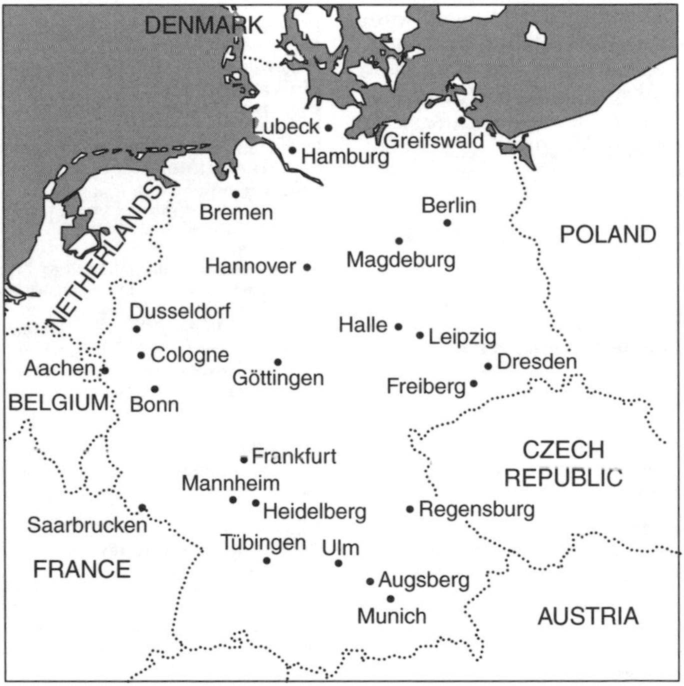

Germany, lying in the heart of Europe, has enjoyed economic growth even while having to support the newly reunited East. It has some vibrant cities and some beautiful countryside. Many people are fluent in English as well as German though at least a basic knowledge of German is highly recommended. Most of the medical terminology, however, is very similar to the English. The European Medical Students' Association runs eurotalks frequently where you learn medical vocabulary and culture over 2–7 days. These are advertised in the student BMJ.

✪ Medicine:

A very comprehensive social security system is set up in Germany with compulsory health insurance paid for by both employer and employee. Most hospitals are state-run; however some are run by Christian organizations. There are 313 people per doctor and the killers of the West (cardiovascular diseases, cancers and accidents) are the big causes of mortality.

In the early 1960s it was decided that there needed to be an expansion in the number of doctors being trained and hence there were proposals for seven new medical schools. For this reason there are a number of institutions that are relatively new, whereas there are others that date back to the early fifteenth century. Most medical schools are listed below, although like most of Europe, exchanges can easily be arranged through Socrates/Erasmus.

◎ Climate and crime:
Typical warm summers and wet winters. Germany is a very safe country.

Aachen

Rheinisch-Westfälische Technische Hoschschule Aachen, Medizinische Fakultät
Goethestraße 27–29, D-5100 Aachen, Germany.

Berlin

Medizinische Fakultät Charité der Humboldt-Universität zu Berlin
Schumannstraße 20/21, Berlin, Germany.
Tel: 30 2802 2391 Fax: 30 2802 3615
www.rz.hu-berlin.de/
www.charite.de/home
Charité, established in the early eighteenth century, gets its name from its humble beginnings as a pest house during the Plague. The medical college, mainly for military personnel, was incorporated into Berlin University in 1806. Initially the new medical college was separate from the Charité and hence built new hospitals (such as the Surgical University Clinic) which is still in use. Today this huge institution is spread over three campuses, Charité Mitte, Virchow-Clinic, Berlin-Buch.

Bonn

Rheinische Friedrich-Wilhelms-Universität Bonn
Medizinischen Fakultaet, Sigmund Freud STR 25 53105, Bonn Tel: 73 7298
http://www.meb.uni-bonn.de/institute/institute.html
Founded in 1818, this large university uses 12 different hospitals totalling 1500 beds.

Cologne

Universität zu Köln, Medizinische Fakultät
Joseph-Stelzmann-Straße 9, Lindenburg, Köln 41, Germany
www.rrz.uni-koeln.de/med-fak
Founded in 1901, the medical college uses 12 hospitals in Cologne and surrounding areas one being:

Kliniken Der Stadt Koln
Kinderkrankenhaus, Amsterdamer Strasse 59, 50735 Köln, Germany.
The hospital: Koln is one of the largest cities in Germany with a population of about a million. The hospital is outside the city centre, but is well-served by the underground. Although a large hospital, very complicated cases get referred to the city's Uniklinik, the main academic teaching hospital. Teaching, at least in paediatrics, is good with afternoon teaching sessions and seminars. As an elective student the ward work is pretty much that of helping the house officer . . . taking blood, siting venflons etc.

Dresden

Medizinische Fackultät Carl Gustav Carus der Technischen Universität Dresden
Fiedlerstraße 27, Dresden, Germany
www.tu-dresden.de/medf/
Originally founded as a military training institute in 1748, it was refounded in 1954 as a medical school. New building

work is trying to locate everything on to one site.

Düsseldorf

Henriche Heine Universität Düsseldorf

Medizinische Fakultät, Univeritätsstraße 1, 40225 Düsseldorf, Germany Tel: 81 12242 Fax: 81 12285 www.uni-duesseldorf.de

The University (founded in the early twentieth century) uses a number of specialist hospitals, including a neurology hospital. In total it has around 2000 beds.

Frankfurt

Klinikum der Johann Wolfgang Goethe-Universität Frankfurt am Main

Theodor-Stern-Kai 7, 60590 Frankfurt, Germany Tel: 069 6301 1
www.uni-frankfurt.de

This huge medical centre (founded in 1914) has 1465 beds with 60 buildings. The medical college also uses another 13 hospitals in Frankfurt itself.

Freiburg im Breisgau

Albert-Ludwigs-Universität Freiburg, Medizinische Fakultät

Werthmannplatz, D-7800 Freiburg im Breisgau, Germany www.uni-freiburg.de/

The school's main hospital is Klinikum der Albert-Ludwigs Universität (Innere Medezin I, Hugstetter Strasse 55, Freiburg im Breisgau D-79106). It's a friendly place where students are given reasonable responsibility and procedures (central lines, bone marrow aspirates) to do. In the oncology/haematology department everyone (from consultants to domestics) has breakfast together to discuss patients.

Language: Obviously a good knowledge of German is necessary.

Giessen

Justus-Liebig-Universität Giessen

Rudolf-Buchheim-Straße 8, D-35385 Giessen, Germany Tel: 641 99-40000 Fax: 641 99-40009 www.med.uni-giessen.de

Founded in 1607, Giessen has had an interesting history, including famous scientists such as Roentgen, inventor of the X-ray. The new medical/surgical centre is on campus hill with good views of the Taunus foothills and Lahn valley. It has all major specialities, including cardiothoracic, trauma and neurosurgery. The university is also affiliated with hospitals in nearby towns. It has a forensic medicine department.

Göttingen

Universität Göttingen, Medizinische Fakultät

Robert Cook STR40, 37075 Göttingen, Germany Tel: 0551 39 6988
www.uni-gottingen.de

Greifswald

Ernst-Moritz-Arndt-Universität Greifswald, Bereich Medizin

Fleischmannstr 8, 17487 Greifswald, Germany Tel: 3834 86 5000 Fax: 3834 86 5002 www.medizin.uni-greifswald.de/

Greifswald (founded 1456) provides all major departments, including three medical departments and forensic medicine (Insitut für Rechtsmedizin Tel: 86-5743 Fax: 86-5752).

Halle/Saale

Martin-Luther-Universität Halle-Wittenberg, Bereich Medizin

Leninallee 5, Halle/Saale, Germany
www.medizin.uni.halle.de

Halle (founded in the early eighteenth century) has everything from paediatric cardiology to trauma surgery. Full addresses and contacts are on their web site.

Hannover

Medizinische Hochschule Hannover
30623, Hannover, Germany Tel: 511 532 1
Fax: 511 532 5550 www.mh-hannover.de/
The Medical School of Hannover, although new (1965), has grown rapidly and now has 1350 beds in its main clinic on campus as well as 18 other medical centres over Hannover. All major departments and sports and forensic departments are here. Specialist research includes that into inflammatory bowel disease, CF and traffic accidents.

Heidelberg

Ruprecht-Karls-Universität Heidelberg, Medizinische Gesamtfakultät
Im Neuenheimer Feld 346, 69120 Heidelberg, Germany Fax: 6221 565404
www.uni-heidelberg.de
Although founded in 1386 the University and medical school had a slow start. In 1523 the entire University had 14 pupils. Today there are seven departments of internal medicine (including sports medicine) and the school uses 15 hospitals providing over 4000 beds in Heidelberg.

Homburg

Universitätskliniken des Saarlandes, Fachbereich Medizin
66421 Homburg/Saar, Germany
Tel: 06841/16 0 www.med-rz.uni-sb.de/
Homburg (in the far south-west of Germany, near France) has its hospital in the south of the town centre situated in 200 hectares of woodland. Originally founded in 1947 the hospital has 1500 beds and all specialities, including forensic psychology and medicine.

Leipzig

Universität Leipzig
Medizinische Fakultät, Liebigstr 27, Leipzig, Germany www.uni-leipzig
Founded in 1414, this is the oldest medical school in Germany. It has recently built a new heart centre with Europe's largest ITU. Leipzig is a beautiful city (population 700,000) and there is a good student life.

Lübeck

Medizinische Universität Lübeck
Ratzeburger avenue 160, 23538 Lübeck, Schleswig-Holstein, Germany
Tel: 0451 5000 Fax: 0451 500 3016
www.mu-lubeck.de/
Founded in 1964, approximately 20 hospitals provide over 1000 beds to the medical school.

Magdeburg

Otto-von-Guericke-Universität Magdeburg
Medizinische Fakultät, Leipziger Str 44, D-39120 Magdeburg, Germany
Tel: (0391) 6701 Fax: (0391) 67 13440
www.med.uni-magdeburg.de/fme/
This relatively new medical college (1954) only became part of a University in 1993. It uses 29 hospitals, 22 institutes and enrols 180 students a year. It has specific interests in neuroscience and immunology research.

Mannheim

Fakultät für Klinische Medizin Mannheim der Universität Heidelberg
Theodor Kutzer Ufer, 68135 Mannheim, Germany Tel: (0621) 3 83 25 27 Fax: (0621) 3 83 38 02 www.uni-heidelberg.de
www.uni-mannheim.de
Mannheim got its own medical school (part of the University of Heidelberg) in 1964. The University hospital is the major teaching facility. Specialist interests include transplant and minimal invasive surgery, psychiatry, imaging and oncology. It has 2600 beds.

Munich

Ludwig-Maximilians-Universität München, Fachbereich Medizin
Goethestraße 29/III, D-8000, München 15, Germany www.med.uni-muenchen.de/
This is a very large faculty founded in 1826. Associated with it is a large cancer centre. One of its peripheral hospitals is Zentralklinikum, D-86009 Augsburg. It is a massive hospital on the outskirts of Augsburg, a medium-sized city in the south of Germany. Here, previous elective students have joined in with Munich student's teaching. There are some excellent pubs and plenty to do in the old town. If you want to get out, Munich and the Bavarian Alps (good weekend skiing) are very close.
Accommodation: Has previously been provided.

Regensburg

Universität Regensburg, Medizin Fakultät
Universitätsstraße 31, Regensburg, Germany www.uni-regensburg.de
This new medical college (1970) uses a large clinical centre just outside the city.

Tübingen

Eberhard-Karls-Universität Tübingen, Medizische Fakultät
Geissweg 3, Tübingen, Germany www.uni-tubingen.de
Founded in the late fifteenth century it has nearly 2000 beds.

Ulm

Universität Ulm, Medizinische Fakultät
Oberer Eselsberg, M23, Ulm, Germany www.uni-ulm.de/uni/fak/medizin
This new medical college (1969) uses large modern hospitals, including the Medical University Clinic. In total it has access to 1500 beds.

ARMY WORK:

Medical Reception Station, Imphal Barracks
Osnabruck, Germany BFPO 36.
General practice: This is an opportunity to see general practice in an army setting, although reports suggest not a particularly good one. You will be expected to be at the 'MRS' between 8 am and 6 pm and they like you to spend as little time with the doctors and most time with 'the other services'. So if you fancy spending days going around as a health visitors 'young trainee' and being allowed to read off a baby's weight from a set of scales . . . this is the elective for you. You will get some time with the GPs, but again experience gained has been very limited.
Accommodation: And food are excellent and provided.

Gibraltar

Population: 30,000
Language: English and Spanish
Capital: Gibraltar
Currency: Pound
Int Code: +350

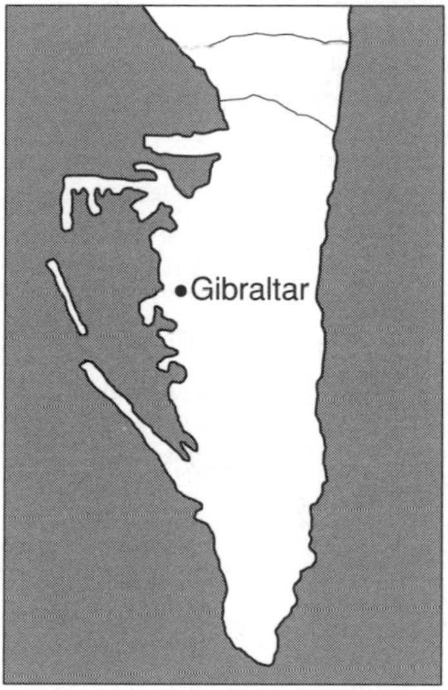

Gibraltar is a two by three mile rock in the southern part of Spain guarding the entrance to the Mediterranean. Its military use has dwindled in recent years; however, it is still very much a British colony with British shops and banks in its main street. There is a National Health Service-type system of care given by an 11-man GP practice and St Bernard's Hospital. Although English is the official language, some people can only speak Spanish so a little knowledge does help. At the time of writing, the Naval GP service and hospital are being transferred to the civilian services.

Casemated Health Centre

Gibraltar.

The practice: An 11-man, well-run, busy GP service. Most conditions are similar to those seen in western Europe.

❍ **Elective notes:** A welcoming friendly practice with great willingness to teach.

St Bernard's Hospital

Gibraltar.

The hospital: The public hospital for Gibraltar. It has the major specialities (medicine, surgery, paeds, O&G, ENT, care of the elderly) but complicated cases have to be transferred to the UK or Spain. There is one surgeon here.

❍ **Elective notes:** Due to the rarity of students the staff are keen to teach. A wide range of conditions is seen.

Hungary

Population: 10 million
Language: Hungarian
Capital: Budapest
Currency: Forint
Int Code: +36

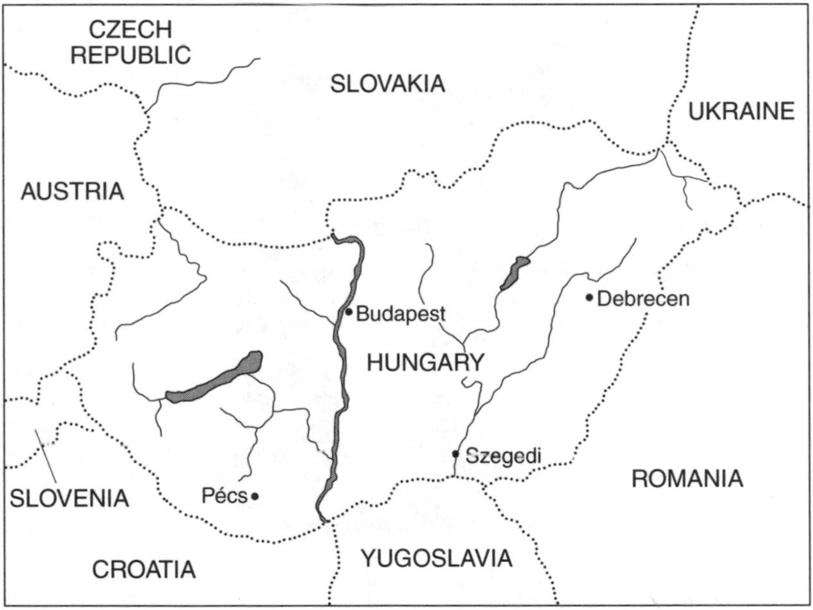

Hungary, a landlocked country in central Europe, has outperformed other Eastern Bloc countries receiving a great deal of overseas investment. It is moving closer to the EU. There is a fair bit to see and do. The capital has baths from the Ottoman period and Lake Balaton is popular with tourists.

✪ Medicine:

A state health system provides free care to everyone, although a 15% charge on prescriptions is made. Like many state systems, however, it is under-funded and hence waiting lists are long. Western diseases are the order of the day.

➲ Visas and work permits

Students from most Western countries (including the UK, USA, Canada and most of Europe) do not need a visa to travel or shadow in a hospital. Australian and New Zealand citizens are exceptions. Contact your local embassy where a visa is easily obtained for a small fee, an application form and a few photos. To work in Hungary, a permit is required.

◎ Climate and crime:
Hungary is warmest between May and August and has a fairly constant level of rainfall. It is a pretty safe country for tourists.

Budapest

Semmelweis University of Medical Sciences

Orvostudományi Egyetem, Üllöi út 26. 2nd Floor H-1085 Budapest VIII, Hungary Tel: 317 9057 www.sote.hu/

Founded in the eighteenth century, Semmelweis has had a long and interesting history. It now has 3100 beds in its affiliated hospital. Most instruction is in English.

Debrecen

University Medical School of Debrecen

4012 Debrecen, PO Box 48 Nagyerdei krt. 98 Debrecen, Hungary Tel: 52 417 571 Fax: 52 419 807 www.dote.hu

Established in 1918, the medical school separated from the university in 1951. Most teaching is in Hungarian but approximately 15% of students are taught in English. Debrecen, in eastern Hungary, has a population of 250,000 and a number of sites such as the great forest and thermal baths. Although English instruction is available, the patients obviously speak Hungarian. Most specialities, including traumatology, are catered for.

Accommodation: US$2–300/month.

Pécs

University Medical School of Pécs

Szigeti ut 12, H-7600 Pécs, Hungary
www.pote.hu/

This is one of Hungary's oldest medical schools (founded in 1367), although it was rebuilt after WWI. It admits 175 students per year and all teaching and clinical activities are in one area.

Szegedi

Albert Szent-Györgyi Medical University

Dugonics tér 13, PO Box 479, H-6701 Szegedi, Hungary Tel: 62 455 007 Fax: 62 455 005 www.szote.u-szeged.hu/

Established in 1921 the university uses a number of hospitals situated between the Cathedral and River Tisza. It has all major specialities and preclinical departments, including forensics. It is a requirement that students can speak English. Szegedi is situated on the banks of the River Tisza of the southern edge of the Great Hungarian Plains. It has 200,000 people and a very pleasant climate.

Iceland

Population: 300,000
Language: Icelandic
Capital: Reykjavík
Currency: New Icelandic króna
Int code: +354

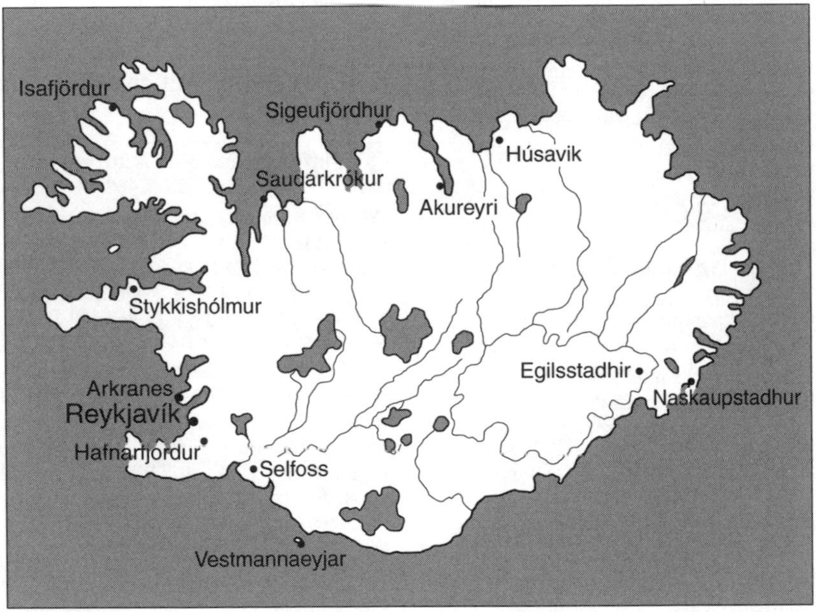

Iceland, just south of the Arctic Circle, is situated between the American and European continental plates which accounts for its numerous volcanoes and geysers. It has some spectacular scenery although obviously gets very cold. There are plenty of natural interest spots such as 'The Golden Waterfall' and the Geysir Geothermal Area near Reykjavik. In the north go to Myvatn with old and new volcanoes, lava fields, boiling mud pots and steam vents on the North Atlantic Ridge. Organized tours cost about £40, but if you're there in the summer (June to September), public transport is good. Although the official language is Icelandic, most people can speak English very well.

✪ Medicine:

Iceland has an excellent record on health with a free healthcare service for all, one of the longest life expectancies and the lowest infant mortalities anywhere. It has one medical school and a number of hospitals across the island.

➲ Visas and work permits:

No visa is required for elective students. EU citizens can spend up to three months looking for work without a visa. Once they have work they do need one. Doctors must apply to one of the hospitals below. Before being allowed to practise medicine in Iceland, confirmation from the Ministry of Health and Social Security has to be obtained. The hospitals are very helpful with that.

Reykjavík

MEDICAL SCHOOL AND MAIN HOSPITAL:

Landspitalinn, The National University Hospital

Baronstigur, 101-Reyjavík, Iceland or Thverholt 18, IS-105 Reykjavík, Iceland Tel: 560 2360 Fax: 560 2359.

The best way to obtain information about medical students exchange programmes is to contact the extremely friendly and well-run Icelandic Medical Students International Committee (IMSIC) via e-mail: imsic@rhi.hi.is or the University of Iceland, Office of International Education, Neshagi, IS-107 Reykjavík Tel: 525 4311 Fax: 525 5850. They can help organize placements, board and lodgings. They even arrange weekend outings. The main hospital used is:

Sjúkrahús Reykjavíkur (The Reykjavík Hospital) (Mark all correspondence: 'Starfsmannathjonusta')

Landakot 5.haed, IS-108, Reykavík, Iceland Tel: 525 1800 Fax: 525 1959.

The hospital: The main teaching hospital in Iceland. It is so big it uses 22% of the health sector budget. It offers most specialities but particularly prides itself in its use of laproscopic surgery, *in vitro* fertilization, paeds and maternity services and cardiac surgery. It has 11 operating theatres and an A&E that sees 10,000 patients a year.

O Elective notes: The staff are very friendly. In the summer there are no other students around so there's plenty of teaching. The surgeons are very heavily into laproscopic surgery. There is a great deal of gastric surgery as Iceland has the second-highest incidence of gastric cancer in the world. The 'general surgeon' really is doing mastectomies and aortic aneurysms on the same list.

Accommodation: Iceland is an expensive place, but the Medical Student Association is well-organized and since they can arrange accommodation and board in the hospital as well as sightseeing trips, it actually works out very reasonable.

OTHER HOSPITALS IN ICELAND:

Fjórdungssjúkrahúsid Akureyri

IS-600 Akureyri, Iceland Tel: 463 0101 Fax: 462 4621.

The hospital: A quiet, friendly place in Iceland's second-largest town (population 15,000). The day starts at 7.45 am with X-ray meetings and a ward round. There's plenty of elective surgery and the days tend to finish about 4 pm. They are quite happy for you to disappear for a bit.

Heilbrigdisstofnun Sudurnesja, Mánagata 9, IS-230 Reykjanesbaer, Iceland Tel: 422 0580 Fax: 421 3471.
Heilbrigdisstofnunin í Vestmannaeyjum, Sólhlíd 10, IS-900 Vestmannaeyjar, Iceland Tel: 481 1955 Fax: 481 1072.
Heilbrigdisstofnunin, Egilsstödum, IS-700 Egilsstadhir, Iceland Tel: 471 1400 Fax: 471 1971.
Sjúkrahús Akraness, Merkigerdi 9, IS-300 Akranes, Iceland Tel: 431 2311 Fax: 431 2319.
Sjúkrahús Húsavíkur, Audbrekku 4, IS-640 Húsavík, Iceland Tel: 464 0500 Fax: 464 0575.
Sjúkrahús Ísafjardar, IS-400 Ísafjödur, Iceland Tel: 450 4500 Fax: 450 4522.
Sjúkrahúsid Neskaupstad, Myrargata 20, IS-740 Neskaustadur, Iceland Tel: 477 1402 Fax: 477 1879.
Sjúkrahús Saudárkróki, IS-551 Saudárkrókur, Iceland Tel: 455 4000 Fax: 455 4010.
Sjúkrahús Siglufjardar, Hvanneyrarbraut, IS-580 Siglufjördhur, Iceland Tel: 467 2172 Fax: 467 1551.
Sjúkrahús Sudurlands, Árvegi, IS-800 Selfoss, Iceland Tel: 482 1300 Fax: 482 2534.
St Fransiskusspítalinn, Austurgata 7, IS-340 Stykkishólmur, Iceland Tel: 438 1128 Fax: 438 1628.
St Jósefsspítali, Sudurgata 41, IS-220 Hafnarfjördur, Iceland Tel: 555 0000 Fax: 565 3255.

Ireland

Population: 3.6 million
Language: Irish and English
Capital: Dublin
Currency: Irish punt
Int Code: +353

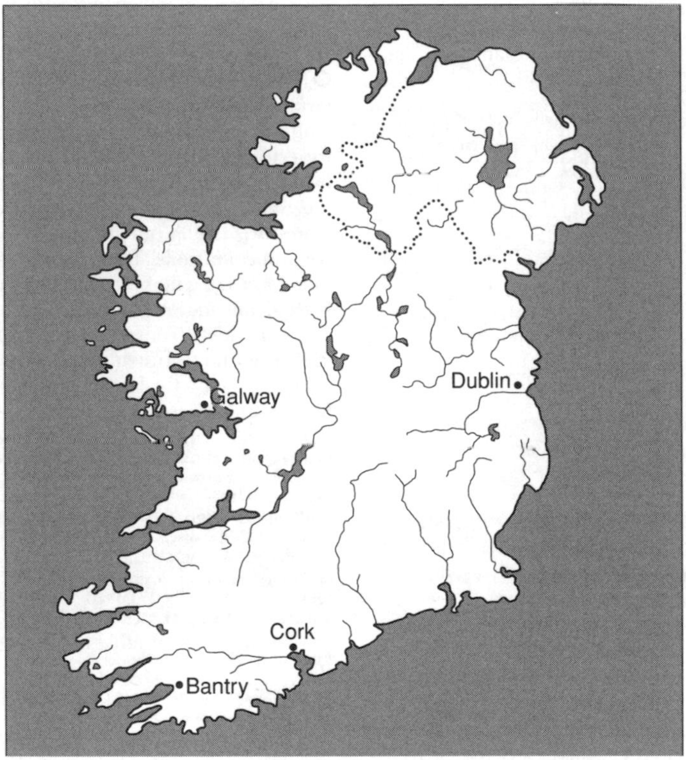

Ireland is a beautiful, friendly country with coastal hills, charming bays in the west and some lovely people. The vast majority simply want peace (so do not let the conflict in the north put you off going). It's a superb place for those easily sunburned.

Medicine:
A free healthcare system (means tested) is in place, although a third of people rely on healthcare insurance. Typical Western pathologies (heart disease, cancers) are the order of the day and

there is a good doctor:patient ratio (1:588). Ireland claims to have the lowest consumption of alcohol in the EU (surely they lost count!).

➲ Visas and work permits:
British citizens do not require a visa to enter Ireland. However, if enrolling in study or actually practising medicine, permits are required. British students doing electives have not reported any needs for visas. Contact the Embassy for more details. Doctors need to register with the General Register of Medical Practitioners, **The Medical Council**, 8 Lower Hatch Street, Dublin 2, Ireland. EEC qualifications give full registration. Others usually grant temporary registration. Another useful address is **Royal College of Surgeons of Ireland**, 123 St Stephen's Green, Dublin 2, Ireland Tel: 1 402 2100. www.rcsi.ie e-mail: info@rcsi.ie

Note: Irish doctors swap around on 1 July and it can therefore get chaotic around then. Many doctors also take their holidays in the first two weeks of August; therefore you can get busy as a student. If going from the UK why not take a car if you have one?

Dublin

A vibrant, lively city, probably most famous for it's Guinness Brewery. There's plenty to do and some beautiful countryside nearby. You won't get bored in the evenings.

MEDICAL SCHOOLS:

Royal College of Surgeons of Ireland, 123 St. Stephen's Green, Dublin 2, Ireland Tel: 1 402 2100. www.rcsi.ie email: info@rcsi.ie (Since 1784, the college has had its own medical school. It also has a school of physiotherapy.)
National University of Ireland, University College of Dublin, Faculty of Medicine, Earlsfort Terrace, Dublin 2, Ireland.
University of Dublin, School of Physic, Trinty College, Dublin 2, Ireland. (The oldest medical school in Ireland.)

If applying to do an elective, enquire whether accommodation can be arranged as it can be expensive in Dublin.

TEACHING HOSPITALS:

The Beaumont Hospital

Beaumont Road, Dublin 9, Ireland Tel: 1 809 3000 Fax: 1 837 6982
www.beaumont.ie

The hospital: A big (620-bed), busy teaching hospital affiliated to the medical school of the Royal College of Surgeons of Ireland situated on the north side of the city. It has all major specialities and has the National Neurology and Neurosurgery Unit. It is also the national centre for renal transplants, pancreatic disorders and cochlear implantation. It has an A&E for its catchment of 250,000.
❍ Elective notes: There are usually around 50 students from the Royal College of Surgeons of Ireland. They have comprehensive daily tutorials and lectures and their weekly departmental meetings. It's a friendly hospital and great for a cheap fun elective.
Accommodation: No hospital accommodation is available but has previously been arranged through the College (lodgings in 1998 cost about £90 (118 IEP)/week).

St James's Hospital

PO Box 580, James's Street, Dublin 8, Ireland Tel: 1 453 7941
www.stjames.ie/address.html

The hospital: Although only built in 1971, St James's is now the largest university teaching hospital in the Republic of Ireland. It is the hospital for Trinity College, Dublin and accordingly has nearly all medical and surgical specialities.
❍ Elective notes: The teaching and clinical experience are usually very good. It is a very friendly hospital.
Accommodation: Not provided.

Mater Misericordiae Hospital

Eccles Street, Dublin 7, Ireland
www.mater.ie

The hospital: An acute tertiary referral university teaching hospital with many specialist services. It is the National Centre for cardiothoracic surgery and spinal injuries and is the major accident and emergency hospital serving Dublin's inner city. It is associated with University College Dublin.

The Coombe Women's Hospital

Dolphins Barn, Dublin 8, Ireland Tel: 1 453 7561 Fax: 2 453 6033
www.coombe.ie e-mail info@coombe.ie
The hospital: (Est. 1826) is the busiest women's hospital in Ireland delivering over 6000 babies a year. It is a centre of excellence with a low C-section rate due their very successful active management of labour. It has a busy ultrasound department, modern homely delivery suite and state-of-the art SCBU. It is affiliated with University College Dublin, Trinity College and the Royal College of Surgeons in Ireland. It has it's own Midwifery School.

The National Children's Hospital

Tallaght, Ireland.
The main paediatric hospital.

Central Mental Hospital

Dundrum, Dublin, Ireland.
The hospital: The only centre for forensic psychiatry in Ireland. Of the 80 or so patients, half are admitted on a short-term basis from the prison system for acute psychiatric crises. The others are long-stay chronic patients who are detained as they are judged unfit to plead. They have usually committed very serious crimes.
O **Elective notes:** The elective consists of shadowing a registrar, assessing patients and going to court. If you're into this it has been a highly recommended elective.

Cork

A lively city in the south if Ireland with plenty of festivals in the summer. It's great if you like hill walking.

MEDICAL SCHOOL:

University College, Cork, Faculty of Medicine, National University of Ireland, Cork, Ireland.

HOSPITALS:

City Hospital

Cork, Ireland.
The hospital: Is the main University Hospital and has all major specialities. Apply through the University to do an elective here.

Mercy Hospital

Cork, Ireland.
The hospital: Is in central Cork and smaller than the University Hospital (City Hospital). It is still used by Cork medical students, and students from elsewhere in Europe, but its smaller size makes it that bit more friendly. Teaching has been reported as excellent.
Accommodation: Not provided but available nearby for approx. £30/week (39 IEP).

Bantry General Hospital

Bantry, Co Cork, Ireland.
The hospital: Has a medical (29 beds), a surgical ward, an ITU and a psychiatric department. It covers West Cork and South Kerry. The medical team has a consultant, a reg, three SHOs and two JHOs. Surgery has one consultant. Bantry itself is a small town right on the Atlantic coast. Outside Bantry there's plenty to do for the outdoors type with a car (mountain biking, hill walking, golf); however, some have found it too isolated for their liking.
O **Elective notes:** Despite its small size there is usually quite a variety of cases and the staff are very friendly, keen to teach and let students do procedures.
Accommodation: Not provided though there is an independent hospital in Bantry.

Galway

THE MEDICAL SCHOOL:

University College, Galway, Faculty of Medicine, National University of Ireland, Galway, Ireland.

Italy

Population: 58 million
Language: Italian
Capital: Rome
Currency: Italian lira
Int Code: +39

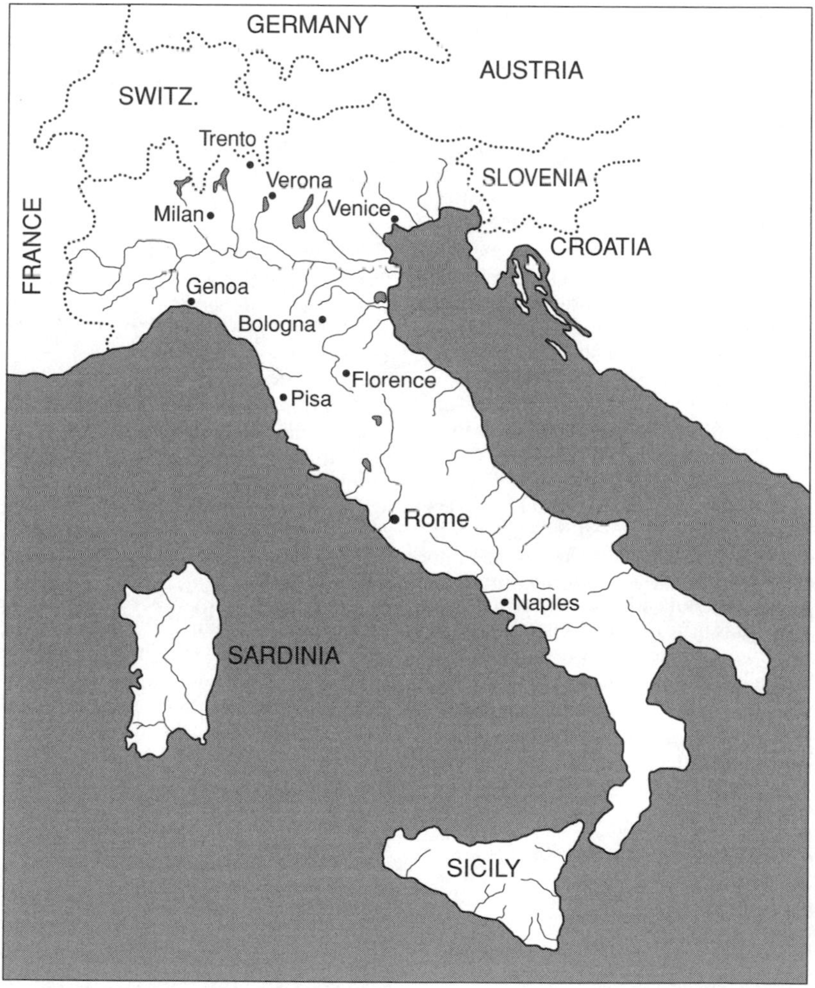

Italy has a great deal to offer from excellent skiing in the Alps, to beautiful sun-drenched Mediterranean beaches. There are many cosmopolitan cities and many sights to see. Italian culture and food are yet more reasons to visit this country. One major drawback, however, is the real need to have fluent Italian in a hospital setting. For this reason (and because it is expensive) Italy is not a popular elective destination. Because of this and the fact that many schools are on the Erasmus/Scorates programme, only a few medical schools and hospitals are listed here. If you can speak Italian there are a number of great resources on the web. Try the Yahoo home page for Italy.

✪ Medicine:

The relaxed lifestyle, daily glass of red wine and Mediterranean food are supposed to make Italians very healthy and indeed it does. They have one of the highest life expectancies. Nonetheless, typical Western diseases get them in the end. There is a state-run healthcare system that varies from region to region. Although it was originally free, patients now have to pay prescription charges, a daily hospital fee and yearly health fee. The state hospitals have been described as pretty poor. This is another reason why they are not popular with elective students. The system for medics is also is a bit odd. Once qualified, you get a job. You then (if you want) never have to apply for another job. You just progress up through the ranks in that job. It can make people a bit lazy. Undergraduate medicine has been described as a bit of a spectator sport and hence is a further deterrent. A useful web address: **The Italian Medical Organization:** Federazione Nazionale Ordine dei Medici www.FNOMCeOit

➲ Visas and work permits:

Citizens of the EU, USA, New Zealand and Australia do not need a visa to stay in Italy for up to 90 days.

Note: Australian, US and a few other citizens may require a Schengen visa if they intend to visit some other European countries as well. For work permits, contact the Embassy.

MEDICAL SCHOOLS:

Instituto Scientifico H san Raffaele

Fondazione Centro San Raffaele del Monte Tabor, Milano, Via Olgettina 60, Italy
Tel: 02 2643.1 www.hsr.it

The hospital: This huge private institution has a worldwide reputation and, it is claimed is *the* place in Italy to do virtually any speciality (very highly recommended for electives). It is the only private medical school in Italy. The main Institute (in Olgettina Street) with 1300 beds has everything from the emergency room to gamma knife neurosurgery. Also associated is the Centro San Luigi, an HIV treatment and research centre with 35 beds, a resus unit to assist terminal cases and a dedicated operating theatre. The Department of Neuropsychic Science is a 280-bed centre for the treatment of mental disorders. There is also a department of biological and technological research.

O Elective notes: If you can't speak Italian, they can organize electives in molecular biology, cellular biology, neuroscience, immunology and radiology. They are on the Erasmus/Socrates system. Write to Luisa Meldolesi, Ufficio Socrates/Erasmus, Universita Vita-Salute San Raffaele via Olgettina 58 20132 Milano, Italy Tel: 2 2643 3813 Fax: 2 2643 4704.

Note: There is a second San Raffaele in Rome with 500 beds providing general services and a spinal unit.

OTHER MEDICAL SCHOOLS:

Università Cattolica de Sacro Cuore, Facoltà di Medicina e Chirurgia 'Agostino Gemelli', Via della Pineta Sacchetti 644, I-00168 Roma, Italy.
Università di Bologna, Facoltà di Medicina e Chirurgia, Via San Vitale 59, I-40138 Bologna, Italy. (Founded in the thirteenth century.)
Università di Milano, Facoltà di Medicina e Chirurgia, Via Festo del Perdonon 7, I-20122 Milano, Italy.

Università di Napoli, Facoltà di Medicina e Chirurgia II, Via Sergio Pansini 5, I-80131 Napoli, Italy.
Università di Pisa, Facoltà di Medicina e Chirurgia, Via Roma 55, I-56100 Pisa, Italy. (This is an old medical school also founded in the thirteenth century.)
Università di Roma-La Sapienza, Facoltà di Medicina e Chirurgia, Cittá Universitaria, Piazzale Aldo Moro 5, I-00185 Roma, Italy. (Founded 1303 making it Rome's oldest.)
Università di Roma-Tor Vergata, Facoltà di Medicina e Chirurgia, Via A Raimondo, I-00173 Roma, Italy.
Università di Verona, Facoltà di Medicina e Chirurgia, Borgo Roma, I-37134 Verona, Italy.

NON-TEACHING HOSPITALS:

Ospedale Santa Chiara

L'Go Medaglie D'Oro, 838100 Trento, Italy.

The hospital: Santa Chiara is a large general hospital serving the city of Trento and the surrounding areas in Trentino, north Italy. The general medical and dermatology departments are at least relaxed and friendly. There is no medical school here, so although the doctors are very friendly, it does lack something in social life. The surrounding areas are beautiful with the lakes and Verona nearby.

Istituto G Gaslini

167147 Genova, Italy.

The hospital: The largest paediatric hospital in Italy and a specialist referral centre for the entire country. It is very friendly.

O **Elective notes:** Teaching is informal. Genova is a small city on the coast of north-west Italy. It is very pretty.

Luxembourg

Population: 400,000
Language: Letzeburgish
Capital: Luxembourg
Curency: Luxembourg franc
Int Code: +352

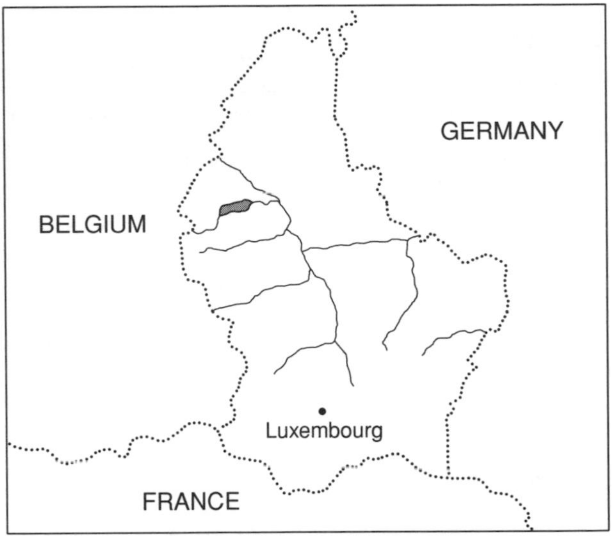

Despite its small size and population, Luxembourg has the highest income per capita in the EU. It borders the industrial regions of France, Belgium and Germany, but today it is its tax haven status and banking that generate its prosperity. The countryside consists of rolling hills and forests.

✪ Medicine:

There are no private hospitals in Luxembourg. They are either state-run or run by nuns. All nationals are covered by the *Caisse de Maladie* (the state sickness fund) from whom any expenses can be reclaimed. The big killers are Western: heart, cerebrovascular diseases and cancers. Doctor: patient ratio is 1:476.

◎ Climate:

It's warmest (20 °C) between June and August. The winter in the Ardennes (south) can get cold and snowy.

USEFUL ADDRESSES:

Ambassaed Du Grand-Duché de Luxembourg, 27 Wilton Crescent, London. SW1X 8SD, UK Tel: 020 7235 6961 Fax: 020 7235 9734.
Ministère de la Santé, 57 et 90 boulevard de la Pétrusse, L-2320 Luxembourg Tel: (352) 4781 Fax: 484903.

Luxembourg has one medical school:

Collège Médical, 90 bd de la Pétrusse, L-2320 Luxembourg Tel: 478 5514.

Macedonia

Population: 2.2 million
Language: Macedonian/Albanian
Capital: Skophe
Currency: Macedonian denar
Int Code: +389

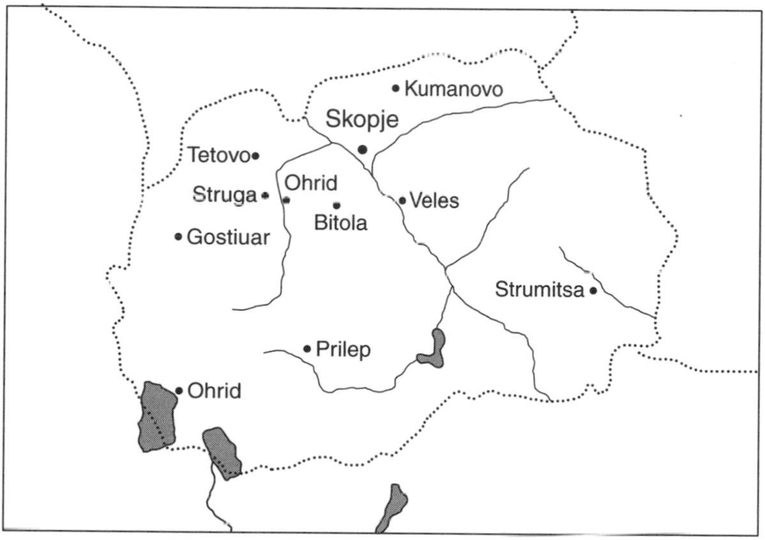

The Former Yugoslav Republic of Macedonia (FYRM) had its economic blockade of Serbia and Montenegro lifted in 1996. However, Greece is still hostile as it worries that the FYRM may try to take over an area also called Macedonia in northern Greece. This is certainly not a popular elective destination at present, although the Sara Mountains offer good skiing.

✪ Medicine:

The state guarantees universal healthcare; however, for quick and reliable treatment people have to go private.

➲ Visas and work permits:

Contact the Embassy of the Republic of Macedonia. No clear information is available.

USEFUL ADDRESS:

Chamber of Doctors of the Republic of Macedonia, Ul 'Naroden Front', BR 21 91009 Skopje, Republic of Macedonia Tel/Fax: 91 124 066.

UNIVERSITY MEDICAL SCHOOL:

Medicinski Fakultet, Univerziteta vo Skopje, Vodnjaanska 15, Skopje, Republic of Macedonia.

HOSPITALS IN SKOPJE:

Army Hospital, Ilindenska BB, Skopje, Macedonia Tel: 362 622 Fax: 250 340.
Bucharest Polyclinic, bul Partizanski odredi BB, Skopje, Macedonia Tel: 364 088.
City Hospital, 11 Oktomvri 53, Skopje, Macedonia Tel: 221 133 Fax: 128 097.
The Main Hospital, Vodnjanska BB Skopje, Macedonia Tel: 114 244.

MEDICAL CENTRES OUTSIDE SKOPJE:

Dr Trifun Panovski Medical Centre, Partizanska BB, Bitola, Macedonia Tel: 251 211, 252 448 Fax: 253 435.
Gevgelia Medical Centre, Slobodan Mitros-Danko BB, Gevgelia, Macedonia Tel: 89 710, 89 351 Fax: 89 693.
Kumanovo Medical Centre, Boris Kidrich 11, Kumanovo, Macedonia Tel: 22 484 Fax: 20 334.
Medical Centre Borka Taleski, Borka Taleski BB, Prilep, Macedonia Tel: 22 450, 22 430 Fax: 22 457.
Ohrid Medical Centre, Sirma Vojvoda BB, Ohrid, Macedonia Tel: 34 144. Fax: 22 749.
Struga Medical Centre, 8 Noemvri BB, Struga, Macedonia Tel: 71 464. Fax: 72 142.
Strumitsa Medical Centre, Mladinska BB. Strumitsa, Macedonia Tel: 24 888 Fax: 26 448.
Shtip Medical Centre, Ljuben Ivanov 25, Shtip, Macedonia Tel: 33 666, 34 099 Fax: 31 357.
Tetovo Medical Centre, 29 Noemvri 16, Tetovo, Macedonia Tel: 32 861, 24 988, 24 419 Fax: 20 148.
Veles Medical Centre, Shefki Sali 5, Veles, Macedonia Tel: 33 322 Fax: 33 322/102.

PRIVATE CLINICS:

Atik Cor, Nikola Trimpare 3, Macedonia Tel: 228 213; 110 341 Fax: 228 213.
Neuromedika, Bul Partizanski Odredi 3/1–4, Macedonia Tel: 215 780, 117 848 Fax: 215 780.

Malta

Population: 400,000
Languages: Maltese and English
Capital: Valletta
Currency: Maltese lira
Int Code: +356

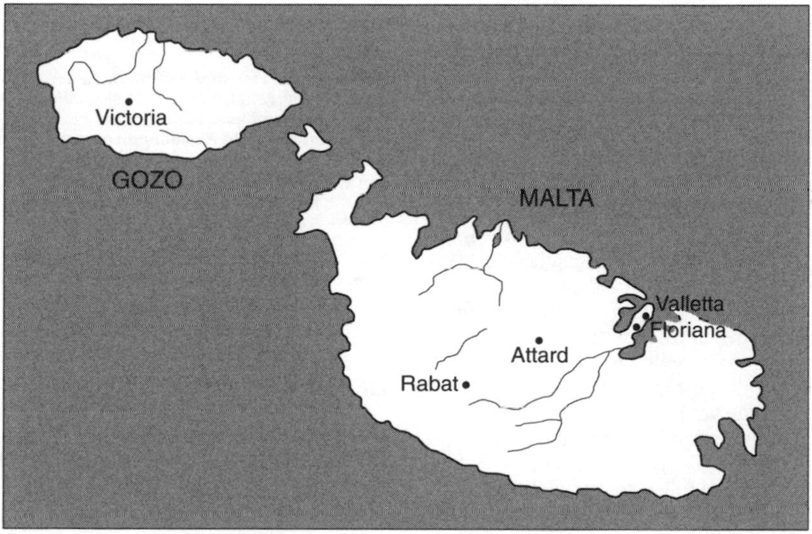

Lying midway between Europe and North Africa, Malta has been controlled by a number of colonial powers until its independence from the UK in 1964. There are a number of islands belonging to Malta but only Gozo and Kemmuna are inhabited. The economy is mainly based around the tourists who visit for the warm climate and beaches. Most people (bar the elderly) can speak both Maltese and English. All doctors' communications are in English.

✪ Medicine:

The Maltese Government provides a comprehensive free health service to all Maltese residents. Government health centres and hospitals provide preventative (both educational and vaccinations), investigative, curative and rehabilitative services. Those on a low income or with a chronic condition are also entitled to free pharmaceuticals. Private healthcare also exists and is becoming more popular. In total there are eight healthcare centres providing primary care and a number of hospitals providing secondary and tertiary care. The main teaching hospitals is St Luke's with 850 beds. Building is underway to replace this with a new (800-bed) hospital next to the University. In total there are about 2000 acute beds in Malta. There is a shortage of nurses.

➲ Visas and work permits:
EU nationals do not require a visa to do an elective. Contact the Maltese Embassy for work permits.

◎ Climate and crime:
The climate is similar to Greece, warmest between July and September (reaching 30 °C). Crime rates are pretty low.

THE MEDICAL SCHOOL AND HOSPITALS:

The Medical School, St Luke's Hospital

MSIDA, Guardamangia, Malta.
This is the only Maltese Medical School and they are very well set up for arranging electives. Write to: **The Maltese Medical Students Association Exchange Committee** at the above address e-mail: mmsa@hotmail.com Visit: www.sunnyislands.com/electives

They operate an 'exchange' programme whereby they try to tie in one of their students going to your country. This is not a problem. If you arrange an exchange your accommodation is free, if not it's £3.75/night. Elective fees work out at £1.50/day. The Medical School provides the following specialities: medicine, neurology, O&G, paeds, cardiology, geriatrics, pathology, community medicine, public health, surgery, radiology, ENT, opthalmology, psychiatry, health information, dermatology, oncology, orhthopaedics, dentistry and casualty. They can be arranged in St Luke's or in one of the other hospitals.

St Luke's Hospital

Guardamangia, Malta Tel: 241251/247860/234101.
The hospital: St Luke's, the teaching hospital (850 beds) of Malta, is at the top of a very large hill, one mile out of the capital, Valletta. Life is very relaxed and you can join in with this and that as you please. Teaching is good although there is little hands on for students. The beaches nearby are not brilliant, but the water sports are good. Days are usually from 8 am until 2 pm.
Accommodation: *See above.*

Gozo General Hospital, Tel: 561600. (This is a general hospital for those on the island of Gozo. It has 159 beds.)
Mount Carmel Hospital, Attard, Malta Tel: 415183/4/5. (Malta's main psychiatric hospital with 625 beds.)
Sir Paul Boffa Hospital, Floriana, Malta Tel: 224491/224581/245019/245091. (A skin cancer, convalescence and fever hospital. It has 110 beds.)
St Vincent de Paule Residence, Luqa, Malta Tel: 224461/2/3. (A residence for the elderly with over 1000 beds.)
Ta'L-Ibragg Hospital, Gozo, Malta. (This is the psychiatric and geriatric hospital for the island of Gozo. It has 100 beds.)
Zammit Clapp Hospital, St Julian's, Malta Tel: 344950 Fax: 344914. (A specialized geriatric hospital. It has 60 beds.)

HEALTH CENTRES:

For primary healthcare contact: Dr Ray Busuttil, 7 Harper Lane, Floriana VLT 14, Malta Tel: 233393 Fax: 233393.

There are eight Health Centres:

Triq FS Fenech, Florina VLT 14, Malta Tel: 243314-5/244340.
Pjazza M Scicluna, Gzira GZR 05, Malta Tel: 337245/344766.
Triq iL-Vitorja/Triq San Dwardu, Qormi, Malta Tel: 484450-3.
Centru Civiku, Paola, Malta Tel: 691314/5.
1 Triq Sofia, Cospicua CSP 02, Malta Tel: 675492/673292/3.
Centru Civiku, Mosta, Malta Tel: 433256/432062/411065.
Centru Civiku, Rabat, Malta Tel: 459082/3.
Dr Enrico, Mizzi Street, Victoria VCT 107, Malta Tel: 561600.

Monaco

Population: 31,000
Language: French
Capital: Monaco
Currency: French franc
Int Code: +377

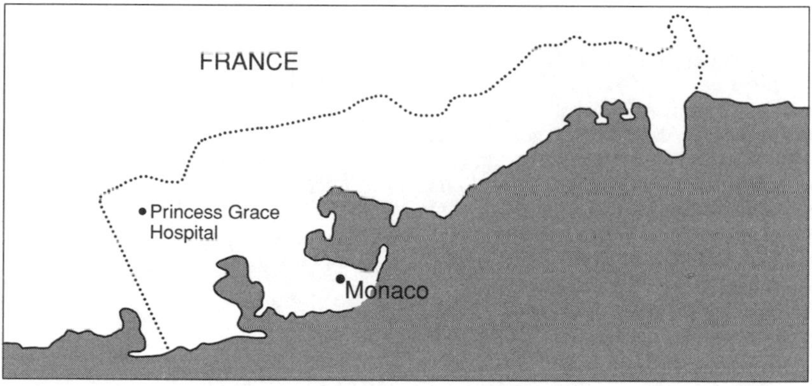

Monaco, on the Côte d'Azur in south-eastern France, is a centre for the international jet-setter. It has a lucrative banking and tourist industry. With this in mind, the healthcare not only provides for its 31,000 citizens but many overseas as well.

Medicine:
A private healthcare system operates to provide a costly, but effective health service. There are no establishments for training doctors. Most come from France. Heart and cerebrovascular diseases with cancers are the big causes of mortality.

Visas and work permits:
Since 1998, no members of the EU state need to obtain a settlement visa to enter Monaco. You will need a 'Carte de Sejour Monegasque'. Write directly to the Police Directorate: **Direction de la Sûreté Publique**, Section des étrangers, 3 Rue Louis Notari, Monaco-Cedex Tel: 93 15 30 17. Contact the embassy in your country for more details.

HOSPITALS:

Princess Grace Hospital
Av Pasteur BP 489, MC 98012 Monaco.
The hospital: The main hospital in Monaco. Officially founded in 1958 it has been at the forefront of medical advances. There is a maternity unit, good surgical facilities, a nursing school, a geriatric and psychiatric unit and a good radiology department. There are many other units; however, this is all very much in a private setting.

The Monaco Cardio-thoracic Centre

CCM 11 bis av D'Ostende-BP 223,
MC 98004 Monaco Tel: 92 168 000
Fax: 92 168 299 http://www.ccm.mc
e-mail: info@com.mc

The hospital: Renowned for its diagnosis and its treatment of cardiac disease of all ages, neonatal to the oldest of patients. Each year about 800 open-heart operations and more than 2000 investigations are performed. In nine years it has operated on 800 children with congenital heart diseases. The permanent team has particular interests in the reconstruction of the left ventricle after myocardial infarction. Again, this is very much in a private setting. Quoting from the brochure 'All types of accommodation [for patients] are available ... from the adaptable suite, a private room with lounge or office area fitted with a fax to the standard room for two patients'.

Netherlands

Population: 15.5 million
Language: Dutch
Capital: Amsterdam
Currency: Dutch guilder
Int Code: +31

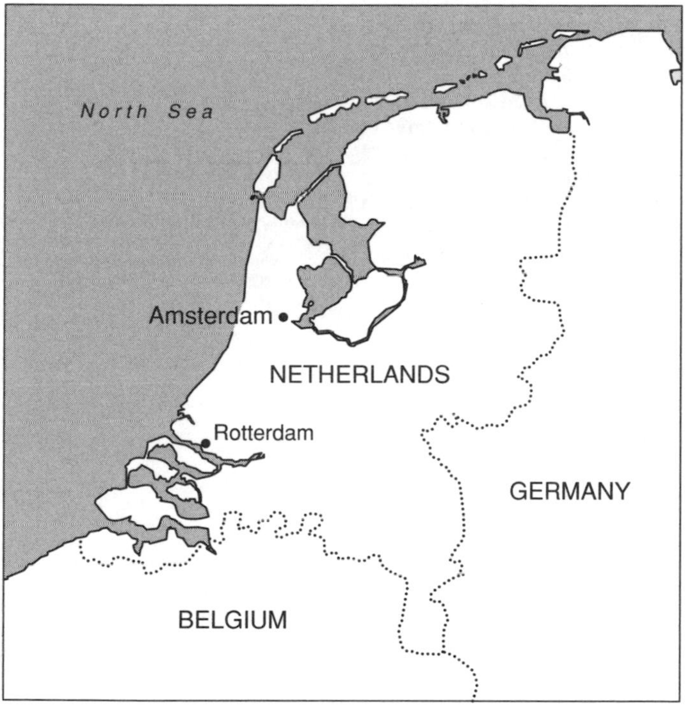

Situated in the north-west of Europe, Holland is best-known for its tulips, clogs and flat reclaimed land. It is not a popular elective destination which is surprising since most Dutch speak English extremely well. A number of hospitals are on the Soctrates/Erasmus programme. For these reasons only a few places are listed below.

Medicine:

Medical practice is typically western with both state and private healthcare systems.

Visas and work permits

EU citizens do not need a visa or work permit to go to or work in the Netherlands.

USEFUL ADDRESSES:

Ministry of Health, Welfare and Sports,
PO Box 5406, 2280 HK Rijswijk, Netherlands
Tel: 340 7911 Fax: 340 7834.
Stichting Federatie van Medisch Wetenschappelijke Verenigingen in Nederland

(FMVV), (Federation of Medical Scientific Associations in the Netherlands), PO Box 9101, 6500 HB Nijmegen, Netherlands Tel: 24 361 3168 Fax: 24 356 5557.

Amsterdam

Universiteit van Amsterdam
Faculteit der Geneeskunde, Jan Swammerdam Institute, Eerste Constantijin Hugensstraat 20, 1054 BW Amsterdam, Netherlands.
This is the oldest medical school in Holland and uses **Academisch Medisch Centrum**, Universiteit van Amsterdam, Amsterdam (Tel: 20 5662509).
The hospital: The Academic Medical Centre (AMC) is a new hospital built in the 1970s. It is on the metro line about 15 minutes out of town. It is a very pleasant hospital to work in and has a well-known intensive care unit. It serves a wider catchment population than the older hospital in town.

Accommodation: Contact University Foreign Relations Offices, Universiteit van Amsterdam, Netherlands.

Free University (Vrije Universiteit)
Faculteit der Geneeskunde, Van der Boechorststraat 7, 1081 BT Amsterdam, uses **Vu Ziekenhuis**, Postbus 7057, 1007 MB Amsterdam, Netherlands Tel: (020) 444 44 44 Fax: (020) 444 46 45. http://azvu.nl/
The hospital: Has 733 beds and provides most specialities. It has a trauma centre and provides a Helicopter Emergency Medicine Service (HEMS).

Rotterdam

Erasmusuniversiteit, Faculteit der Geneeskunde, Postbus 1738, Dr Molewaterplein 50, 3015 CN Rotterdam, Netherlands uses Academisch Ziekenhuis Rotterdam, a 1304-bed hospital.

Norway

Population: 4.5 million
Language: Norwegian
Capital: Oslo
Currency: Norwegian krone
Int code: +47

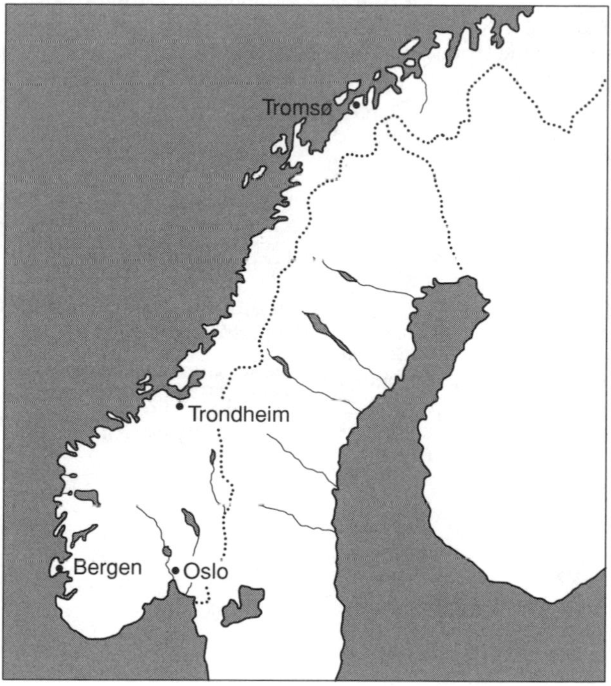

Norway, the furthest west of the Scandinavian countries, is a beautiful land of fjords and coastline. Fishing and oil are the mainstays. All doctors can speak English as there are few Norwegian textbooks. Most patients can also speak at least a little.

✪ Medicine:

Norway has an excellent healthcare system. It is very efficient and even though only 8% of the GDP is spent on it, Norway has one of the lowest infant moratalities and highest life expectancies of any country. Recently tele-medicine has been introduced so that people in the far north do not have to travel to get specialist consultations.

A full list of Norwegian Hospitals is available on: http://aetat.no/english/

UNIVERSITIES:

There are four universities that teach medicine in Norway. All bar the Norwegian University of Science and Technology also teach nursing.

University of Bergen

N-5020 Bergen, Norway Tel: 55 58 90 22 Fax: 55 58 90 25 www.uib.no

Situated in Norway's second-largest city (population 220,000) this sea-port is surrounded by mountains. The school uses: **Haukeland Sykehus**, 5021 Bergen, Norway, a modern hospital near the centre of Bergen.

O **Elective notes:** There's lots to do with a very busy procedures unit. It comes recommended.

University of Oslo

Postboks 107 Blindern N-0316 Oslo, Norway Tel: 22 85 50 50 Fax: 22 85 44 42 www.uio.no

The capital of Norway (population 500,000) is surrounded by hills and forests. Write to the medical faculty at the above address for elective details. A couple of its hospitals are:

The National Hospital (Rikshospitalet)

Pilestredet 32, 0027 Oslo, Norway Tel: 22867010 Fax: 22867580.

The hospital: A state-run hospital acting as both a regional and national referral centre. The hospital encompasses the 'old' National Hospital, the Oslo Rheumatism Hospital (Akersbakken, Oslo) and the National Centre for Orthopaedics (Carl Berners plass, Oslo). It provides a national centre for transplantation, epilepsy surgery, bone marrow transplantation, haemophilia and transsexualism. The only things it doesn't do are geriatrics, psychiatry and a few cancer treatments. **Aker University Hospital:** a 806-bed hospital serves the north-east portion of Oslo and includes Gaustad Hospital, Norway's oldest psychiatric hospital.

University of Tromsø

N-9037 Tromsø, Norway Tel: 77 64 40 00 Fax: 77 64 49 00 www.uit.no

The world's most northern university is in Tromsø (population 50,000) and was founded in 1972.

Norwegian University of Science and Technology, NTNU, N-7034 Trondheim, Norway Tel: 73 59 50 00 Fax: 73 59 80 90 www.unit.no (Trondheim is Norway's third-largest city.)

Romania

Population: 23 million
Language: Romanian
Capital: Bucharest
Currency: Leu
Int Code: +40

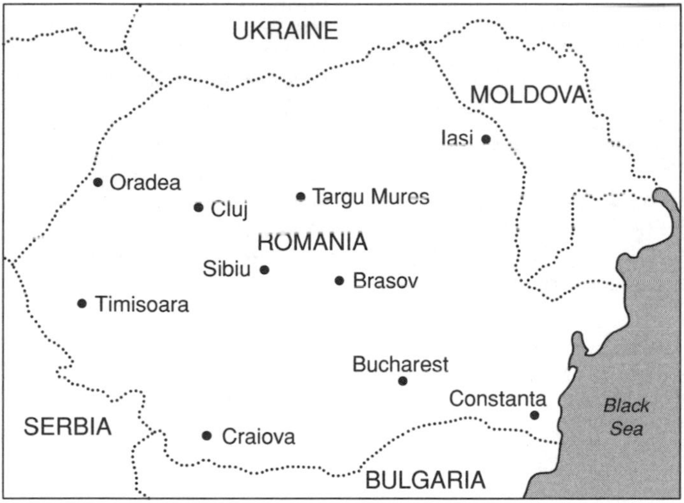

Romania left Communism in 1989 after a coup and has slowly developed a free market economy. It is, however, still very poor. It does have some beautiful countryside, the Danube, the Carpathian Mountains and lies on the Black Sea. Like most of Eastern Europe and Russia, it is not a common elective destination.

✪ Medicine:

Romania's health is probably the worst in Europe, with TB being highly prevalent. Developed country diseases are also common. HIV has become a real problem leaving many HIV-positive orphans. Despite a lack of resources, there is no shortage of doctors. This means that an elective here is not really the same as a deprived country in Africa. You don't get to do as much as you're not needed.

➲ Visas and work permits:

A visa is required to enter Romania (contact the Embassy), but the fee can be reduced if there is an official exchange. Work permits can only be obtained in Romania.

◎ Climate:

Romania has a continental climate in the summer, but can get bitterly cold with snow in the winter.

MEDICAL SCHOOLS:

Brasov-Universitatea Transilvania (Transilvania University), Bd Eroilor 29, Romania Tel: (068) 14 15 80 Fax: (068) 15 02 74.
Bucharest-Universitatea de Medicinã si Farmacie Carol Davila (Carol Davila University of Medicine and Pharmacy), 70183 Bucharest, Str Dionisic Lupu 37, Romania Tel: (01) 210 31 08 Fax: (01) 211 02 76.
Cluj-Napoca-Universitatea de Medicinã si Farmacie Iuliu Hateaganu (Iuliu Hateganu University of Medicine and Pharmacy), Str Emil Isac 13, Romania Tel: (064) 19 65 85 Fax: (064) 11 72 57.
Constanta-Universitatea Ovius (Ovidus University) Bd Mamaia 124, Romania Tel: (041) 61 45 76 Fax: (041) 61 83 72.
Craiova-Universitatea Craiova (University of Craiova) Str Al. I, Cuza 13, Romania Tel: (051) 41 45 48 Fax: (051) 41 16 88.
Iasi-Universitatea de Medicinã si Farmacie Grigore T Popa (Griore T Popa Universit of Medicine and Pharmacy), Str Universitãtii 16, Romania Tel: (032) 11 61 04 Fax: (032) 21 35 73.
Oradea-Universitatea Oradea (Oradea University) Str Armatci Romane 5, Romania Tel: (059) 13 28 30 Fax: (059) 43 27 89.
Sibiu-Universitatea Lucian Blaga (Lucian Blaga University) Bd, Victorici 10, Romania Tel: (069) 41 62 21 Fax: (069) 21 78 87.
Timisoara-Universitatea de Medicinã si Farmacie (University of Medicien and Pharmacy) Piata Etimie Murgu 2, Romania Tel: (056) 13 40 96 Fax: (056) 19 06 26.
Târgu Mures-Universitatea de Medicinã si Farmacie (University of Medicine and Pharmacy) Str Gh Marinesu 38, Romania Tel: (065) 21 31 27 Fax: (065) 21 04 07.

A couple of hospitals in Bucharest that take elective students directly:

Fundeni Hospital

258 Fundeni Road, Bucharest – Z, Romania.

Spitalul de Copii 'Victor Gowoiv'

(Bd Basarabrei ur 21), Bucharest, Romania.
The hospital: A paediatric hospital with a great deal of poverty and very limited resources (no gloves, few drugs). Children get dumped here by their parents who don't come back to pick them up. It is the one commonly featured on the news.

Russia

Population: 150 million
Language: Russian
Capital: Moscow
Currency: Rouble
Int Code: +7

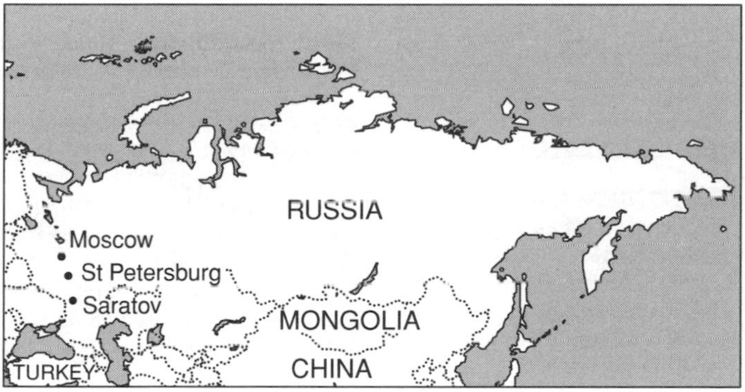

Russia is huge, nearly twice as large as China or the USA. Despite this, it is not a popular destination for Western doctors, nurses or medical students. This is probably mainly due to the language barrier, but the country's economic and political problems (and climate!) don't really help its appeal. That said, there is a desperate need within the healthcare system and reports from those who have worked with organizations and hospitals have found it very worthwhile.

✪ Medicine:
With Communism a comprehensive healthcare system was provided by employers; however, since its collapse, the now-privatized companies do not have to provide such cover. This is just one way Russian people have suffered as they attempt to leave their Communist past. The state itself simply does not have the resources to provide an adequate National Health Service and the costs of private healthcare are way beyond the pocket of most Russians. For that reason bribery within the profession has become common. There is a shortage of all bar the very basic medications. Patients keep costs down by supplying their own food and relatives often act as nurses. There is not, as you might imagine, a shortage of doctors (1:220 people). An unusual combination of medical conditions is relatively common. On the one hand, Western diseases are prevalent (cardiovascular disease, accidents), but so are infectious diseases (TB and diphtheria). With the Chernobyl disaster oncological pathology has increased.

Medical students choose at the outset whether they want to do adult, paeds or preventative medicine and are trained in it specifically.

➲ Visas and work permits:

You will need to contact the embassy. They have so few elective students they don't really understand what it is. As regarding paid work, no one goes to do that unless through an Aid agency.

◎ Climate:

Cold going down to –15 ºC in winter. The summers can get up to +20 ºC. It obviously varies across such a huge country.

MAIN MEDICAL SCHOOLS:

I Moskovskij Ordena Lenina I' Ordena Trudovogo Krasnogo Znameni Medicinskij Institut im

IM Secenova, Ulica Bol'saja Pirogovskaja 2/6, 119435 Moskva, Russia.

This is Russia's oldest medical school, founded in 1765 in Moscow. The two paeds hospitals used are the **Russian Republic Children's Hospital** and the **Filatov Children's Hospital**, 15 Sadovaya-Kurdinskaya Street, Moscow 103001.

Lomonosov Moscow State University

Vorobjevy Hills, MSU Main Building, Room 1029, Moscow, 119899, Russia Tel: (7-095) 939 5600 Fax: (7-095) 939 0015 www.fbm.msu.ru

This medical school teaches foreigners as well as local Russians and hence is better if your Russian is poor.

Leningradskij Ordena Trudovogo Krasnogo Znameni Medicinskij Institut im

Akad IP Pavlova, Ulica L'va Tolstogo 6/8, 197089, St Petersburg, Russia.

This is the main adult medical school in St Petersburg.

Saratovskij Ordena Trudovogo Krasnogo Znameni Medicinskij Institut

410710 Saratv Russia ul Bolshaya Kazachia, 112, Russia Tel: 7 (8452) 51 16 17 Fax: 7 (8452) 24 35 31.

Saratov State Medical University has become one of the largest medical institutes in Russia and admits 400 medical students a year. Since the early 1990s they have also been training Indian, Pakistani, Nepalese and African students.

An institution that has previously taken Western volunteers is:

New Life Drug Rehabilitation Centre

47 Karl Marx St, 188450 Kingisepp, St Petersburg, Russia.

This is a very friendly group who go into the community to aid drug rehabilitation.

Slovakia

Population: 5.5 million
Language: Slovak
Capital: Bratislava
Currency: Slovak koruna
Int Code: +421

The 'other half' of the former Yugoslavia is less-developed and is struggling to break into Western-style industry-based economy. It does, however, have some beautiful areas and historical cities.

✪ Medicine:

Despite the relative poverty, healthcare is fairly good and Western diseases are the most common causes of death. It has three well-organized medical schools. Possibly because of the language barrier, Slovakia is not visited commonly.

➲ Visas and work permits:

Visas are not required for many countries if visiting for less than 30 days. Most EU country and Canadian citizens can stay for 90 days. US and Italian citizens have a 30-day upper limit. UK citizens have a 180-day maximum. For official study or work you need a residence permit. For this you need confirmation of work or place of study, a medical (including HIV test), confirmation of accommodation and a criminal record check both in your home country and Slovakia. All this has to be in Slovak and can take up to 60 days.

USEFUL ADDRESS:

The Slovak Medical Students Association (Slovenská asociácia študentov medicíny (SloMSA))
c/o BSM, Sasinkova 2, 813 72 Bratislava, Slovakia Tel: 07/59357 458

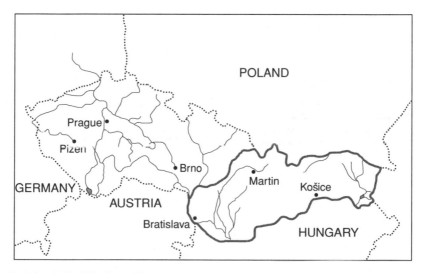

http://crick.fmed.uniba/sk/slomsa/activi.html
SloMSA, as well as representing their own students, can help arrange exchanges in Bratisvala, Martin or Košice. They offer a vast array of electives in each of them. Shared accommodation in a student hostel can usually be provided. Full details are on the web.

MEDICAL SCHOOLS/MAIN HOSPITALS:

Comenius University, Faculty of Medicine

(Universita Komenskeho, Lékarská Fakulta) Špitálska 24, 811 08 Bratislava, Slovakia Tel: +421 7 59357111 Fax +421 7 59357201 e-mail sd@fmed.uniba.sk
The medical faculty was founded in 1919 and has 1500 students making it the largest and oldest in Slovakia. It uses the Faculty Hospital in Miciewiczova Street, the Faculty Hospital of Academian L Derer and Paediatric Hospital in Limbova Street, Ruzinov Hospital in Ruzinovska Street and the Hospital of St Cyril and Metod and the Oncological Institute of Al Beta in Heydukova Street.

PJ Safarik University

(Universita PJ Šafarika) Lékarská Fakulta, Dekanát LFUPJS Košice, Tr. SNP è1, 041 80 Košice, Slovakia.
The second-largest medical school in Slovakia has a new large University Hospital as well an old one.

Comenius University

(Universita Komenskeho) Jesenius Medical Faculty, MaláHora C4, 036 01 Martin, Slovakia.
The University uses the teaching hospital in Martin, a town in central Slovakia below Low Fatra Mountains, 40 minutes from excellent skiing and tourist facilities.

Spain

Population: 40 million
Languages: Spanish, Galician, Basque and Catalan
Capital: Madrid
Currency: Peseta
Int Code: +34

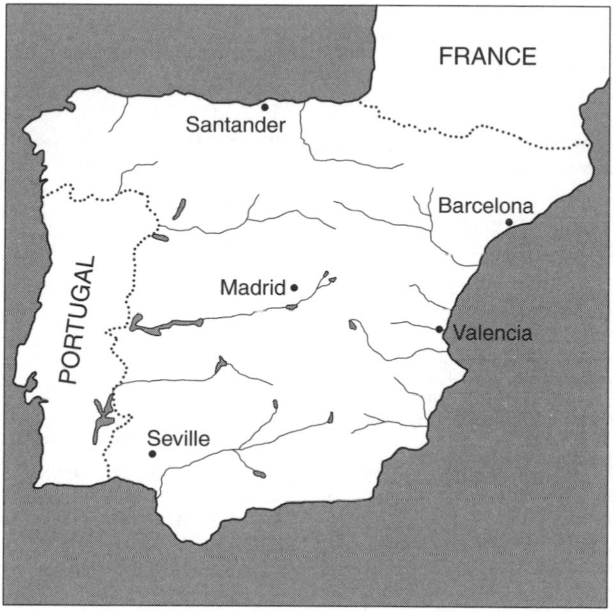

Situated in the south-west corner of Europe, Spain has a beautiful Mediterranean coast and the Pyrenees in the north. There is plenty to see and do as it has a very rich history. However, because it is not a popular elective destination and because the Socrates/Erasmus exchange programme makes it easy to organize electives here, this chapter will not go into much detail. A comprehensive list of hospitals is available from the Spanish Embassy or by looking on the Yahoo Spain Home Page. Fluent Spanish is needed to work or do an elective in most parts of Spain.

✪ Medicine:

The public health service is actually very good and the Spanish tend to be a healthy population. However, HIV has crept in and Spain has the second-highest rate in Europe.

➲ Visas and work permits:

No visa is required for other EU

nationals to enter Spain. Contact the Spanish Consulate if requiring a work permit.

USEFUL ADDRESS:

For a full list of Spanish hospitals and medical organizations contact the Ministry of Health in Madrid: **Ministerio de Sanidad y Consumo**, Paseo del Prado 18–20, 28071 Madrid, Spain Tel: 420 0000.

MAIN MEDICAL SCHOOLS AND THEIR HOSPITALS:

Madrid

Universidad Autónoma de Madrid, Facultad de Medicina, Arzobispo Morcillo 4, Madrid-34, Spain.

Its associated hospitals include:
Hospital De La Princesa, C/Diego de León No 62 28006, Madrid, Spain Tel: 520 22 20 Fax: 520 23 44.
Hospital Del Niño Jesús, Avda/ Medéddz Pelayo No 65, 28009, Madrid, Spain Tel: 504 61 93 Fax: 504 46 12.
Fundacion Jimenez Diaz, Clinica de la Concepcion, Avda De Los Reyes Católicos No 2, 28040, Madrid, Spain Tel: 543 10 71 Fax: 543 10 71.
Hospital Puerta De Hierro, 28040 Madrid, Spain. Tel: 316 23 40.
Hospital Universitario la Paz, C/ Arzobispo Morcillo No 2 y 4, Facultad de Medicina 28029, Madrid, Spain Tel: 397 54 95 Fax: 91 729 22 80.

Universidad Complutense de Madrid, Facultad de Medicina, Ciudad Universitaria, Madrid-3 is the other big medical school in Madrid. It's associated with:

Clínica Puerta de Hierro (Hospital Universitario), C/San Martín de Porred, 4/ 28035 Madrid, Spain Tel: 91 316 22 40 Fax: 91 316 05 35 www.cph.es

Barcelona

Universidad de Barcelona, Facultad de Medicina, Casanova 143, 08036 Barcelona. As well as the university hospital, the University of Barcelona also uses: **Vall d'Hebron Hospitals**, 119–129 08035 Barcelona. Tel: 93 489 30 00 www.ar.vhebron.es The Vall d'Hebron hospitals are a group of four large centres in Catalonia: **The General Hospital**, the **Maternity and Children's Hospital**, the **Traumatology and Rehab Hospital** and the **Adrià Surgical Clinic** totalling 1400 beds.

Seville

Universidad de Savilla, Facultad de Medicina, Sevilla, Spain.

Valencia

Universidad de Valencia, Facultad de Medicina, Valencia. One of their hospitals is: **Hospital de Sagunto,** Avda. Ramón y Cajal, s/n-46520 Puerto de Sagunto (Valencia) Tel: 962659400 Fax: 962659420. It provides general medical and surgical services to part of Valencia.

Universidad de Santander, Facultad de Medicina, Polígono de Casañas s/n, Santander. This school uses: **Hospital Universitario 'Marques De Valdecilla'**, 39008 Santander, Cantabria, Spain.
The hospital: 'Marques de Valdecilla' is the major teaching hospital in Santander, a town on the Spanish north-west Atlantic coast. Santander is a compact city with an abundance of good cafes and bars and a superb nightlife. There are good beaches and occasional good surf. The nearby Picos de Europa offer superb walking and climbing.

Málaga

Universidad de Málaga, Facultad de Medicina, Málaga, Spain.

Canary Islands

Universiario de Canarias, 38320 La Laguna, Santa Cruz de Tenerife, Canary Islands Tel: (34) 922 678091 Fax: (34) 922 660433. (This school uses the University hospital in Santa Cruz as well as other hospitals throughout the Canaries.)

Sweden

Population: 8.8 million
Language: Swedish
Capital: Stockholm
Currency: Krona
Int Code: +46

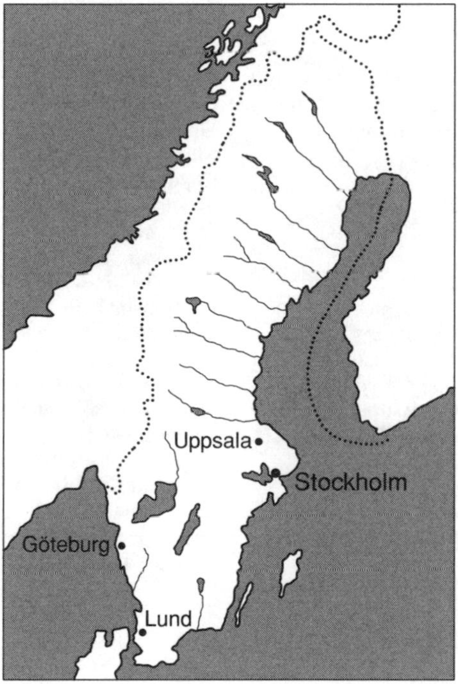

Sweden (a member of the EU since 1995) reaches high into the Arctic Circle and is situated between Finland and Norway. Most of the country is dense forest. Many people can speak English, but despite that it is not a common elective destination. Electives can be arranged through the Socrates/Erasmus programme.

⊕ Medicine:
Sweden spends less of its GNP on healthcare (8.8%) than nearly every other country in Europe and is trying to reduce it further. Despite this it manages to have the second-lowest infant mortality and fifth-highest life expectancy in the world. This says a great deal about their well-run

comprehensive healthcare system. A consultation costs100SEK (£10). For chronic disorders there is a ceiling of 1500SEK (£150). Private practice has only recently become available.

➲ Visas and work permits:

EU passport holders do not require a visa to stay or work in Sweden for up to three months. If staying or working longer a residence permit and working permit are required. Other nationals, including those from Australia, NZ and the USA, also do not require a visa to visit.

◎ Climate:

It's pretty cold all the time but really cold in winter and freezing cold in the north where the Baltic Sea often freezes.

MEDICAL SCHOOLS AND HOSPITALS:

Karolinska Institutet

SE-171 77 Stockholm, Sweden
http://info.ki.se/ki/index_en.html

Founded in 1810, the medical school of the capital has a good research reputation. The University only does medicine and uses **Södersjukhuset Hospital**, 118 83 Stockholm, Sweden.

Universitetet I Lund

Medicinska Fackulteten, Box 1703, S-221 01 Lund, Sweden.

Founded in 1666, Lund uses **Lund University Hospital**, S-22100, Lund, Sweden.

The hospital: The medical school and hospital (built in 1968) are large institutions with a great deal of history. Most diseases are typical of the West. Lund can arrange electives in more peripheral hospitals as well. There are no general medical wards. Patients are admitted to an acute ward then transferred to the relevant speciality. Write to the Elective Committee to do an elective here. They can also sort out accommodation.

Universitetet I Göteborg

Medicinska Fakulteten, Fack, S-400 44, Göteborg 33, Sweden.

Gothenburg University uses the massive **Sahlgrenska University Hospital** (Sahlgrenska Universtetssjukhuset S-413 45 Göteborg, Sweden Tel: 31 342 10 00). This is one of the biggest hospitals in Europe and has been created by the fusion of six hospitals. You will be very hard-pushed to find a speciality not catered for.

Universitetet I Uppsala

Medicinska Fakulteten, Box 256, S-751 05, Uppsala, Sweden.

Uppsala uses **Uppsala University Hospital** (S-751 85 Uppsala, Sweden Tel: 18 663000 Fax: 18 508127 www.uas.se). This is a large 924-bed hospital with a vast array of specialities.

Switzerland

Population: 7.2 million
Official Languages: German, French, Italian
Capital: Bern
Currency: Swiss francs
Int Code: +41

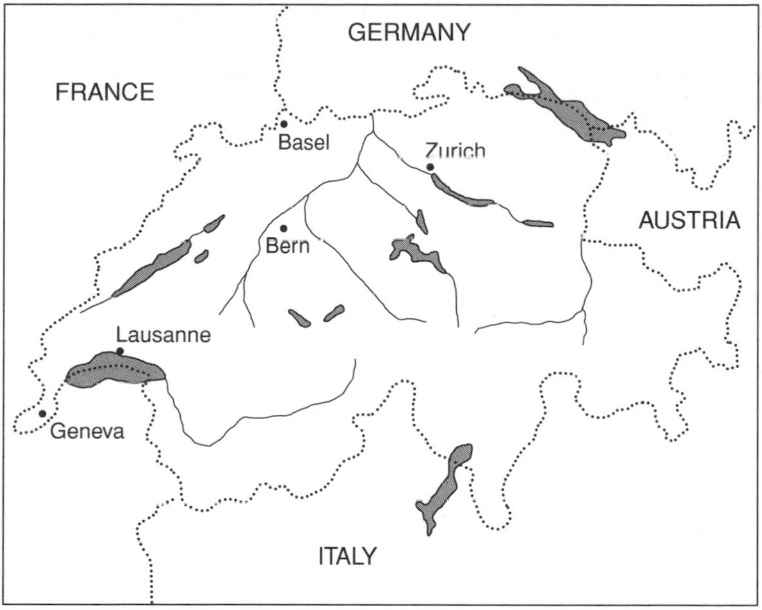

Despite being right in the middle of Europe, Switzerland has managed to avoid European politics and remained neutral in all conflicts. It has many rivers and the Alps in the south with some excellent ski resorts. Like much of Europe, it is surprisingly not a popular elective destination. The universities and many of the hospitals, however, are on the web.

✪ Medicine:

The healthcare costs of Switzerland are covered by compulsory insurance schemes (amounting to 8% of the GNP). From this the Swiss have built up a very efficient and advanced health service.

➲ Visas and work permits:

The embassy states that full-time students require a residence permit. Send a CV, proof of acceptance by the University, proof of finances and three photographs to the Swiss Embassy. It is unclear as to whether it is really necessary just for an elective. To work in

Switzerland as a medical practitioner you need the Swiss Qualifications and a work permit.

◎ Climate:

Obviously depends on altitude. The Alps can get extremely cold, but away from them it is considerably warmer.

USEFUL ADDRESS:

The Federation of Swiss Medical Doctors, Verbindung der Schweizer Aerzte, Fédération des médecins Suisses, Elfenstrasse 18, 3000 Bern 16, Switzerland.

MEDICAL SCHOOLS:

Universität Basel, Medizinisch Fakultät, Hebelstrasse 25, 4031 Basel, Switzerland.

Universität Bern, Medizinisch Fakultät, Murtenstrasse 11, CH-3010 Bern, Switzerland Tel: 31 632 35 53 Fax: 31 632 49 94 www.unib.ch

Université De Genève, Faculté de Médecine, Anée d'Etudes à Option, CMU, 1 rye Michel Street, 1211 Genève, Switzerland. (The exchange office is contactable on the net at www.medecine.unige.ch).

Université de Lausanne, Faculté de Médecine, Centre hospitalier universitaire vaudois, Rue du Bugnon 9, 1011 Lausanne, Switzerland.

Universität Zürich, Medizinische Fakultät Rämistrasse, 8091 Zürich, Switzerland.

HOSPITAL ASSOCIATIONS:

H+Die Spitäler der Schweiz, H+ Les Hôpitaux de Suisse, Rain 32, 5001 Aarau, Switzerland.

Schweizerische Vereinigung der Privatkliniken. Association Suisse des cliniques privées, Moosstrasse 2, 3073 Gümligen, Switzerland.

Turkey

Population: 62 million
Language: Turkish
Capital: Ankara
Currency: Turkish lira
Int Code: +90

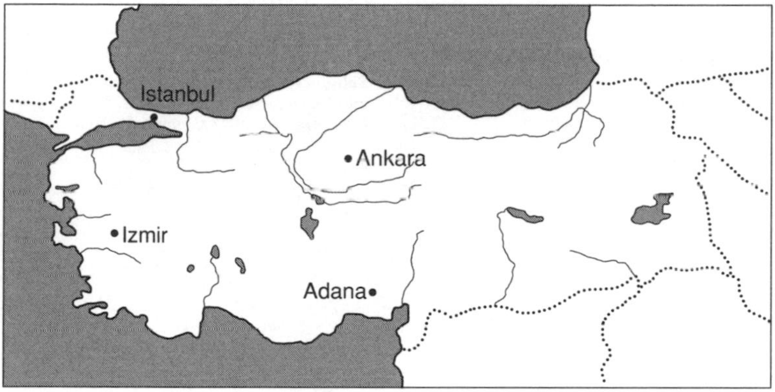

Turkey is in an unusual situation. It's 'nearly Europe', but its Islamic status pulls it Eastward. Most people live in the west, whereas the east and south-east are Kurdish areas. It has recently had a number of tremendous earthquakes, which has put an incredible strain on both hospitals and the economy. Work and electives here (apart from help during the recent troubles) are relatively unusual and hence only major institutions are listed.

✪ Medicine:
A National Health Service provides care for all; however, it is under-equipped. The recent troubles have made this a great deal worse.

SOME MEDICAL SCHOOLS:

Adana

Çukurova Üniversitesi
Tip Fakültesi, 01330 Balcalý, Adana, Turkey
Tel: (322) 3386084 Fax: (322) 3386945
www.cu.edu.tr

Ankara

Gazi Üniversitesi
Tip Fakültesi, Balgat, Ankara uses **Ankara Numune Hospital**, Ankara, Turkey.

Founded in 1881, the Ankara University Hospital is the biggest postgraduate service hospital (1250–1700 beds) and offers a full range of specialities. The Accident and Emergency sees 200,000 patients a year.

Istanbul

Istanbulüniversitesi
Tip Fakültesi, Istanbul, Turkey.

Marmara Universitesi
Tip Fakültesi, Haydarpasa, Istanbul, Turkey.
The medical school uses **Haydarpap Numune Hospital**, which was established in 1903 and has grown to house 700 beds and level 1 trauma and tertiary referral centres.

Izmir

Ege University
Medical School, Bornova, Izmir, Turkey
http://medicine.ege.tr
Founded in 1955 it uses the 1733-bed hospital of Ege University.

Dokuz Eylul Universitesi
Tip Fakültesi, Incirati, Izmir, Turkey uses **Dokuz Eylul University Hospital**, Dokuz Eylul Universitesi Tip Fakültesi Arastrima Ve Uygulama, Hastanesi, Bilgi Islem Merkezi Izmir. This is a relatively modern medical school founded in 1982.

United Kingdom

Population: 58 million
Language: English
Capital: London
Currency: Pound
Int Code: +44

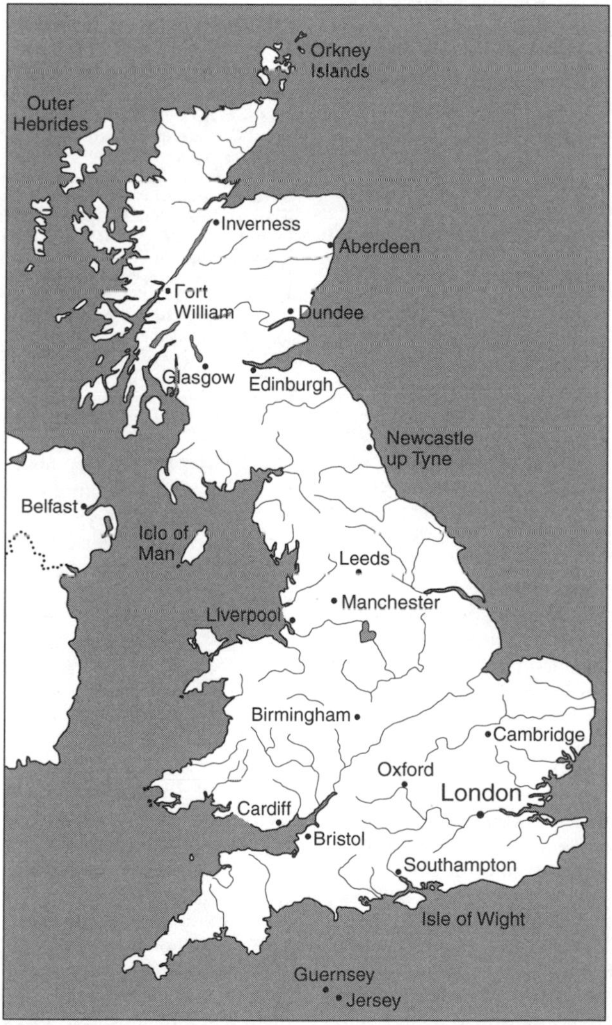

The UK (England, Wales, Scotland and Northern Ireland) to many people reading this is 'home'. A land in, but slightly separated from, the rest of Europe. Many medics from overseas spend some time here and many students stay here for their elective period. Why? In the UK there are no safaris, no sun-drenched beaches and no natural wonders. There's also little risk of heat stroke, no risk of rabies or malaria and you are unlikely to break any bones skiing. It is however a great place to see some historic institutions and experience one of the many vibrant cities. If it's home and you're broke, staying here can keep things cheap. It can also be a safety net if other plans fall through. If you're visiting, however, it can be expensive. Always enquire about the cost of accommodation when applying.

✪ Medicine:

The UK uses the National Health Service, a system whereby the state provides (nearly) all healthcare needs for everyone. This includes both GP and hospital treatment, although patients have to pay a modest charge for prescriptions. Because of the increasing demand on hospital services, waiting times for non-urgent cases are getting very long. This is encouraging more and more people to go private. Common conditions are those of any developed nation, cardiovascular diseases and cancers.

◎ Climate and crime:

It doesn't rain all year, just the winter (mainly). There is quite a variation between north Scotland and the south coast. Crime is mainly confined to inner-city areas. Due to the paucity of guns, penetrating trauma is comparatively rare compared to many other countries.

➲ Visas and work permits:

Requirements vary greatly depending on nationality. Those coming from New Zealand or Australia to work can easily obtain a two-year working holiday visa if under 26. Most hospitals, however, would rather you had a training permit. The conversion is usually not a problem once in the UK. For medical qualification enquiries contact the **General Medical Council** (78 Great Portland Street, London W1N 6JE Tel: 020 7580 642 Fax: 020 7915 3641). If coming from a non-English-speaking country you may well have to sit the PLAB (a language test) before you can do much else. Another group to contact is the **British Medical Association** BMA House, Tavistock Square, London WC1H 9LP Tel: 020 7383 6177 Fax: 020 7383 6220.

OTHER USEFUL ADDRESSES:

Royal College of Physicians of Edinburgh, 9 Queen Street, Edinburgh EH2 1JQ Tel: 0131 225 7324 Fax: 0131 225 2053 www.rcpe.ac.uk
Royal College of Surgeons of Edinburgh, Nicholson Street, Edinburgh EH8 9DW Tel: 0131 527 1600 Fax: 0131 557 646 www.rcsed.ac.uk
Royal College of Physicians and Surgeons of Glasgow, 242 St Vincent Street, Glasgow G2 5RJ Tel: 0141 221 6072 Fax: 0141 248 3414.
Royal College of Physicians of London, 11 St Andrew Place, Regent's Park, London NW1 4LE Tel: 020 7935 1174 Fax: 020 7486 4514.
Royal College of Surgeons of England, 35/43 Lincoln's Inn Fields, London WC2A 3PN Tel: 020 7405 3474 Fax: 020 7973 2179.
Northern Ireland Council for Postgraduate Medical Education, 5 Annadale Avenue, Belfast BT7 3JH Tel: 01232 491731 Fax: 01232 642279.

Note: The UK is a very popular destination for overseas elective students. Apply VERY EARLY (a year in advance is often necessary). Most places will only take you for a maximum of eight weeks and only if in your final year. Some places charge, whereas others don't and give free accommodation.

England

Birmingham University Medical School

Edgbaston, Birmingham B15 2TT, UK
Tel: 0121 414 6888 Fax: 0121 414 7159
www.bham.ac.uk

The University and medical school are about 6 miles from the centre of Birmingham. **Queen Elizabeth Hospital** (Edgbaston Tel: 0121 472 1311) is the main teaching hospital although others, both in and around Birmingham, are also used. These include **Birmingham Women's/Maternity Hospital** (Edgbaston Tel: 0121 472 1377), **The City Hospital** (Dudley Rd, B18 Tel: 0121 554 3801), **Children's Hospital** (Steelhouse Lane, B4 Tel: 0121 333 9999) and the **Royal Orthopaedic Hospital** (The Woodlands, Bristol Rd Tel: 0121 685 4000). There is not a great deal to do in the centre (shops, a few theatres), but around the hospital there is a good young social life. Outside you can explore the Midlands. Electives can be arranged in any department. There is an administration charge of £100. Some hospitals provide free accommodation, others charge around £35/week.

Bristol University Medical School

Clinical Dean's Office, Dolphin House, BRI, Bristol BS2 8HW Tel: 0117 9282335
www.bris.ac.uk

Bristol is a fairly compact town and the medical school and its hospitals have some pioneering departments. The main teaching hospital is the **Bristol Royal Infirmary** (Marlborough St BS2 Tel: 0117 923 0000), but there are a couple of others (including **Bristol General**, Guinea St BS3 Tel: 0117 926 5001) in the city and many DGHs outside that are also used. Electives can be arranged in most subjects depending on availability (the school has to see if any consultants are able to take you). There are no elective fees and accommodation is provided free. This is a popular elective destination. Apply at least a year in advance.

University of Cambridge, Addenbrooke's Hospital

Faculty of Medicine, Hills Road, Cambridge CB2 2QQ, UK Tel: 01223 336700
www.cam.ac.uk.

Cambridge has a reputation for academic excellence. **Addenbrooke's Hospital** (address as above Tel: 01223 245151) reflects this being a large (900-bed), well-run hospital with nearly all specialities provided on site. It is particularly known for its liver and kidney transplant services, but other specialities, including paediatrics, are also very highly regarded. Cardiothoracic surgery is done at **Papworth Hospital** (Papworth Everard, Cambridgeshire Tel: 01480 830541) about 30 minutes away by car. The town itself (two miles from the hospital) is very much a university town. There's an excellent college social life, so get involved with the local students. Other hospitals include: **Hinchingbrooke Hospital**, Hinchingbrooke Park, Huntingdon Tel: 01480 416416, **West Suffolk Hospital**, Hardwick Lane, Bury St Edmunds Tel: 01284 713000. Electives can be arranged in most subjects. There is a £150 administration charge and accommodation can be provided on the Addenbrooke's hospital site for £25/week.

Leeds University School of Medicine

Worsley Medical and Dental Building, University of Leeds, Leeds LS2 9JT, UK Tel: 0113 233 4362 www.hci.leeds.sc.uk

Leeds is a hilly city in the north of England. The main hospital, **St James' University Hospital** (Beckett Street, Leeds LS9 7TF Tel: 0113 243 3144) has been famed through the long-running TV series 'Jimmy's'. This has every speciality under the sun. The other main hospital is **Leeds General Infirmary** (Great George St LS1 Tel: 0113 243 2799). The University of Leeds will only permit visiting students between June and October and attachments outside this will not be considered. They will, however, try to provide hospital accommodation free of charge. A £50 non-refundable fee is charged to cover the cost of a blood test on arrival to ensure Hep B status. Applications should be made six months in advance and no later than February. The minimum stay is four weeks, maximum is 10.

Leicester University Medical School

Morris Shock Building, PO Box 138 Leicester, UK Tel: 0116 252 2295 or 2522
www.le.ac.uk

This is one of the UK's youngest medical schools situated just a few minutes' walk from the city centre. Its main hospital is **Leicester Royal Infirmary** (Infirmary Close, Leicester LE1 5WW Tel: 0116 254 1414 www.lri.org.uk), but others used include **Leicester General** (Gwendolen Rd, Leicester Tel: 0116 249 0490), the **Glenfield** (Groby Road, Leicester LE3 9QP Tel: 0116 287 1471) and a number of DGHs. Leicester itself is a fairly small town but has plenty of pubs and restaurants. Electives can be done in most subjects. There is no elective charge and accommodation is provided free.

The University of Liverpool

The Faculty of Medicine, 1st Floor, Duncan Building, Daulby Street, Liverpool L69 3GA
Tel: 0151 706 2000 Fax: 0151 709 2601
www.liv.ac.uk

The medical school is very large with nearly 1000 students. It is part of the **Royal Liverpool University Hospital** (Prescot St Tel: 0151 706 2000). This hospital offers most specialities and has a very busy A&E (possibly the largest in Europe). There are a number of specialist hospitals within Liverpool. The **Broadgreen** (Thomas Dr, L14 Tel: 0151 282 6000) and **Alder Hey Children's Hospital** (Eaton Rd, Liverpool L12 2AP Tel: 0151 228 4811) are in the suburbs. Specialist hospitals include **The Liverpool School of Tropical Medicine** (Pembroke Place L3 Tel: 0151 708 9393), **Liverpool Women's Hospital** (Crown St, L8 Tel 0151 708 9988) and the **Walton Centre for Neurology and Neurosurgery** (Rice Lane L9 Tel: 0151 525 3611). The Alder Hey is a very large paediatric hospital with 25 wards catering for everything from medicine and surgery to intensive care, psychiatry and A&E. There are many specialized clinics.

The University is a keen player on the Socrates exchange programme, but unfortunately says that this restricts it to only accepting elective students from the UK and the rest of the EU. It is still worth asking if from outside, but if they can't take you, try applying to the hospital/NHS trust directly. Some hospitals (such as the Alder Hey) have previously been able to provide free accommodation. Liverpool is a vibrant city with plenty of nightlife (home to the Beatles) and a world-famous football team. The people are genuine and friendly. There is, however, quite a bit of crime about. Just be careful with valuables.

London

London, the capital of the UK has everything to offer a visiting medic. There are some world-class institutions set in a vibrant, busy city. There are many attractions from the usual tourist traps to the many and varied bars and clubs. London is known for being expensive, and with good reason. However, if you budget carefully, there is no reason why it need be any more expensive than anywhere else. Accommodation can be costly, so try and arrange this as early as possible.

London is home to a very diverse range of people and this has a big impact on the type of medicine seen. The West End tends to be relatively well off while the East End has areas of real poverty and many immigrants. Only a few years ago there were 10 medical schools that were principally affiliated with one hospital each (e.g. **Bart's Medical School** was at **Bart's Hospital**). For better or worse, it was decided that all medical schools should merge and join multi-faculty universities. Today this means that there are technically only five medical schools in London. The original hospitals, however, are all still present. It has been worked so that there is a north, south, east and west school. **St George's** is a little further out in the southern suburbs. Whichever you visit, they are all on the Tube and hence give easy access to the nightlife and attractions of central London.

Royal Free and University College Medical School

Gower Street, London WC1E 6BT, UK
www.ucl.ac.uk (Or on the Royal Free site: Rowland Hill Street, London NW3 2PF
Tel: 020 7830 2686 Fax: 020 7435 4359)

In the early 1990s **UCH Medical School**

merged with the **Middlesex Hospital Medical School**. In the last couple of years, the **Royal Free** has also been engulfed. The new medical school is based in the heart of the London's West End, near Oxford Street. It is now huge using smaller hospitals such as the **Whittington**, many specialist hospitals such as **Great Ormond Street** and the **National Hospital for Neurology and Neurosurgery** as well as its original teaching hospitals. Because of the merger, the situation regarding electives is currently a bit up in the air. Apply to one of the above addresses. If you have no luck, write directly to one of the hospitals. Hospitals affiliated include:

University College Hospital

Grafton Way, London WC1E 6AU, UK
Tel: 020 7387 9300.

This is the acute admitting hospital for the UCH/Middlesex partnership. It has a busy A&E which gets a variety of customers from the business men and media types, to the down'n'outs and IVDUs.

The Middlesex Hospital

Mortimer Street, London W1N 8AA, UK
Tel: 020 7636 8333.

Once admitted from UCH patients are transferred to the Middlesex. It has many medical and surgical specialities, but obs & gynae, paeds and neuro go to the relevant specialist centres (*see* below).

The Royal Free Hospital

Rowland Hill Street, London NW3 2PF, UK
Tel: 020 7794 1876 Fax: 020 7435 5803.

The Royal Free has only very recently joined the huge UCL jungle. It is situated in Hampstead which sets it a little bit out of the hustle and bustle of the rest of UCH. It has many highly regarded departments and areas of research.

The Obstetric Hospital

Huntley Street, London WC1E 6AU, UK
Tel: 020 7387 9300.

This is the main obstetric hospital for North/Central London.

Great Ormond Street Hospital for Children

Great Ormond Street, London WC1N 3JH, UK Tel: 020 7405 9200 Fax: 020 7829 8643 www.ich.bpmf.ac.uk/center.htm

Probably the most famous paediatric hospital in the UK, Great Ormond Street has all specialities and many research areas in paediatrics. It has very large cardiac and oncology departments. Accommodation for students has previously been provided but is expensive.

Hospital for Tropical Diseases

4 St Pancras Way, London NW1 0PE, UK
Tel: 020 7387 4411.

The hospital's history extends back to the Seaman's Hospital Society wanting to care for returning sailors. They first set up hospital on board *HMS Grampus* on the River Thames. The medical conditions were obviously orientated towards diseases brought in from the tropics and sub-tropics. In 1899 the **London School of Tropical Medicine** was founded and in 1929 the **London School of Hygiene and Tropical Medicine** in Keppel Street was established. It was in 1951 that the HTD was built. The HTD has an 18-bed inpatient facility, travel clinic, outpatients and casualty for people who are ill having just returned from abroad. Note: tropical diseases include typhoid, cholera and typhus, all of which were in Britain in the nineteenth century so it may see more than what you simply imagine to be tropical. The hospital is at the forefront of research against new strains of drug-resistant malaria.

O Elective notes: The HTD charges £200 for a four-week elective. There is no student teaching but you join the SHO teaching and teaching for the Tropical Medicine Diploma. Ward rounds are very good learning points. The wards often have chloroquine-resistant malaria and schiostosomiasis and leishmaniasis may be seen in OPD.

The National Hospital for Neurology and Neurosurgery

Queen's Square, London WC1N 3BG
Tel 020 7837 3611 Fax: 020 7278 5069.

This is an international centre of

excellence for neurology and neurosurgery. Every aspect is catered for with very good teaching from people who are passionate about this subject. It's popular with American, German and Australian students and therefore there's a good social life. Contact the student office at the above address.

The Elizabeth Garrett Anderson Hospital and Hospital for Women, Soho 144, Euston Road, London NW1 2AP, UK Tel: 020 7387 2501.
The Eastman Dental Hospital, 256 Gray's Inn Road, London WC1X 8LD, UK Tel: 020 7915 1000.

Imperial College School of Medicine

London SW7 2AZ, UK Tel: 020 7594 3598 Fax: 020 7594 8004 www.med.ic.ac.uk

The **Imperial College School of Medicine** was formed in 1995 by the merger of St Mary's Medical School and the National Heart and Lung Institute. It then increased further absorbing Charing Cross and Westminster Medical Schools and the Royal Postgraduate Medical School in 1997. Each of these original institutions still has its own hospital in various parts of west London. Each has a long history of its own. All this merging has now made ICSM one of the largest medical schools in the UK. It has the following campuses:

St Mary's Hospital, Praed St Paddington, London W2, UK Tel: 020 7530 3500. (This is a large teaching hospital providing most specialities.)
Charing Cross Hospital, Fulham Palace Road, London W6, UK Tel: 020 8846 1234. (Again, this is also a large teaching hospital.)
Chelsea and Westminster Hospital, 369 Fulham Rd, London SW10, UK Tel: 020 8746 8000. (This is a very plush hospital in a very nice area of London. It has a state of the art new A&E.)
The Hammersmith Hospital, 150 DuCane Rd, London W12, UK Tel: 020 8743 2030. (The Hammersmith is a postgraduate teaching hospital. It is highly regarded for its acaedemic and clinical excellence.)
The Royal Brompton Hospital,Sydney Street, London SW3 6NP Tel: 020 7352 8121 Fax: 020 7351 8473 www.rbh.nthames.nhs.uk (The Royal Brompton is a large cardiothoracic unit in the West End.)

Hospitals throughout Middlesex and Surrey are also associated. Because of the recent merger, at the time of writing they are not accepting elective students. This will change. Previously electives have been possible at all hospitals free of charge. Write to the elective co-ordinator at the above addresses.

St Bartholomew's and The Royal London School of Medicine and Dentistry

Queen Mary and Westfield College, Turner Street, London E1 2AD, UK Tel: 020 7377 7611 Fax: 020 7377 7612
www.mds.qmw.ac.uk

Bart's and the London merged with QMW in 1993. Bart's is situated within the square mile of the city of London in an attractive courtyard setting. The London is in Whitechapel, a pretty deprived area of London with many Asian and Muslim immigrants. The hospitals therefore span the full breadth of social classes. Hospitals in Hackney (**The Homerton**), Whipp's Cross, Newham and Southend are also used as are a number of specialist units, including the **London Chest** (Bonner Road, London E2). A well-organized elective package in subjects from ITU to cardiothoracic surgery is available. Dental electives are also possible. There is no elective fee and you should apply six to 18 months before your intended date. A list of sources of accommodation is provided.

The Royal London Hospital

Mile End Road, Whitechapel, London E1 1BB, UK Tel: 020 7377 7000.

'The London' is a busy teaching hospital in the rough East End of London. Nearly all specialities are catered for. The Accident and Emergency department (level 1 trauma unit) is highly regarded. It has a Helicopter Emergency Medical Service (HEMS) on the roof which deals with all major trauma within the M25. In the A&E is a five-bed resus area and a paediatric A&E. There is plenty for students to see and do. In addition students get to spend time on the helipad and at the '999' ambulance control centre (unfortunately students are not allowed on the helicopter for insurance reasons).

St Bartholomew's Hospital
West Smithfield, London EC1A 7BE, UK
Tel: 020 7601 8888.
'Bart's' is a beautiful hospital in the heart of London. It has a great history and many famous old boys. Today, most acute care (A&E) has been transferred to the London. Bart's has now become a specialist centre for cancer, endocrine and a number of other specialities.

Guy's, King's and St Thomas' Medical School
Guy's Campus, London Bridge, St Thomas's Street, London SE1 9RT, UK Tel: 020 7955 4127 Fax: 020 7955 4425 www.kcl.ac.uk
'Guy's' and 'Tommy''s merged a number of years ago to form UMDS. In the last couple of years they have merged with the other big south-east London medical school, **King's College**. All have retained their original hospitals, but organization has been centralized. **Denmark Hill Hospital** and hospitals throughout south-east England are associated. The **Maudsley Hospital** in Lewisham is a specialist psychiatry centre.

St Thomas's Hospital
Lambeth Palace Rd, London SE1, UK
Tel: 020 7928 9292.
Situated on the River Thames right opposite the Houses of Parliament. Tommy's has a busy A&E department and many specialities. It's in an excellent location for getting into the West End.

Guy's Hospital
St Thomas St, London SE1, UK Tel: 020 7955 5000.
Situated nearer the financial city at London Bridge, 'Guy's, also has an A&E (not as busy) and medical and surgical specialities. Some departments are moving over to St Thomas's.

King's College Hospital and School of Medicine and Dentistry
Bassemer Road, Denmark Hill, London SE5 9PJ, UK Fax: 020 7346 3589.
King's is a large hospital, again with a busy A&E. It is also the regional liver unit for the whole of London and the south of England. It also has an affiliated hospital in Dulwich.

St George's Medical School
Crammer Terrace, London SW17 ORE, UK Tel: 020 8725 5992 Fax: 020 8725 5919 www.sghms.ac.uk
The last standing London medical school not to have been engulfed. It is in Tooting, South London. Although away from the city it has an interesting range of patients with diverse needs. Central London is a few stops away on the northern line. **St George's Hospital** (Blackshaw Rd, London SW17 Tel: 020 8672 1255) is the main teaching hospital but the school also has links with the **Atkinson Morley** (31 Copse Hill, London SW20 Tel: 020 8992 2277 (a specialist neurology hospital in Wimbledon)) and **St Helier's** in Sutton. There is a forensic medicine unit on the main site (Tel: 020 8725 0015) which has previously been popular with visiting (UK) students. Electives can be arranged in most departments. Accommodation is provided cheaply. German students must apply under the DAAD scheme. Write to the electives co-ordinator for more details.

OTHER SPECIALITY HOSPITALS:

Moorfield's Eye Hospital
City Road, London EC1V 2PD, UK Tel: 020 7253 3411 www.moorfields.org.uk
Moorfield's was founded in 1805 as a postgraduate teaching hospital and national centre for ophthalmic care. It is a centre of quality care, research and teaching. It has eight outreach centres and a mobile unit.

The Royal National Ear, Nose and Throat Hospital
330 Gray's Inn Rd, London WC1, UK Tel: 020 7837 8855.

The University of Manchester
Faculty of Medicine, Stopford Building, Oxford Road, Manchester M13 9PT, UK
Tel: 0161 275 5025 Fax: 0161 275 5697
www.medicine.man.ac.uk
Manchester has a large medical school.

The principal hospital is the **Manchester Royal Infirmary** (Oxford Road, M13 Tel: 0161 276 1234); however, it also uses hospitals in a 50-miles radius around Manchester. These include: **St Mary's** (Whitworth Park, M13 Tel: 0161 276 1234 – for obs, gynae and paeds), the **Hope**, the **Withington Christie** (Nell Lane, M20 Tel: 0161 445 8111), **North Manchester General** (Tel: 0161 740 1444), **Stepping Hill** and **Tameside General Hospitals**. **Booth Hall Children's Hospital** (Charlestown Rd Tel: 0161 795 7000) and **Royal Manchester Children's Hospitals** (Pendlebury Tel: 0161 794 4696) are the specialist paeds centres. The city itself has 50,000 students, hence there are always places to go.

There are many pubs, clubs and curry houses. Ask people where to go as some areas aren't all that safe for wandering around at night. There is no formal procedure for electives. You need to write to the Undergraduate Tutor in the Postgraduate Department of the subject you wish to do. A full list of names is in the third volume of the *British Medical Directory*. They can sometimes arrange accommodation. If you need a form signed by the Dean of the medical school you must enrol as a Manchester medical student and pay fees.

Newcastle University Medical School

Framlington Place, Newcastle upon Tyne NE2 4HH Tel: 0191 222 7034 Fax: 0191 222 6139 www.ncl.ac.uk

Situated right at the north end of England, Newcastle is a medium-sized, friendly city. The Medical School is situated in the centre and is on the same site as its principle teaching hospital, the **Royal Victoria Infirmary** (Victoria Rd Tel: 0191 232 5131). The school also uses a number of other hospitals in and around Newcastle. Write to the elective co-ordinator. All subjects bar dermatology, O&G and radiology can be catered for. There is currently no fee and accommodation can be provided for approx £120/month in the doctors' residence.

Nottingham University

Medical School Faculty Office, Queen's Medical Centre, Nottingham NG7 2UH Tel: 0115 970 9379 Fax: 0115 970 9922 www.nott.ac.uk

Nottingham is a pleasant city towards the north of England. It uses **University Hospital** (**Queen's Medical Centre**) on campus as well as **City Hospital** and **Derby Hospital**. Queen's Medical Centre has most specialities and is highly regarded for paeds surgery.

Oxford University

Medical School Offices, John Radcliffe Hospital, Headington, Oxford OX3 9DU Tel: 01865 221689 www.ox.ac.uk

Oxford, renowned for its academic excellence, has more to offer than just highbrow clinicians. The main teaching hospital, the **John Radcliffe** (Headley Way, Headington Tel: 01865 741166) is huge and caters for most needs. The **Churchill** (Old Road, Headington Tel: 01865 741 841) and **Radcliffe Infirmary** (Woodstock Rd Tel: 01865 311188) are older hospitals that are also used. The city has a pleasant centre and there is abundant student life. It is not just a university town though. London is only an hour away by train. Electives can be arranged in most subjects. The school has limited accommodation for a reasonable rent. There is no elective fee.

University of Sheffield Medical School

Faculty of Medicine, Medical School, Beech Hill Road, Sheffield S10 2RX Tel: 0114 271 1910 Fax: 0114 271 3960 www.shef.ac.uk

Sheffield conjures up images of mining, steel works and unemployed male strippers. The reality (apparently) is very different. The hospitals are in a nice part of town and the surrounding countryside is great if you like hill walking/rock climbing. The University has two main hospitals, the **Royal Hallamshire** (Glossop Road S10 2JF Tel: 0114 271 1900 Fax: 0114 271 1901) where the school is situated and the **Northern General** on the other side of town (about 20 minutes away). Together with the

Jessop Hospital for Women (Leavygreave Rd, S3 7RE Tel: 0114 226 8000) these cover all specialities. A number of DGHs in Humberside and South Yorkshire are also affiliated. There is a well-known Forensic Pathology department on the main site.

University of Southampton Medical School

www.medschool.soton.ac.uk

Southampton has the medical school for the south coast of England. It has better weather than the north of England and there's a beach on which to appreciate it. There's pleasant countryside to see and a trip to the Isle of Wight to make. The school is modern and students get patient contact from day one of the course. **Southampton General** (Tremona Rd Tel: 01703 777222) and the **Royal South Hampshire** (Brintons Terrace Tel: 01703 634288) are the main teaching hospitals, but hospitals in Bournemouth and Portsmouth are also used.

Royal United Hospitals Bath

Conbe Park, Bath Tel: 01225 428331.

Also a popular elective destination although not attached to a specific medical school.

ISLANDS NEAR ENGLAND:

Guernsey

Guernsey has a population of 66,000, 30 miles of coastline and beautiful beaches. Healthcare is private; there is no NHS. There are no junior doctors either, only consultants, specialists and GPs. Primary care is provided by GPs and islanders have to pay (£16) to see them. The GPs also run A&E and patients also have to pay to be seen there (around £40 depending on treatment). The people of Guernsey pay a compulsory premium giving access to secondary healthcare (specialists) for free. The specialists run wards in **Princess Elizabeth Hospital** and clinics in **Alexandra House**. If a treatment is not available they are transferred to the mainland, usually Southampton. Consultants sometime visit.

The Princess Elizabeth Hospital

Le Vanquiedor, St. Martins, Guernsey GY4 6UU, Channel Islands.

The hospital: Has all major specialities and an A&E. There are five physicians with speciality interests who rotate on a 1:5 on-call. To arrange an elective here write to the postgraduate tutor at the above address. There is a £25 administration cost and they need a CV. Tour all the specialities, meet some GPs and go out to their practice.

Accommodation: Available, but may cost around £12/night.

Two other hospitals on the island are: **King Edward VII Hospital** (geriatrics) and **Câtel Psychiatric Hospital**.

Jersey

General Hospital

Gloucester Street, St Helier, Jersey JE2 3QS, Channel Islands.

A similar system to that in Guernsey exists, although junior doctors are present (a popular job). Again, write to the postgraduate tutor at the above address.

Isle of Wight

St Mary's Hospital

Newport, Isle of Wight PO30 5TG Tel: 01983 524081.

This is the main acute hospital on the Isle of Wight. It caters for all basic and some advanced specialities.

Isle of Man

Noble's Isle of Man Hospital

Westmoreland Road, Douglas, Isle of Man Tel: 01624 642642.

The hospital: Is actually a teaching hospital for Manchester University but also takes elective students in medicine or surgery for maximum of 4–6 weeks. There is a relaxed atmosphere and you are not expected to be on-call though there is a bleep if you want. Accommodation is free in the nurses' home directly opposite the hospital. There is a lively mess for doctors and nurses. Douglas is a short walk away and has a few shops. The island has beautiful scenery and ancient heritage.

Ramsey Cottage Hospital, Cumberland Rd, Ramsey, Isle of Man Tel: 01624 811811.

Scotland

Aberdeen University

Faculty of Medicine, Aberdeen Royal Infirmary, Forresterhill, Aberdeen AB29 2ZB Tel: 01224 681818 www.abdn.ac.uk

On the east coast of Scotland, Aberdeen has a great deal of history, but now plays a major role in the oil industry. Although cold, the city is friendly and there is plenty to do. The multi-faculty university is about two miles from the hospital. The medical school and infirmary are on the same site. The teaching hospital (**Aberdeen Royal Infirmary**, Fosterhill) is large with a busy A&E that admits from a large area, including the Shetland and Orkney Isles as well as the oil rigs and shipping in real emergencies. All major specialities are on-site, including neurosurgery. Elective students have found they have had good practical experience in A&E. Aberdeen students are very nice (!).

Dundee University

Medical School, Level 10, Ninewells Hospital, Dundee DD1 9SY Tel: 01382 632247 www.dundee.ac.uk

Three hospitals in Dundee (**Ninewells**, a very large purpose-built teaching hospital), **Dundee Royal Infirmary** (Barrack Rd) and **Kings Cross Hospital** (Clepington Road) all on Tel: 01382 660111 and a number of hospitals outside the city are all used. Dundee itself may not have the best weather and there may not be much to do in the centre, but there is easy access for skiing and hill walking. Electives can be arranged for a £100 administration fee in any subject depending on availability. Rotations are available all year. There is a £25 per week compulsory hospital accommodation fee. Contact the electives co-ordinator.

University of Edinburgh

Faculty of Medicine, Teviot Place, Edinburgh EH8 9AG Tel: 0131 650 1000 Fax: 0131 650 6525 www.med.ed.ac.uk

Edinburgh University itself has a great history and very well-known medical school. It is situated in the centre of town and uses a number of hospitals in and around the city. Although you can apply to departments directly, the faculty much prefers that you apply through them (£25 administration charge). They have a quota system so apply early. They can arrange electives at central and peripheral hospitals. If you apply through a department the school may not recognize you as a student and therefore won't provide certificates of attendance (you'll need to get the Consultant to do it). Hospitals affiliated include: the **RIE**, **The Royal Hospital for Sick Children**, **The Western General**, **The Eastern General**, **Princess Margaret Rose**, **City Hospital** (Greenbank Drive, Edinburgh) and **St John's** (Livingston, Howden Road, West Livingston EH54 6PP). Accommodation is not provided by the school although peripheral hospitals may. There is also a **Community Drug Problem Service** (Spittal Street Centre, 22–24 Spittal Street, Edinburgh EH3 9DU) which has previously taken students.

The Royal Infirmary of Edinburgh

Lauriston Place, Edinburgh, EH3.

The RIE is the main teaching hospital of the University of Edinburgh. It has a great deal of history and is in a beautiful building. It is has a busy A&E and all specialities (bar neurosurgery and infectious diseases at the Western). Many departments are world-renowned for their excellence (e.g. orthopaedics, surgery) and it is home to the **Scottish Liver Transplant Centre**. The hospital is very close to the Royal Mile (main area of Edinburgh) and next to the University.

Note: In the next 4–5 years the hospital is due to move to a new site outside the city in a place called Little France.

The Western General Hospital

Crewe Road, Edinburgh EH4 2XU.

The Western is a busy hospital with many specialities including neurosurgery. A large HIV unit has just moved here from **City Hospital**. It has the **National Surveillance Unit for Creutzfeldt–Jakob disease**. There is a limited supply of accommodation in the nurses' home.

Law Hospital

Carluke, Lanarkshire ML8 5ER.

Law is a rural hospital used by Edinburgh, Glasgow and Dundee students. It is a friendly DGH with some good teaching.

University of Glasgow

Faculty of Medicine, Glasgow G12 800 Tel: 0141 330 4424 Fax: 0141 330 5440
www.medicine.gla.ac.uk

Glasgow is a very lively, cultural city with plenty to do both day and night. It also has some very poor areas affecting the population's health (drug abuse and TB problems being relatively common). The medical school is based in the West End of the city and uses six large hospitals and 13 DGHs in the region. Its main teaching hospitals include **Glasgow Royal Infirmary** (84 Castle St G4 Tel: 0141 211 4000), the **Western Infirmary** (Dumbarton Rd, G11 Tel: 0141 211 2000), **Gartnavel General** (1053 Great Western Road, Glasgow G12 0YN Tel: 0141 211 3600) and **Stobhill** (Balornock Rd G21 Tel: 0141 201 3000) hospitals. All tend to be very friendly and welcoming. The **Royal Hospital for Sick Children** (Yorkhill, Glasgow G3 8SJ) is the main paeds hospital in Glasgow with many specialists and a dedicated A&E. It has previously provided free accommodation to students. Electives can be arranged in most subjects for six weeks in term time. There is a £20 admin fee and no elective charge. Electives of eight weeks are only available in the summer holidays, and because of the length of time, you have to enrol as a Glasgow student (£357). The university requires proof of certain vaccinations to do an elective in one of its hospitals. You have to arrange accommodation with the accommodation officer at whichever hospital you are placed in. Those in Glasgow itself often do not provide accommodation which then has to be arranged through the University (charging up to £100/week). Those on the outskirts can sometimes provide it free.

When you've 'done' Glasgow there is plenty of beautiful countryside to the north, Loch Lomond and the highlands. Skiing is about two hours away.

OTHER INTERESTING HOSPITALS IN SCOTLAND:

Glasgow Homeopathic Hospital

1000 Great Western Road, Glasgow G12 0NR.

This is an NHS hospital that treats with conventional medicines as well as alternatives. It has 16 beds and an extensive outpatients department. It is very friendly and reasons for doing things are explained. It has a very holistic approach ('*What side of the bed do you sleep on?*' is not a question many of us normally ask). Apparently the results are 'astounding'. Recommended as an elective both for homeopath fans and total sceptics.

Raigmore Hospital

Perth Road, Inverness IV2 3UJ (Highland Acute Hospitals NHS Trust Tel: 01463 704000 Fax: 01463 711322).

Raigmore is the main trauma centre for the region. It is a busy hospital and used by Aberdeen students. It provides good teaching and a very friendly setting.

Belford Hospital
Fort William PH33 6BS.
A friendly hospital with a medical and surgical ward, A&E and maternity unit. Excellent for mountain climbers (Ben Nevis is just around the corner). All the docs are outdoor types. Good skiing nearby (when it snows) and the A&E and ski-patrols get busy as a result.

SCOTTISH ISLANDS:

Western Isles Hospital
Macaulay Road, Stornoway, Isle of Lewis HS1 2AF Tel: 01851 704 704.
The hospital is in Stornoway on the Outer Hebrides. It has general and orthopaedic surgery, medicine, O&G, geriatrics and psychiatric services. There is an HDU but no ITU. CT scanners/MRI/ mammograms/neuro/cardiothoracic surgery are all on the mainland. This is an incredibly friendly hospital is a beautiful area. There are outreach clinics to other islands. An elective here has been highly recommended though it is not for high-powered city types. On Sundays the only things open are the hospital and churches. There's no cinema, just some quiet pubs. However, the hospital is great and there are plenty of wildlife to places to see. This is an excellent cheap elective (if you have a car take the ferry from Ullapool).
Accommodation: On site (very good) has previously been available.

GP work on the islands is also popular. Rather than writing a great list, GPs (who will be bombarded with letters) for **GP work/electives in the Outer Hebridies**, contact the Primary Care Manager, Western Isles Health Board, Health Board Offices, 37 South Beach Street, Stornoway, Isle of Lewis, Western Isles HS1 2BN. Previously they have contacted GPs to arrange electives. A small GP/minor ops unit is **The Griminish Surgery**, Griminish, Benbecula, Western Isles HS7 5QA which has two GP/anaesthetists and one locum surgeon allowing them to do an elective list a week and also emergency surgery. If it can't be done a helicopter transfers to the mainland.

Gilbert Bain General Hospital, Shetland Isles Tel: 01595 695678.
Balfour and Eastbank Hospitals, Orkney Tel: 01856 885400.

Northern Ireland

Queen's University Belfast
Faculty of Medicine and Health Sciences, Ground Floor, Whitla Medical Building, 97 Lisburn Road, Belfast BT9 7BL Tel: 01232 245133 Fax: 01232 330571 www.qub.ac.uk
Queen's Belfast is situated in the heart of Belfast and uses the **Royal Victoria** and **Belfast City** (Lisburn Rd, L9 Belfast, N Ireland Tel: 01232 329241) hospitals as well as a number of smaller peripheral sites. Despite its reputation, Belfast is a safe, friendly city and there is certainly plenty to do, both in and outside. Dublin is only two hours away and there is beautiful countryside nearby. Electives can be arranged here in any subject between June and December. There is no charge and accommodation is provided free (and is fine). Write to the Elective Co-ordinator at the above address.

The Royal Hospitals
Grosvenor Road, Belfast BT12 6BA Tel: 01232 894702.
The group comprises the **Royal Victoria** (Grosvenor Rd, Belfast BT12 Tel: 01232 240503), **Royal Maternity** (Grosvenor Rd BT12 Tel: 01232 240503), **Royal Belfast Hospital for Sick Children** (Falls Rd BT12 Tel: 01232 240503) and a dental hospital. Almost two-thirds of N Ireland's population lives within 40 minutes of these hospitals which are a few minutes out of Belfast centre. The Royal Victoria is a large busy central teaching hospital with all specialities. The A&E is the trauma centre for Northern Ireland seeing 118,000 patients a year. It has a world-wide reputation. The cardiology department set up the world's first mobile CCU and played a

major role in the development of the defibrillator. Electives here come thoroughly recommended. A&E sees quite a bit of trauma, some related to the conflict. There is the opportunity to see patients first and do minor procedures. The Royal Belfast Hospital for Sick Children is the only dedicated paediatric hospital in Northern Ireland.

OTHER INTERESTING HOSPITALS IN NORTHERN IRELAND:

The Ulster Hospital

Dundonald, Belfast BT16 DRH.

This is a general hospital on the outskirts of Belfast. It can get very busy. Belfast students are also present so visitors may not always get into theatre or specialist clinics. Orthopaedic trauma can be very interesting.

Tyrone County Hospital

Hospital Road, Omagh, Co Tyrone.

Tyrone County is a 200-bed hospital and very friendly. Elective reports show students are a bit of a rarity and hence teaching is enthusiastic and good. A few Queen's University, Belfast students are around.

Colerane Hospital

Mount Sandle Road, Colerane,
Co Londonderry.

Colerane has three medical, two surgical, one geriatric ward and an A&E. It's popular with Dundee students so apply early. It's a friendly place and you are fairly free to do as much or as little as desired.

Antrim Area Hospital

45 Bush Road, Antrim, Co Antrim.

This is a relatively new DGH providing care for a large area of Co Antrim. It has a friendly A&E and the staff are very helpful. It is used as a teaching hospital by Queen's University, Belfast and hence there are quite a few other students around. Apply early. There's a good bus and train service into Belfast. Accommodation is available.

Wales

University of Wales

College of Medicine, Heath Park, Cardiff
CF14 4XN Tel: 01222 743436
www.uwcm.ac.uk

This is the only medical school in Wales and is situated in the capital. The **University Hospital of Wales** is the principle teaching hospital, but the faculty has links with many hospitals throughout Wales. With a student population of over 20,000, Cardiff is great for young people. There are lovely pubs and theatres. Outside there are the Brecon Beacons and some beautiful coastal sites to explore. Electives here can be arranged in most subjects. There is a £200 administration fee per eight weeks and a charge for accommodation.

SOMETHING DIFFERENT:

Motor racing

The Medical Centre, Silverstone Circuit

Silverstone, Nr Towcester, Northants
NN12 8TN.

The centre: Arranges provision of medical support for motorsport events. Learn how to get drivers out and the priorities after a crash.

Diving

Diving Diseases Research Centre,

Deriford Hospital, Plymouth, Devon.

PACIFIC ISLANDS

The Cook Islands

Population: 20,000
Language: English and Maori
Capital: Avarua
Currency: New Zealand dollar
Int Code: +682

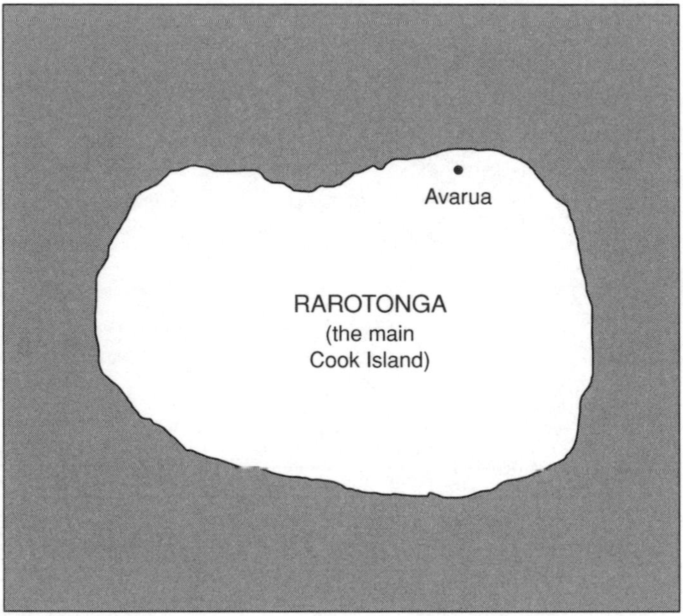

The Cook Islands are over 2000 miles into the Pacific from the coast of New Zealand and consist of 24 volcanic and coral islands. Tourism and banking are now their main economy, although clam and pearl farming are still very important. The capital is Avarua on Rarotonga in the south.

Rarotonga

Avarua Hospital

Avarua, Cook Islands Tel: 22664.

The hospital: The main hospital for the Cook Islands. It offers all major specialities. They can also arrange attachments in other hospitals.

Mauke

Mauke is a small Island (population 639) in the middle of the South Pacific, one hour's flight from the main Cook Island, Rarotonga.

Mauke Hospital

Mauke, Southern Cook Islands, South Pacific.

The hospital: The hospital has one doctor, two nurses and three beds and supplies all the healthcare needs for the island!

Elective notes: In 1998 the doctor on the island was allegedly dismissed for negligence and general drunkenness. Since then there has been the odd newly qualified doctor from Bulgaria, but nothing particularly well-organized. An elective here may well result in you being the island doctor. With a population of 639 you are unlikely to be wildly busy but organizing the hospital and basic childcare is very much needed. Any emergencies are very worrying. The perfect remote elective! Write to the hospital in Rarotonga for more details.

Fiji

Population: 800,000
Language: English
Capital: Suva
Currency: Fiji dollar
Int Code +679

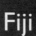

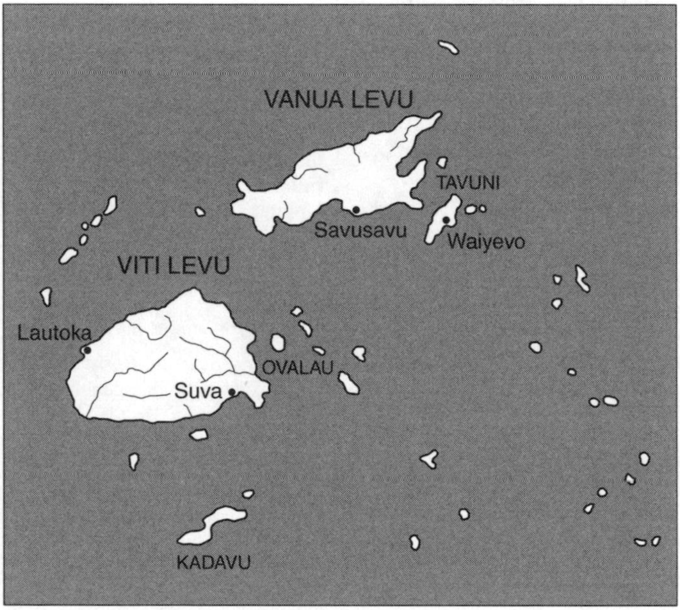

Fiji comprises a number of volcanic islands in the South Pacific. The two largest islands are Viti Levu and Vanua Levu. There are 880 smaller islands. Indians were brought in as slaves by the British and now the numbers of natives and Indians are about equal (although there was a mass exodus of Indians after the 1987 coup). The islands, especially the smaller ones, are beautiful and offer a host of water sports, including scuba diving. The Fijians (including the local medical students) are very friendly and keen to feed visitors and make sure you get kava (the national drink, a mild opiate!). Elective students normally get into the country by saying they are tourists.
Note: At present there is political unrest and there have been violent clashes. Check with the Foreign Office before going.

✪ Medicine:
The Fiji health service is pretty poor and, although it covers most things, some drugs have to be paid for by the patients and anyone needing major operations (such as transplants) has to raise funds (or have private insurance) to get themselves to Oz or New Zealand. Rural areas have a number of nursing stations. Despite what

you may imagine, there are actually few tropical diseases on the islands and there is no malaria. Leading causes of death include cardiovascular disease, cancers and accidents. The doctor to patient ratio is one per 2000 people.

◎ **Climate and crime:**
New Year and Christmas are good times to visit as it is warm and sunny every day. The east side of the islands gets more rain than the west. Hurricanes and cyclones are not uncommon.

Viti Levu

Suva

MEDICAL SCHOOL:

Fiji School of Medicine
Private Mail Bag Suva, Fiji Islands Tel: 311700 Fax: 303469 www.fsm.ac.fj
There is also a dental and nursing school within the health sciences complex. To arrange electives on Fiji, either write to the hospital itself or the Electives Co-ordinator at this address. It takes about two months to get an application form, but is relatively well-organized.

The main teaching hospital is:

The Colonial War Memorial Hospital
GPO Box 115 Suva, Fiji Tel: 313444 Fax: 303232
The hospital: A very well-equipped hospital. It is the largest and most high-tech hospital in Fiji. Excellent for training as it has good facilities and a wide range of pathologies. It is friendly and relaxed. Occasionally 'mercy missions' to outlying islands are carried out in emergencies.
O Elective Notes: Excellent opportunity for experience and some responsibility. If applying through the University ask to do some community medicine in Taveuni and/or Savusavu to get some touring done at the same time.
Accommodation: Not provided but South Seas motel is £3 (9.8 FJD)/night.

Lautoka

Lautoka is a port for many of the small boats that visit the nearby islands this makes it easy to get off the mainland, go to the Yasawa Islands and to Abaca to trek in the rainforest. Scuba diving, windsurfing etc. is a must. Lautoka is not touristy but there is a cinema and Internet café. There are wonderful beaches once you get out of Lautoka (which is otherwise quite a sleepy and not an attractive town).

Lautoka Hospital
PO Box 65, Lautoka, Viti Levu, Fiji Islands.
The hospital: A 400-bed, 1970s hospital in a city on the west coast of Viti Levu. Lautoka is the second-largest city (after the capital Suva), and is populated by Fijians and Indians in equal number. The languages therefore consist of English, Fijian and Hindi. The hospital is funded largely by voluntary aid and is relatively primitive for Western standards. Diabetes (1:5 prevalence), TB, rheumatic fever (and its heart complications) and SLE are fairly common.

The hospital has general medical and surgical wards (divided into male and female), a paediatrics, O&G and TB ward.
O Elective notes: The teaching from the medical staff has had good reports (you can move around to find the best) with many opportunities for lumbar punctures, aspirates etc. Those who have done A&E and orthopaedics have found it busy (TB, many RTAs and the occasional shark bite!) but interesting and well worthwhile. Paeds tends to have diseases of deprivation ... malnutrition, gastroenteritis and infectious diseases. Spending some time in the outpatients is good experience as you get to see and treat people on your own. People present late, often because they may have to pay for treatment, but also because they are a very uncomplaining race. They also run 'mercy missions' in a helicopter to rescue people from neighbouring islands. Try to get to any clinics on other islands. The staff are

very keen that you get out and see more of the main island as well as some of the smaller islands. The two medical house officers work a 1:2 rota and are grateful for any help you can give. Attendance requirement is low but you need to be in at 8 am. Take long weekends to see the islands.

Accommodation: An accommodation block is just being built; however, the Cathay Hotel (PO Box 239) is a 10-minute stroll away and comes highly recommended. Prices vary from $9 (dormitory with fan) to $22 (single room) with negotiable reductions for three sharing a room. Across the way from the Cathay is the Northern Club, a colonial establishment serving good (cheap) food, tennis and squash courts, a swimming pool and snooker tables. Membership is mere $10 (£5) a month. There are usually many elective students here.

Vanua Levu

Savusavu Hospital

Savusavu, Vanua Levu, Fiji.

The hospital: A small district hospital with very limited resources. It has only three doctors and so they are grateful for any help they can get. They are very friendly but there is not much to do in the town (it's not really on the tourist route). There is a local dive centre. It can get lonely. You may also have language problems although there is often a Fijian medical student to help.

Taveuni

Taveuni is Fiji's third-largest island, but having said that there are no roads, mains electricity or (more importantly) bars. It does have three shops.

Taveuni Hospital

Waiyevo, Taveuni, Fiji.

The hospital: A collection of wooden huts (built in the 1920s) run by a husband and wife team. It has four wards (women's, men's, O&G and paeds, each with eight beds. The lack of people means that you will get heavily involved running your own clinics. The main problems on the island are hypertension and diabetes. There are also many antenatal clinics. Take comfort if you have any fears of running clinics in the fact that there are very few facilities and so it's pretty difficult to kill anyone. Days start early (8 am) but finish by 1 pm so there's plenty of time for swimming/sunbathing (there's not a lot else to do!) Repeatedly highly recommended as an elective.

Ovalau

Levuka Hospital

Levuka, Ovalau, Fiji Islands.

The hospital: A small, almost cottage, hospital with male, female and 'paying' wards and an outpatients department that acts as a general practice. It covers the villages of Ovalau and some of the surrounding islands.

O Elective notes: They are very grateful for the extra pair of hands and so this is actually a hard-working elective. They may well be relying on you to turn up, do your own clinics and ward rounds. Throw yourself into it and you will be rewarded with the Fijians' great kindness. You will meet the chiefs and be considered a guest of honour at dinners. It can get lonely if you're on your own but it is a beautiful country and the beaches are amazing.

Kadavu

Kadavu Hospital

Kadavu, Fiji Islands.

The hospital: Another small cottage hospital on an island about 40 miles long catering for the scattered population of around 4000.

Kiribati

Population: 79,000
Languages: English and Gilbertese
Capital: Bairiki
Currency: Australian dollar
Int Code: + 686

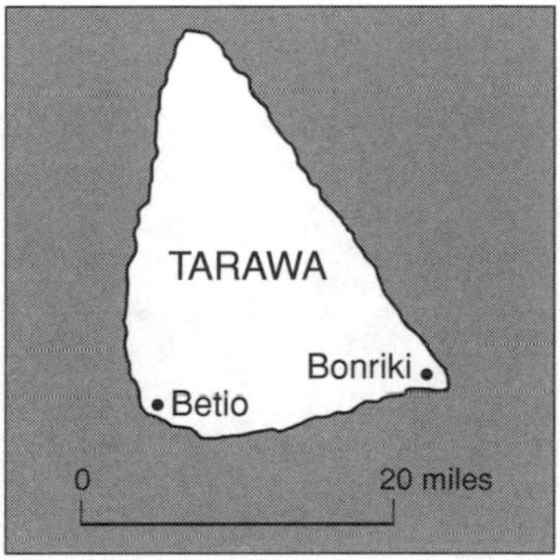

The Republic of Kiribati is a collection of 33 very isolated islands in the South Pacific. They gained independence from the UK in 1979. Most of the 79,000 Gilbertese population live in thatched huts. Previously the British had extensively phosphate-mined Banaba (one of the islands). Now the islands are very poor and coconut growing and fishing are the main livelihoods. Most of the islands are coral reefs and surround a lagoon. Due to their remoteness it may not rain for months and droughts have occurred.

✪ Medicine:

Until recently the locals have had a healthy diet, although this has changed as canned food has been imported. There is an incredibly high death rate. Of the 192 countries in the world it comes in at 154 for poor life expectancy. TB, measles, diabetes and heart conditions are all very common.

◎ Climate and crime:

It is hot all year round (30 °C) with variable rainfall. Apart from the odd pub brawl, there's not much for the police to do (only around 70 prisoners in total!).

Tungaru Central Hospital

Nawerewere, Tarawa, Republic of Kiribati
Tel: 28100 Fax: 28152.

The hospital: On Tarawa (80 km north of the equator and next to the International Date Line). The Japanese built it in 1989 for the care of all the central Pacific islands that were too far from Papa New Guinea or Australia. It is a modern 120-bed hospital with medicine, surgical, paeds, O&G, TB and private wards and well as an A&E.

O Elective notes: It is a friendly hospital but a real pain to get to (Air Marshall or Air Nauru from Fiji). Accommodation is not provided and can be a real problem. You need someone to put you up or it'll cost more than £30/night in a guesthouse. It's not all palm trees, some of the island is very polluted. Highly recommended if you can get there.

The Solomon Islands

Population: 400,000
Language: English
Capital: Honiara
Currency: Solomon Islands dollar
Int Code: +677

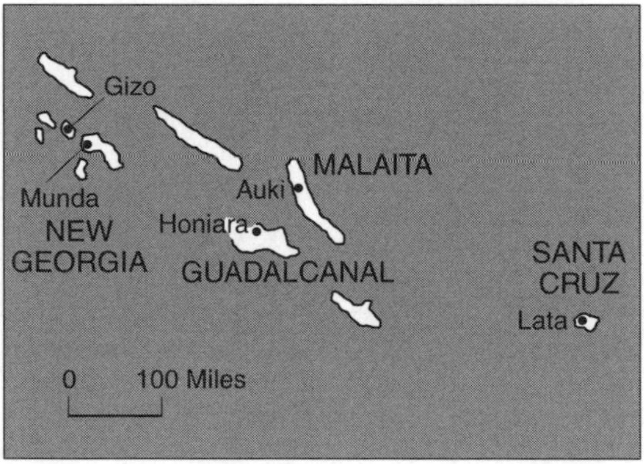

The 922 Solomon Islands form an archipelago in the south-west Pacific. They have been independent from the UK since 1978. The six main islands are Choiseul, Guadolcanal, Malaita, New Georgia, San Cristobal and Santa Isabel. The capital is Honiara on the island of Guadalcanal. There are 80 languages, but most speak Pidgin (a variant of English) in addition to their local language. Ninety-three per cent of the population are of Malaysian origin. There are many beautiful beaches and sites for the best in diving. Note: There has been civil unrest. Check with the Foreign Office before you go.

✪ Medicine:

It's tropical medicine in a developing country. There are many infectious diseases: TB+++, malaria and many pyrexias of unknown origin.

➲ Visas and work permits:

No visa required for Solomon electives. You will have to enquire with the embassy for the need for work permits.

◎ Climate:

It has tropical climate, temperatures averaging 28 °C, 70% humidity. Jan–Feb is the rainy season.

USEFUL ADDRESS:

Ministry of Health and Medical Services, PO Box 349, Honiara, Solomon Islands Tel: 23600 Fax: 24243. (The Ministry is based in the main hospital. The Director of Medical Services is also based at this address.)

Guadalcanal

Honiara is the capital on the main island of Guadalcanal. It makes an excellent base from which to explore the other islands.

Central Hospital (Numbaneen)/ National Referral Hospital

Box 349, Honiara, Solomon Islands Tel: 23600.

The hospital: The main hospital for the islands. Originally known as 'Number 9' it was built as a military hospital by the US army during World War II. It is mainly tropical diseases (malaria, TB, pyrexia of unknown origin, tropical splenomegaly) that are seen. It is very busy.

O Elective notes: It has friendly staff with excellent teaching. Very highly recommended for medicine or surgery. There's lots of assisting and opportunities for procedures with supervision (but can vary depending on the number of doctors around). O&G has a similar story.

Accommodation: Can be provided in 'Kiwi House' (approx £30 for as long as you want (SI$15). It can get fully booked and is not great).

New Georgia

Munda is the name given to the largest settlement on the island of New Georgia. It comprises six villages in the Roviana lagoon. The largest village is Lambete with three grocery stores, a baker and a bank that changes travellers' cheques. There is also Agnes Lodge, a pub/restaurant. Most people live in leaf huts. There is a Japanese-built railway, a remnant from the war. There was a great deal of heavy fighting here during WWII which now provides some excellent diving and snorkel opportunities.

Helena Goldie Hospital

PO Box 82, Munda, Solomon Islands.

The hospital: A 55-bed general hospital in the village of Kokkngolo in Munda. It serves a population of 25,000 spread over 10,000 sq km of ocean. It is a mission hospital financed by the United Church and overseas donations. It has male, female, maternity and paeds wards and an air-conditioned operating theatre. There is a Nurse Aide Training School on site taking 20 self-funding nurses a year. The hospital is run by two doctors, seven registered nurses, a radiographer–pharmacist and two lab techs. The most common cause of admission and death is malaria. TB, abscesses and obstetric problems are also common. Surrounding islands are visited by motorized canoe to run clinics (giving immunizations and weighing children).

O Elective notes: After prayers at 7.30 am there is a ward round and outpatients at 9.00 am (very busy). Then there may be theatre. Student on-call is 1:3. The medical student is often the anaesthetist (mostly under ketamine). You can do clinics in the hospital and are often sent out on the remote clinics with just a nurse. Swimming and diving are excellent (sunken ships and planes). Traditional dancing, bush walks and crocodile spotting are other pastimes.

Accommodation: A student flat is available for around £20 (159 SBD)/ week.

Gizo

Gizo Hospital

Gizo, Gizo Province, Solomon Islands.

The hospital: Opened by the Duke of Edinburgh in 1959, Gizo has 55 beds and around four doctors. The four wards are male, female, paeds and maternity and there's an outpatients/A&E service. All are well run. Many patients travel great distances by canoe to get here. Nurses see patients first and can prescribe. If concerned they can refer to the doctor. Malaria and TB are common, as are bush knife injuries. There is a well-equipped theatre.

O Elective notes: There are very few students and so less teaching but lots more opportunity to do practical procedures. Excellent scuba diving nearby.

Accommodation: Not available so stay at Paradise Lodge (£5 (40 SBD)/night).

Santa Cruz Island

Lata Hospital

Lata, Santa Cruz Island, Temotu Province, Solomon Islands Tel: 53044/5 Fax: 53044.

The hospital: A 40-bed hospital with eight Antenatal (one delivery room), eight male and eight female, eight paeds beds, one TB ward (four beds), one isolation bed, an operating theatre and a minor ops room. They do about 20 minor cases a month. Lots of paeds, TB, STDs (though not HIV), malaria and scrub typhus. It's good for general medicine and minor surgery (most major surgery is at the central hospital).

O Elective notes: Doctors and nurses are both friendly and speak English. Patients speak Pidgin. Every 2–3 months a coconut ship tours surrounding islands for a week from which staff do clinics. You may have to canoe to some clinics. There's excellent snorkelling from here. Temotu is very remote and can be very hot (35 °C). Electricity and water are in short supply.

Accommodation: Has to be arranged on arrival.

Malaita Island

Auki Hospital

Malaita Island, Solomon Islands.

The hospital: This is the hospital for a large island just north of Guadalcanal.

Tonga

Population: 98,000
Language: Tongan
Capital: Nuku'alofa
Currency: Pa'anga
Int Code: +676

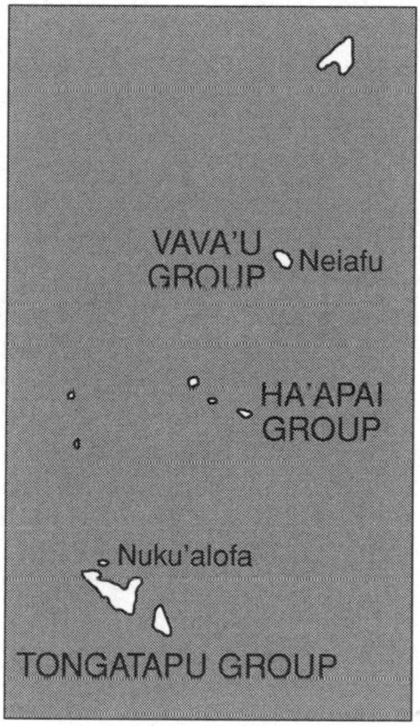

The Kingdom of Tonga consists of 170 islands in an idyllic location in the South Pacific. Only 39 are inhabited. Tongatapu is the main island with Nuku'alofa as its capital. The main language is Tongan but nearly all Tongans speak some English. Tonga has never been colonized by a European power and hence has maintained its own identity. It is also not yet a tourist destination. The people are very sincere and hospitable. There is no TV, negligible crime rate and no deadlines. It's Royal family has one of the world's oldest dynasties and Tonga is probably the smallest Kingdom in the world. Although the main island is only 60 feet above sea level, the seabed around Tonga is up to six miles deep. Things to do include Kava drinking (a brew from mixing dried and powdered root of a pepper plant – Pipermethysticum*). It has many medicinal properties from antifungal to anticonvulsive! See the flying foxes in Kolovai, blow holes in Houma, go to the Royal Palace, the national centre, the beaches (Keleti and Oholei) the churches and temples. Definitely snorkel, but wear something on your feet (coral cuts).*

✚ Medicine:

All medical care in Tonga is free except small private clinics and the Tongan witchdoctors. It's pretty modern, but specialist services are only available in New Zealand or Australia. Diabetes from the Westernization of their diet and infectious diseases are common.

➲ **Visas and work permits:** The procedures for medical students taking their electives in Tonga are as follows:

- The medical student applies to the Director of Health, Nuku'alofa, Tonga for the possibility of undertaking an elective in Tonga (allow months for a reply).
- They will then be sent a letter of approval from the Director of Health that is handed to the Immigration Officer at the point of entry in Tonga for endorsement of the appropriate visa.
- Medical students usually make their accommodation reservation in Tonga with the help of the Ministry of Health, Tonga Visitors Bureau and Sela's guesthouse.
- Where possible, the Ministry of Health assists with the transportation of the medical student.

USEFUL ADDRESSES:

The Ministry of Health, Nuku'alofa, Tonga Islands Tel: 23 200 Fax: 24 291.
Tonga Visitor's Bureau, Vuna Road, Nuku'alofa, Tonga Islands Tel: 25 334 Fax: 23 507.
Sela's Guest House, Pahu Kolofo'ou, Nuku'alofa, Tonga Islands Tel: 21 430 Fax: 22 755.

Nuku'alofa

The city can be a bit of a disappointment if you're expecting a tropical paradise and it can be quite hard to get to some of the islands. However, it does make a good base.

Vaiola Hospital

PO Box 59, Nuku'alofa, Tonga Tel: 23 200 Fax: 24 291.

The hospital: This is the main hospital (200 beds) and is situated in the capital city of Nuku'alofa. It has medical and surgical, paeds, O&G, ophthalmological, psychiatric and A&E services run by 10 consultants and a similar number of junior staff. The medicine is pretty basic, but the hospital is very clean and well-run. The outpatients also functions as a GP service. X-ray and ultrasound facilities are available. Major problems include diabetes (and subsequent wound sepsis), rheumatic fever, Hep A and B, dengue fever, STDs, asthma (increasing) and gastroenteritis. HIV is not yet a major problem.

❍ **Elective notes:** Medical students are encouraged as much as possible and there's the opportunity to do minor procedures such as lumbar punctures and assisting in theatre. Because of limited resources there is no complex surgery but there is good surgical teaching. There are also clinics to do. Occasionally, attendance is discouraged offering ample opportunity to explore. It's very popular with the Aussies. There are three other hospitals (which are more like clinics) in Tonga, but attachment to these can be arranged once in Vaiola. You won't see much at these, but they give a good excuse for visiting other islands.

Accommodation: Not provided. Not a problem to get though (around £5/night). Tonga is not a well-known tourist spot yet ... whereas this has advantages, it does mean there aren't many leisure activities. Toni's Guesthouse in Nuku'alofa comes recommended as does The Beach House (PO Box 18, Nuku'alofa). The food may not be that good. One month here may be enough.

NGU Wellington Hospital

Neiafu, Vava'u, Tonga

The hospital: Has around 60 beds and is situated on Vava'u, 200 km north of Tongatapu. It caters for the northern islands and is run by about five doctors. The waters around here are especially beautiful. Anything major gets sent to Tongatapu.

Hapaa'i Hospital

Hapaa'Island, Tonga.

The hospital: A 28-bed hospital with one doctor and very limited resources.

Vanuatu

Population: 160,000
Languages: Bislama, English
Capital: Efaté
Currency: Vatu
Int Code: +678

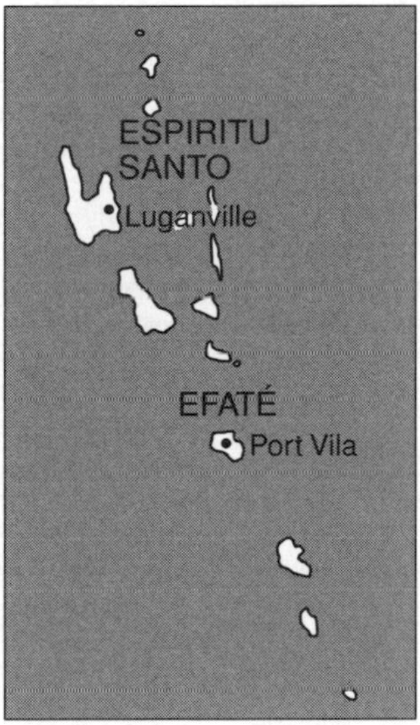

Vanuatu is a cluster of 80 small islands in the South Pacific. They lie between a triangle formed by the Solomon Islands, Fiji and New Caledonia. Until 1980 they were governed jointly by the French and English. Now they are independent. Most people speak English, some speak French as well but the most widely spoken is Bislama, *a creole based on English (e.g.* Hed blong yu I goroan = Does your head go round?, Taem yo slip wetem wuman kok blong yu i go slak = are you impotent!*). It is pretty easy to learn and within a couple of weeks you'll be able to take a good history. The main island is Efate (the third-largest). The others have mainly small villages with leaf huts. Vanuatu is a developing nation that has preserved its traditional heritage and is largely unspoilt by Western tourism (although the capital is a port for Australian cruise ships). The ni-Vanuatu people are very warm and welcoming. Unfortunately, since independence the government has mismanaged the economy and there is a great deal of poverty (although a number of Westerners have settled as it is a tax haven). As alcohol has become commonplace so has abuse to women. The islands were originally populated in around 3000* BC *and christened as the New Hebrides by Captain James Cook in 1774. There is loads of spectacular diving and snorkelling. The sister ship of the* Titanic, the Star of Russia, *which sank in Vila harbour*

is a popular dive as are the USS Coolidge *and* Semle Federson. *Some of these are very deep (55 m) and hence diving accidents are not uncommon. The nearest recompression chamber is Sydney. Don't have any accidents. Tanna is a nearby island that still has an active volcano. Pentecost has the famous land-diving sport (bungee jumping with linola vines instead of rope). There is also plenty of bush-walking.*

➲ Visas and work permits:
No visa is required with a common-wealth passport. You will have to contact the hospital regarding the need for work permits.

◎ Climate:
November to April is the wet season with temperature around 30 °C and high humidity. May to October (winter) is the best time to go as its cooler and dryer. When it rains, it really rains. The odd hurricane can do a lot of damage.

Vila Central Hospital

Private Mail Bag 013, Port Vila, Efaté, Vanuatu Tel: 22100 Fax: 27618/27621.

The hospital: The hospital is in the city (Port Vila) on the main island (Efaté). It's set on the side of a hill overlooking a lagoon and is 10 minutes' walk to the town centre. It has medical, surgical, delivery and paediatric wards totalling 150 beds. There are two theatres, a radiology department (with ultrasound) and a very busy outpatients. Lab facilities are mainly for malaria, although basic blood tests are available. There are usually six or seven doctors, but much of the work is done by Nurse Practitioners. Pathology in outpatients can be somewhat poor as many people just want sick notes, but there is malaria, measles, diabetes, Hep B, rheumatic fever and GI upsets. Reactive arthritis and trauma (including wife-beating) are relatively common. TB (drug-resistant) is common and all the rare presentations are seen. Pathology is commonly advanced as people tend to try traditional medicines first.

The nurses and the 60 nursing student here are exceptionally friendly and helpful with language problems. They have a football team and commonly invite students out to play volleyball.

❍ Elective notes: The doctors there in previous years have varied from being exceptionally good, very experienced medics and surgeons to very poor with no interest in teaching. Fortunately, the most recent reports have had very friendly and knowledgeable staff. Students get to run their own clinics. If you want to catch babies, this is the place. One hundred deliveries a month and the midwives encourage you. Medical students also do on-calls as the admitting doctor working 4.30 pm to 7.30 am on a 1:5 rota. This is very rewarding. As the hospital is relatively well-staffed, the doctors tend to encourage students to get out and about and the island. Book early as this is becoming a popular destination. Write to the medical student co-ordinator.

Accommodation: And food are provided but costs around 1000VT (approx £5.50) a night.

Luganville Hospital

Luganville, Espirito Santo Island, Vanuatu.

This is home to the world's largest accessible recreational diving wreck, the *USS Coolidge* and hence is probably better for diving medicine.

Western Samoa

Population: 10,000
Languages: Samoan and English
Capital: Apia
Currency: Tala
Int Code: +685

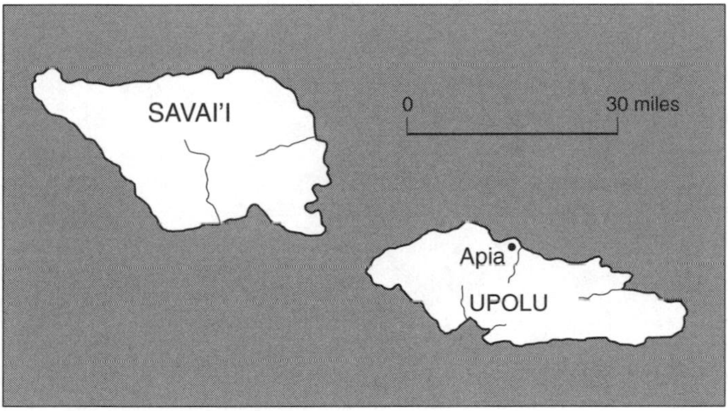

The nine islands that make up Samoa lie in the middle of the South Pacific between Fiji and the Cook Islands. Only four of the volcanic islands are inhabited and most of the population is on Upolu. There are beautiful beaches, rainforests and coconut plantations. The people are very welcoming and hospitable. It is now officially Samoa since the east (formally US-controlled) and the west (formally governed by New Zealand) became fully independent in 1962.

✪ Medicine:

Just take a look at their rugby team. Samoans are big. This was fine when on the natural diet, but now that it has become heavily Westernized, diabetes, hypertension and cardiovascular disease are common.

◎ Climate:

It is hot all year round (30 °C) but rains most around Christmas time.

Western Samoa National Hospital

Apia, Upolo, Western Samoa.

The hospital: The national hospital is 15 minutes' walk from the centre of the capital. All the major specialities are present (medicine, surgery, O&G, orthopaedics and paeds). Facilities are pretty basic with very few lab resources. There are only a limited amount of drugs and no crash trolley. The medical staff are enthusiastic and work very hard. Diabetes is a major problem here.

O Elective notes: Students have found this a wonderful elective, lots of hands on experience and the opportunity to run clinics. It's a beautiful and very friendly place. Work is not too strenuous and weekends are always free. Lots of Aussie and NZ students. Thoroughly recommended.

Note: There is the opportunity to go to small hospitals on other islands. Savai'i (the next main one) has only two doctors so there's an opportunity to do a bit more.

Accommodation: Sometimes provided; however, previous students have stayed with Samoan families and had a wonderful time.

THE MIDDLE EAST

Israel

Population: 5.6 million
Language: Hebrew
Capital: Jerusalem
Currency: New shekel
Int Code: +972

Although Israel has become better known for its Gaza Strip and West Bank disputes, it still offers a great deal of history and mixed cultures. Jerusalem, Nazareth, the Dead Sea and Bethlehem are commonly visited. It is a popular destination for both Christian and Jewish medics. Doctors trained in Israel can speak English as it is taught in school from the age of ten and many of the textbooks are in English. Many patients also speak English, but rarely enough to give a history. It may well be worth doing a basic course in Hebrew before you go.

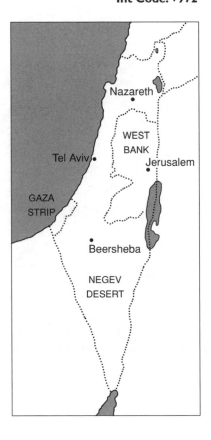

✪ Medicine:
Healthcare is available to all people in Israel and is pretty good. Indeed, many hospitals have pioneered new treatments. Conditions of developed countries (cardiovascular disease and cancers) are common.

Note: Israel has the second-highest litigation rate in the world after the USA and medicine is practised with this in mind.

➲ Visas and work permits:
Officially, to study in Israel you need to apply for a student visa. Once you have a confirmed place of study, you can apply, with the help of your destination, to the Ministry of Interior in Israel for one. Despite this Tel Aviv University say that elective students only need a tourist visa and many students visiting other institutions also don't bother. It would be worth asking your host institution directly whether they require a study visa; if not, a tourist visa should suffice for an elective. In order to be able to do paid work in Israel you have to have a work permit. This has to be applied for in Israel, directly to the Ministry of Interior, by the person who would be employing you.

◎ Climate:
Between June and September it can get very hot (30 °C) and dry.

USEFUL ADDRESS:

The Israel Medical Association in Britain, c/o Dr David Katz, Secretary, 6 Lawn Road, London NW3 2XS, UK.

Note: SHABBAT AND HOLIDAYS: Shabbat begins at sunset on Friday evening and finishes at sunset on Saturday evening. Many Jewish families attend the synagogue on Friday and Saturday. It is traditionally a time for the family to be together, especially for the Friday night meal. All buses stop running and shops close for the period.

There are several holidays during March and April, including *Pesach* (Passover), Holocaust Memorial Day, Remembrance and Independence Day. All the Jewish holidays begin at sunset. *Pesach* lasts a full week (the medical students have two weeks off) and Moroccan Jews celebrate its end by feasting.

Jerusalem

In this capital with such an extensive religious history there are plenty of places to visit. If on elective, the Jerusalem Society of Medical Students organizes parties and excursions to the local sights. These include: Jerusalem-old city (Muslim Quarter, Dome of the Rock, Western Wall, the Mosque of Asqa), Zion square and the new city, Jewish Market (haggle!), Israel Museum, Knesset and gardens, Yad Vashem (Holocaust Museum), Talpiot Promenade, Hebrew University on Mount Scopus, Mount of Olives and any of the historical districts (Meah Shearim, Russian Compound, American Hill). Outside Jerusalem you must get to the Dead Sea (get a bus from the central bus station to Ein Gedi), Tel Aviv, Jaffa, Golan Heights and Sea of Galilee, Negev Desert, Eilat and Sinai. That's enough for the first few weeks!

To do an elective in Jerusalem you can either write to the hospital or, more easily, contact:
The Exchange Officer, **Jerusalem Society of Medical Students (JSMS)**, Hebrew University-Hadassah School of Medicine, Ein Kerem, POB 12272, Jerusalem 91120, Israel.
For this society to find you a place you have to send a letter 'certifying your good standing as a medical student' from your Dean and $50 US.

Accommodation is not provided by the University or hospitals and can often only be arranged on arrival. There are plenty of hostels in Jerusalem but two that come particularly recommended are: Ein Kerem Youth Hostel, POB 16091, Jerusalem, Israel Tel: 02 416282 and Beit Shmuel Youth Hostel, King David 13, Jerusalem, Israel Tel: 02 203466. The one in Ein Kerem is a 15-minute walk from the University and Haddash Hospital in a quiet location (with beautiful views) 20 minutes' bus ride from the city centre. Many medical students stay here as it is near the hospital and cheaper than those nearer the city. Allow $4–600 for eight weeks. The JSMS provides cheap lunchtime food.

A few tips:

- Buy a monthly bus pass (£35) but note it is only valid until the first of the next month not the day you bought it (so don't buy it at the end of a month).
- Also change money at the Post Office in The University Hospital to save commission.

The Hebrew University, Hadassah Medical School

PO Box 12272, Jerusalem 91120, Israel
www.md.huji.ac.il

Established in 1946, the Faculty of Medicine has five schools, including medicine and nursing. Based on the Ein Kerem campus, the major hospitals used are the **Ein Kerem** and **Mount Scopus Hadassah** University Hospitals (both run by the Hadassah Medical Organization, Kiryat Hadassah POB 12000, Jerusalem 91120 Tel: 2 677 6078 Fax: 2 677 7013). These provide over 1000 beds. The Kaplan hospital in Rehovot and the Shaare Zedek and Bikur Cholim hospitals in Jerusalem are also affiliated. The University is the oldest in Israel and is world-renowned for its research into brain function, cancer, biotechnology and AIDS.

Hadassah Teaching Hospital

Ein Kerem, POB 12272 Jerusalem 91120, Israel.

The hospital: The Hadassah is a 700-bed tertiary referral hospital situated on the south-western side of Jerusalem on the hillside above the village of Ein Kerem. It has departments covering all the major specialities plus the medical school and research laboratories. The Emergency room consists of 28 beds, four of which are in the trauma unit and six for high-risk patients. There is also a paediatric emergency facility. Every patient admitted comes through the ER. IVF, bone marrow, lung and liver transplantation, laproscopic and cold laser surgery are examples of its advanced specialities. The working week begins on Sunday morning, the working day is 8 am to 4 pm. Hadassah is one of four major hospitals in Jerusalem and takes part in an 'On Duty' rota between them.

O Elective notes: This is a friendly teaching hospital. You can join their students teaching which is usually in Hebrew with English slides. Many lecturers will speak in English for you; if not the other students are more than happy to translate. In the ER practical procedures of suturing, central lines and chest drains can all be practised. RTAs are very common, but alcoholic injuries are not seen. The neurosurgery department is well recommended with good teaching that rotates on a two-weekly bases with the new group of students. They also encourage you to go out and explore the country.

Accommodation: *See above*.

Mount Scopus Haddash University Hospital

Jerusalem, Israel.

The hospital: Has 300 beds and serves the Jewish and Arab neighbourhoods of north and eastern Jerusalem. It has most specialities and an ER (but neuro goes to Ein Kerem). It also runs a 'hospice on wheels'.

Shaare Zedek Medical Centre

POB 3235, Jerusalem, 91031, Israel
Tel: 02 6555316 (or 6555111) Fax: 02 6540744.

The hospital: A large modern hospital affiliated with the Hebrew University. It has a busy ER. Patients have a wide variety of backgrounds and consultations can be in Hebrew, English, Arabic, Russian, Yiddish, French or Spanish. Most major specialities are catered for.

O Elective notes: You should have good command of Hebrew here as all notes and many consultations are in it. If you do it is a very worthwhile elective. Quite a lot of responsibility and practical skills. Write to the director of Foreign Medical Student's Programme.

Accommodation: Not provided (*see above*).

Also in Jerusalem is the **St John Ophthalmic Hospital**, PO Box 19960, Sheikh Jarrah, Jerusalem 97200 Tel: 02 5828325 Fax: 02 5828327 e-mail: stjohn@palnet.com

Nazareth

Nazareth is the largest Palestinian settlement in Israel with a population of around 60,000 people. A lot of building work has occurred for the new millennium. From Nazareth, excursions to the Golan Heights and Sea of Galilee are relatively easy and there are good bus connections to Tel Aviv and Jerusalem.

The Nazareth Hospital (EMMS)

71501–71502 PO Box 11,16100 Nazareth, Israel Tel: 0 6657 1501. Fax: 06 657 5912 e-mail: nazhosp@rannet.com

The hospital: Is a Christian mission institution (owned by the Edinburgh Medical Missionary Society) and is the oldest hospital in Israel today. It is small (136 beds), but offers medical, surgical, emergency, paediatric, psychiatric, obstetric and gynaecological services. In the last decade it has become integrated in the Israeli State Health Service as a District General Hospital. Recently a new wing has been constructed and plans for further expansion exist. Currently it has 6000 inpatients and 37,000 outpatients a year. Most staff are local Nazarenes, although a few medics and paramedics are expatriates. There is an unusual mix of cultures, Jewish, Muslim and Christian. Communication is not always easy: the patients speak in Arabic, but the doctors communicate with each other and write notes in Hebrew regardless of their background. Fortunately, many of them also speak English.

The hospital serves the ever-growing community of Nazareth and the surrounding Gallilean villages. Arab–Israeli relationships in this area are entirely peaceful, but the Jewish communities use other hospitals.

O Elective notes: There's no formal teaching, but most doctors (mainly expatriates) are happy to teach on ward rounds and in clinics. O&G is very busy (and some of the staff a bit volatile!) and there is very little time for teaching. However, there is a 'muck in' approach and you'll get great hands on experience. There are a higher number of congenital defects as there are many first-cousin marriages. If the prognosis is poor, the child is often rejected by its parents. Overall, at least in other departments (ER, respiratory medicine and paediatrics) it's a fairly relaxed atmosphere (the hospital day is from 8.30 am to 3.30 pm). This elective has been highly recommended by some as an excellent way to see some common conditions, some Arabic culture and some very genuine people.

Accommodation: Can be arranged. There are single-sex flats where many young people stay – carpenters, gardeners etc. It is important to get involved as otherwise you'll just 'pass through' this experience. There are plenty of evening activities such as sport, cinema and eating out. Regardless of personal belief, attendance at religious ceremonies (although not compulsory) and respect is recommended.

For more details write to **The Edinburgh Medical Missionary Society**, 7 Washington Lane, Edinburgh EH11 2HA (Tel: 0131 313 3828).

Beersheba

Ben Gurion University of the Negev

School of Medicine, 84 105 Beer-Sheva, Israel http://medic.bgu.ac.il/ (Part of the **Soroka Medical Centre,** PO Box 151, Beersheba 84101, Israel Tel: 07 640 0909 Fax: 07 627 4096.)

The Negev Desert makes up 60% of Israel (6000 square miles) and is home to a number of different ethnic peoples many of whom are still semi-nomadic. The hospital (1200 beds) serves the entire population of the Negev. Community medicine is obviously important in this area and the medical school (founded 1974) takes great pride in that it trains good generalists rather than specialists.

Tel Aviv

Tel Aviv University

Sackler Faculty of Medicine, PO Box 39040, Tel Aviv 69978, Israel Tel: 03 640 9657 Fax: 03 640 9103
www.tau.ac.il/medicine/

The medical faculty was founded in 1963 to cope with the increasing population. It is now based on the Ranat Aviv campus and uses 14 hospitals (totalling 6000 beds) in the greater Tel Aviv area (providing care for 40% of Israel's population). All the hospitals are state-owned. Hospitals include the **Assaf Harofeh Medical Center** (800 beds, 12 miles south-east) which is renowned for its orthopaedics and paediatrics; **Rabin Medical Center** (1650 beds in two hospitals six miles east); **Sapir Medical Center** (672 beds in the Sharon region) with excellent spinal and max-fax departments; **Schneider Children's Medical Center of Israel** (224 beds) – a very advanced paeds centre (transplants, MRI); **Chaim Sheba Medical Center** (1600 beds and a busy ER); **Tel Aviv-Sourasky Medical Center** (second-largest hospital in Israel, 1100 beds) with all departments and **Dana Paediatric** and **Serlin Maternity** Hospitals in the same complex.

○ **Elective notes:** The Tel Aviv University Medical Students' Organization sorts out electives. You need your own travel insurance and malpractice insurance is recommended though not obligatory. You only require a tourist visa (check their web site).

Haifa

Technion-Israel Institute of Technology, The Bruce Rappaport Faculty of Medicine

PO Box 9649, 31 096 Haifa, Israel
www.technion.ac.il

Founded in 1969, the newest medical faculty in Israel uses **The Rambam Medical Center** (a 900-bed hospital receiving from northern Israel and southern Lebanon (Jews, Muslims and Christians). It is at the base of Mount Carmel on the shores of the Med; **Bnai-Zion Medical Center** and **Carmel Hospitals** in Haifa; **Haemek Medical Center** in Afula, **West Galilee Medical Center** in Naharia and **Hillel Yafe Hospital** in Hadera.

Jordan

Population: 5.5 million
Language: Arabic
Capital: Amman
Currency: Jordanian dinar
Int Code: +962

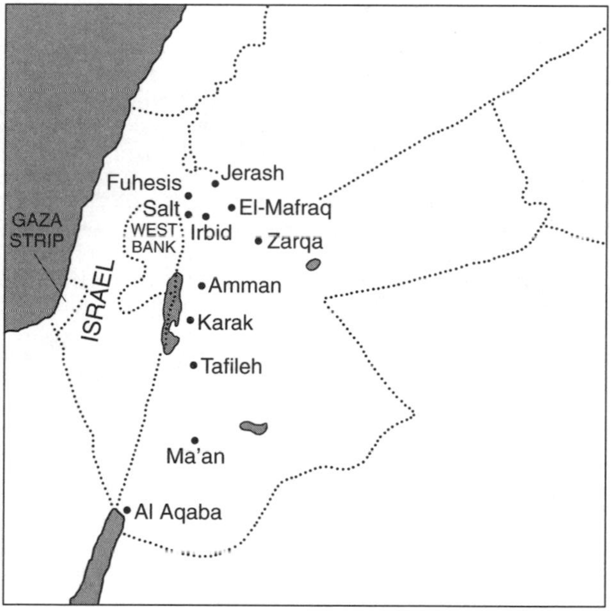

Jordan has some good beaches (with scuba diving) in Al Aqaba and the ruins of Petra. It is, sadly, now more famous for the dispute with Israel over the West Bank. It is not a popular destination for elective students (possibly because of the need for fluent Arabic) and information is difficult to come by. For this reason only the main hospitals (and the medical school) are listed below.

✪ Medicine:
The government provides a subsidized healthcare system and reasonable hospitals are widely available. Cardiovascular and respiratory diseases and cancers are common causes of mortality.

➲ Visas and work permits:
A three-month visa for British, French, German, US, Australian and New Zealand citizens is available, usually within 48 hours from the Embassy (two weeks by post) by filing in a simple form.

GOVERNMENT HOSPITALS:

Aqaba Hospital, Aqaba, Jordan Tel: 2465-Aqaba (50 beds).

Ashrafieh Hospital, Jabal El-Ashrafieh, Amman, PO Box 10005, Jordan Tel: 75111.
El-Mafraq Hospital, El-Mafraq, Jordan Tel: 213/176/El-Mafraq (50 beds).
El-Ramtha Hospital, El-Ramtha, Jordan Tel: 338 El-Ramtha (13 beds).
Fuhesis Hospital, Fuhesis, Jordan (118 beds).
Government Hospital, Zerka, Jordan Tel: 03 83323 (90 beds).
Jerash Hospital, Jerash, Jordan Tel: 90-Jerash 50 beds).
Jordan University Hospital, University Road, Amman. PO Box 13046, Jordan Tel: 845 65 841841 (550 beds).
Karak Hospital, Karak, Jordan Tel: 98-Karak (60 beds).
King Hussein Hospital, Salt, Jordan Tel: 2957 (100 beds).
Ma'an Surgical Hospital, Ma'an, Jordan (78 beds).
Princes Basma Hospital, Irbid, Jordan Tel: 3665/7 (168 beds).
Tafileh Hospital, Tafileh, Jordan Tel: 90-Tafileh (32 beds).

SOUTH AND CENTRAL AMERICA

Argentina

Population: 34.6 million
Language: Spanish
Capital: Buenos Aires
Currency: Argentine peso
Int Code: +54

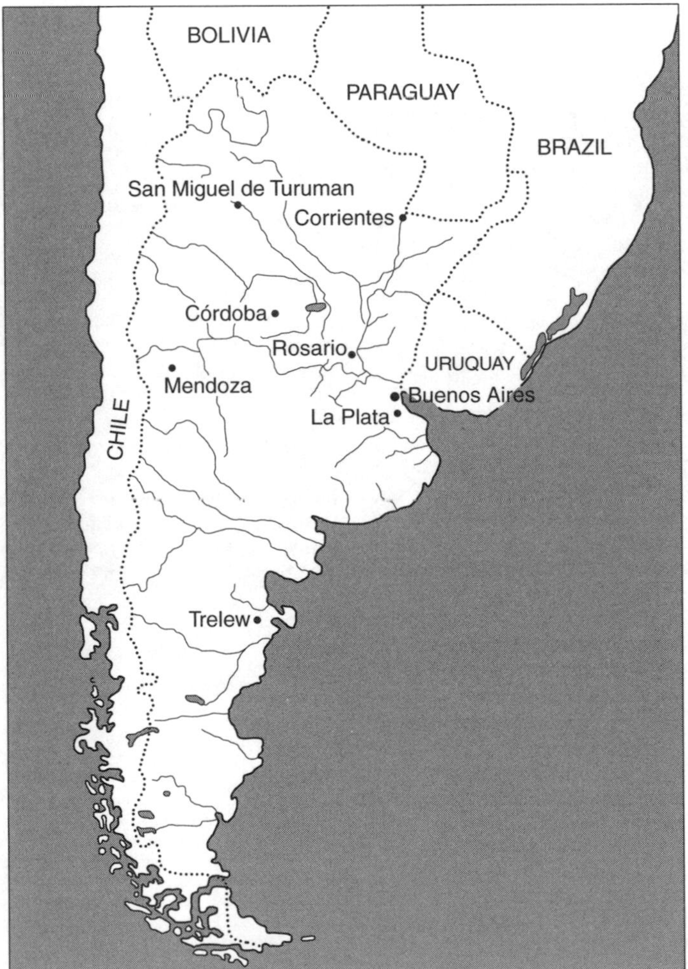

*The 2145 miles of Argentina extends from Bolivia to Cape Horn. The Andes separate it from Chile in the west. Farming forms the main source of income and, since 1983, Argentina has had multiparty democracy. To get anything out of and enjoy working here you will have to speak very fluent Spanish. Few people speak English. The only way around it is to go to Patagonia in the south where you'll need to speak fluent Welsh! (*see below*). This language barrier makes it an unusual place for electives/work.*

Medicine:

Access to medical healthcare is available throughout Argentina. Proportionally, there are more doctors than in the USA (one doctor per 330 people). The big killers include heart disease, cancers and accidents. Most nationals rely on health insurance as doctors charge. Indeed, in state hospitals you tend to only see the poor. The Menem administration introduced a Worker's Health Plan system to improve healthcare for the poor.

Visas and work permits:

A visa is required to enter Argentina. Contact the embassy for more details. As a foreign medic you need to get your degree validated and contact the provincial health authorities or the **Dirección de Control del Ejercicio Profesional y Establecmientos Sanitarios**, Defensa 120, 5° piso, 1345 Buenos Aires which is attached to the Ministry of Health.

Climate and crime:

Covering such a great length means whole ranges of climates can be encountered. In the north-east it is virtually tropical, becoming semi-arid in the Andes. In the south it can get very cold and snowy. The lowlands in the west are desert, the pampas are mild. South America is not generally regarded as safe; however, Buenos Aires is one of the safest cities in Latin America. Beware of the small shanty towns where crime is rising.

THE MAIN MEDICAL SCHOOLS:

Universidad de Buenos Aires

Facultad de Medicina, Paraguay 2155, 1121, Capital Federal, Buenos Aires, Argentina Tel: (54 11) 4 508-3702 www.fmed.uba.ar

This, the nation's oldest medical school, is situated in the capital and has links with over 50 hospitals in Argentina (a full list is available on their web site). The main hospitals are: **Hospital de Clínicas José de San Martín**, Avenida Córdoba 2351, Buenos Aires, Argentina Tel: (+4) 1 5083994. The hospital founded in 1877 is a major centre with an A&E and many specialist departments; **Hospital Municipal de San Miguel** in the north-west of Buenos Aires is a 236-bed general hospital catering for a poor population where only half have running water and 15% don't have a toilet.

Universidad Nacional de Cordoba

Facultad de Ciencias Médicas, Pabellón Argentina-Ciudad Universitaria 1° Piso a la izquierda, 5000 Córdoba, Argentina Tel: 54 351 4334065 Fax: 433 4083
www.unc.edu.ar
e-mail aci-web@seu.unc.edu.ar

This, Argentina's second oldest medical school, uses **Hospital Nacional de Clínicas** (Tel: 337025 337014) and **Hospital Universitario de Maternidad y Neonatologia** (Tel: 331053 1050 1052) in Córdoba.

OTHER MEDICAL SCHOOLS:

Universidad Católica de Córdoba, Facultad de Medicina, Jacinto Rios 571, 5000 Córdoba-CBA, Argentina.
Universidad del Salvador, Facultad de Medicina, Tucumán 1859, 1050 Buenos Aires-CF, Argentina.
Universidad Nacional de Cuyo, Facultad de Ciencias Médicas, Parque General San Martin, Casilla de Correo 3, 5500 Mendoza-MZA, Argentina Fax: (5461) 380232.
Universidad Nacional del Nordeste, Facultad de Medicina, Moreno 1240, 3400 Corrientes-CTS, Argentina.
Universidad Nacional de La Plata, Facultad de Ciencias Médicas, Calle 60 y 120, 1900 La Plata-BS.AS, Argentina.

Universidad Nacional de Rosario, Facultad de Medicina, Santa Fe 3100, 2000 Rosario-SF, Argentina.
Universidad Nacional de Tucumán, Facultad de Medicina, Casilla de Correo 159, Lamadrid 875, 4000 San Miguel De Tucuman-T, Argentina.

Patagonia

Patagonia is the huge wasteland of southern Argentina. On July 28, 1856, the sailing ship Mimosa *landed on the coast of Patagonia. Aboard were 150 Welsh emigrants. They had sailed from Liverpool in search of a new land where their culture would be safe. Between then and 1911, 3000 Welsh men, women and children endured the three-month voyage to Patagonia. For many years Welsh culture flourished. Even now there is a lively (though diminishing) Welsh community and outside the hospital, the language can be pure Welsh. The Welsh community is strongest in the province of Chubut (which is about the size of Spain) and especially in the town of Trelew (Tre = town in Welsh, 'Lew' is after Lewis Jones, one of the community's founders). This is where Trelew's Zonal Hospital lies.*

Hospital Zonal Trelew

9100 Chubut, Patagonia, Argentina.

The hospital: State-funded with 150 beds serving a population of 80,000. Welsh is the language of the hospital but it is advisable to take some Spanish lessons before arriving. NO ONE SPEAKS ENGLISH. Lots of the nurses can speak Welsh, however.

Since it is a state hospital, it tends to only see the poor Chilean immigrants. Treatment is free and so theoretically are all prescriptions (subject to means testing). Expensive drugs are simply not available. Chubut is renowned throughout Argentina for the progress it has made in combating two major diseases and the work has been centred in Trelew. These two diseases are hydatid disease and tuberculosis. Chubut has the world's highest incidence of hydatid disease (Wales has the highest in Europe!). This is probably because of the many sheep and clogs (known as the 'poor man's blanket') that live in close proximity to the people. The incidence has declined by a programme of public education and the treatment of all dogs with the anti-parasitic prasiquantel.

O Elective notes: You can follow the physicians, neonatologists, paediatricians, neurologists or casualty officers. There are also peripheral clinics and a psychiatric hospital to attend.

Aruba

Population: 69,000
Language: Dutch
Capital: Oranjestad
Currency: Dutch guilder
Int Code: +297

Aruba, an autonomous part of the Netherlands, 15 miles off the coast of Venezuela, is a small island whose economy is built on offshore finance and oil refining. At present it is building a medical school and new hospital. Teaching is in English. Contact **Universidad di Aruba**, Dr Schaepman Street, Sint Nicolaas, Aruba Tel: 011 297 8 4587 Fax: 011 297 8 48118 ArubaUniversity@hotmail.com

Belize

Population: 216,000
Language: English
Capital: Belmopan
Currency: Belizean dollar
Int Code: +501

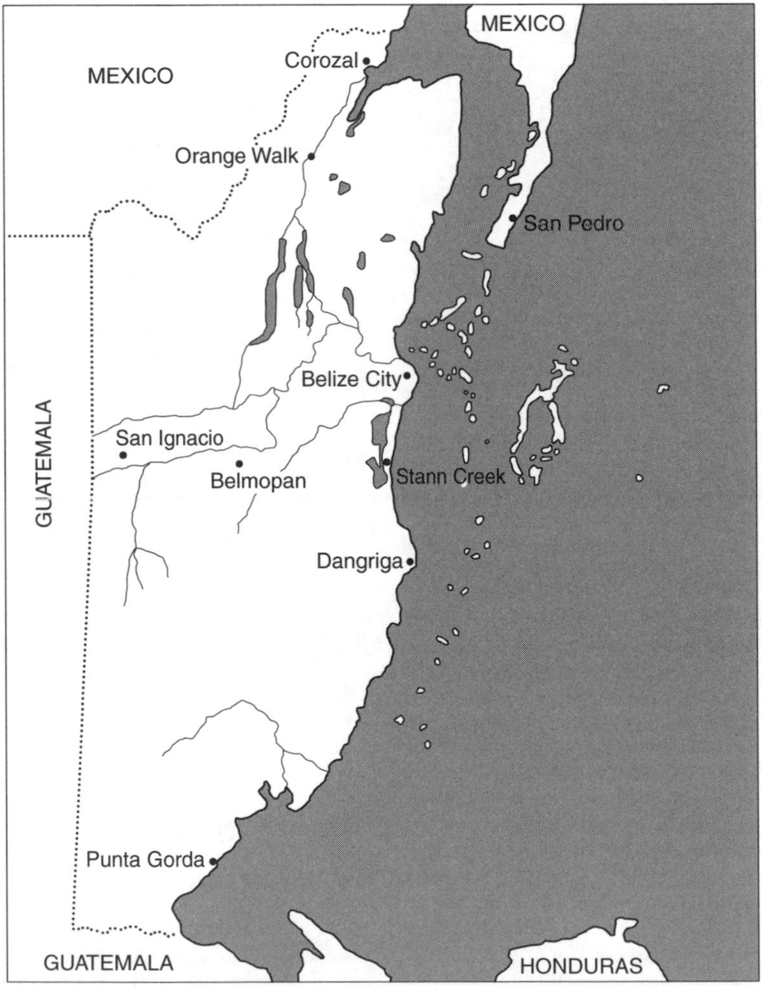

Belize lies on the eastern shores of the Yuctan Peninsula and is bordered in the west by Guatemala and Mexico. Since its independence in 1981, Belize (formerly British Honduras) has slowly increased in prosperity. It is the least populous country in Central America with over half of the land still covered in dense forest. The coast has the world's second-largest barrier reef giving protection from flooding. The population is diverse in nature but there is still great poverty. Spanish speaking black Creoles now make up over half with the rest of the population being Maya groups, black Caribs and immigrants from Mexico. Due to a successful education system there is a high literacy rate. This is a good central American country to go to as so many people speak English. There's plenty to do in Belize, excellent diving and beautiful coastlines. You can trek into the jungle and when finished, visit a Caribbean Island.

Medicine:

There are eight hospitals and many mobile clinics in Belize to which around 75% of the population has access. Basic sanitation and water supplies have been a priority and now over half the houses in Belmopan have both. Respiratory, heart and cerebrovascular diseases are the big killers. HIV rates in Belize City are pretty high due to drug abuse. The doctor to patient ratio is also rather high, 1:1809. They'll appreciate any old *BNF*s/textbooks here.

Visas and work permits:

European, American and British Commonwealth citizens (bar India and Nigeria) do not need visas to enter Belize. If gaining employment you need a temporary employment permit, an HIV negative certificate and a certificate showing no criminal convictions. Application forms can be obtained in any labour department office in Belize. Contact the High Commission for more information.

Climate and crime:

Hot and humid weather is normal throughout the year. However, hurricanes can often cause havoc in the coastal regions. Belize is a route for Colombian cocaine and there are a few drugs gangs in Belize City. The city is not a safe place at night. Rural Belize is usually fine.

PUBLIC HOSPITALS:

Karl Huesner Memorial Hospital

Princess Margaret Drive, Belize City, Belize, CA Tel: 2 31584.

The hospital: Is the main hospital and brand new. Although it caters for nearly all specialities, it does lack some facilities. There's a very busy A&E department.

Elective notes: Students play an active role in the A&E, lots of suturing of machete/knife wounds. There's good supportive staff. O&G and surgery are also highly recommended.

Belize City Hospital, Eyre Street, Belize City, Belize, CA Tel: 2 77251.
Belmopan Hospital, Belmopan, Belize, CA Tel: 8 22263/64.
Corozal Hospital, Corozal, Belize, CA Tel: 4 22081.
Dangriga Hospital, Dangriga, Belize, CA Tel: 5 22084.
Orange Walk Hospital, Orange Walk, Belize, CA Tel: 3 22143.
Punta Gorda Hospital, Punta Gorda, Belize, CA Tel: 7 2026.
San Ignacio Hospital, Hospital Street, San Ignacio, Belize, CA Tel: 92 2066.

SMALL CLINICS:

To do community work write to the Chief Medical Officer, Ministry of Health, Belmopan, Belize.

RURAL CLINICS:

San Pedro Health Centre

San Pedro, Belize.

It is possible to spend some time doing clinics on one of Belize's cayes (islands), e.g. Ambergris Caye. You need to get a boat to San Pedro and then once a week they fly you in a tiny plane to the neighbouring island. There are no hospitals on these islands so you are the only medical care.

The Independence Health Centre

Independence, Stann Creek, Belize.

Mongo Creek on the edge of the jungle is a rural village also with a clinic. You do home visits on a bike. This is a great place to go to experience developing medicine in a beautiful country.

PRIVATE HOSPITALS:

Fort George Medical and Dental Clinic, 6 Eyre Street, Belize City, Belize, CA Tel: 234504.
Medical Centre, 1, Marquet Square, Belize City, Belize, CA Tel: 272727.
Myo'on Clinic Ltd, 40 Eve Street, Belize City, Belize, CA Tel: 2-45616 Fax: 2-31557.
Northern Medical Center, 50 North Front Street, Belize City, Belize, CA Tel: 231371.
St Michael's Clinic and Hospital, 43 Barrack Road, Belize City, Belize, CA Tel: 235148.
The Belize Medical Assoc Ltd, 5791 St Thomas Street, Belize City, Belize, CA Tel: 230302. Fax: 233837.

Bolivia

Population: 7.4 million
Languages: Spanish, Aymará, Quechua
Official Capital: Sucre
Administrative Capital: La Paz
Currency: Boliviano
Int Code: +591

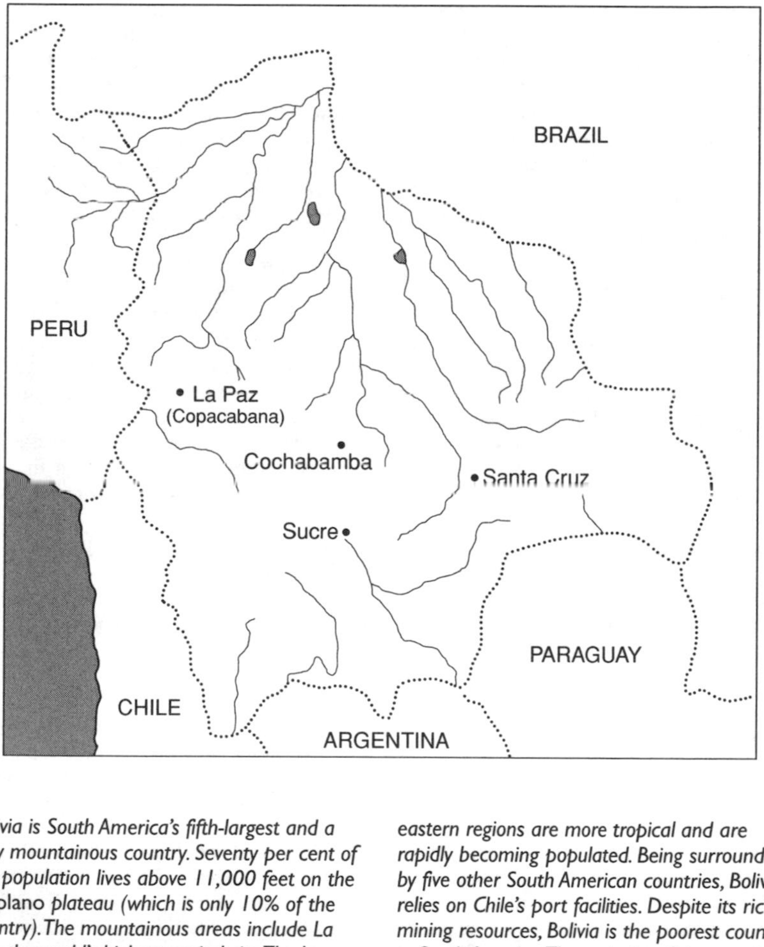

Bolivia is South America's fifth-largest and a very mountainous country. Seventy per cent of the population lives above 11,000 feet on the altiplano plateau (which is only 10% of the country). The mountainous areas include La Paz, the world's highest capital city. The lower eastern regions are more tropical and are rapidly becoming populated. Being surrounded by five other South American countries, Bolivia relies on Chile's port facilities. Despite its rich mining resources, Bolivia is the poorest country in South America. The majority of the popula-

tion rely on agriculture, although many ascend even higher into the mountains to mine. Bolivia's third-largest economy is coca leaves. These have a huge importance in traditional medicines, but also generate around $1 billion in illegal trafficking. It has a great cultural heritage. Things you must do in Bolivia include: Valle du Luna (the 'Valley of the moon'), Chacaltaya the 'World's highest ski area', Tiahuanaco (Tiwanaku) ancient ruins, The Yungas the beginning of the tropical rainforest and Lake Titicaca the world's highest navigable lake. It's also worth going to Copacabana, staying the night and going to the Isla del Sol and Isla de la Luna. After that, cross the border and do Peru. Although two-thirds of the population is of pure Indian descent many of the remainder are mestizos *(mixed Spanish). The national languages are Aymará and Quechua, but Spanish is taught in the schools (although outside the cities many cannot speak Spanish). To get on in working out here you must have a basic knowledge of Spanish. The local money is Boliviano (B$) but US$ are used everywhere (B$5= about US$1).*

✪ Medicine:

Because of their isolation, many people do not have access to Western medicine and basic provisions such as clean water and sanitation are only available to half of the population. Many children do not receive immunizations and hence preventable infectious diseases are common causes of death. Big killers are influenza, tuberculosis and malaria. TB vaccination is free, but mothers don't want it for fear it may do harm. TB treatment is also free, but TB is still a problem because the diagnostic test is not free and so people don't find out if they have it. Although 95% are Roman Catholic they still have traditional beliefs such as guidance from witches. Doctor to patient ratio is one per 1971. TB, rheumatic fever and malaria are common as in many developing countries, African or American. Chagas' disease and its complications are more confined to South and Central America. *Trypanosoma cruzi* is carried by the Reduvid bug which lives in the roofs of mud houses. This makes it difficult to eradicate and hence this is a common 'unusual' disease. Its prevalence is as high as 80% in some populations. Chronic diseases of the West are not really seen as the life expectancy is about 60. Infant mortality is also outrageously high from 92 per 1000 to 300 per 1000 in some areas.

Acute mountain sickness (nausea, vomiting, headache, pulmonary and cerebral oedema and retinal haemorrhage) is also seen in natives, but more commonly tourists. For treatment *see* Section 1, 'Your Health Whilst Overseas'. In chronic mountain sickness, polycythaemia (complications include thrombosis, haemorrhage, cardiac failure), drowsiness, cyanosis, clubbing, right ventricular enlargement, cor pulmonale and hypertension are seen.

There are three types of hospitals: General, Caja Nacional de Salud (CNS) and private. The general hospitals are accessible to everyone for a small fee for all diagnostic tests and treatment. The facilities are very limited here. The CNS hospitals (house of the nation's health), which is for people who pay social security, give them free treatment. These are the most common. The third type are private. Doctors train at either government or private medical schools. There are three preclinical years, two clinical then an intern year after which they sit exams and then have to do a year in a rural hospital.

◎ Climate and crime:

Climate varies greatly. The plateau between the Andes has a tropical highland climate and is very cold at night. The eastern regions are lower and therefore tend to be warmer. Bolivia has had a very good crime record and it is still a very safe place for tourists. Drug-related crime is, however, on the increase especially in the east and in Santa Cruz.

➲ Visas and work permits:

Elective students have previously entered on a tourist visa. The official line from the consulate is that a student visa can be obtained from them once the student provides the necessary documents certifying his registration with a university or any other education institution. Work visas can only be obtained at the Immigration Office in Bolivia and the applicant should enter Bolivia with a Business Visa issued by the Consulate. The requirements to obtain a working visa are: passport valid for one year from the date of entry into Bolivia and a working certificate or a business contract.

To work in any city here write to the General Hospital, City Name, Bolivia. Note: You may well get AMS here, especially if you fly straight in. Follow the guidelines at the beginning of this book (rest, no smoking, no drinking etc.). The locals sell Soroche pills in most pharmacists in La Paz which allegedly help in the first few days. *Mate de coca* (coca leaf tea) is another remedy the locals swear by.

La Paz

La Paz is the highest capital in the world at 3636 m and is the largest city in Bolivia. It is the centre of commerce and finance, but Sucre remains the judiciary capital. La Paz has more than a million people. The weather is very changeable even within a single day. Daytime temperatures are about 20 °C and 10 °C at night. There's plenty to do: San Francisco Cathedral, four museums and a couple of markets (Mercado de Heciceria (witches market) and Linares market which sells herbs, seed and llama skeleton remedies). The local cinema shows a number of English films.

UNIVERSITY AND MEDICAL SCHOOLS IN LA PAZ:

Colegio De Enferemeras De Bolivia, Calle Batallon Colorados Ed, El Condon P-14, La Paz, Bolivia Tel: 2 322713.
Colegio Departmental De Enferemeras, Ave 16 De Julio Ed, San Pablo P-10 Oficina 6, La Paz, Bolivia Tel: 2 314940.
Colegio Medico De Bolivia, Calle Balivan 1266, La Paz, Bolivia Tel: 2 315404/369961/341575.
Colegio Medico De La Paz, Calle Balivian 1266, La Paz, Bolivia Tel: 319113/319121.
Universidad Boliviana Mayor de San Andrés, Facultad de Ciencias de la Salud, Avenida Saavedra 2246, La Paz, Bolivia (Founded 1834).

Hospital Obrero

La Paz, Bolivia.

The hospital: Hospital Obrero (hospital of the workers) is the best CNS hospital in Bolivia. It has good facilities (e.g. a CT scanner), but only few patients get scanned because of the cost. It sees all the diseases above. The surgical department performs not only your standard Western list, but also the unusual such as bowel resection due to megacolon caused by Chagas. Many cholecystectomies are done as the locals have a high fat diet. Gynae is busy with cancers (due to poor screening) and illegal abortion complications.

Hospital du Mujer

La Paz, Bolivia.

The hospital: The 'Hospital of Women' (O&G only), about five minutes' walk from Hospital Obrero. It is much poorer and patients' treatment is governed by what they can afford. To the Western eye it can seem brutal. On the delivery suite there are eight beds, no curtains, no relatives, no midwives. The only staff are doctors. The women are given an enema and shaved. In the delivery room aparous women get an episiotomy. No analgesia. When its all over they get monitored and a night on the ward. This costs £10, and so, not surprisingly, 80% of women deliver at home.

Cochabamba

Universidad Mayor de San Simon

Facultad de Medicina, Av Aniceto, Arce, No 0371, Casilla 3119, Cochabamba, Bolivia Fax: 42 31690.
Uses:

Hospital Viedma

Av Aniceto Arce E-0257, Cochabamba, Bolivia Tel 28106.

The hospital: Viedma is the main public hospital in Cochabamba (there are many surrounding clinics/small hospitals) serving a population of 1,100,000. It is poorly equipped (the only ECG is in ITU). Gloves and needles are resterilized (take your own). It's a friendly place with a lot of respect for foreigners. Unusual pathologies that are more common here include Chagas, TB, rheumatic heart disease and Fournier's gangrene.

O Elective notes: It's very busy but enjoyable. The final year students work as interns doing 96-hour weeks on call 1:2 or 1:3. They get paid $15/week for the privilege. The patients and hospital are very poor. They may ask for a blood donation while you are there ... students have said it's fine just make sure they use a new set. You get a lot of hands of experience. Few patients can afford a plastic surgeon and hence you'll be doing facial lacerations.

Accommodation: A dorm block if on-call in A&E otherwise it is not provided. Hotel Elisa (SO 834 Calle Agustin Lopez) is recommended (about £4 (38 BOB)/night).

UNIVERSITY IN SUCRE:

Universidad Boliviana Mayor de San Francisco Xavier de Chuguisaca, Facultad de Ciencias se la Salud, Casilla 233, Sucre, Bolivia. (Founded 1846.)

Medical Colleges in Santa Cruz:

Colegio Departmental de Medicos-Veterinarios, Avenida Irala 603, Santa Cruz, Bolivia Tel: 3321941.
Colegio Medico Departmental, Ave 3er anillo Interno, Santa Cruz, Bolivia Tel: 3425582.

HOSPITALS AND CLINICS IN BOLIVIA:

La Paz

Clinica Adventista La Paz, C. Carrasco 1405, Miraflores, La Paz, Bolivia.
Clinica Alemana, Av 6 de Agosto 2821, La Paz, Bolivia (Tel: 320355/323023).
Clinica Americana, Av 14 de Septiembre, Obrajes, La Paz, Bolivia (Tel: 783371/783372).
Clinica Boston, Av Ecuador 2475, La Paz, Bolivia.
Clinica Britanica, Av Mscal Santa Cruz, Edif Esperanza, La Paz, Bolivia.
Clinica de Neurocirugia, C Genaro amarra 1887, La Paz, Bolivia.
Clinica del Sur, Av Hernando Siles 5353, Obrajes, La Paz, Bolivia.
Clinica el Alto, Urb. Boris Banzer, El Alto, La Paz, Bolivia.
Clinica Radiologica, Av Arce 2081, La Paz, Bolivia.
Clinica Rengel, C Victor Sanjines 2762, La Paz, Bolivia.
Clinica Santa Maria, Av 6 de Agosto 2487, La Paz, Bolivia.
Hospital de Psiquiatria, Av Villalobos 1477 Miraflores, La Paz, Bolivia.
Hospital Juan XXIII, Av Naciones Unidas, Munaypata, La Paz, Bolivia.
Hospital Metodista, Av 14 de Septiembre, Obrajes, La Paz, Bolivia (Tel: 783509/10/11).
Hospital Neumologico, Av Vicente Burgaleta V, Copacabana, La Paz, Bolivia.
Hospital Obrero, Av Brasil, Miraflores, La Paz, Bolivia (Tel: 350101).

Cochabamba

Clinica Boliviano Americano, Av San Martin S-1023, Cochabamba, Bolivia (Tel: 56316).
Clinica Cochabamba, c Lanza S-0931, Cochabamba, Bolivia (Tel: 29433).
Clinica Copacabana, Av Potosi N-1253, Cochabamba, Bolivia.
Clinica de Especialidades Pediatricas, Av Heroinas E-1024, Cochabamba, Bolivia (Tel: 54133).
Clinica del Nino Cochabamba, C Bolivar E-1113, Cochabamba, Bolivia (Tel: 31839).
Clinica del Valle, Av Tadeo Haenke O-1171, Cochabamba, Bolivia (Tel: 82228).
Clinica Geriatrica Dorian, C Felix Del Grando N-1251, Cochabamba, Bolivia (Tel: 45009).
Clinica Iriarte, C Victor Cabrera Lozada E-023, Cochabamba, Bolivia (Tel: 33780).
Clinica La Paz, Plza Barba de Padilla E-0233, Cochabamba, Bolivia (Tel: 45998).
Clinica Maternologica Santa Ines, C La Merced O-1585, Cochabamba, Bolivia (Tel: 46768).
Clinica Policial No 2 Virgen de Copacabana, Plza. Sucre 206, Cochabamba, Bolivia (Tel: 50374).
Clinica Pronto Socorro de Fracturas Laser C Pasteur N-0210, Cochabamba, Bolivia (Tel: 52424).
Clinica Recolete, Av Potosi N-1326, Cochabamba, Bolivia (Tel: 44235).
Clinica Saavedra, C Calama O-0380, Cochabamba, Bolivia (Tel: 22776).
Clinica San Francisco Ltda, C Sucre E-0987, Cochabamba, Bolivia (Tel: 21379).
Clinica San Joaquin, Av Del La Fuerza Aerea 2433, Cochabamba, Bolivia (Tel: 53875).
Clinica San Pablo, Av Simon Lopez O-0375, Cochabamba, Bolivia (Tel: 46009).
Hospital Albina Patino, C Jordan E-0886, Cochabamba, Bolivia (Tel: 26161).
Hospital Antituberculoso, Av Aniceto Arce E-0257, Cochabamba, Bolivia (Tel: 21120).
Hospital Clinico Viedma, Av Aniceto Arce E-0257, Cochabamba, Bolivia (Tel: 28106).
Hospital Cuschieri, Plza 15 de Abril Cocap 17, Cochabamba, Bolivia (Tel: 61891).
Hospital Elizabeth Seton, Av Blanco Galindo Km 5, Cochabamba, Bolivia (Tel: 41889/40201).
Hospital Militar No 2, Av Ramon Rivero s/n, Cochabamba, Bolivia (Tel: 21086).

Hospital San Vicente, C Baptosta N-0541, Cochabamba, Bolivia (Tel: 54321 Fax: 54352).

Santa Cruz

Clinica Angel Foianini, Av Irala, Chuquisaca, Santa Cruz, Bolivia (Tel: 362211–366005 Fax: 365577).
Clinica Baldivieso, 764 Av Viedma, Santa Cruz, Bolivia (Tel: 337868).
Clinica Cristo Rey, Av Roca y Coronado, Chilon, Santa Cruz, Bolivia (Tel: 533914).
Clinica de Cirugia Plastica, 489 C Junin, Santa Cruz, Bolivia (Tel: 351915).
Clinica de Emergencias Bilbao, 482 Av Mons Rivero, Santa Cruz, Bolivia (Tel: 322255).
Clinica de Emergencia Cardenal Maurer, 103 Av Melchor Pinto, Santa Cruz, Bolivia (Tel: 335558).
Clinica de Ojos Santa Cruz, Av Centenario, Pasillo Barbery, Santa Cruz, Bolivia (Tel: 332478 Fax: 327327).
Clinica del Accidentado, 6 C/1 Oeste Pasillo 1, Barrio Hamacas, Santa Cruz, Bolivia (Tel: 425988).
Clinica del Reposo Monte Sinai, 3er Anillo Ext/Radial 19, Santa Cruz, Bolivia (Tel: 520895).
Clinica Dr Torres, Km 3½ Carr al Norte, Santa Cruz, Bolivia (Tel: 426710).
Clinica Incor, Av 26 Febrero/Caranda, Santa Cruz, Bolivia (Tel: 529236).
Clinica Infantil San Patricio, Libertad/Canoto, Santa Cruz, Bolivia (Tel: 341190).
Clinica Instituto de Gastroenterologia, 265 Av Mons Rivero, Santa Cruz, Bolivia (Tel: 342385 Fax: 343430).
Clinica Medica Sirani, 667 Rene Moreno, Santa Cruz, Bolivia (Tel: 352200).
Clinica Odontogica Integrada, 216 Campero, Santa Cruz, Bolivia (Tel: 323827).
Clinica Pereira, Radial 26, Final Barr Oriental, Santa Cruz, Bolivia (Tel: 426368).
Clinica Saavedra, 382 A Saavedra, Santa Cruz, Bolivia (Tel: 364688).
Clinica San Prudencio, Km6 Carr a Cochabamba, Santa Cruz, Bolivia (Tel: 529664).
Clinica Santa Cruz, 140 Av Busch, Santa Cruz, Bolivia (Tel: 366111).
Clinica Santa Maria, 754 Av Viedma, Santa Cruz, Bolivia (Tel: 352001 Fax 324288).
Clinica Urkupina, 550 Av El Trompillo/O Chavez, Santa Cruz, Bolivia (Tel: 527081).
Clinica Virgen de Lourdes, 352 Rene Moreno, Santa Cruz, Bolivia (Tel: 325518).
Clinica Virgen del Carmen, 163 Piriti, Santa Cruz, Bolivia (Tel: 527502).
Hospital de Nino Dr Mario Ortiz, C Santa Barbara/Buenos Aires, Santa Cruz, Bolivia (Tel: 336841).
Hospital Japones, Av 3er Anillo Ext 747, Calle Ballivian, Santa Cruz, Bolivia (Tel: 332516).
Hospital Modelo San Lucas, 747 Ballivian, Santa Cruz, Bolivia (Tel: 32514).
Hospital San Juan de Dios, C Cuellar/Espana, Santa Cruz, Bolivia (Tel: 332222).
Hospital Urbari, Calle Igmiri, Santa Cruz, Bolivia (Tel: 534000).

Brazil

Population: 161.8 million
Language: Portuguese
Capital: Brasília
Currency: Real
Int Code: +55

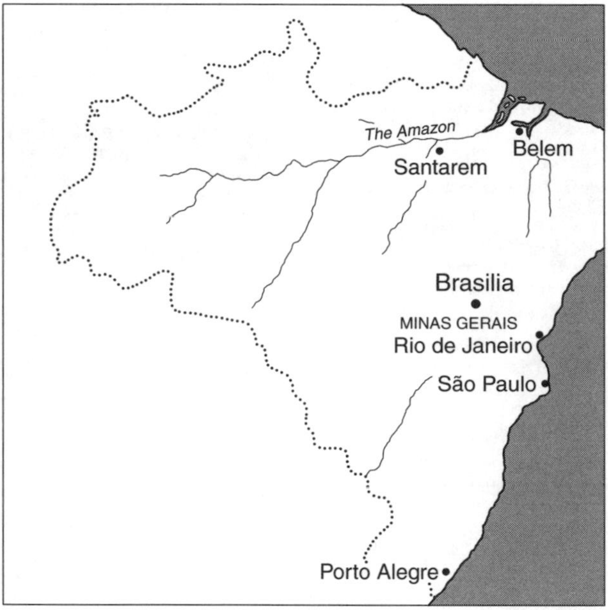

Brazil, the largest country in South America, is famous for its rainforest, the huge Amazon river, its coffee, gold and diamonds. It has 1243 miles of Atlantic coastline. Brazil has a diverse population based on the original Indians, Portuguese colonizers and the African slaves brought to work in the sugar plantations. Over the last century many of the Indian villages have been wiped out by disease or by Western force. The total number of Indians is now only 200,000. The history and the annual Mardi Gras in Rio de Janeiro make it a popular tourist destination; however, probably because of language difficulties (which is a variation on the European Portuguese), Brazil is not a popular elective destination at all. Nor is it a popular work destination. For this reason only a brief outline will be given here. Contact the NGOs listed in Section 3 for more ideas.

✪ Medicine:

For Brazil's rich, the private healthcare is good. However, for the vast majority healthcare is sparse or non-existent. Only 20% of the country's hospitals are state-run. Infectious diseases are increasing, in particular malaria, leprosy and parasitic skin infections. This is because of the lack of preventative medicine for which Brazil has been strongly criticized.

➲ Visas and work permits:
A visa is required to enter as is a work permit to work. Consult the embassy for more details.

◎ Climate and crime:
High temperatures and relatively constant rainfall are usual in the Amazon basin. The north-east of the country has little rainfall and over recent years has suffered episodes of drought. The Brazilian plateau has wider temperature ranges and most rainfall between October and April. The south has a temperate climate of warm summers and cool winters. Over the last couple of decades crime has risen sharply. This is particularly so in the shanty towns and urban conurbations where street children have been murdered by uncontrolled death squads. Drug-related crime is also on the increase. The displacement of original people and land workers is still occurring.

There are over 70 medical schools in Brazil and since Brazil is not a common elective or work destination they are not all listed here. A full list can be obtained through the World Health Organization (WHO) or visit www.epm.br/dhsp/dhsplik9.htm. A number of charities and NGOs also do a considerable amount of work in Brazil. (*See* Section 3: The Appendix.) **Action In International Medicine**, 125 High Holborn, London WC1V 6QA Tel: 020 7405 3090 Fax: 020 7405 3093 has been particularly recommended for primary care work and arranges work with **Fundacao Esperanca** (*see below*).

MEDICAL SCHOOLS IN BRAZIL:

Brasília

Fundação Universidade de Brasília, Faculdade de Ciências da Saúde, Campus Universitário, Asa Norte Residencial 70919, Brasília, Brazil.

Minas Gerais

Universidad Federal de Minas Gerais, Faculdade de Medicina, Av Alfredo Balena 190, Belo Horizonte-MG CE: 30.130–100 PO Box 340, Minas Gerais, Brazil Tel: 31 274 6267 Fax: 31 273 4985.

Rio de Janeiro

Universidade Federal do Rio de Janeiro, Faculdade se Medicina, Centro de Ciências da Saúde, Ilha da Cidade Universitária, 21910-Rio de Janeiro, Brazil.

São Paulo

Escola Paulista de Medicina, Universidade Federal de São Paulo, Rua Botucatu 740, 5° andar, Caixa Postal 7144, 02023, São Paulo, Brazil www.epm.br. (The medical school uses the huge 654-bed São Paulo Hospital. Clinics are also run into rural communities.)

PRIMARY CARE WORK:

Fundacao Esperanca

Rua Coaracy Nunes, 3344, Caixa Postal 222, Santarem, Para CEP 68040–100 Brazil
Tel: 91 522 2726 Fax: 91 522 7878
fesperan@ax.apc.org or
fesperan@ax.ibase.org.br

The clinic: *Fundacao Esperanca* (Hope Foundation) is a non-profit organization run largely by North Americans and is based in Santarem in the mid-Amazonian basin. It is a primary health-care facility that runs clinics. Santarem is a short flight or a three-day boat trip down the Amazon from Belem. The region is poor with very deficient health services. Esperanca serves the town's 30,000 inhabitants and rural people scattered through the municipality (about the size of Belgium). There is a great deal of tropical medicine (leprosy, leishmaniasis, malaria) and general medicine (diabetes, hypertension, TB). Paeds and O&G are also busy. The main doctor in charge is very friendly and there are a number of volunteers who work here. The elective surgery programme brings volunteer orthopaedic, plastic and ophthalmological teams to the Fundacao every three months.

○ Elective notes: This is an excellent place to see medicine in a developing world. It is not the place if you want loads of trauma and chest drains. At the

education centre (good library), training is provided at various levels and in different areas of health work. It is demanding, but rewarding. A typical day starts at 7.30 am with a two-hour tutorial and goes through to 5.30 pm with a two-hour lunch break. In the clinics students consult patients. There are very few acute cases, but many tropical diseases, gynae and paeds problems. Students can also go out with a health worker on a four-day journey into the jungle to check on remote communities, immunize and weigh children. Being able to speak Portugese is a big advantage though not necessary due to the American presence.
Accommodation: Provided free to volunteers. Some elective students have had to pay $10 (17.5 BRL)/day, but this includes food and laundry. There are plenty of opportunities at weekends to go off with the Americans and explore the beauties of the region.

Porto Alegre

Porto Alegre, with its 1.5 million inhabitants, is the capital of Brazil's southernmost states in the most affluent and developed part of the country. Many southerners are descended from Germans and Italians and take pride in their 'non-Third-Worldism'. They are famed throughout Brazil for their 'work-ethic' mentality, their barbeques, their money and their lack of Brazilianess (carnival and chaos).

Hospital Nossa SRA da Conceicao

Rua Francisco Trein, 556, Porto Alegre, Brazil.

The community health service: Has been in existence for almost 20 years. It is modelled on the UK GP system and is one of the only services of its kind in the country. It started from within a public hospital and gradually, through demand from local communities, spread outwards so that today there is the largest and original 'post' with 13 others scattered throughout the north of the city. Originally financially independent, it is now government-subsidized and offers primary healthcare, free of charge, to anyone within ill-defined catchment areas. Working at one of these posts means you can get to see the rich diseases (similar to the UK) as well as those of the terrible conditions in the shanty towns.

Instituto Matern Infantil de Pernambuco, Rua Dos Coelhos, 300 Boa Vista, CEP 50070–550, Recife, Brazil.

Chile

Population: 14.3 million
Language: Spanish
Capital: Santiago
Currency: Chilean peso
Int Code: +56

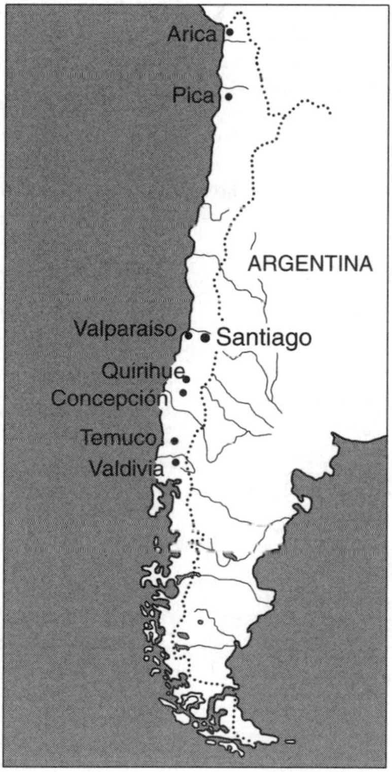

Chile stretches some 2697 miles down the west coast of South America. In the east it is bordered by the Andes. The length and variation in altitudes gives Chile a wide range of climates. During the Pinochet years a dramatic decline in tourism occurred; however, since democracy in 1993 tourism to the Andes, the Elqui Valley wine region and Easter Island has increased. Very few doctors and even fewer locals speak English. If you are thinking of going here it is vital that you have at least some basic Spanish. This is especially true in rural hospitals. If you can at least try most people will be sympathetic and keen to help.

✪ Medicine:
There is a public health service that covers 80% of the population. However, it does not reach the rural areas. The overcrowding of the capital, Santiago, is also a major health problem. Doctor to patient ratio is 1 per 2150. Heart diseases and cancers are the big killers.

➲ Visas and work permits:
A visa is required to enter Chile; however, as it is not a popular elective destination, no clear information on the need for a visa specifically for electives is available. You should be OK with a tourist visa, but contact the embassy for more details or if intending to work.

◎ Climate:
The climate varies widely from a wet south and the glaciers of the Andes to the pleasant central region.

Santiago

Santiago, the nation's capital has two medical schools. The largest two hospitals are also listed.

Universidad de Chile, Facultad de Medicina, Avenida Independencia 1027, Casilla 13898, Santiago, Chile.
Pontificia Univeridad Católica de Chile, Facultad de Medicina, Lira 40, Santiago, Chile.

Hospital Clinico, Universidad de Chile
Santos Dumont 999, Independencia, Santiago, Chile Tel: 678 81 34 Fax: 777 13 73.
The hospital: Has 614 beds and all major specialities. It is situated just north of downtown. Although Spanish is the primary language, some staff do speak a little English, French or German. It is privately funded. It has a major trauma centre and is advanced with cardiothoracic and neurosurgery.

Hospital del Salvador
Av Salvador 364, Santiago, Chile.
The hospital: One of the main public hospitals in Santiago (and it's enormous). The facilities for such a large hospital are pretty basic, but the standard of clinical care is high. Despite poor amenities, renal transplants and other major operations are often carried out.
❍ Elective notes: There's not much hands on work for students as they tend to use their own junior doctors. There are many consultants, but most tend to do private clinics in the afternoons which are therefore quiet. There is a very relaxed atmosphere and they are very keen to teach. Some doctors do speak English but you really must speak Spanish to survive here.

Valparaiso

Chile's third-largest city is on the coast, just two hours by car from Santiago. It is a picturesque and colourful city.

THE MEDICAL SCHOOL:

Universidad de Valparaiso, Facultad de Medicina, Casilla 92-V, Hontaneda 2653, Valparaiso, Chile.

Hospital Carlos van Buren
Servicio de Salud Valparaiso y San Antonio, Valparaiso, Chile.
The hospital: A large teaching hospital with excellent facilities in Valparaiso. The internal medicine department occupies one very large ward on one floor. In it are a number of specialities. There is a much higher staff:patient ratio compared to provincial hospitals in north Chile.
❍ Elective notes: There is good support and teaching. The medical students are very friendly and may well take you out around the city.
Accommodation: Not provided but you can stay in 'pensiones'.

OTHER MEDICAL SCHOOLS:

Universidad Austral de Chile, Facultad de Medicina, Isla Teja, Casilla 567, Valdivia, Chile Fax: 212953.
Universidad de Concepción, Facultad de Medicina, Barrio Universitario s/n, Casilla 60-C, Concepción, Chile.
Universidad de la Frontera, Facultad de Medicina, Casilla 54-D, Temuco, Chile.

Arica

Arica is a large coastal town near the Peruvian border in northern Chile. It is surrounded by desert but does have some beautiful national parks and good beaches. It has one state hospital and numerous private practices.

Hospital de Arica

1 Region de Tarapaca, Arica, Chile

The hospital: The main city hospital in Arica, the most northern city in Chile. It serves a large population, including many immigrants from Peru. There is a paediatric department run by 12 consultants. There is a lot of TB and childhood leukaemias. There are many morning clinics in a number of specialities such as respiratory and neurology. Many of the doctors do private clinics in the afternoon. The staff are keen to teach and take you on day trips to the local communities in the mountains.

Accommodation: Not provided.

Hospital Dr Juan Noe

18 de September 1000, Arica, Chile.

The hospital: A relatively large state hospital. It covers all specialities. The doctors do ward rounds and clinics in the mornings but tend to disappear in the afternoons to their private clinics. Accident and Emergency is often busy but usually with minor complaints ('flu) as there is no GP service. Internal medicine has all the subspecialties. TB is common and there is a surprising amount of SLE, Chagas' disease and gallstones. Obstetrics and gynaecology can be very interesting and different to the West. Abortion is illegal so most of their workload is dealing with the often sinister complications of back street abortions. The plastic surgeon is the only one in north Chile so if plastics what you want to see, there's plenty of it. It's mainly skin-grafting for diabetic and deep varicose ulcers. There's no on-call anaesthetist so after hours the nurses step in.

Accommodation: Not provided, but lunch is! There are many cheap hostels and student places.

RURAL HOSPITALS:

Hospital de Quirihue

Quirihue, Chile.

The hospital: A small, basic public hospital in a rural town located in the north of the Lake District region of Chile. It provides the surrounding area with A&E, paediatric, obstetric and gynaecology, medical and minor surgical facilities. However, most serious cases get sent to nearby cities. It is run by newly qualified doctors (there are only six) and the most senior is usually only a few years out of medical school. They work in such hospitals before specializing. There are often Chilean medical students doing attachments here; they tend to run the A&E department.

O Elective notes: You can do as much or as little as you want. There are many procedures (suturing, plastering and helping in Caesars) to get involved in. They are keen to teach and there is plenty of opportunity to go on rural clinics. You can also spend a week with a GP in a nearby coastal village.

Consultorio de Pica

Balmaceda Sin Numero, Pica, Chile.

The hospital: Not a hospital, just a 'Consultorio' run by a doctor with a resident dentist. There are also one midwife and six nurses. It provides medical and dental services to the town and also a large area of the Altiplano in the Andes. Clinics are run daily and the doctor's role is very much that of a GP. However, they do also provide an A&E service which is run by the paramedics. There are superb clinics to go on in the Altiplano.

O Elective notes: Make sure you're all right at altitude as these indigenous Indian villages are up above 5500 m and hence clinics can be physically exhausting. There is an extensive vaccination campaign (MMR) in the local communities. Back down in Pica, there's plenty of suturing and minor surgery to be done. The medicine may not be cutting edge, but you get to see and do more than at the major hospitals in Chile. No one will speak English.

Accommodation: Food has previously been provided by the Consultorio in the local hotel. The doctor and midwife live in the hospital.

Columbia

Population: 36 million
Language: Spanish
Capital: Bogotá
Currency: Colombian peso
Int Code: +57

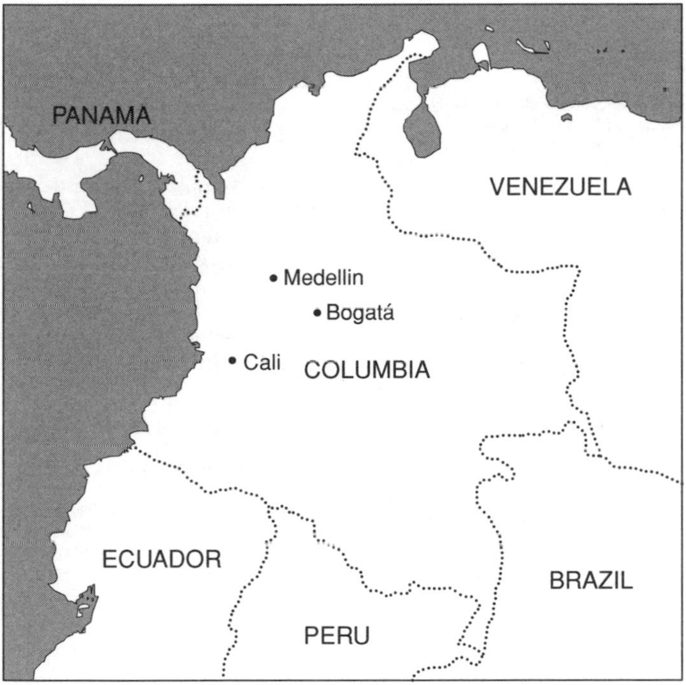

Lying at the top of South America, Columbia is better-known for its drug trafficking than its healthcare. All language of instruction is in Spanish and hence the hospitals are not commonly visited by English-speaking medics.

✪ Medicine:

Only a small minority are covered by the state healthcare system and they are usually in remote areas where it is physically impossible for them to get help. Depending on where you are, trauma, both through deliberate violence and RTAs, is common.

✪ Climate and crime:

The Caribbean side tends to be dry and hot while the Pacific side is wet and hot.

The Andes are obviously cool and Bogotá seems to have an everlasting spring. Violent crime and kidnappings are a real problem and a reason for the lack of tourism and lack of interest in overseas medics. These incidences are usually drug-related and usually confined to Bogotá, Mendellín and Cali.

Columbia has a number of medical schools. Some of the main ones are included below. If planning work it is best to approach NGOs (*see* Section 3).

Bogotá

Universidad Nacional de Columbia, Facultad de Medicina, Ciudad Universitaria, Bogotá, Columbia. (This is the oldest and largest medical school in the capital.)

Centro Medico Cristiano

Avenida Caracas, No 46–26, Santafe de Bogotá, Columbia.

The hospital: The Centro Medico Cristiano is run by a Columbian Christian organization which for the past 10 years has been establishing a wide network of services aimed at alleviating the suffering of the city's poorest, especially the large population of drug abusers and street children. The medical arm of the organization involves clinics and education programmes as well as vaccination schemes. There is obviously a great deal of work to be done by the paediatricians; however, investigation and treatment facilities are severely limited. There is a mobile clinic which goes into many of Bogotá's 'no-go' areas where there is a great deal of deprivation pathology.

Cali

Universidad del Valles

División de Ciencias de la Salud, Apartado Aéreo 2188, Cali, Valle, Columbia. (This is Cali's oldest school and has its own University teaching hospital.)

The hospital: The Central Hospital is the university's main hospital and from A&E there are 50 admissions a day. There's plenty of violent trauma. There are also associated smaller family heath clinics.

O Elective notes: Many procedures can be done in A&E as the turnover is so great. It's almost a 'war setting'. Time can also be spent at the smaller clinics. You must speak Spanish ... not necessarily fluent, but enough to get by. Write to the **Directora Promocion Academica y Asuntos Internacionales** at the above address.

Antioquia

Universidad de Antioquia, Facultdad de Medicina, Apartado Aéreo 1226, Medellín, Antioquia, Columbia. (This is the main medical school in Columbia's second-largest city.)

Ecuador

Population: 12 million
Language: Spanish
Capital: Quito
Currency: Sucre
Int Code: +593

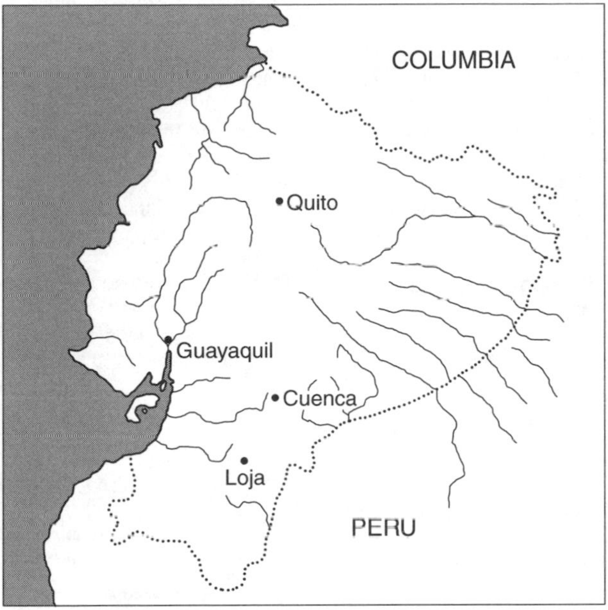

Ecuador is a country with amazing diversity – from coastal mangrove swamps and beaches to the high Andes and the rainforest in the Amazon basin. Flights are relatively cheap and frequent buses mean that no place is more than a day's journey from Quito. Very few people speak English and so fluent Spanish is pretty much essential.

✪ Medicine:
Basic healthcare provisions are being established throughout Ecuador with rural clinics. Malaria and other infectious diseases are common, as is stomach cancer.

Quito

MEDICAL SCHOOL AND HOSPITALS:

Universidad Central del Ecuador
Escuela de Medicina, Facultad de Ciencias Médicas, Sodiro e Iquique, Quito, Ecuador.
This is the oldest medical school of

Ecuador founded in the early nineteenth century. It is situated in the capital and uses a number of hospitals totalling 3000 beds. These include:

Hospital de Niños Baca Oritz, N 6 de diciembre y Colon, Quito, Ecuador.
Hospital, Gineo-Obstetrico, 'Isiror Ayora', Quito, Ecuador.
Hospital voz Andes, Desarrollo Comunidad, Villa Lengua 267, Casilla 691, Quito, Ecuador.

Cuenca

Cuenca, situated at 2530 m above sea-level with over 300,000 inhabitants is the third-largest city in Ecuador. It has a compact, central 'old town' area with cobbled streets and colonial buildings. There are plenty of restaurants, bars and cinemas. Nearby there are national parks, Inca ruins and a spar town (Banos). It has two medical schools.

MEDICAL SCHOOLS AND HOSPITALS:

Universidad Católica de Cuenca, Facultad de Medicina y Ciencas de la Salud, Car Tomás Ordoñez No 6–41, Casilla 19A, Cuenca, Ecuador.
Universidad de Cuenca, Facultad de Ciencas Médicas, Avenida El Paraíso s/n, Casila Letra 'X', Cuenca, Ecuador.

Hospital de IESS (Instituto Ecuaro-riano De Seguridad Social)

Avenida Guayna-Capac, Cuenca, Ecuador.
The hospital: Affiliated to Cuenca University with over 200 beds and all surgical specialities (bar cardiac surgery). The A&E department is extremely busy and well worth spending time in.
O Elective notes: This offers a wonderful opportunity to observe many procedures, although you may not actually get to do much. Seek out the very friendly coloproctol surgeon who will provide excellent one-to-one teaching (and introductions to most people in Cuenca). There are loads of parties and fiestas to go to as well.

Hospital Vicente Corral Moscoso

Casilla 418, Cuenca, Ecuador.
The hospital: A regional hospital for Cuenca and surrounding areas and has about 500 beds covering all specialities. It cares for the majority of the population who cannot afford to pay either social security or private health insurance. It is government-funded, but very poorly equipped compared to the Hospital de IESS.
O Elective notes: There's plenty to see and cases such as malnutrition and infectious diseases tend to present very late, so you often see them at there worst. You'll be busy ... ward rounds start at 7 am.

OTHER MEDICAL SCHOOLS:

Universidad de Guayaquil, Facultad de Ciencias Médicas, Ciudad Universitaria, Avenida Kennedy, Guayaquil, Ecuador.
Universidad Nacional de Loja, Escuela de Medicina Humana, Casilla No 349, Loja, Ecudaor.

Falkland Islands

Population: 2000
Language: English
Capital: Stanley
Currency: British pound
Int Code: +500

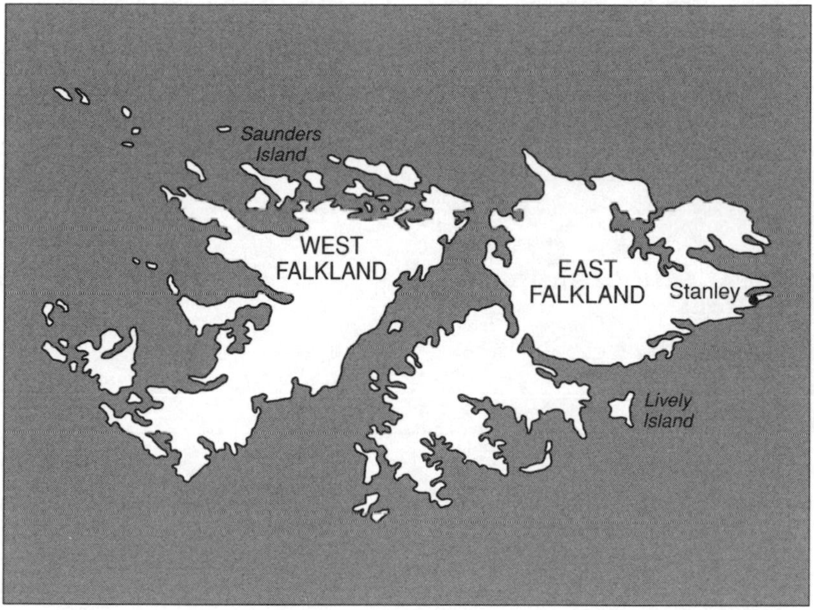

Southernmost in the South Atlantic, the Falkland Islands consist of hundreds of little islands surrounding the main east and west islands. They are famed for the dispute they caused between Argentina and the UK. They have a large agricultural and fishing industry. The recent discovery of oil could transform their economy and may cause further disputes. It's usually pretty damp and windy.

Stanley

King Edward (VII) Memorial Hospital (KEMH)

Stanley, Falkland Islands, South Atlantic.
The hospital: KEMH is a small hospital that caters for the 2000 civilians and 2000 military personnel that live on the Falkland Islands. It is run by four GPs

and a military field surgical team (one surgeon and one anaesthetist) providing GP, A&E, medical inpatient, emergency and some elective surgery services. Despite its size it can get quite busy, especially when there are visiting Antarctic cruise ships and fishermen.

Most of the population lives in Stanley. However, due to the large size of the Falklands, many of the outside settlements can only be reached by a 'flying doctor' service. As a medical student, you can participate in this, setting up surgery in someone's lounge before returning the next day. There may also be the opportunity to join the RAF in their search and rescue helicopter. As there are no medical students around, the doctors are very keen to teach. Most of the medicine is fairly similar to that in the UK and this is a very British elective; however, there is plenty to do with some great scenery, penguins and remnants of the 1982 conflict to visit. There are sports facilities and if you have time, Chile is in reach. Beer is cheap and Stanley has a night-club!

Accommodation and transport: Flights to the Falklands, by RAF TriStar from Brize Norton, can be arranged through **FI Government** in London. A student rate is available. KEMH provides accommodation. Considering the distance, this can be relatively inexpensive elective.

Guatemala

Population: 10.6million
Official language: Spanish
Capital: Guatemala City
Currency: Quetzal
Int Code: +502

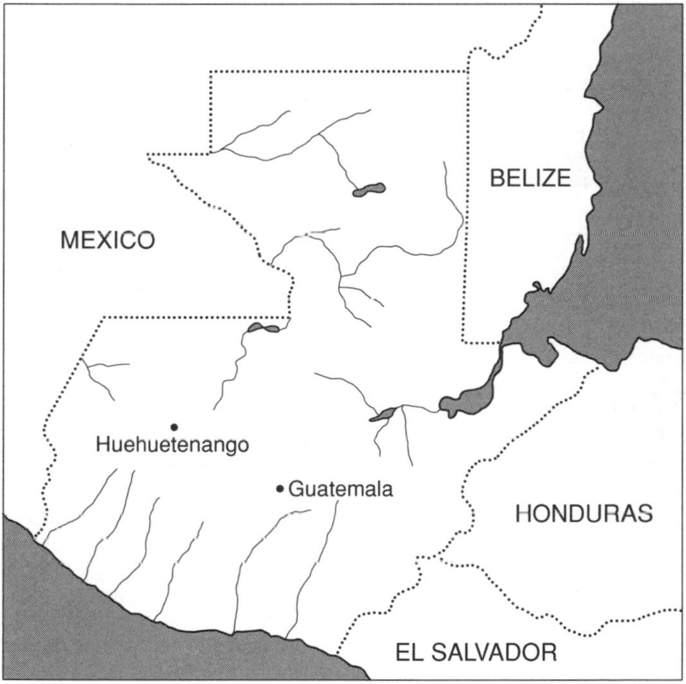

Guatemala is the largest, most populous and poorest of Central American states. Although it has been independent since 1838, military rule between 1954 and 1986 means that 90% of people are now below the poverty line. It's not a popular destination, presumably because of the need for fluent Spanish.

Medicine:
Very little is spent on healthcare as a nation, as demonstrated by the small number of hospitals (there are actually a number more private than there are public hospitals). Mortality rates are the highest in Central America. Seventy per cent of health funding goes to the capital

where 80% of the doctors work. Many deaths are poverty linked with common causes being heart disease, violence, TB and accidents. There is only one doctor per 2200 people.

➲ Visas and work permits:

As a British citizen, no visa is required if you are staying less than 90 days and your passport is valid for six months from the time of entry. If you wish to stay longer or work contact **Direction General de Migracion**, 41C–17–36, Zona 8, Ciudad de Guatemala Tel: 475 13 90/02. To work you also need to register with the **Colegio de Médicas y Cirujanos de Guatemala,** 17 Calle 1–61, Zona 1, Guatemala.

UNIVERSITIES:

There are two universities teaching medicine in Guatemala.

Universidad Francisco Marroquin

Facultad de Medicina, 6a Avenda 7–55, Zona 10, Guatemala.

This private university, based in Guatemala City, uses among others, **Esperanza** (a private hospital) in the city. For rural healthcare the medical students run clinics on their own. San Juan Sacatepequez is a market town 15 miles outside Guatemala city and clinics are also held here. There are next to no facilities but it gives a superb insight into how the locals live. Most consultations are antenatal or paeds. You will need good Spanish in the clinics but most of the medical students will translate if you get stuck.

Universidad de San Carlos, Facultad de Ciencias Médicas, Edifico M-2, Ciudad Universitaria, Zona 12, Guatemala.

MAIN PUBLIC HOSPITALS:

Hermeroteca Nacional,'Lic Clemente Marroquin Rojas', 5 Av 7-26 Z-1 Niv 2, Guatemala Telefax: 232 7625.
Hospital de Gineco-Obstetrica, 14 Av y 4 C Z-12 Col Colinas de Pamplona, Planta Telefónica, Guatemala Tel: 471 0249.
Hospital de Infectologia, Z-7 Fca La Verbena, Guatemala Tel: 471 2790.
Hospital de la Polcia Nacional, 11 Av 4-49 Z-1, Guatemala Tel: 232 6467/7633.
Hospital de Rehabilitacion, 14 Av y 4 C Z-12 Col Colinas de Pamplona, Guatemala Tel: 472 1678.
Hospital de Salud Mental, Z-18 Col Atlántida, Guatemala Tel: 256 1486.
Hospital General de Accidentes, 13 Av y Calz, San Juan Z-4 Mixco, Guatemala Tel: 597 9626.
Hospital General Del Igss, 9 C 7-55 Z-9, Guatemala Tel: 332 1009.
Hospital General San Juan de Dios (The main hospital), Av Elena 9 y 10 C Z-1, Guatemala Tel: 232 3741/3744/0423/3764 Fax: 253 6604.
Hospital Infantil de Infectologia y Rehabilitacion, 9 Av 7-01 Z-11, Guatemala Tel: 472 3532.
Hospital Roosevelt, Calz Roosevelt Z-11, Guatemala Tel: 471 1441/6380/3384/6390 Fax: 471 5071.

There are also a number of private hospitals. Enquire with the Embassy for a list.

A RURAL HOSPITAL:

Hospital de Jacal Tenango

Jacaltenango, Huehuetenango, Guatemala.

The hospital: Jacaltcnango is a rural town in the Chucumantes mountains. It is a very beautiful area. The hospital is a 50-bed mission hospital run by Mexican nuns. The three doctors (a medic, surgeon and obstetrician) who work there cover a vast population and are generalists in themselves since they do a 1:3 rota (i.e. the medic does appendectomies etc.). It's a friendly place and has a residential nutrition centre for malnourished children. You will definitely need to speak Spanish.

Guyana

Population: 800,000
Official Language: English
Capital: Georgetown
Currency: Guyana dollar
Int Code: +592

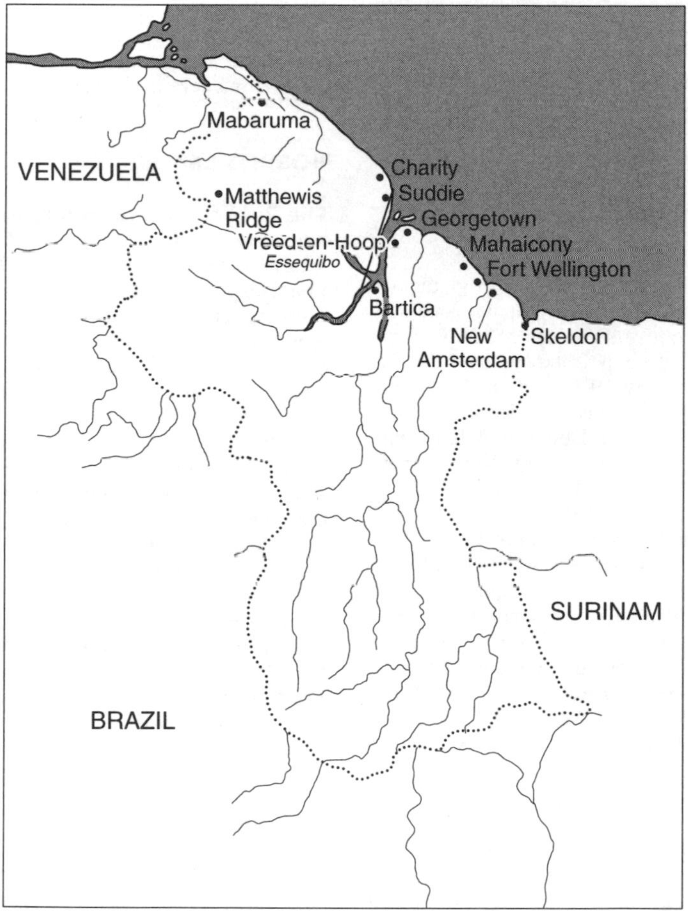

Eighty-five per cent of Guyana's 83,000 square miles consists of its dense rainforest interior and hence virtually all of its population lives on the coast (which itself is partially reclaimed land). It gained independence from the UK in 1966 and since then its economy has relied on the export of bauxite, gold, rice and sugar. There are still border disputes with

Surinam and Venezula. In the north-east (the coastal belt) sugar and rice are grown. In the inner forest, bauxite, diamonds, gold and manganese are found. 'Guyana' means 'land of many waters' – with the rivers Demerara, Berbice, Essequibo and Potaro and the Kaieteur falls (222 m high = five times Niagara) you can see where it gets its name. Georgetown is famous for its Dutch-inspired wooden architecture, street layouts and drainage canals. Fifty-one per cent of people are East Indian, 30% African, the rest European, Chinese and Amerindians (living in the west, south or on the reserves).

Note: Be sensible in Georgetown as it's not all that safe. Girls get chatted up but it is non-threatening. Guyana is still a developing country with poor transport facilities. If you're on for an adventure it has some of the world's most unexplored rainforests and largest waterfalls.

Medicine:

The Guyana state-run health system (on a National Insurance scheme) is actually pretty good and covers 95% of the population. Life expectancy is over 70. The main causes of death include heart diseases, violence, accidents, cancers and tuberculosis. Doctor:population ratio is around one per 3000. Nurse:population is one per 500.

Visas and work permits:

British nationals and nationals of other EEC countries do not require a visa to visit Guyana, just a passport valid for six months and a return ticket. Since no doctors are trained in Guyana, they have to accept those from a recognized medical school outside. Contact the **Guyana Medical Board**. As regards work permits, contact the **Guyana High Commission**.

Also Visit Guyana on the web! **Tourism Association of Guyana** www.interknowledge.com. General Information www.guyana.org

Climate and crime:

It is hot all year round (20–30 °C) with most rain between April and August and again over December and January. The Highlands are cooler. Crime is rife in the poorer areas and care should be taken not to enter these at night. The police are pretty ineffectual.

UNIVERSITIES:

University of Guyana

The Admission Office, Turkeyen Campus, East Coast Demerara, Guyana Tel: 22 5406 Fax: 22 3356.

Although this does have some health-related subjects, medicine itself is not taught anywhere in Guyana.

HOSPITALS*

The Public Hospital Georgetown

New Market Street, Georgetown, Guyana Tel: 2 56900 or Tel: 2 62687/59673/78224.

The hospital: Tries to provide most major specialities. The hospital has just been rebuilt in the last couple of years and, although it looks spanking brand new, there is an obvious lack of facilities (drugs and nursing staff). TB and cardiovascular disease are relatively common. AIDS is also a major problem. In A&E a great deal of violent trauma can be seen.

Elective notes: There is loads to see and do in A&E (though few practical procedures on the wards).

Bartica Hospital

Second Road, Bartica, Essequibo, Guyana Tel: 5 2339.

The hospital: Reached by forest track or boat. It has 40 beds and poor facilities. Rural clinics are run.

* (P) = Private

Best Hospital, Best, West Coast Demerara, Guyana Tel: 64 702.

Charity Hospital, Charity, Essequibo, Guyana Tel: 71 204.

Davis Memorial Hospital (P), 121 Durban Backlands Lodge, Georgetown, Guyana Tel: 2 72041.

Fort Wellington Hospital, Public Road, New Amsterdam, Berbice, Guyana Tel: 3 2396.

Jesus Rescue Mission Children's Hospital (P), 67 Croal Street, Stabroek, Georgetown, Guyana Tel: 2 54090.

Leonora Hospital, Leonora, West Coast Demerara, Guyana Tel: 61 2502.
Mabaruma Hospital, Mabaruma Compound, North West District, Guyana Tel: 77 205.
Mahaica Hospital, Mahaica Village, East Coast Demerara, Guyana Tel: 28 211.
Matthew's Ridge Hospital, Matthew's Ridge, North West District, Guyana Tel: 75 205.
Medical Arts Centre (P), 265 Thomas Street, North Cummingsburg, Georgetown, Guyana Tel: 2 57402 Fax: 2 65220.
New Amsterdam Hospital, New Amsterdam, Berbice, Guyana Tel: 3 2266.
Port Mourant Hospital, Corentyne, Berbice, Guyana Tel: 37 2883.
Prashad's Hospital Ltd (P), 258–9 Middle and Thomas Streets, North Cummingsburg, Geogetown, Guyana Tel: 2 67214 Fax: 2 67213.
Skeldon Hospital, Corriverton, Berbice, Guyana Tel: 39 2211.
St Joseph's Mercy Hospital (P), 130–2 Parade Street, Kingston, Georgetown, Guyana Tel: 2 72070 Fax: 2 502260.

Suddie Hospital

Suddie, Essequibo, Guyana Tel: 74 227.

The hospital: A small (50–100-bed) rural hospital on the coast. Rural outreach clinics are done into the remote interior.

West Demerara General Hospital, Best Village, Vreed-en-Hoop, West Coast Demerara, Guyana Tel: 64 271.
Woodlands Hospital (P), 110–11 Carmichael Street, North Cummingsburg, Georgetown, Guyana Tel: 2-54050 Fax: 2 55865.

Guyana

Honduras

Population: 6 million
Language: Spanish
Capital: Tegucigalpa
Currency: Lemipra
Int Code: +504

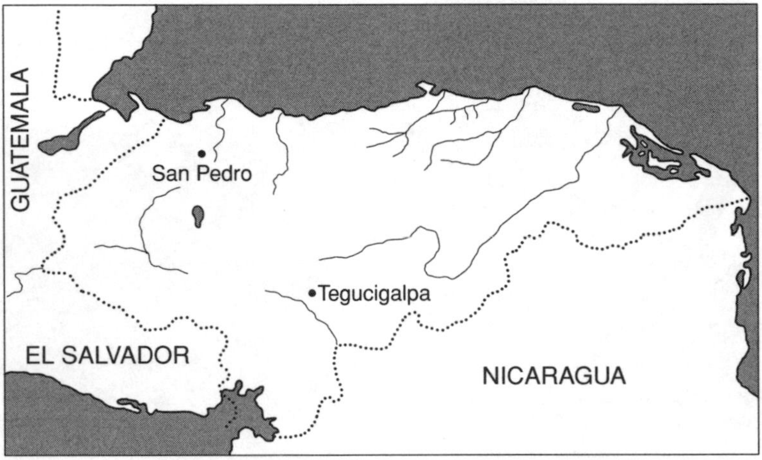

Despite being one of the world's biggest banana exporters, Honduras is very poor. It has been independent from Spain since 1821 but military dictatorships prevented democracy until 1984. The land itself spans Central America with some beautiful, virtually uninhabited coasts. The centre is mountainous.

✪ Medicine:

The healthcare system is not comprehensive and is only available to two-thirds of people. Infectious diseases, including malaria, are common. There is only one doctor per 2000 people.

➲ Visa and work permits:

To visit, British citizens do not require a visa. However, if gaining employment, work visas through the Embassy can take up to six months to obtain. For more information contact: **The Ministry of Health**, 3 Calle, 4 Avenida Tegucigalpa MDC, Honduras Tel: 222 8518 Fax: 238 4141.

There is only one medical school:

Universidad Nacional Autónom de Honduras, Facultad de Ciencias Médicas, Atras del Hospital Escuela, Tegucigalpa, Honduras.

The two main hospitals are:

Hospital General San Felipe, Boulevard San Felipe, Avenida Los Prceres, Tegucigalpa, MDC, Honduras Tel: 336 7698
Hospital Leonard Martinez, 9–10 Avenida, 7 Calle, SO No 56, San Pedro Sula, Honduras.

Mexico

Population: 94 million
Language: Spanish
Capital: Mexico City
Currency: Mexican new peso
Int Code: +52

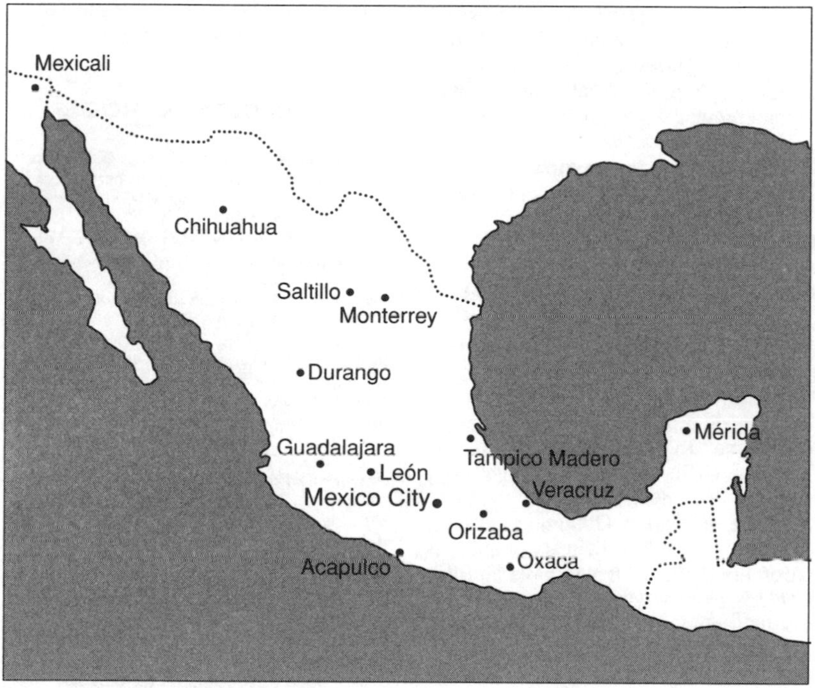

Mexico has been independent from Spain since 1836 but still retains a great deal of Spanish as well as its own culture. It straddles the whole of Central America. There are enormous wealth disparities. The slums of Mexico are some of the poorest in the world, 16% live in extreme poverty. On the other hand, there are a number of billionaires who don't even pay tax. Mexico has some amazing beaches (Acapulco, Yucatán) and a great deal of Aztec history making it a popular tourist destination. It is not, however, a popular elective destination. This is probably because of the definite need for fluent Spanish. For this reason only a few hospitals and the major medical schools are outlined below.

Medicine:

There are two main healthcare institutions; the **Mexican Institute of Social Security (IMSS)** which has recently been privatized, and the **Institute of Social Service and Security for State Employees (ISSSTE)**. ISSSTE is the public welfare system and is government-funded. It provides health services, gives loans, pensions and sets health and safety standards. Mexico is renowned for having good surgery and dentistry, but this is really only in the private sector. There is a mixture of 'developed country' diseases amongst the rich and infectious diseases, including TB, amongst the poor. What you see will depend on where you go.

Visas and work permits:

The Embassy states that students need a Student Entry Permit requiring:

- Passport (valid for more than one year)
- Application form completed
- Letter of acceptance from a University in Mexico
- Letter indicating you can fund yourself (minimum US$500/month)
- Photographs (six full-face and five right-side profile)

You have to go personally to the Consular Office to sign and fingerprint the entry document.

Working in Mexico: Obtaining a visa for short-term work (less than six months) is extremely difficult. If you have an offer of work from a Mexican Institute they should apply to the immigration authorities in Mexico City to issue a working visa. This can take some time. Contact the Mexican embassy for more details. Visit: http://mexico.web.com.mx/ and www.trace-sc.com/

USEFUL ADDRESS:

The International Relations Department of the Health Ministry: Secretaría de Salud, Dirección General de Asuntis se Asuntos Internacionales, Dr Rafael Alvarez Cordero, Director General, Francisco P Miranda No 177–4o piso 06100 Mexico, DF Tel: (525) 651 0828 Fax: (525) 583 0833 www.ssa.gob.mex

THE MAIN MEDICAL SCHOOLS:

Mexico City

Escuela Nacional de Medicina y Homeopatia, Arroyo de Guadelupe No 239, Fraccionamiento 'La Escalera', Colonia Ticomán, 07320 México.

Universidad Autónoma Metropolitana, División de Ciencias Biológicas y de la Saud, Unidad Zochimilco, Calzada del Hueso No 1100, Colonia Villa Quietud, Delegación Coyoacán, 04960 México 21.

Universidad La Salle, Escuela Mexicana de Medicina, Fuentes 31, Tlalpan, Apartado Postal 22271, 14000 México.

Universidad National Autónoma de México, Facultad de Medicina, Ciudad Universitaria, México 20. (This is the oldest and probably the largest medical school in Mexico, founded in 1572.)

OTHER MEDICAL SCHOOLS:

Universidad Autónoma de Baja California, Escuela de Medicina, Calle los Misioneros, Centro Civico Comercial de Mexicali, 21000 Mexicali, Baja California Norte, Mexico.

Universidad Autónoma 'Benito Juárez' de Oxaca, Escuela de Medicina y Cirugía, Calzada Porfirio Díaz, Oxaca de Juárez, Oxaca, Mexico.

Universidad Autónoma de Chihuahua, Facultad de Medicina, Avenida Colón y Rosales, Apartado Postal 1090, Chihuahua, Mexico.

Universidad Autónoma de Coahuila, Escuela de Medicina, Francisco Murguia Sur No. 205, 25000 Saltillo, Coahuila, Mexico.

Universidad de Guadalajara, Facultad de Medicina, Centro Médico, Colonia Independencia, Guadalajara, Jalisco, Mexico.

Universidad de Guanajuato, Facultad de Medicina de León, 20 de Enero 929, 37000 León, Guanajuato, Mexico.

Universidad Autónoma de Guerrero, Escuela de Medicina, Avenida Ruz Cortinez, Acapulco, Guerrero, Mexico.

Universidad Autónoma de Nuevo León, Facultad de Medicina, Apartado Postal 1563, Avenida Francisco I, Madero 64460 Monterrey, Neuvo León, Mexico.

Universidad Autónoma de Tamaulipas, Facultad de Medicina, Centro Universitario Tampico Madero, Apartado Postal C-33, 89339 Tampico, Veracruz, Mexico.

Universidad de Yucatán, Facultad de Medicina, Avenida Itzáez No. 498, Apartado Postal 1225, Mérida, Yucatán, Mexico.

Universidad Juáeez del Estado de Durango, Escuela de Medicina Humana, Avenida Universidad y Fanny Anitúa, Apartado Postal 229, 34000 Durango, Mexico.

Universidad Valle del Bravo, Escuela de Medicina, Hospital Universitario, Calle Septima y Rio Mante, Colonia Longoria, Ciudad Reynosa, Tamaulipas, Mexico.

Universidad Veracruzana, Facultad de Medicina, Sedán e Iturbide, Veracruz, Mexico.

RURAL WORK:

Programa de Ampliacion de Cobertura (PAC)

Jurisdiccion, Orizaba, Veracruz, Mexico

PAC is an initiative founded in 1996 by the Mexican Secretariat of Health to take basic health services and health education to the most isolated indigenous communities of the country. The initiative started in just one state (Veracruz). From a base in the city of Orizaba, ten 'modules', each consisting of about 6 individuals – doctors, nurses, dentists and social workers, disperse each Monday morning to their own substation, often many hours' drive up into the mountains. One such settlement is a tiny community called Tehuilango. From here each morning the team walks for 2–3 hours to little Indian settlements on the hills to hold a clinic and various education seminars. These rural people are incredibly tough and most of the time is spent educating, vaccinating, pulling teeth and suturing. As secondary referral is virtually impossible, serious but otherwise treatable conditions (such as obstetric complications) are often fatal.

Nicaragua

Population: 4.5 million
Language: Spanish
Capital: Managua
Currency: Córdoba oro
Int Code: +505

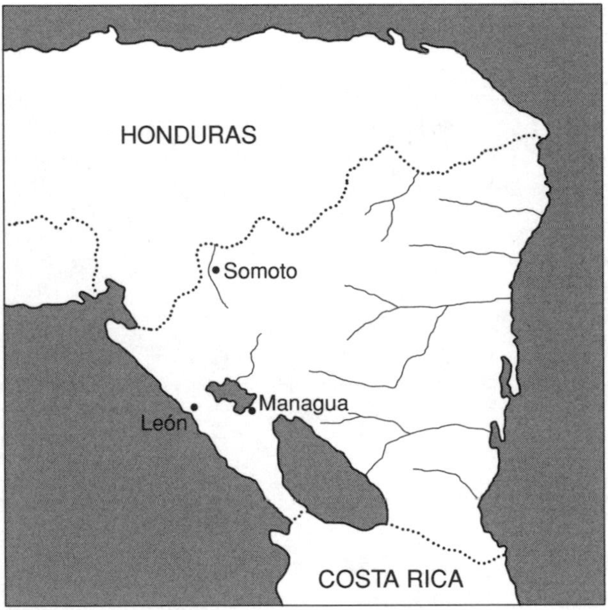

Nicaragua lies in the heart of Central America and has ocean to the east and west. It is the poorest country in Central America (some places won't be able to afford a stamp to write back to you) as a result of 40 years of dictatorship then an 11-year civil war. Despite that, Nicaragua is a beautiful place and well worth visiting. You must be very confident in your Spanish as no one speaks a word of English. It is not a common elective destination because of this. The Nicaragua Health Fund (83 Margaret Street, London W1N 7NB) can arrange electives with the medical school in Managua and also work in rural health centres.

Medicine:

Infectious diseases, especially TB, are common. Violence and accidents also provide plenty of work. Nicaragua has two medical schools, one in León, one in Managua.

Climate:

Nicaragua has a tropical climate, being particularly hot between March and

May. The occasional hurricane and earthquake make it that bit more exciting.

Managua

Universidad Nacional Autónoma de Nicaragua

Facultad de Ciencias Médicas, Managua, Nicaragua.

This is the medical school for the capital. (*see above* for electives here).

León

Universidad Cacional Autónoma de Nicaragua

Facultad de Ciencias Médicas, León, Nicaragua.

This is an old medical school that uses:

Hospital Escuela Dr Oscar

Danilo Rosales Arguello, León, Nicaragua.

The hospital: An extremely busy tertiary referral centre in Nicaragua's second-largest city. Conditions are very grim but it is an incredible experience. Lots of tropical pathology and practical procedures for students. Not many investigations. Doctors get paid $30/month here. León is 20 mins from the coast.

RURAL WORK:

Centro de Solvo

'Jaro Bismark Moncada', Somoto Madriz, Nicaragua.

The hospital: A health centre in the mountains on the border with Honduras. It is in Madriz, the poorest area of Nicaragua and it is incredibly poor. The medicines are provided by charity and the doctors do very well with their limited resources. Many patients have to walk for three days to get here. Lots of malaria, TB, dengue fever and other tropical diseases. It's very busy. There are also mobile clinics to surrounding areas. An excellent elective experience. Highly recommended if you have good Spanish.

Paraguay

Population: 5 million
Languages: Spanish and Guaraní
Capital: Asunción
Currency: Guaraní
Int Code: +595

Paraguay has only recently struggled out of a military dictatorship. It is a landlocked country with the River Paraguay dividing it. In the east are hills and fields that are home to 90% of the people. In the west (Chaco) it is virtually uninhabited. It is not a popular elective destination presumably because of the need for fluent Spanish.

✪ Medicine:

Basic sanitation is still not available with only a third of people being able to access safe drinking water. Resources are really only available in Asunción where over half of the county's hospital beds are. Infectious diseases (including TB) and obstetric complications are commonly seen.

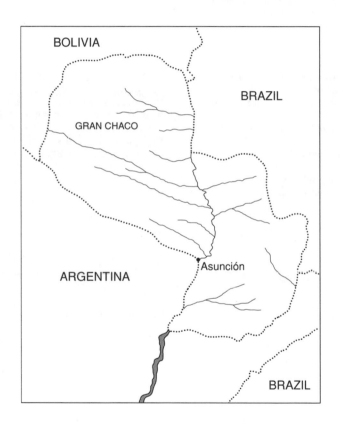

Visas and work permits:
No clear information on requirements for electives can be obtained. A tourist visa at least will be needed. The embassy then states the following: To permanently reside in Paraguay you would need:

- A passport
- Good Conduct certificate from your police
- Birth certificate
- Marriage certificate
- A special certificate from the Department of Informatica if over 18
- A good conduct certificate from INTERPOL in Asunción (Cnel Gracia 468 y Tte Rodi)
- A health certificatc
- A certificate of life from the local police (!)
- Proof of legal entrance issued by customs
- Two passport photos
- A tourist visa from the Paraguayan Consulate.

If there temporarily, the embassy claims you need all the above plus a letter from the employer or a copy of the labour contract with the Certificate of Studies or degree. You are best to contact the embassy yourself.

USEFUL ADDRESS:

The Ministry of Health, Ministerio de Salud Publica y Bienestar Social, Av Pettirossi y Brasil, Asunción, Paraguay Tel: 21 207 328 Fax: 21 206 700.

MEDICAL SCHOOL:

Universidad Nacional de Asunción, Facultad de Ciencias Médicas, Casilla de Correo No 1102, Avenida Dr Montero 658, Asunción, Paraguay. (Founded 1898.)

HOSPITALS:

Barrio Oberero, Yegros y 11 Pdta, Asunción, Paraguay Tel: (21) 72 989.
Cruz Roja, Brasil 216 or José Berges c/Brasil, Asunción, Paraguay Tel: (21) 200 004/22 797/208 199.
Hijas de la Caridad, Dr Montero y Lagerenza, Asunción, Paraguay Tel: (21) 42 0868.
Hospital Bauista, Rca Argentina y Campos Cervera (RA), Asunción, Paraguay Tel: (21) 600 171 Fax: 21 602212.
Hospital de Clinicas, Dr Montero y Lagerenza, Asunción, Paraguay Tel: (21) 420 982/420 983.
Hospital Nacional de Itagua, Itagua, Paraguay Tel (24) 450 Fax: (24) 459.
Hospital Privado Frances, Brasilia e/Insurralde, Asunción, Paraguay Tel: (21) 295 250.
Hospital Privado Salem, Colon y Holanda, Asunción, Paraguay Tel: (21) 80 199/80 532.
Instituto del Cancer y del Quemado, Paraguay Tel: (291) 227/242.
Lacimet, Avda, Venezuela, Asunción, Paraguay Tel: (21) 292 652.
Metropolitano SRL, Tte Ettiene c/Ruta Mcal Estigarribia, Asunción, Paraguay Tel: (.21) 501 270.
Militar Central, Gral Diaz y Don Bosco, Asunción, Paraguay Tel: (21) 494 601.
Pediatrico, Taruma 1038, Asunción, Paraguay Tel: (21) 552 459.
Primeros Auxilios, Brasil e/FR Moreno y M Dominguez,. Asuncion, Paraguay Tel: (21) 203 113.
Samaritano, Fdo de la Mora 2248 (RA), Asunción Paraguay Tel: (21) 550 121.
Sanatorio Juan Max Boettner, Avda Venezuela y Sol, Asunción, Paraguay Tel: (21) 290 288.
Universitario NTRA SRA de fa Asunción, Lilio y E Miranda, Asunción, Paraguay Tel: (21) 602 236.

Peru

Population: 24 million
Languages: Spanish, Quechua and Aymará
Capital: Lima
Currency: New sol
Int Code: +51

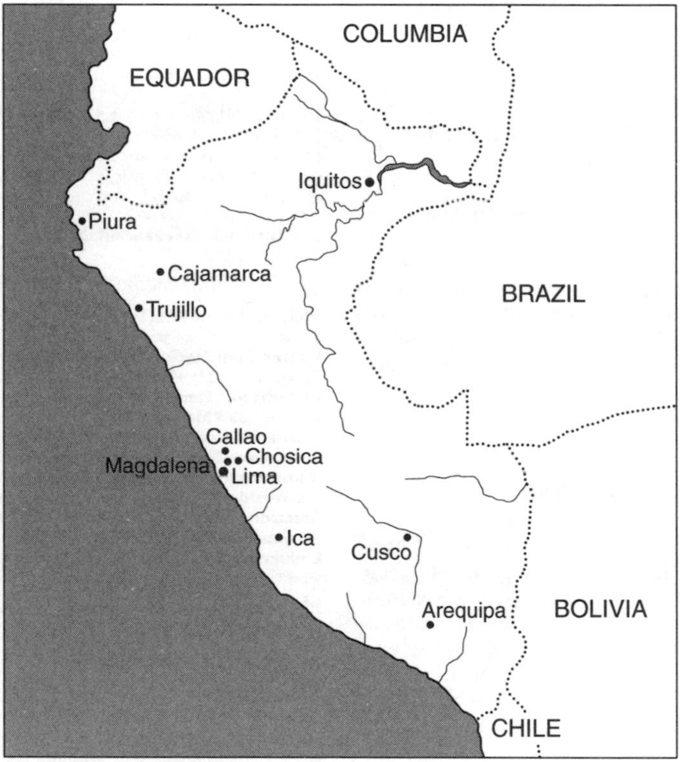

Situated on the west coast of South America, Peru has fame from themes as diverse as its great Inca Empire to Paddington Bear. Until relatively recently it has had a turbulent economic and political history, although since the election of Alberto Fujimori in 1990 the situation has improved greatly. Fifty per cent of Peru's 24 million live in rural areas. Seven million live in Lima. The population structure contains 50% Indian, 33% Mesi. Food is cheap but dangerous. Travelling around Peru is best by air. A trip to the Andes is a must. The two official languages are Spanish and Quechua; however, there are a number of

different dialects in the jungles and highlands. You must have a good knowledge of Spanish, especially if going anywhere remote.

✪ Medicine:

Peru's public healthcare system has really gone to pot. There is no free cover and no GP service. On top of that, as social deprivation increases, infectious diseases are becoming more and more prevalent. Cases are often very advanced by the time they get to hospital. Malaria and TB are widespread and in recent years cholera has returned to epidemic proportions. You really need to go to a private clinic if you want good treatment. The lack of iodine in the mountains has also meant that between 40% and 90% of children get goitres.

➲ Visas and work permits:

Nationals of countries, including the UK, Australia, NZ, USA and most of Europe can stay for 90 days without a permit. They are required to have a return ticket. British volunteer workers should obtain a visa either before they go or once in Peru. Student visas can be easily obtained with a letter from the institution in Peru, a couple of photos, passport and a copy of your last bank statement. To work for pay, the institution has to apply to their department of immigration. If working for a charity their sponsors must apply to the **Secretaria Ejecutiva de Coperacion Technica International** of the **Ministerio de la Presidencia**. The Peruvian Immigration Service can then authorize a visa. Alternatively, you can go out as a tourist and apply for a visa when there. The Embassy can provide a list of clinics and hospitals across Peru.

✪ Work:

Most Westerners work through an international organization. Some that work in Peru include:

Comite Internacional de la Cruz Roja (CICR) (Red Cross International Committee). Av Juan d Aliaga 620, Magdalena, Peru.
Organizacion Panamericana de la Salud (Pan-American Health Organization), Los Cedros 269, Lima 27, Peru.
UNICEF, Parqe Melitón Porras 350, Lima 18, Peru.

USEFUL ADDRESSES:

Instituto Peruano de Seguridad Social (IPSS) (Social Security Institute), Av. Domingo Cueto 120, Lima 14, Peru.
Ministry de Salud (Ministry of Health), Av Salaverry Cuadra 8, Lima 11, Peru.

◎ Climate and crime:

There are a number of different climates, an arid desert with cool winters, the chilly Andes and the tropical Amazon Basin. It is warmest around Christmas time. Peru is not that safe and there are several no-go areas in Lima. There is the odd kidnapping.

MEDICAL SCHOOLS:

There are nine medical schools/universities in Peru, three of which are in Lima:

Universidad Nacional Federico Villarreal, Programa Académico de Medicina Humana, Colmena 412, Lima, Peru.
Universidad Nacional Mayor de San Marcos, Programa Académico de Medicina Humana, Casilla 529, Avenida Grau 755, Lima, Peru. (This is the oldest one, founded in 1856.)
Universidad Peruana Cayetano Heredia, Apartado 5045, Programa Académico de Medicina, Avenida Honorio Delgado 932, San Martin Porres, Lima, Peru.

Medical Schools outside Lima are:

Universidad Nacional de la Amazonía Peruna, Programa Académco de Medicina, Apartado 496, Iquitos, Peru.
Universidad Nacional de San Agustin, Programa Académico de Medicina, Siglo XX No 227, Apartado 23, Arequipa, Peru.
Universidad Nacional de Trujillo, Programa Académico de Medicina Humana, Independencia 431, Of 203, Trujillo, Peru.
Universidad Nacional San Antonio Abad, Programa Académico de Medicina Humana, Avenida de la Cultura s/n, Apartado 367, Cusco, Peru.
Universidad Nacional Técnica de Piura, Programa Académico de Medicina Humana, Prolongación Avenia Grau s/n, Apartado 295, Piura, Peru.
Universidad 'San Luis Gonzaga', Programa Acaedémico de Medicina Humana, Jr Dos de Mayo 187, Ica, Peru.

Lima

*Lima has suffered with overpopulation since the 1920s. It has become polluted, noisy, dirty and rife with theft. There are many shanty towns (*pueblos jovenes*) in poorer areas. These have come about as migrants have come in trying to find jobs. In some of these there is no electricity, water or adequate sanitation. This is a great contributing factor to spread of diseases. In recent years cholera has become endemic.*

The most popular elective destination in Peru is to the tropical medicine institute (**Instituto de Medicina Tropical Alexander von Humboldt**) which is associated with the Universidad Peruano Cayetano Heredia.

Instituto de Medicina Tropical Alexander von Humboldt (Universidad Peruana Cayetano Heredia)

Apartado 5045, Postal 4314, Lima 100, Peru Tel: (14) 823401 Fax: (14) 823404.

The hospital: In the outpatients department of this tropical diseases hospital you'll see leishmaniasis, brucellosis, typhoid, viral hepatitis, bartonellosis and other rarer conditions such as spider bites and free living amoebiasis. Hep B and HIV are also very common. The ward has 30 beds dedicated to tropical diseases and HIV. Facilities are sparse, but there are opportunities for practical procedures such as lumbar puncture.

O Elective notes: Conditions around the hospital, which includes many slums, are extremely poor, to the extent that interns often have to supply their own syringes and needles. Despite this, the staff are incredibly friendly and encourage you to get involved. They charge a fee of $300 per month for teaching. This is well worth it as you are unlikely to know much about the diseases otherwise. A good understanding of Spanish is essential. They can also arrange for you to spend a week in Iquitos in the Amazon jungle ($170 rtn flight, two hours north-east of Lima). There you'll see many cases of leprosy, snake bites and leishmaniasis. The hospital here (**Hospital Regional de Loreto**) again is very ill equipped, but the staff are welcoming.

Accommodation: Difficult unless you have relatives in Peru.

Hospital del Niño

Av Brasil 600, Lima, Peru.

One of the big general hospitals.

Instituto de Salud del Niño (Children's Hospital of Lima)

Av Brasil 600, Breña, Lima 5, Lima, Peru Tel: 424 1996 Fax: 425 1840.

The hospital: The first paediatric hospital in Peru. It has 600 beds and receives children from all over the country.

Cajamarca

Cajamarca is an Andean town in Peru's northern highlands 2700 m above sea level. It has a population of 70,000 and, although not a tourist spot, it is rich in Inca and pre-Inca history.

Hospital Regional de Cajamarca

Avenida Mario Urteaga No 500, Cajamarca, Peru Tel/Fax: 44 922414.

The hospital: Has 170 beds and serves a widely dispersed population of 150,000. There are regional outposts with nurses and junior doctors. There is no GP service so everything has to come to one of these. This may mean a few days' walking. Common conditions are TB (the national TB programme does free tests and treatment for anyone with a persistent cough to try to eliminate this), malnutrition and infectious diseases. There is very poor antenatal health care as even that has to be paid for.

Accommodation: One of the hospital secretaries has previously rented a room for around US$50/month (Jiron San Sebastian 332, Cajamarca Tel 0051 44 821660). Meals are free in the hospital.

Moyobamba

Moyobamba is a Spanish-speaking town of 25,000 people in the Peruvian jungle in the region of San Martin. It is on a plateau and therefore has a pleasant climate.

Asociación San Lucas

Apartado #2, Moyobamba, San Martin, Peru.

The hospital: Run by the Asociación San Lucas which is a medical missionary organization running a GP-type consultation service in the town with healthcare workers in surrounding villages. It provides a free service to under-fives and their mothers and gives basic advice on sanitation and nutrition. The medical/nursing team also visits the villages from time to time. There is a great deal of parasitic infection, nutritional problems, skin, chest, GI and urine infections. There is very much a Christian emphasis in the way things are done.

Accommodation: Usually arranged with one of the church in Moyobamba families.

OTHER PLACES IN PERU:

Asociacion Cristiana Femenina (YWCA), B Herrera 157B, Lima 14, Peru.

Clinica San Juan de Dios, Plaza Garibaldi s/n, Lima, Peru.

Comp Hijas de la Caridad San Vicente de Paul, S/n Hospital Dos de Mayo, San Martin, Lima, Peru.

Ejercito de Salvacion (Salvation Army), Colón 138, Callao, Peru.

Hermanitas de los Ancianos Desamparados (For old people), La Florida 339, Chosica, Peru.

Hijas de Maria Immaculada, Av El Polo 350, Monterrico, Lima 33, Peru.

Hogar Clinica San Juan de Dios, Km 1 Carr Central, Lima, Peru.

Hospital de Beneficencia de Maternidad, Clinica Sta Maria S/n AM Quesada, Lima, Peru

Iglesia Anglicana Episcopal del Peru, Chacaltana 114, Lima, Peru 18. Tel: 14 453044.

Obras Misioales Pontificias, Mrcal Miller 1524, Lima 14, Peru.

Puericultorio de Beneficencia Perez Aranibar, Av del Ejército, Lima 17, Peru.

Sociedad Francesa de Beneficencia, Centro Hospitalario Maison de Sante, M Aljovin 208, Lima, Peru.

Union Nacional de Ciegos del Peru (For blind people).

Venezuela

Population: 22 million
Language: Spanish
Capital: Caracas
Currency: Bolívar
Int Code: +50

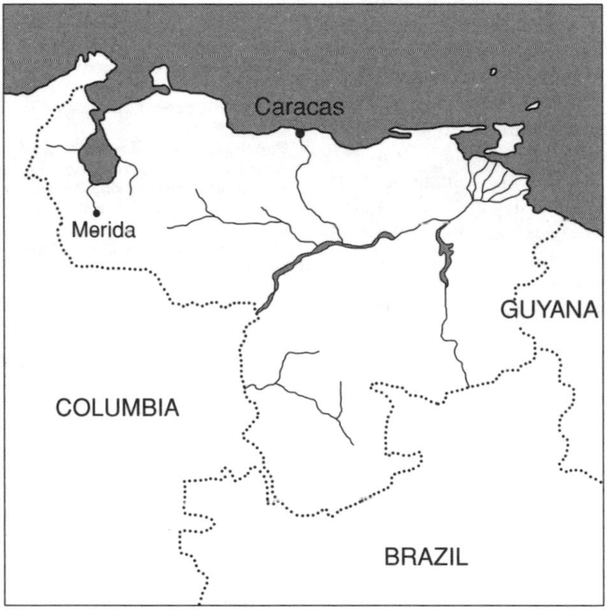

Venezuela is not a common destination. Most of its population lives in very poor conditions in shanty towns. It does, however, have large oil reserves so the economic situation may change over the next few decades. There's a lot to do in Venezuela: trekking and biking in the Andes, Los Llanos (the Plains), the Amazon basin, Gran-Sabana, Angel Falls, diamond mines and the Orinoco delta. Very fluent Spanish is absolutely necessary to work or do an elective here.

Medicine:
Most healthcare is concentrated in the towns and people from indigenous communities often have to travel long distances to receive treatment. Because of this, many conditions present very late. Venezuela has a reputation for innovative plastic surgery.

PLACES OCCASIONALLY VISITED:

University de Los Andes
Fac De Medicina, Calle 35, Edificio Palomon, Merida, Venezuela.
The hospital: A teaching hospital with

good teaching. They can also arrange trips to remote medical centres. There's plenty of tropical medicine. Public health is another strong point of the University.
Accommodation: In Merida guest-houses is $4–8 (2670–5340 VEB)/night.

Centro Medico Dolente La Trinidad (CMDLT)

Av Interlomunal El Hatillo, Apdo Postal 80474, Caracas 1080A Venezuela
The hospital: CMDLT is a plush private clinic run as an outpatients. All specialities up to plastics and ophthalmological surgery are catered for.

○ **Elective notes:** There are no other medical students and so you get a great deal of attention You can run exercise ECGs, pulmonary function tests, outpatients and help in theatre. There are many outpatients to be seen. Previously staff have helped arrange trips down the Amazon to help supply medication to rural communities.

Hospital de Los Niños

'JM De Los Rios', Caracas, Venezuela.
Although many have previously enjoyed time here, reports say they are not keen on elective students.

USA, BERMUDA and CANADA

United States of America

Population: 274 million
Language: English
Capital: Washington DC
Currency: US dollar
Tel Code: +1

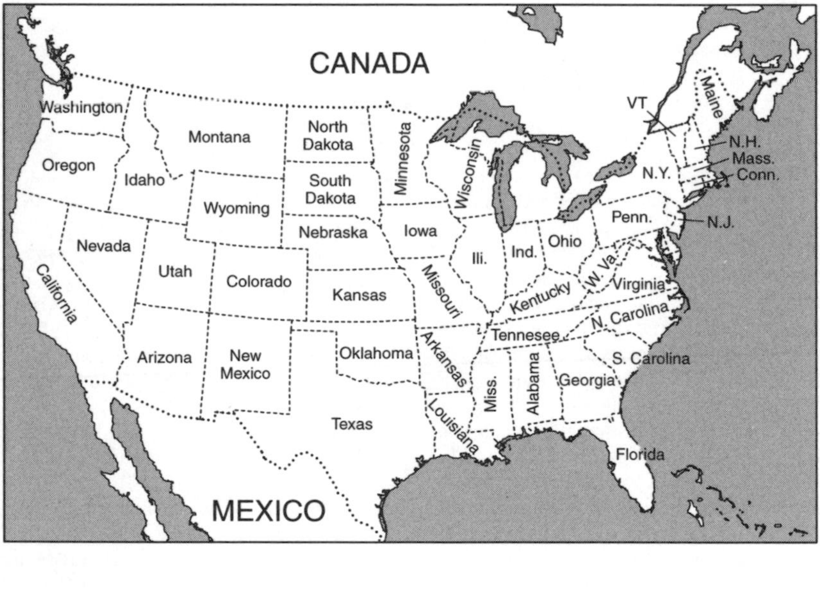

Little needs to be said about the USA. It's big. It offers many sites and activities in a high-tech First World setting. From California to New York, it has something for everyone. You probably already know if American-style medicine is for you. All 126 medical schools and the hospitals commonly visited are listed below. It is a popular elective destination and information is easily available on the net. That said, it doesn't make it easy to decide where to go. Each claims to be the biggest and best in everything. Every hospital and doctor has been named in a magazine (such as Home and Garden*) as being one of the top 10 in America. How will you choose? Look at the speciality you want to do and what there is*

to do in the vicinity. For nurses and other health specialists, virtually every single medical school listed also has a nursing school so just write to the head of nursing at the appropriate address.

Medicine:

The state of medical care in the US is well-known and is a constant problem for successive administrations. It has been described as a paradox of excess and deprivation. Although 11% of the GDP is spent on healthcare, 30 million Americans can't afford fees or insurance. There are four sources of funding:

- Patient fees (the very rich)
- Private insurance, with many clauses and limits
- Federal-funded Medicare insurance for the elderly and disabled which is not comprehensive
- State-funded Medicare insurance for low income families, although single people are not eligible (therefore one-third of children below the poverty line have no insurance).

The **Veterans Affairs Medical Centers** (VAMC) are a group of government-run hospitals (similar to the NHS) established to serve ex-service men, although they now also serve the general community. Despite these, three-quarters of US hospitals are privately owned. US physicians are renowned for using high-tech medicine and many investigations. The use of such tests is high principally because of the high rate of litigation. Patients also tend to be quite knowledgeable and can demand tests and since they (or their insurance company are paying) it's no skin off the doctor's nose. In some cases, the more tests done, the more the doctor gets paid. It really is a huge market. An 'accountant' in the ER counting up the number of cannulae and drugs used in a resus situation is not uncommon but seems strange to those from outside. All this does paint a rather bad picture. There are, however, many small hospitals outside the cities. Some are mentioned below, but a good list of hospitals in America is available on http://www.internets.com/mednets/hospitalsusa.htm

Overall, if you want first-class medical experience with cutting edge technology, the US is probably the place to be.

Visas, work permits and exams:

ELECTIVES:

Many students going to America only fill in the visitor's waiver on the plane that lets you stay there as a tourist for three months. Be very careful if thinking of doing this. The official line from the US Embassy is that you need a J1 visa (currently costing £30). There are a couple of reasons why it is a good idea to get a visa. Some institutions (especially large research places such as NASA) need to see the visa to give you a security pass. No visa will therefore ruin any elective plans. Another reason is if you get caught, you'll jeopardize your chances of ever being allowed to work there. For detailed information contact the United States Embassy (*see* Section 3: The Appendix). The Visa Information line is: 0891 200290 (50p/min to listen to it reeled off as slowly as possible) or 0991 500590 (a criminal £1.50/minute to speak to someone). They don't make life any easier if you try to visit them. You'll need an appointment (take everything with you, letters from the hospital etc.). For all these reasons think about getting a visa early.

A few students have been requested to have medical examinations before going to specific hospitals. This is on the whole unusual, but ask the hospital directly if you need to bring any documents. (A copy of your Hep B certificate and immunizations will always stand you in good stead).

WORKING IN AMERICA:

If wanting to work in America, then main problem is not getting in, but getting exams done to obtain licensure. The following are needed before you apply for a work permit:

- You must pass the United States

Medical Licensing Examinations (USMLE) (three steps, *see below*).
- Pass an English Language Proficiency test
- Pass a Clinical Skills Assessment
- You need all the appropriate documents from your country stating that you can practise medicine unrestricted
- The Educational Commission for Foreign Medical Graduates (ECFMG) will also need to confirm your medical credentials with your medical school

The USMLE itself does not give licensure, but the results are given to the appropriate state medical board who can then grant such licenses. Step one concerns basic biomedical science with emphasis on principles and mechanisms of health, disease and modes of therapy. Step two assesses the application of your medical knowledge to clinical science, including health promotion and disease prevention. Step three assesses how you combine your knowledge of biomedical science and clinical medicine to unsupervised patient care. All steps should be completed within seven years. A number of medical students are now doing the USMLE exams whilst doing their undergraduate course (steps one and two can be done before qualification). This has the obvious advantage that it's all fresh in your mind. If you didn't do them don't panic. There are excellent revision courses available specifically for them. A good time to consider doing them is after MRCP/MRCS, but you will also need to revise preclinical medicine and all the specialities, including paeds, psychiatry etc. For detailed information contact: the **Educational Commission for Foreign Medical Graduates**, 3624 Market Street, Philadelphia, PA 19104 USA Tel: 215 386 5900 or visit www.usmle.org or www.ecfmg.org

Contact the Embassy for information regarding work permits, but by far the biggest hurdle is getting licensed. This licensing makes short-term work opportunities near impossible, although there are plenty of research opportunities since no licence is needed for this.

MALPRACTICE INSURANCE:

For electives the best and simplest option is to ask the institution accepting you whether they can provide cover as they do their own students. Some will do this automatically, others may charge you for it. Some may give you an address of a local provider and a few will say that they don't take foreign medical students at all as they won't accept any cover you can get. With threats of '*Well, we take your students*' they may say that they will take you so long as your University takes full liability (which they won't). Another way around it is to ask for a purely observational elective (no touching!); this may be fine in psychiatry but is pretty stupid if doing trauma. Recently the MDDUS has provided cover. Contact your defence union to see if they can and enquire with your host institution as to whether they will accept their cover.

For working it's pretty simple. You need to either get insurance through the hospital or a recommended broker. The MPS and MDDUS recommend **Physicians Insurers Association of America (PIAA)**, 2275 Research Boulevard, Suite 250, Rockville, MD 20850, USA.

IMPORTANT NOTE ON ELECTIVES:

Some universities in America are incredibly elective-friendly ... no tuition fees and they cover malpractice insurance. Others are completely obstructive and charge exorbitant tuition fees no matter how long or short your elective. For example, Harvard charges over $2000 for a four-week elective. Although some students have said they have found the teaching worth it, many have found it a complete rip-off. If this becomes a problem, don't panic. There are ways around it. If you are threatened with extortionate fees try to find the name of someone in the department you want to visit (either through a hospital contact or from the www). Write DIRECTLY to them. They may then say that you have to go through the school. Try someone else. If you have real problems and a friendly Dean, ask them to write (they may say that they will charge their students silly figures to stop them coming to your medical school).

Note: Do try the medical school in the first instance as this makes it official and they can help with accommodation. There is one medical school that actually gives you a grant if you do an elective with them ....

◎ Climate and crime:
Climate varies considerably across this huge country from the sunny beaches of LA to the constant rain in Seattle. Crime rates also vary. Washington, New York and L.A. are the worst (or best if you want to do trauma).

Alabama

University of Alabama School of Medicine

VH100, Birmingham, Alabama 35294-0019, USA Tel: (205) 934 2330 Fax: 934 8724
www.uab.edu/uasom/
Initially founded in Mobile in 1859, the school moved to Birmingham (via Tuscaloosa) in 1945. Birmingham is now the main campus with medical divisions in Tuscaloosa and Huntsville.

University of South Alabama College of Medicine

Mobile, Alabama 36688-0002, USA Tel: (334) 460 7176 Fax: 460 6278.
Although the school was not running until 1973, the South Alabama Medical Centre has existed since 1831. This is the largest site of the university and has a level one trauma centre. Other associated institutions are the **USA Springhill Campus**, Cancer Centre, Health Services building, the **Searcy Hospital, Knollwood and USA children's and women's hospitals**.

Arizona

University of Arizona College of Medicine

1501N Campbell Ave, PO Box 245018, Tuscon, Arizona 85724-5018, USA
Tel: (520) 626 7383 Fax: 626 4884
www.medicine.arizona.edu
The college was established in 1967 and the main 30-acre complex (Arizona Health Sciences Center) comprises a number of facilities. Of specialist interest here are centres for cancer, cardiac care (they're big in transplants, especially pioneering artificial ones), arthritis and paediatric research.

POPULAR HOSPITALS IN ARIZONA:

St Joseph's Hospital Trauma Unit

West Thomas Road, Phoenix, Arizona, USA.
The hospital: A major trauma centre. It is very busy with many penetrating injuries.
O Elective notes: There's plenty of procedures to do and very friendly staff. Highly recommended. ATLS courses are run regularly and there are chances to go out with paramedics/firefighters.

Mayo Clinic Scottsdale

13400 East Shea Boulevard, Scottsdale, Arizona 85259 USA Tel: 1 602 301 4338 Fax: 1 602 301 8323.
The hospital: High-tech and advanced. Look under the Mayo Clinic Rochdale for more information.

Arkansas

University of Arkansas College of Medicine

4301 West Markham Street, Little Rock, Arkansas 72205-7199, USA Tel: (501) 686 5354 Fax: 686 5873 www.uams.edu
UAMS is the principal biomedical research centre for Arkansas. The college comprises the University Hospital (350

beds, state of the art ICU and ITU) and State hospitals, a Cancer Research Centre, the **Harvey and Bernice Jones Eye Institute**, the **Donald Reynolds Centre on Ageing, Arkansas Children's Hospital**, the **VA Medical Centre** and **Arkansas Rehabilitation and Radiation Therapy Institutes**.

California

University of California School of Medicine

One Shields Avenue, Davis, California 95616–8661, USA Tel: (530) 752 2717 www.med.ucdavis.edu

The school has existed since 1973. It mainly uses the 455-bed **UC Davis Medical Centre** (with level one trauma department) but has connections with the **Shriners Hospital for Children** and the **Ellison Ambulatory Care Centre**.

University of California, Irvine College of Medicine

Medical Education Building, Irvine, California 92697–4089, USA Tel: (949) 824 5388 Fax: 824 2485 www.com.uci.edu

The medical college of Orange County has existed since 1896 but became part of UCI in 1965. It consists of the UCI medical centre (with level one trauma, cancer, burns, transplant and neuropsychiatric centres) on-site and many affiliated hospitals. Research areas include neurosciences, oncology, imaging, neonatology, CVS, genetics and geriatrics. They have a well-organized elective programme on the web but charge $200 to international students.

University of California, Los Angeles School of Medicine

Box 957035, Los Angeles, California 90095–7035, USA Tel: (310) 825 6081 www.medsch.ucla.edu

Running since the 1950s, UCLA is associated with: the **University Medical Centre** (600 beds), **UCLA Ambulatory Medical Plaza** (with level one trauma centre and specialist intensive care and operating suites), **Mater Children's Hospital** (120 beds), the **Stein Eye Institute**, the **VA**, **Cedas–Sinai** and **Olive View Medical Centres** and the **Santa Monica Hospital**. UCLA has recently acquired the **Santa Monica UCLA Medical Center** (1250 Sixteenth Street, Santa Monica, 90404 Tel: (310) 319 4000) with 363 beds, an emergency centre, ITU, NICU and a facility for sexually abused children.

University of California, San Diego School of Medicine

Medical Teaching Facility, 9500 Gilman Drive, La Jolla, California 92093–0606, USA Tel: (619) 534 3880 Fax: 858 822 3067 www.medicine.ucsd.edu

The Medical School is surrounded by a wonderful variety of laboratory teaching and research facilities. Along with the UCSD Medical Centres (**Hillcrest** at 200 West Arbor Drive, San Diego, CA 92103 Tel: 619 543 622 and **La Jolla** at 9300 Campus Point Drive, La Jolla, CA 92037 Tel: 619 657 7000) it is associated with the **VA**, the **Naval Regional Medical Centre** and eight other hospitals and clinics. Details of their elective programme (costing $250.00 per four-week clerkship) are on their web site. Excellent research opportunities exist here.

University of California, San Francisco School of Medicine

Box 0408, San Francisco, California 94143, USA Tel (415) 476 4044 www.som.ucsf.edu

UCSF Medical Center (505 Parnassus Avenue, San Francisco, CA 94122, USA Tel: (415) 476 1000) is a 560-bed hospital near Golden Gate Park spilt between **Moffitt** (built in 1956) and **Long** (built in 1983).

Hospitals: Cardiac, neurosurgery and many other specialities are provided and the hospital has a great history for pioneering medical advances. **UCSF/ Mount Zion Medical Center** (1600 Divisadero St, San Francisco, CA 94115 Tel: (415) 567 6600) is a 365-bed hospital and is best known for its cancer center. UCSF is also linked to **San Francisco General Hospital** (724 beds) and **San Francisco VA Medical Center** (500 beds). UCSF has a commitment to increasing the number of doctors from minority groups and has links with Berkeley.

Loma Linda University School of Medicine

Loma Linda, California 92350, USA Tel: (909) 558 4467 Fax: 422 4558
www.llu.edu

Loma is a very Christian medical school founded in 1909. The campus has the **LLU Medical Center** (11234 Anderson Street, Loma Linda, CA 92354 Tel: (909) 558 4000) including a children's hospital. It has close links with the **LLU Behavioural Medical Center**, the **VA**, **San Bernardino County General Hospital** and the **Glendale Adventist Medical Center**.

University of Southern California School of Medicine

1975 Zonal Avenue (KAM 100-C) Los Angeles, California 90033, USA Tel (323) 442 2552 Medadmit@hsc.usc.edu

USC is a private, non-religious co-ed university that established its medical school in 1885. It is opposite the main teaching hospital, the **Los Angeles County and USC Medical Center**. There is also the 284-bed **USC University Hospital**, **USC Cancer Centre**, **Doheny Eye Institute**, **House Ear Institute**, an orthopaedic and the **Children's Hospital LA**.

Stanford University School of Medicine

851 Welch Road, Palo Alto, California 94304–1677, USA Tel: (415) 723 6861 Fax: 725 4599 www.stanford.edu

Teaching institutions include **Stanford University Hospital** (663 beds), **Lucile Packard Children's Hospital** (214 beds, 725 Welch Road, Palo Alto, CA 94304 Tel: 650 497 8000), **Palo Alto VA Hospital** (1000 beds), **Santa Clara County Valley Medical Center** (791 beds). The University Library has one of the most impressive medical collections anywhere.

POPULAR HOSPITALS IN CALIFORNIA:

San Francisco

With its Golden Gate Bridge and rich culture, San Francisco is often considered the most pleasant part of California. A sharp contrast to its nearest neighbour LA.

San Francisco General Hospital (SFGH)

1001 Potrero Avenue, San Francisco, CA 94110, USA.

The hospital: SFGH is a county hospital with the only trauma centre in San Francisco serving a population of 1.5 million. The Emergency department treats 70,000 patients a year from a diverse background, many homeless, IVDUs and alcoholics. It is world-renowned for having the first-ever inpatient ward for HIV/AIDS. This unit receives awards year after year and is leading AIDS research. There is also a large paediatric and genetics department.

O **Elective notes:** Like everywhere in California, medicine here is very serious ... you'll be expected to work long and hard. Four weeks in the ER is well-organized with (monitored) eight-hour shifts (4–5 days on, one day off), good teaching and a paramedic ride along. Plenty of procedures (suturing, central lines and manipulations under supervision) exist. Each day starts at 7 am with breakfast and a tutorial. You are treated as an integral part of the team and as such expected to conduct 'consults'. The HIV unit is repeatedly highly recommended. This is a 24-bed ward dedicated to the care of patients with HIV/AIDS. The friendly team on this ward provides an AIDS consult service. The function of this service is to assess and make recommendations on any hospitalized patient with HIV/AIDS. There are daily ward rounds and excellent tutorials. Outpatient clinics include dermatology (mainly Kaposi's sarcoma), ophthalmology for CMV retinitis and general follow-up. To get more involved in the AIDS programme in SF you can write to UCSF medical school but they may say you can't work there for insurance reasons. In that case write directly to the department: UCSF AIDS Program, Building 80, Ward 84, San Francisco General Hospital, 995 Potrero Avenue, San Francisco, CA 94110, USA Tel: 415 206 8313 Fax: 415 476 6953.

Accommodation: Tuition is free but accommodation is near impossible (try to make friends). The university can give advice but it's all expensive. You'll also need insurance.

If you just want to do paramedic work in SF try contacting **SF Dept of Public Health**, Paramedic Division, 2789 25th Street, San Francisco CA 94110, USA.

Los Angeles

Famed for 'Baywatch', a huge movie industry and a population of health freaks that jog every morning, you may wonder why LA needs hospitals at all. Fortunately there are also a lot of overweight couch potatoes providing the need for more cardiologists in one city than there are in the entire UK. There is also a huge (often illegal) Hispanic immigrant population that lives in poverty and in whom many diseases are far more prevalent. It really is a land of dichotomy, from the incredibly rich to the exceedingly poor.

There are two main teaching hospitals in LA, **LAC & USC Medical Center** and **UCLA Medical Center**.

LAC and USC Medical Centre

University of Southern California GNH 11900, 2025 Zonal Avenue, Los Angeles, CA 90033, USA.

The hospital: LAC and USC Medical Center is a state-run hospital and one of the largest acute-care hospitals in the US. It provides a huge range of medical and surgical services and it is a level one trauma centre with a busy ER.

Harbour-UCLA Medical Center

1000 West Carson Street, Torrance, California, USA.

The hospital: Harbour UCLA Medical Center is a friendly county hospital just south of central LA. If you can't pay, treatment is free and therefore it is mainly the disadvantaged that are seen. Many patients from Mexico have never seen a doctor before and hence it provides an interesting range of medicine. The hospital has 500 beds and most specialities are catered for.

O Elective notes: You are well-looked after in a medical consult team being given a couple of patients to assess and manage (with supervision). There are two interactive teaching rounds a day with afternoon lectures every day and many seminars so you're always busy. Don't walk around here at night as it's just outside South-Central. All doorways have metal detectors which tells you something.

Accommodation: Free and in the hospital grounds. There is, however, no heating, no kitchen and nowhere to wash clothes. Three generous meals a day are also provided. It is therefore a relatively cheap elective (until you go touring).

The Kaiser Sunset Facility

Sunset Boulevard, Los Angeles, California, USA.

The hospital: The tertiary referral centre for cardiothoracic surgery and interventional cardiology catering for a population of 2.5 million. It is run as a 'not for profit health management organization' which means you still need insurance to go there. It is an excellent place for an elective if you know you want to do cardiology.

Colorado

Most people who go to Colorado on elective are really looking for a place to go skiing. With that said the following places are recommended. See 'Something different' at the end of this chapter as well.

University of Colorado School of Medicine
4200 East 9th Avenue, C-297, Denver, Colorado 80262, USA Tel: (303) 315 7361 Fax: 315 8494 www.uchs.edu
Founded in 1883, the school now uses a number of hospitals throughout the Denver region and clinics throughout Colorado.

POPULAR HOSPITALS IN COLORADO:

University of Colorado Health Sciences Center
4200 East North Avenue, Denver, Colorado 80262, USA.
The hospital: The hospital complex caters for most specialities and has a busy ER, although the major trauma centre is at Denver General Hospital.
O Elective notes: Organizing electives here has been difficult in the past. In the ER students do four 10-hour shifts a week and there is plenty to do. Lots of procedures. They'll let you off to go skiing. Stay in Summit county where there are free buses up to Copper Mountain.

St Anthony Central Hospital
4231 West 16th Avenue, Denver, Colarado 80204, USA.
The hospital: One of a group of three private hospitals in Denver (there is another in the city and one at Frisco in the Rockies). It has a level one trauma centre (which isn't that busy) and a helicopter emergency service.
O Elective notes: The hospital does expect you to turn up (try to do four days on, three off) but it is excellent for skiing. You may well need a car though to get to some of the resorts. Allow £200/week for this.

BOULDER HOSPITALS:

Boulder is a unique enclave of science, research, education, sports and outdoor pursuits. At an altitude of 5300 feet and with 350 days of sunshine a year it attracts a great number of athletes for altitude training. The town has a population of 94,000 served by one large community hospital. The Rockies are on the doorstep with unlimited trails. Definitely the place if you like the outdoors. It is a university town (though there's no medical school).

There are a number of institutes as well as the main hospital. **Boulder Orthopedics** (933 Alpine Avenue, Boulder CO 80304) sees a great deal of sports injuries and is run by four orthopods. **Boulder Heart Institute** (2750 Broadway, Boulder CO 80304) is a private practice run by two invasive cardiologists. As it's private there are no waiting lists. Chest pain on Monday – angiogram on Tuesday – CABG by Friday. **Boulder Valley Oncology LLP** (1155 Alpine Avenue, Suite 360, Boulder CO 80304 Tel: (303) 449 9500) is a large private practice right next to the main hospital.
Accommodation: As it is a university town, there is plenty available. Expect to around $350–$400/month.

Connecticut

University of Connecticut School of Medicine
263 Farmington Avenue, Farmington, Connecticut 06030–1905, USA Tel: (860) 679 4713 Fax: 679 1282 www.uchc.edu
Founded in 1968 the school is part of the University of Connecticut health center consisting of a 204-bed hospital, an ambulatory unit and large library. It is affiliated with eight hospitals in Hartford and 11 community hospitals.

Yale University School of Medicine
367 Cedar Street, New Haven, Connecticut 06510, USA Tel: (203) 785 2643 Fax: 785 3234
http://info.med.yale.edu
The school was established in 1810 and forms part of the **Yale–New Haven Medical Center** with the nursing school and hospital. The local **VA**, the

Connecticut Mental Health Center, **St Raphael** and **Waterbury Hospitals** and **Yale Psychiatric Hospitals** are associates. It has a huge library.

POPULAR HOSPITALS IN CONNETICUT:

Yale is a particularly well-known university and hence attracts many students. Skiing in Vermont is also accessible and Boston and Washington are easy train rides away. To arrange an elective in any of their hospitals write to the Office of International Medical Studies, Yale University School of Medicine, 60 College Street, PO Box 208034, Newhaven, CT 06520–8034 or the address above. Visit http://info.med.yale.edu There is a $500 administration fee ($350 if only doing four weeks), but this gives use of all the academic and social facilities. Electives here have been highly recommended.
Accommodation: Can be provided in a dormitory adjacent to the school and New Haven Hospital for $110/week. It has good facilities. Many other students live here too so it's also good socially.

Yale–New Haven Hospital

New Haven, Connecticut, USA.
The hospital: A spacious modern (900-bed) teaching hospital with a large children's hospital attached. All specialities are catered for with high-tech facilities.

Washington DC

George Washington University School of Medicine

2300 Eye Street, Washington DC 20037, USA Tel: (202) 994 3506 www.gwumc.edu
The University Hospital has a number of research opportunities as well as providing teaching. **The National Naval Medical Center**, **Washington Hospital Center** and the **Children's**, **Fairfax**, **Holy Cross**, **St Elizabeth's** and **VA** Hospitals are also linked.

Georgetown University School of Medicine

3900 Reservoir Road, NW Washington DC 20007, USA Tel: (202) 687 1154 www.dml.georgetown.edu/schmed
The medical school (part of the oldest Catholic- and Jesuit-sponsored University in the US) works with the University hospital (389 beds) and nine federal and community hospitals. The Medical Center (the largest in the capital) has a concentrated care centre providing emergency, outpatients, surgery, X-ray and transplant facilities. The **Lombardi Cancer Research Center** is near and there are good sports and dining facilities close by.

Howard University College of Medicine

520 W Street, NW Washington DC 20059, USA Tel: (202) 806 6270 Fax: 806-7934 www.med.howard.edu
When founded in 1868 with seven students, Howard was the only black medical school in the US. Today it trains men and women from all backgrounds. Twenty-five per cent of black American doctors are from Howard. The University hospital has 321 beds. Other hospitals used are: **District of Columbia General Hospital**, **St Elizabeth's Hospital**, **US Naval Medical Center**, **Walter Reed Medical Center**, **Washington VA**, the **Providence**, the **National Rehab**, the **Washington** and **Prince George's** Hospitals.

POPULAR HOSPITALS IN WASHINGTON:

Washington Hospital Center

110 Irving Street, NW, Washington DC 20010–2975, USA Tel: 202 877 5190 Fax: 202 877 3173.
The hospital: The Washington Hospital Center is a large general hospital within a campus comprising the National Children's, the Washington Heart, the National Rehabilitation and the Veterans' Administration. Washington has the dubious privilege of being the most

violent city in the USA. Much of this trauma is still drugs-related (despite a clean up campaign) and commonly involves the poorer black population. **MedSTAR** (Medical Shock, Trauma and Acute Resuscitation) is the level one trauma centre within the hospital and it deals purely with major trauma such as gunshot wounds (20%), stabbings, beatings, RTAs (= MVAs, motor vehicle accident, 50%) falls and burns. It consists of seven patient bays and two helicopters. There are three surgical trauma teams (one civilian, one US Army, one US Navy) who work a 1:3 rota.

O Elective notes: Medical students make an essential part of the team with specific roles and jobs. These jobs are very varied, but can be mundane from stabilizing c-spines to writing the history and exam. The reward for this is being allowed to perform procedures from suturing to chest tubes, central lines and removing bullets for the truly keen. You'll be expected to be a house officer to 3–4 patients. Normal working hours are 7 am (ward round with the junior members of the team) until late afternoon and one night in three you'll be expected to assist (and don't expect any sleep ... they average 14 trauma responses a day). BEWARE OF THE AMOUNT OF WORK YOU HAVE TO DO (this cannot be overemphasized). You are there every day (including weekends) and average 80 hours a week. Despite this, there is time to see the city. The other students are from George Washington and Uniformed Services medical schools. This elective comes thoroughly recommended to anyone wishing to pursue a career in A&E or surgery. All specialities are catered for in other departments. Malpractice insurance is provided by the hospital.

Accommodation: Includes a swimming pool and satellite TV for $130/month although the rooms are shared and not that great. There is an excellent canteen (with Pizza Hut!). The area around the hospital is fairly dodgy and at night a taxi from the hospital to Georgetown or downtown DC is a good idea. During the day, the Metro to downtown is good. Washington is an incredible city with lots of tourist things to do as well as some good bars and clubs in Georgetown and at Du Pont Circle. There are usually a lot of elective students around and the American interns are very sociable, although they apparently insist on wearing white trainers to the pub!

Veterans Affairs Medical Center

(George Washington School of Medicine)
50 Irving Street NW, Washington DC 20422, USA.

The hospital: The VA is a large general hospital with most specialities.

O Elective notes: Expect to work hard, but it is a rewarding experience. Again, there is a great deal of responsibility. The endocrinology unit is friendly but will work you, expecting papers to be reviewed for journal clubs etc. In return you do see a great deal of medicine, diabetes, thyroid problems, Klinefelter's, Paget's, osteoporosis etc. You will be expected to write a six-page essay (remember this if applying for grants). Busy but highly recommended.

Accommodation: A major drawback. A retired couple rent out rooms (2045 Park Rd NW, Washington DC 20010). It's 20 minutes from the hospital and too dangerous a neighbourhood to walk through so a bus is needed. The accommodation itself is a room in a house. The couple are pleasant, and there are no other students. Go in a pair if you can.

Florida

University of Florida College of Medicine

UF Health Sciences Center, Gainsville, Florida 32610–0216, USA Tel: (352) 392 4569 Fax: 846 0622 www.med.ufl.edu

Founded in 1956, the University Health Center comprises the Stetson Medical Science Building, an academic and cancer research building, Shands Hospital, the Brain Institute and the VA Jacksonville.

University of Miami School of Medicine

PO Box 016159, Miami, Florida 33101, USA Tel: (305) 243–6791 Fax: 243 6548 www.miami.edu

This, the largest and oldest medical school in Florida, is next to the **Jackson Memorial Hospital** (3000 beds) in Miami (50,000 admissions/year). This, with the VA, provides most patients. There are also the **Mailman Center for Child Development**, the **Bascom Palmer Eye Institute**, the **Applebaum MRI Center**, the **Ambulatory Care Center**, the **UM Hospital**, **Diabetes Research Institute**, the **Sylvester Comprehensive Cancer Center** (the only one in Florida) and the **Ryder Trauma Center**.

University of South Florida College of Medicine

12901 Bruce B Downs Boulevard, Tampa, Florida 33612 4799, USA Tel: (813) 974 2229 Fax: 974 4990 www.med.usf.edu

Founded in 1971, the main clinical areas are the USF Medical Clinics, **Tampa General Hospital**, **Haley Veterans Hospital**, **Shriners Hospital for Children**, **Moffitt Cancer Center**, **Genesis Clinic**, **USY Psychiatry Center** and **Eye Institute**. It also has links with the **All Children's Hospital**, **Bayfont Medical Center**, **Bay Pines Veterans Hospital** (St Petersburg) and the **Orlando Regional Medical Center**.

Georgia

Emory University School of Medicine

Woodruff Health Sciences Center, Atlanta, Georgia 30322 4510, USA Tel: (404) 727 5660 Fax: 727 5456 www.emory.edu/WHSC/

Founded in 1915, the medical school has access to over 3000 beds in its teaching hospitals.

Medical College of Georgia School of Medicine

Augusta, Georgia 30912 4760, USA Tel: (706) 721 3186 Fax: 721 0959 www.mcg.edu

Founded in 1828 it is the eleventh-oldest medical school in the US. The main hospital used is the **Medical College of Georgia Hospital** with 80 speciality clinics and regional trauma centre. Elective details here and in rural hospitals are on their web site.

Mercer University School of Medicine

1550 College St, Macon, Georgia 31207, USA Tel: (912) 301 2600 Fax: 301 2547 www.mercer.edu

MUSM (founded 1982) uses Mercer Health Systems consisting of an ambulatory care facility, the **Medical Center of Central Georgia** in Macon, the **Memorial Center** in Savannah as well as the Medical Centers in Rome, Albany and Columbus.

Morehouse School of Medicine

720 Westview Drive, SW Atlanta, Georgia 30310–1495, USA Tel: (404) 752 1500 Fax: 752 1512 www.msn.edu

Founded in 1978 Morehouse is historically black. The affiliated hospitals include **Grady Memorial Hospital**, the **Tuskegee VA** (Alabama) and the **Southwest Community Hospital**.

Hawaii

University of Hawaii at Manoa John A Burns School of Medicine

1960 East-West Road, Honolulu, Hawaii 96822, USA Tel: (808) 956 8300 Fax: 956 9547 www.medworld.bomed.hawaii.edu

The school is on the Manoa campus and the **Leahi Hospital**. It uses hospitals and facilities throughout the state. Their web page has details of elective arrangements.

POPULAR HOSPITALS IN HAWAII:

Since full details of electives on Honolulu are given on the web page, it is not discussed here. If you fancy something a bit smaller try another hospital or another island:

Kaiser Permanente Medical Center

3288 Moanalua Road, Honolulu HI 96819, USA Tel: 808 834 5333.

The hospital: A fairly small, friendly, advanced hospital with 260 beds, a 30-bed CCU, six theatres, a cardiac catheterization suite and a very busy ER. It provides care for Kaiser Insurance Members throughout the Hawaiian Islands.

O Elective notes: Because of the insurance situation in the US you have to sign a contract saying that you won't do anything to patients. This immediately limits practical procedures. There are, however, plenty of patients to clerk and meetings to attend. It is very friendly and many people are keen to teach.

Hilo Medical Center

1190 Waianuenue Avenue, Hilo, Hawaii, 96720, USA.

The hospital: Hilo is a small place on a big island. The hospital is pretty small and probably less well-run than you might expect from an American hospital. It does, however, provide most basic specialities.

O Elective notes: The staff are generally friendly and there's lots of pathology to be seen, but don't expect everyone to be up-to-date with the latest technologies. Travel around the island, although public transport is incredibly limited. Check out the volcanoes, Waipio Valley, Kona side of the island (stay in Patey's place – cheap and cheerful), do some snorkelling and swim with the dolphins. At night you can whale watch too! It really is the travelling that makes this elective worthwhile. Hilo is pretty quiet … if it's nightlife you want go to Honolulu or Waikiki.

Accommodation: Do NOT let them put you in the hospital accommodation – apparently it's not up to much. Find a student flat with low rent. If you arrive early stay at Arnott's Lodge – a really friendly hostel. While you're there you can sort out the accommodation for the rest of your stay.

Illinois

University of Chicago, Pritzker School of Medicine

924 E 57th Street, BLSC 104, Chicago, Illinois 60637 5416, USA Tel: (773) 702 1937 Fax: 702 2598

http://pritzker.bsd.uchicago.edu

The University is in south Chicago (12 min from downtown) in the Hyde Park area. The school prides itself in producing academic physicians. The university is a hive of biomedical research. Hospitals used include the **University of Chicago**, the **Weiss** and the **MacNeal** hospitals.

Finch University of Health Sciences, Chicago Medical School

3333 Green Bay Road, North Chicago, Illinois 60064, USA Tel: (847) 578 3200 Fax: (847) 578 3284 www.finchcns.edu

Founded in 1912 and based in north Chicago, the school uses **Cook County Hospital**, **Edward Hines VA Medical Center**, **North Chicago VA**, **Illinois Masonic Medical Center**, **Swedish Covenant Hospital**, **Norwalk Hospital**, **Lutheran General Hospital**, **Mt Sinai Hospital** and **Henry Ford Health Sciences Center** (Detroit).

University of Illinois at Chicago College of Medicine

808 South Wood Street, Chicago, Illinois 60612–7302, USA Tel: (312) 996 5635 Fax: 996 6693 www.uic.edu/depts/mcam

Since its foundation in 1881, the University of Illinois College runs two parallel medical school programmes over four sites. The **College of Medicine at Chicago** is in the Health Sciences Center of the University. The **College of Medicine at Urbana–Champaign** is on a large campus with many academic and multi-faculty contacts. The **College of Medicine at Peoria** has many community hospitals and a modern campus and the **College of Medicine at Rockford** is central and has a number of hospitals.

Loyola University of Chicago Stritch School of Medicine

2160 South First Avenue, Maywood, Illinois 60153, USA Tel: (708) 216 3229.

Founded in 1870, this is a private and the largest Catholic university in the US. The medical school was organized in the 1920s and in 1969 the **Loyola University Medical Center** was built in Maywood, 12 miles west of the Chicago Loop. The centre has the school and the 570-bed **McGaw Hospital**. They also use the 1022 bed **Hines VA Hospital**.

Northwestern University Medical School

303 East Chicago Avenue, Chicago, Illinois 60611, USA Tel: (312) 503 8206 www.nums.edu

The Medical School (founded 1859) is on the University's lakefront Chicago campus and uses **Glenbrook** (100 beds), **Evanston** (420 beds), **Children's Memorial** (248 beds) and **Northwestern** (659 beds) hospitals as well as the **Rehabilitation Institute of Chicago** and the **Chicago VA**.

Rush Medical College of Rush University

600 South Paulina Street, Chicago, Illinois 60612, USA Tel: (312) 942 6913 Fax: 942 2333 www.rushu.rush.edu

Originally founded in 1837, **Rush Medical College** was closed between 1942 until 1971 when it was made part of the University of Chicago. Today it uses a number of institutions, including the **Rush–Presbyterian–St Luke's Medical Center** (1653 W Congress Parkway, Chicago, Illinois 60612, USA Tel: 312 942 5000) serving two million people.

Southern Illinois University School of Medicine

PO Box 19624, Springfield, Illinois 62794–9624, USA Tel: (217) 524 6013 Fax: 785 5538 www.siumed.edu

Founded in 1969, the college uses the **Springfield Memorial Medical Center** and **St John's Hospital**.

POPULAR HOSPITALS IN ILLINOIS:

Cook County Hospital

Chicago, Illinois, USA.

The hospital: A public hospital. The trauma department is famed as the basis for the ER TV series and is one of the best in the US. The staff are very friendly. There is a great deal of penetrating trauma (gunshots, stabbings) and motor vehicle accidents in this very busy department.

O Elective notes: There are excellent opportunities for many practical procedures. Teaching is also very good.

Accommodation: A list is provided. Note; The YMCA in downtown is full of drug-addicts. Try to arrange to stay with someone from the hospital.

Alexian Brothers Medical Center

800 Biesterfield Road, Elk Grove Village, Illinois 60007, USA.

The hospital: Alexian Brothers Medical Center is a private hospital situated about 10 miles west of Chicago. The hospital has about 500 beds and a staggering 470 physicians/surgeons on staff. The world of American private medicine is undoubtedly dominated by matters financial, but the Alexian Brothers has succeeded as a non-profit making organization to become only one of three hospitals in Illinois to be accredited with commendation by the AMA. Medical students are few and far between so people are keen to teach and there are many practical procedures to do, especially in the ER. Facilities are state of the art. This elective is thoroughly recommended.

Accommodation: And meals in the hospital (with own Pizza Hut) are provided free, but the lack of other students does limit your social life to those twice your age.

Indiana

Indiana University School of Medicine

1120 South Drive, Indianapolis, Indiana 46202–5113, USA Tel: (317) 274-3772 www.medicine.iu.edu/welcome.html

This is the medical school for Indiana (founded 1903) having centres in: Bloomington, Fort Wayne, Gary, Evansville, Muncie, Lafayette, Terre Haute and South Bend. The University is also a major research centre and has the University Hospital.

Iowa

University of Iowa College of Medicine
Medicine Administration Building, Iowa City, Iowa 52242–1101, USA
Tel (319) 335 8052 Fax: 335 8049
www.medicine.uiowa.edu/osac/osca.htm
Since its foundation in 1868 the college has become a major part of the state's health. The health sciences campus comprises: the University of Iowa Hospitals and Clinics, the VA and the Hardin Health Sciences Library. A new research/education facility is being built.

Kansas

University of Kansas School of Medicine
3901 Rainbow Boulevard, Kansas City, Kansas 66160 7301, USA Tel: (913) 588 5245 Fax: 588 5259
www.kumc.edu/som/som.html
Founded in 1899 the Medical Center campus includes the Leid Biomedical Research Building, the Dykes Library and the University Hospital (with 485 beds). A separate campus is allied to four Wichita hospitals.

Kentucky

University of Kentucky College of Medicine
Office of Academic Affairs, Chandler Medical Center, 800 Rose Street, Lexington, Kentucky 40536–0298, USA Tel: (606) 323 6161 Fax: 323 2076
www.comed.uky.edu/medicine
The college (founded 1956) is part of the University of Kentucky Chandler Medical Center on the university campus in Lexington. Hospitals used include the **University of Kentucky Hospital** (473 beds), the **VA** (662 beds) and hospitals throughout Lexington and Kentucky. The campus also has critical care, cancer, ageing and MRI centers.

University of Louisville School of Medicine
Abell Administration Center, 323 East Chestnut, Louisville, Kentucky 40202–3866, USA Tel: (502) 852 5193
www.louisville.edu
Founded in 1833 the school is part of the Health Sciences Center in downtown Louisville. Hospitals used include the 404-bed acute and trauma **University Hospital**, **Kosair-Children's Hospital**, **Jewish Hospital**, **Norton Hospital** and the **VA**. Also affiliated are the **Kentucky Lions Eye Research Institute**, **James Brown Cancer Center**, the **Child Evaluation Center** and the **Fazier Rehabilitation Center**.

Louisiana

Louisiana State University School of Medicine in New Orleans
1901 Perdido Street, New Orleans, Louisiana 70112–1393, USA Tel: (504) 568 6262 Fax: 568 7701
www.medschool.lsumc.edu
Since its establishment in 1931, the school has grown and now uses a number of buildings and hospitals principally the **Medical Center of Louisiana** and **University Hospital**. Outside, the **Medical Center** in Lafayette and the **Long Hospital** in Baton Rouge are used.

Louisiana State University School of Medicine in Shreveport
PO Box 33932, Shereveport, Louisiana 71130–3932, USA Tel: (318) 675 5190 Fax: 675 5244 www.sh.lsumc.edu/
Founded in 1969, the school uses two main hospitals, the **Louisiana State University Hospital** (650 beds) and the affiliated **Shreveport VA Hospital** (450 beds).

Tulane University School of Medicine

1430 Tulane Avenue, SL67, New Orleans, Louisiana 70112–2699, USA Tel: (504) 588 5187 Fax: 988 6735 www.mcl.tulane.edu

Established in 1834, this private non-sectarian school is in downtown New Orleans near the Superdrome and Vieux Carre (French Quarter). It uses the **Charity Hospital of New Orleans**, the **VA** and the **Tulane University Hospital**. There are also Public Health, Tropical Medicine, Bioenvironmental, Children's, Neurological, Cardiovascular, Geriatric, Cancer, Transplant, Women's and Sports centres.

Maryland

John Hopkins University School of Medicine

720 Rutland Avenue, Baltimore, Maryland 21205–2196, USA Tel: (410) 955 3182 www.med.jhu.edu

The school is a private non-denominational institution founded in 1893 which uses the **John Hopkins Hospital,** 600 N Wolfe Street, Baltimore MD 21287–4606. There is a school of hygiene and public health and a number of affiliated centres such as the **Krieger Institute** for children with brain disorders. Currently to do an elective in John Hopkins Hospital, the elective fee is £156 and insurance with them costs around £102. **The Sinai Hospital**, 2401 West Belvedere Avenue, Baltimore, Maryland, 21215–5271 is a 500-bed community hospital with strong links to John Hopkins School of Medicine. Teaching is of a high quality and it's recommended for electives.

University of Maryland School of Medicine

655 West Baltimore Street, Baltimore, Maryland 21201, USA Tel: (410) 706 7478 www.som1.ab.umd.edu

Being founded in 1808, this school is the fifth oldest in the US. It is on the Baltimore City Campus of the University (with law, science and other facilities) and next to the downtown Charles Center, Inner Harbour and Oriole Park. It has access to 2300 beds through various hospitals.

Uniformed Services University of the Health Sciences F Edward Herbert School of Medicine

4301 Jones Bridge Road, Bethesda, Maryland 20814 4799, USA Tel: (301) 295 3101/3720/30191(800) 772 1743 Fax: 295 3545 www.usuhs.mil

The USUHS was founded in 1976 to prepare health workers for the services. The school is in the Naval Hospital in Bethesda. It collaborates with federal health resources in Washington DC and serves to select medical officers. It's the same address for school of nursing. A few people who have done electives here have done intensive courses in ATLS, ALS and military medicine.

Massachusetts

Boston University School of Medicine

715 Albany Street, Boston, Massachusetts 02118, USA Tel: (617) 638 4630/5300 Fax: 617 638-5258 www.bumc.bu.edu

Originally the **New England Female Medical College** (founded 1848), the school became part of the University in 1873. The School with the University Hospital and other departments make up the **Boston Medical Center** (1 Boston Medical Center Place, Boston, MA 02118 Tel: 1 800 841 4325 Fax: 617 638 8000) a 547-bed private hospital and level one trauma centre in Boston's South End. It also uses Boston VA.

Harvard Medical School

25 Shattuck Street, Boston, Massachusetts 02115–6092, USA Tel: (617) 432 1550 Fax: 432 3307 www.hms.harvard.edu

The School (which has had 12 Nobel Laureates) has been based in the Longwood Avenue Quadrangle since 1906 although it was actually established in 1782. A number of hospitals are used. These include: **Massachusetts General**,

Children's, Brigham and Women's, Beth Israel Deaconess Medical Center, Mount Auburn, the **Dana-Farber Cancer Institute, Massachusetts Eye and Ear** and **Cambridge** hospitals. The **Massachusetts Mental Health Center** and the **McLean Hospitals** provide psychiatric services. Harvard Vanguard Medical Associates and others provide community facilities. Other institutions include: the **Shriners Burns Institute**, the **West Roxbury** and **Brockton VA Medical Centers** and the **Spaulding Rehab Hospital**. There are close links with the Massachusetts Institute of Technology.

University of Massachusetts Medical School

55 Lake Avenue, North Worcester, Massachusetts 01655, USA Tel: (508) 856 2323
www.ummed.edu

Established in 1962, UMass Medical School uses the UMass Memorial Medical Center comprising 761 beds over two acute hospitals and a number of community hospitals for its clinical teaching. UMass Worchester is next to the Biotechnology Research Park with a molecular medicine and cancer center.

Tufts University School of Medicine

136 Harrison Avenue, Boston, Massachusetts 02111, USA Tel: (617) 636 6571
http://tufts.edu/med

The University was established in 1852 although the medical school was founded in Boston in 1893. Thirty hospitals are associated and a number of departments, including the **New England Medical Center** (750 Washington Street, Boston MA 02111, a specialized diagnostic and referral hospital with paeditric trauma institute), the **Baystate Medical Center** (759 Chestnut Street, Springfield, MA 01199), a 700-bed centre providing comprehensive care to the million people in west Massachusetts, and **Faulkner Hospital** in Jamaica Plain, are used.

POPULAR HOSPITALS IN MASSACHUSETTS:

Boston

Boston is a great city, with good shops, public transport and nightlife. Most people go here because of the reputation of Harvard and the many world-renowned institutions.

To arrange an elective in any Harvard-associated hospital you're supposed to write to Harvard Medical School at the above address. The application form is available on the net: www.harvard.edu Alternatively, e-mail exclerks@warren.med.harvard.edu The application form gives you five or six choices. The big three hospitals are MGH, the Beth Israel and The Brigham and Women's. To apply you need to send $100 with a medical and a report of a clear CXR in the last six months.

The current fee to do a four-week elective here is a mindblowing $2100, and this goes up year on year. This gives full Harvard Student privileges (such as e-mail … woopy doo!) You also get a certificate to state that you've been to Harvard. It has previously also included malpractice insurance. If you happen to have this spare cash lying around or rich relatives, great. A number of people have said that the teaching is so good it is worth every dollar. Realistically though this is way out of most people's reach. There are ways around it although it is becoming increasingly difficult. A few scholarships exist. Ask Harvard or your own medical school for information on these. The most common tactic is to use a contact that someone in your hospital has. You need to apply directly to a consultant there. Many will turn around and say that you must apply through the school. Try someone else. There are lists of consultants in every department on the web. Don't give up. This is, of course, unofficial advice as the University expects students to apply directly though them. However, with charges as high as they are and while their students can visit other hospitals free, they should expect people to try to get round it. In general, an elective in any hospital here is hard work, but you don't pay that kind of money just to swan about Boston.

Note: Massachusetts General, the Brigham and Women's, the Children's, the Beth Israel and the New England Deaconess Hospitals as well as Harvard Medical School are in the Longwood area of Boston (*see* map on web site). It's a great area for academics, but there's not much else close by.

Accommodation: Usually provided in Vanderbilt Hall. Add another $700 to your bill for rent here. (It's a room with a desk but no sink or bedding). The hall is a good 15 mins from the city centre but is next to HMS and close to the Brigham and Women's, Beth Israel and the Children's Hospital. If you want a sink and a heated room, for the same $700 you can stay at Mrs Weinstein's Guesthouse, 48 Temple Street, Boston MA 02214 (Tel: 617 227 4062). Also try the YMCA in Charlestown (free shuttle bus to the MGH).

Full details of all the hospitals are given on the **excellent** web site www.hmcnet.harvard.edu and hence only addresses (and occasional notes) are given below.

Massachusetts General Hospital

55 Fruit Street, Boston MA 02114–2696, USA.

The hospital: Founded in 1811, the MGH now provides 820 beds and is renowned for being at the forefront of technology with nearly all medical and surgical subspecialities. Its emergency centres are on the main campus and in Chelsea.

O Elective notes: The ER has extremely good teaching and is well timetabled. Once the attending physician has seen you with a few patients you are allowed to see patients on your own and then just get them to review things. The trauma team is extremely well-trained and impressive to watch. In anesthetics the surgical ICU has good teaching and is very enjoyable. If interested in ICU this is worthwhile.

Beth Israel Deaconess Medical Center

330 Brookline Avenue, Boston, Massachusetts, MA 02215, USA Tel: 617 667 7000.

This is another large Harvard teaching hospital. It has excellent reports for cardiothoracic and plastic surgery, although both are very busy.

The Children's Hospital

300 Longwood Avenue, Boston MA 02115, USA. (This is the major paeds referral centre.)

Brigham and Women's Hospital

221 Longwood Avenue, Boston, MA 02115, USA.

The Shriners Hospital for Crippled Children Burns Institute

St Blossom Street, Boston MA 02114–2699, USA.

Some people have found they won't provide indemnity cover and there are few patients and so not much teaching.

Mount Auburn Hospital

330 Mount Auburn Street, Cambridge, MA 02238. Tel: 617 492 3500, USA.

A smaller, highly specialized community hospital in Cambridge but still under Harvard Medical School.

Whitehead Institute

Nine Cambridge Center, Cambridge, MA 02142, USA.

The Whitehead Institute has seven different research groups, including oncology. It is linked to **Massachusetts General Hospital** where clinics can be attended.

Accommodation: Book early as Boston is expensive.

Joslin Diabetes Centre

This centre offers good opportunities for those who want to do research.

Lahey Hitchcock Medical Center

30 Mall Road, Burlington, Massachusetts MA01803, USA.

The hospital: Very high-tech with good cardiology dept.

O Elective notes: There's the opportunity to see advanced procedures, but very little hands on (ECHO rather than auscultate).

Accommodation: Can be arranged usually in a private house.

The Veterans Administrative Hospital

1100 VW Parkway, West Roxbury, Boston, Massachusettes, USA.

The hospital: A very busy hospital about eight miles from the centre of Boston.

O Elective notes: It is associated with Harvard and hence there are many medical students around. It's hard work, seeing your own patients in clinic which you then discuss with a senior.

Accommodation: Has not been provided in the past.

Schepen's Eye Research Institute

20 Staniford Street, Boston, MA 02114, USA Tel: (617) 912 0100.

Schepen's is a major eye research centre, now pioneering retinal transplantation research.

The Massachusetts Eye and Ear Infirmary

243 Charles Street, Boston, Massachusetts 02114, USA Tel: 617 573 5520 Fax: 617 573 344.

Michigan

Michigan State University College of Human Medicine

East Lansing, Michigan 48824–1317, USA Tel: (517) 353 9620 Fax: 432 0021 www.chm.msu.edu

The CHM was originally designed to create more primary care physicians in 1964. The first two years of training are on the East Lansing campus then students are sent to one of six community hospitals (Flint, Grand Rapids, Lansing, Saginaw, Kalamazoo of the Upper Peninsula).

University of Michigan Medical School

Ann Arbor, Michigan 48109–0611, USA Tel: (734) 764 6317 Fax: 763 0453 www.med.umich.edu/medschool/

Covering 84 acres with 30 buildings, the medical centre claims to be the worlds largest one-site complex devoted to health education, research and clinical care. The university hospitals have 888 beds in total and treat over half a million patients a year. In addition to the University Hospitals, **St Joseph Mercy Hospital**, the **VA**, **Oakwood Hospital** and the **William Beaumont Hospital** are used.

Wayne State University School of Medicine

540 East Canfield, Detroit, Michigan 48201, USA Tel: (313) 577 1466 Fax: 577 1330 www.med.wayne.edu

The **Detroit Medical Center** houses the medical school, the Lande Medical and Elliman Clinical Research Buildings, the Harper-Grace, Hutzel and Children's hospitals, the University Health Center (ambulatory care), the Detroit Receiving Hospital, the Rehabilitation Institute and VA Hospitals. Outside, **SInai**, **Saint John**, **Oakwood**, **William Beaumont**, **Providence** and **Saint Joseph Mercy** hospitals are used.

POPULAR HOSPITALS IN MICHIGAN:

Providence Hospital

16001 West Nine Mile Road, 3rd Floor Fischer Centre, Southfield, Michigan 48075 USA.

The hospital: A world-leading institute for craniofacial and reconstructive surgery.

O Elective notes: It is very hard work but very rewarding. They show a great deal of interest in students. This is highly recommended to anyone interested in plastics, ENT or max-fax.

Minnesota

Mayo Medical School

200 First Street, SW Rochester, Minnesota 55905, USA Tel: (507) 284 3671 Fax: 284 2634 www.mayo.edu/education/mms/intro.htm

The Mayo Foundation and Mayo Clinic is the world's largest group practice and the medical school is an important part of it. The clinics (run as outpatients) are in three locations, Rochester (Minnesota), Jacksonville (Florida) and Scottsdale (Arizona). Four hospitals (St Mary's Rochester, Rochester Methodist, St Luke's, Jacksonville and Mayo Clinic

Hospital, Scottsdale, are linked for tuition and referral of patients (*see below*). All offer very high tech subspecialities. There are also rural health centres. There are great research opportunities with Mayo and due to the small class size, one-to-one teaching is common.

University of Minnesota–Duluth School of Medicine

10 University Drive, Duluth, Minnesota 55812, USA Tel: (218) 726 8511 Fax: 726 6235 www.d.umn.edu/medweb/

UMD provides two years' preclinical training before students are transferred to the University of Minnesota Medical School for the clinical component. Links are with the **St Mary's/Duluth Clinic**, **Miller–Dwan Medical Centers** and **St Luke's Hospital**.

University of Minnesota Medical School – Minneapolis

420 Delaware Street, SE, Minneapolis, Minnesota 55455–0310, USA Tel: 612 625 3622 Fax: 612 626 6800 www.med.umn.edu

The school is on the Minneapolis campus of the University of Minnesota and part of the University of Minnesota Academic Health Center with which all the major hospitals in the Minneapolis–St Paul area are associated (*see* University of Minnesota Hospital below).

POPULAR HOSPITALS IN MINNESOTA:

Mayo Medical School and its Hospitals

200 First Street SW, Rochester, Minnesota 55902, USA Tel: (507) 284 3671 Fax: 284 2634.

The medical school has only 40 places/year, but 4000 applicants. This tells you what type of institution it is.

The hospital: The Mayo clinics are renowned for their excellence all over the world. The Rochester was the first but two others (Jacksonville, Florida and Scottsdale, Arizona) have followed. It has a multidisciplinary approach and is an international forerunner for thoracic surgery. One-third of patients seen are under Medicare. The Rochester site encompasses the clinic (OPD), **St Mary's Hospital**, 1216 Second Street, SW Rochester, MN 55905 and **Rochester Methodist Hospital**, 201 Center St W, Rochester, MN 55905. St Mary's Hospital was founded in 1883 by Mother Mary Alfred Moes on the condition that the Mayo family provide the medical care. It had 27 beds. The 1157-bed hospital today is leading the way in many fields and many specialities: neurosurgery, cardiac and lung transplants and rehab to name a few. It has a trauma unit with Mayo One, Minnesota's air ambulance. There are eight ICUs! Rochester Methodist Hospital, with 794 beds and 34 operating rooms, provides liver, kidney, pancreas and bone marrow transplant services, O&G and dermatology departments among other specialities.

O Elective notes: The facilities and doctors are outstanding, though surprisingly not intimidating. No one tries to impress you . . . they don't need to. There are opportunities to do research if you wish. You are a total team member and that includes beers after work, ice-skating, skiing etc. This is an excellent package although the hours can be very long. Thoracics has excellent staff and teaching although you start around 6 am. The patients get superb care. The major setback is that Rochester doesn't have much entertainment. Try to meet up with friends. There is an application fee of $US50 but no elective fees, and malpractice insurance is covered by the Mayo.

Accommodation: The Mayo compiles a list of private homes that elective students can stay at for very reasonable rates. Alternatively, you can stay at the Kahler hotel for a very reduced rate.

University of Minnesota Hospital

Minneapolis, Minnesota, USA.

The hospital: The major teaching hospital for the university and accordingly has all specialities.

O Elective notes: To come here write to the **Office of Curriculum Affairs** at the medical school address. Like many American Hospitals, electives here tend to consist of long days and hard work although it is very friendly and they understand you want to go sightseeing. Indemnity cover is provided for around £70.

Accommodation: The university is very helpful in organizing this.

Mississippi

University of Mississippi School of Medicine

2500 North State Street, Jackson, Mississippi 39216–4505, USA Tel: (601) 984 5010 Fax: 984 5008 www.umsmed.edu

Since 1955, the school has used the University of Mississippi Medical Center in Jackson which comprises the 593-bed University Hospital. The **Guyton Research Building** and **Batson Children's Hospital** are also on campus. The **VA** and **McBryde Rehab Center for the Blind** are also linked.

Missouri

University of Missouri–Columbia School of Medicine

One Hospital Drive, Columbia, Missouri 65212, USA Tel: (573) 882 2923 Fax: 884 4808 www.hsc.missouri.edu

Established in 1872, the school is on the Columbia Campus with the Health Sciences Center comprising: the **University Hospital**, the **Truman VA**, the **Mid-Missouri Mental Health Center**, **Rusk Rehab Center**, **Mason Institute of Ophthalmology**, **Cosmopolitan International Diabetes Center** and the **Ellis–Fischel Cancer Center**. In total there are 1000 beds. Affiliations with clinics and hospitals outside are also maintained.

University of Missouri–Kansas City School of Medicine

2411 Holmes, Kansas City, Missouri 64108, USA Tel: (816) 235 1870 Fax: 235 5277 http://research.med.umkc.edu

The Medical School (established in 1969) is on the Hospital Hill campus and is near other colleges in the University and community hospitals.

Saint Louis University School of Medicine

1402 South Grand Boulevard, St Louis, Missouri 63104, USA Tel: (314) 577 8205 Fax: 577 8214 www.slu.edu/colleges/med/

The school was initially privately endowed by the Jesuits in 1818. The **University Hospital**, the **Wohl Memorial Mental Health Institute**, **Busch Eye Institute** and **Cardinal Glennon Hospital for Children** are on-site. Affiliations are with the Deaconess, DePaul, St John's Mercy and St Mary's Medical Centers and the St Louis VA.

Washington University School of Medicine

660 South Euclid Avenue, #8107, St Louis, Missouri 63110, USA Tel: (314) 362 6857 Fax: 362 4658 http://medschool.wustl.edu

Since its establishment in 1891, the Washington University Medical Center has grown to 230 acres housing the **Barnes-Jewish Hospital** (1737 beds), the **St Louis Children's Hospital** (a leading hospital) and the **Central Institute for the Deaf**.

Nebraska

Creighton University School of Medicine

2500 California Plaza, Omaha, Nebraska 68178, USA Tel: (402) 280 2799 Fax: 280 1241 www.creighton.edu

The School, founded by Jesuits in 1892, uses St Joseph's Hospital (403 beds) as its main teaching hospital. The **Children's Memorial**, **VA** and **Alegent Health System** hospitals are also used.

University of Nebraska College of Medicine

986585 Nebraska Medical Center, Omaha, Nebraska 68198–6585, USA Tel: (402) 559 2259 Fax: 559 4148 www.unmc.edu/UNCOM/index.html

Founded in 1880, the college uses the Nebraska Health System (**University Hospital** and **Clarkson Hospital**), **University Geriatric Center**, **Eppley Cancer Research Institute** and the **Meyer Children's Rehab Institute** as well as the **VA** and eight private hospitals. In total it has access to 2800 beds.

Nevada

University of Nevada School of Medicine

Mail Stop 357, Reno, Nevada 89557, USA
Tel: (775) 784 6063 Fax: (784 6194)
www.unr.edu/unr/med.html

This is a state-supported, community-based, university-integrated school that uses community medicine and primary care physicians as its teachers.

New Hampshire

Dartmouth Medical School

7020 Remsen, Hanover, New Hampshire 03755–3833, USA Tel: (603) 650 1505 Fax: 650 1614 www.dartmouth.edu/dms/

The School (the fourth-oldest in the USA, 1797) is part of the **Dartmouth Hitchcock Medical Center** (housing the Mary Hitchcock Memorial Hospital, Cotton Cancer Center and the White River Junction VA). The **Dartmouth–Hitchcock Clinic** is very large serving 1.5 million people with 372 beds. **Brattleboro Retreat** (VT), the **Family Medical Institute of Augusta** (ME), **Hartford Hospital** (CT) and **Tuba City Indian Health Service Hospital** (AZ) offer further instruction.

POPULAR HOSPITALS IN NEW HAMPSHIRE:

Littleton Regional Hospital

262 Cottage Street, Littleton, New Hampshire NH 03561, USA,.

The hospital: Littleton is a town in the north-east consisting of 12,000 people. The hospital serves this and the nearby small towns. Although it is small it is amazingly well-equipped in terms of both machines and people (25 consultants). For example it has a mobile lithotripsy unit, an MRI and a CT scanner. Their consultant staff cover many specialities (family practice, internal medicine, cardiology, radiology, oncology, gastroenterology, neurology, anaesthetics, ER, general surgery, orthopaedics, obs and gynae, paeds, path, ophthalmology, urology and psychiatry).

O Elective notes: There are no other medical students here, so the staff are keen to teach. You can organize what you want to do on a day-to-day basis and do as much (or little) as you want. Teaching is mainly in an outpatient setting although some consultants (e.g. in neurology) may well take you further afield to places such as the Dartmouth–Hitchcock Medical Centre for lectures and grand rounds. Everyone is very friendly ... if you're outgoing, people will always be asking you round for dinner. In the summer there are many outdoor sports and in the winter this is one of the great skiing resorts on the east coast. Public transport isn't very good, but there is a regular bus to and from Boston (airport) and other nearby major cities. It's four hours south to Boston, two hours north to the Canadian border. There's lots to do if you like outdoor pursuits. This elective has been highly recommended if you want to see a not-so-famous part of America which is nothing like the cliché of superficiality and commercialism often associated with the country.

Accommodation: And meals have been free; however, don't expect much as they have no proper accommodation for staff. There is usually an empty room on the medical floor. It's not too bad, with your own bathroom and cable TV.

New Jersey

UMDNJ-New Jersey Medical School

185 South Orange Avenue, Newark, New Jersey 07103, USA Tel: (973) 972 4631 Fax: 972 7986 www.umdnj.edu/njmsweb

The University of Medicine and Dentistry medical school moved to Newark in 1977 to be part of a huge centre containing preclinical buildings, the University Hospital, an ambulatory care centre and community health centre. **East Orange VA**, **Hackensack University Medical Center**, **Morristown Memorial Hospital**, the **Children's Hospital of NJ**, **Kessler Institute** and **Bergen Pines Hospital** are also used.

UMDNJ-Robert Wood Johnson Medical School

675 Hoes Lane, Piscataway, New Jersey 08854–5635, USA Tel: (732) 235 4576 Fax: 235 5078
http://www2.umdnj.edu/rwjms.html

The Robert Wood Johnson University Hospital (named after the president of the Johnson and Johnson company) is the major teaching facility. The **Cooper Hospital** and the **University Medical Center** in Camden also provide training. There are also the Institute of Mental Health, Environmental and Occupational Health Science.

A POPULAR HOSPITAL IN NEW JERSEY:

St Barnabas Medical Center

Old Short Hills Road, Livingston, New Jersey 07039, USA.

The hospital: A medium-sized private hospital with most specialities and an ER. Although not a level one trauma centre it is busy. It is well-known for its burns and renal transplant unit. The O&G and neonatal units also have a good reputation. This is a very safe area and Livingston is a nice suburb of New Jersey about a one-hour drive from Manhattan.

O **Elective notes:** There are plenty of opportunities to see whatever interests you. It is what you make it. From the ER you can go out with the paramedics and see the inner city hospitals.

Accommodation: Not available within the hospital itself.

New Mexico

University of New Mexico School of Medicine

Albuquerque, New Mexico 87131–5166, USA Tel: (505) 272 4766 Fax: 272 8239
http://hsc.unm.edu

Founded in 1964, the medical school facilities are on the North Campus housing biomedical research buildings, **UNM Mental Health Center**, a cancer center, **UNM Children's Psychiatric Hospital** and **Center for Non-Invasive Diagnosis**. The University of New Mexico Hospital has 421 beds and the **Regional Federal Medical Center** in Albuquerque (257 beds) is also used.

New York

Albany Medical College

47 New Scotland Avenue, Albany, New York 12208, USA Tel: (518) 262 5521 Fax: 262 5887 www.amc.edu

Albany was founded in 1839 and is therefore one of the oldest schools in the US. It is non-denominational and privately supported. The **Albany Medical Center** (43 New Scotland Av, Albany, NY 12208) contains a 631-bed hospital that serves the local community and acts as a tertiary referral centre for two million residents in east New York and west New England. Other hospitals are also linked.

Albert Einstein College of Medicine of Yeshiva University

Jack and Pearl Resnick Campus, 1300 Morris Park Avenue, Bronx, New York 10461, USA Tel: (718) 430 2106 Fax: 430 8825 www.aecom.yu.edu

This is a privately endowed, non-denominational college in the residential area of north-east Bronx. It serves populations from the Bronx, Queens and Manhattan using the **Jacobi Medical Center** (a municipal hospital) and four private voluntary hospitals, **Bronx Lebanon**, **Montefiore**, **Beth Israel** and **Long Island Jewish Medical Centers**. There are also biomedical research institutions and accommodation near and on campus.

University of Buffalo School of Medicine and Biomedical Sciences
45 Biomedical Education Building, Buffalo, New York 14214–3013, USA Tel: (716) 829 3466 Fax: 829 3849
http://wings.buffalo.edu/smbs
Initially founded in 1846, it joined the State University of New York (SUNY) system in 1962. Its campus is north-east Buffalo and uses nine hospitals in the area, including **Buffalo General Hospital** (742 beds with high-tech cardiac surgery facilities).

Columbia University College of Physicians and Surgeons
630 West 168th Street, New York, New York 10032, USA Tel: (212) 305 3595
www.columbia.edu/dept/ps/
Founded in 1767, the college was the first in the US to give official doctor of medicine degrees. It is part of the Columbia–Presbyterian Medical Center. This provides clinical teaching along with **Roosevelt–St Luke's Hospital** and **Harlem Hospital Centers** in Manhattan, **Bassett Hospital** in Cooperstown, New York and **Overlook Hospital** in New Jersey.

Mount Sinai School of Medicine of the City University of New York
Annenberg Building, One Gustave L Levy Place, Box 1002, New York, New York 10029–6574, USA Tel: (212) 241 6696 Fax: 828 4135 http://www.mssm.edu
Privately endowed and non-denominational the school was founded in 1968. The Medical Center has the **Mount Sinai Hospital** (1300 beds) and research laboratories. Additional clinical sites are throughout New York City, New Jersey, Westchester County and Long Island. Many institutions including centres for gene therapy, Jewish genetic diseases, neurobiology of ageing, transplantation and cardiovascular disease are associated.

New York Medical College
Sunshine Cottage, Valhalla, New York 10595, USA Tel: (914) 594 4507 Fax: 594 4976 www.nymc.edu
Founded in 1860 (originally as the New York Homeopathic Medical College), the College has a strong Catholic background. The campus is in Westchester, 25 miles from New York City. It uses hospitals throughout urban and suburban New York and regional hi-tech tertiary referral centres.

New York University School of Medicine
PO Box 1924, 550 First Avenue, New York, New York 10016, USA Tel: (212) 263 5290
www.med.nyu.edu
Founded in 1841, NYU now has many associated hospitals. The NYU Hospitals Center comprises the **Tisch Hospital** and the **Rusk Institute of Rehabilitation** (*see below*). **Bellevue Hospital** (First Av at 27th Street, NY 10016 Tel: 212 562 4141) is the original school hospital with many specialities. The **Hospital for Joint Diseases** (301 East 17th St, NY 10003 Tel: 212 598 6000) and **NYU Downtown Hospital** (170 William St, NY 10038 Tel: 212 312 5000) and many others are also associated.

University of Rochester School of Medicine and Dentistry
Rochester, New York 14642, USA Tel: (716) 275 4539 Fax: 273 1016
www.urmc.rochester.edu/smd
The School was founded in 1920 and the on-site facilities include the **Strong Memorial Hospital**, an **Ambulatory Care Center**, research centres and clinics. Five affiliated hospitals are also used.

State University of New York Health Science Center at Brooklyn College of Medicine
450 Clarkson Avenue, Brooklyn, New York 11203, USA Tel: (718) 270 2446 Fax: 270 7592 www.hscbklyn.edu
The college is a descendant of the Long Island College Hospital founded in 1860. It became part of the University in 1950.

It uses a number of major hospitals, including its own 406-bed **University Hospital of Brooklyn** (445 Lenox Rd, Brooklyn, NY 11203-2098).

State University of New York at Stony Brook School of Medicine Health Sciences Center

Stony Brook, New York 11794–8434, USA
Tel: (516) 444 2113 Fax: 444 6032
www.hsc.sunysb.edu/som/

Founded in 1971, the Health Sciences Center uses the 540-bed University Hospital.

State University of New York Health Science Center at Syracuse College

155 Elizabeth Blackwell Street, Syracuse, New York 13210, USA Tel: (315) 464 4570 Fax: 464 8867.

Initially the College was founded as the Geneva Medical College in 1834 and joined Syracuse University in 1872. It then joined SUNY (the State University of New York) in 1950.

Weill Medical College of Cornell University

1300 York Avenue, Box 144, New York, NY 10021, USA Tel: (212) 821 0560 Fax: (212) 821 0576 www.med.cornell.edu

The college, founded in 1898, is in New York, whereas the University is in Ithaca. Many hospitals are used including **The New York Presbyterian Hospital**, **New York Hospital Medical Center of Queens**, the **Hospital for Special Surgery**, **St Barnabas Hospital**, the **New York Community Hospital of Brooklyn**, **Memorial Sloan–Kettering Cancer Center**, **Flushing Hospital** in Queens, **Lincoln Medical and Mental Health Center**, **United Hospital** in Port Chester and **Cayuga Medical Center** in Ithaca.

POPULAR HOSPITALS IN NEW YORK:

To do an elective in New York, either apply directly to the hospital or the medical school (Columbia and New York University are popular choices and well-organized).

The New York Presbyterian Group comprises the Columbia Presbyterian Center and the New York Weill Cornell Center with the nation's busiest burns unit. Electives in this group of hospitals require quite a bit of paperwork, but their electives catalogue can be found on http://cpmcnet.columbia.edu/dept/ps. Currently elective fees are around $500.

Columbia Presbyterian Medical Center

710 West 168th Street, New York, NY 10032, USA.

The center: Well-known for its transplant programme (especially heart transplants) and its Neurology Department. There is a busy ER. It is a level two trauma centre (which can upgrade to level one if necessary) but tends to concentrate on acute medical emergencies. (St Luke's–Roosevelt and Harlem hospital are the level one trauma centres).

Note: Many people in the area only speak Spanish and a knowledge of some is a great help.

O Elective notes: At the time of writing it was found that Columbia University didn't cover for malpractice insurance and hence hands on experience for some has been limited. Teaching (in neurology) though is excellent with the opportunity to do research. The ER has long (12-hour) shifts where students get to clerk their own patients. They are pretty flexible though about when you work. The centre also has an Urban Medicine and Immigrant Health Care Programme. They run medical clinics for the homeless and provide palliative care. Write to the Dean (Office for Student Affairs, College of Physicians and Surgeons, 630, West 168th Street, New York, NY 10032) if interested.

Accommodation: Contact Accommodation Office, Health Sciences Block, 50 Haven Avenue, New York, NY. The Bard Hall (160 St, Manhattan) is a hall for science students and is pretty basic (bring your own sheets). It costs between $270 and $500/month. There's a gym on site and phone in your room. It's not the nicest area of town but close to the subway.

The Babies and Children's Hospital

(Part of the Columbia–Presbyterian Medical Center) 3959 Broadway, New York, NY 10032, USA.

The hospital: A major paediatric centre. It has friendly staff and sees a wide range of pathologies.

O Elective notes: You are treated like a US student and it comes recommended.

Accommodation: Provided free for one month.

Harlem Hospital

Harlem, Manhatten, New York, USA.

The hospital: One of the major level one trauma centres in New York and accordingly receives all major trauma for the area. It does have many other specialities as well.

O Elective notes: It is a popular destination for trauma. Apply through Columbia or directly.

St Luke's–Roosevelt Hospital

New York City, New York, USA.

The hospital: A new hospital with level one trauma centre associated with Columbia University.

NY Hospital Cornell Medical Centre

1300 York Avenue, New York NY 10021, USA Tel: 1 212 746 0780.

The hospital: Large but best known for its A&E and burns unit.

O Elective notes: In ER students are recognized as part of the team. There is a fair bit of responsibility but good supervision.

Accommodation: Good.

The NYU Hospitals Center

500 First Avenue, NY 10016, USA Tel: 212 263 7300.

The group: Part of the NYU Medical School and comprises the **Tisch Hospital** (same address, 726 beds with cardiovascular, neurosurgery, AIDS, cancer, transplant and reconstructive surgery services) and the **Rusk Institute of Rehabilitation** (400 East 34th St, NY 10016 Tel: 212 263 7300 Fax: 212 263 6675) with 174 beds.

O Elective notes: The University has a very well-structured elective programme from forensic medicine to neurosurgery. There is a $25.00 registration fee and you need malpractice insurance. For information on other hospitals associated with NYU and for comprehensive elective details visit their web site.

Mount Sinai Hospital

One Gustave L Levy Place, Box 1002, New York, NY 10029-6574, USA.

The hospital: A 1171-bed premier tertiary referral facility. Areas of particular speciality include spinal cord and brain injury rehabilitation, Jewish genetic diseases, AIDS, geriatrics, neonatal and paeds respiratory diseases. It is affiliated with the Mount Sinai School and NYU. Apply through either of these to do an elective here.

Maimonides Medical Center

4802 10th Avenue, Brooklyn, NY 11219, USA.

The hospital: A very large well-equipped DGH. It is very busy and has all major specialities.

O Elective notes: This is a good place to go if you don't want to work directly in one of the central big teaching hospitals. There is plenty to see and do. Other students are from NY and Grenada. Apply directly to the department you want to work in.

RESEARCH OUTSIDE NEW YORK:

Cold Spring Harbor Labortories

1 Bungtown Road, Cold Harbor, New York, NY11724, USA.

The labs: This is a very large world-renowned research centre with world leaders such as David Beach, Scott Lowe and Bruce Stillman. The director is Dr James Watson (as in Watson and Crick, DNA double helix discoverers). It is very busy in the summer with visiting scientists. This also makes it very sociable. The institute has two 30 ft yachts, *The Double Helix* and *The Transposon* on its beach where they often hold summer parties. The labs are very isolated: 2–3 miles from the nearest town (Huntington) and an hour from Manhattan.

Elective notes: This is an excellent place to visit if you are interested in molecular research. It is very friendly but also very hard work.

North Carolina

Duke University School of Medicine

PO Box 3710, Durham, North Carolina 27710, USA Tel: (919) 684 2985 Fax: 684 8893 www.mc.duke.edu/depts/som

The College, founded in 1930, uses **Duke Hospital** (a private teaching hospital with 1000 beds at the same address) as well as the **Durham VA** (508 Fulton Street, Durham NC 27705 with 489 beds). The money for the University came from tobacco and many of the patients in the hospital still work for tobacco companies. DUMC is a very high-tech hospital and the university has quite an Oxbridge feel. Nightlife is fairly low key.

East Carolina University School of Medicine

Greenville, North Carolina 27858–4354, USA Tel: (252) 816 2202 www.med.ecu.edu

Founded in the 1970s, the 100-acre Health Sciences Center campus houses the preclinical building and the 731-bed Pitt County Memorial Hospital. Other services used include the **Jenkins Cancer Center**, **Child Development Evaluation Clinic**, **Mental Health Center**, **Rehab Centers** and **Neonatal ICU**.

University of North Carolina at Chapel Hill School of Medicine

121 MacNider Hall, Chapel Hill, North Carolina 27599–7000, USA Tel: (919) 962 8331 www.med.unc.edu/

Founded in 1879 it uses the University of North Carolina Hospitals, Cancer Research Center and Biological Sciences Center, all of which are on-site. A number of hospitals outside are also used.

Wake Forest University School of Medicine

Medical Center Boulevard, Winston-Salem, North Carolina 27157–1090, USA Tel: (336) 716 4264 Fax: 716 5807 www.wfubmc.edu

The School was founded in 1902 and is part of the Wake Forest University Baptist Medical Center. It uses the 806-bed **North Carolina Baptist Hospitals** and the 896-bed **Forsyth Memorial Hospital**.

North Dakota

University of North Dakota School of Medicine and Health Sciences

501 North Columbia Road, Grand Forks, North Dakota 58202–9037, USA Tel: (701) 777 4221 Fax: 777 4942 www.med.und.nodak.edu/

When founded in 1905, the college offered a two-year course in basic sciences. Clinical years had to be done elsewhere. In 1981 the school started its own clinical course in North Dakota using community clinics, hospitals and physicians.

Ohio

Case Western University Reserve School of Medicine

10900 Euclid Avenue, Cleveland, Ohio 44106–4920, USA Tel: (216) 368 3450 Fax: 368 6011 http://mediswww.cwru.edu

Case Western is a private, independent university with a very green 600-acre campus five miles east of downtown

Cleveland. Teaching hospitals used include: **University Hospitals of Cleveland**, **St Luke's**, **MetroHealth Medical Center**, **Mount Sinai Medical Center**, the **Veterans Affairs Cleveland Medical Center** and the **Henry Ford Health System** in Detroit.

University of Cincinnati College of Medicine

PO Box 670552. Cincinnati, Ohio 45267–0552, USA Tel: (513) 558 7314 Fax: 558 1165 www.med.uc.edu/

The college offers extensive clinical and research facilities. It uses the huge University of Cincinnati Medical Centre where all specialities are catered for. Full elective details are available on-line and you actually submit your request directly.

Medical College of Ohio

3045 Arlington Avenue, Toledo, Ohio 43614, USA Tel: (419) 383 4229 Fax: 383 4005 www.mco.edu

Founded in the early 1970s, this very academic institution offers good teaching and plenty of research. It is located on a 475-acre campus in south Toledo. Hospitals on campus include: the **Medical College of Ohio Hospital** (258 acute-beds with level one trauma center and transplant specialities), **MCO/ Mercy Rehab Hospital** (36 beds) and the **Kobaker Center** for emotionally disturbed children.

Northeastern Ohio Universities College of Medicine

PO Box 95, Rootstown, Ohio 44272–0095, USA Tel: (330) 325 2511, 1(800) 686 2511 Fax: 325 8372 www.neoucom.edu

NEOUCOM is publicly supported and has its preclinical campus in Rootstown, three major public universities and 16 community hospitals in Akron, Youngstown and Canton areas. In total 6500 beds.

Ohio State University College of Medicine and Public Health

370 West Ninth Avenue, Columbus, Ohio 43210–1238, USA Tel: (614) 292 7137 Fax: 292-1544 www.med.ohio-state.edu

The University is one of the largest in the country and the medical college was founded in 1914. The main campus in Columbus uses university hospitals, the **Arthur James Cancer Hospital** and **Research Institute** as well as rural hospitals.

Wright State University School of Medicine

PO Box 1751, Dayton, Ohio 45401–1751, USA Tel: (937) 775 2934 Fax: 775 3322 www.med.wright.edu/

The school, on the university campus in Fairborn, was established in 1973. It uses seven teaching hospitals totalling 3823 beds.

POPULAR HOSPITALS IN OHIO:

Cleveland Clinic Foundation

9500 Euclid Avenue, Cleveland, OH 44195, USA.

The hospital: The hospital is very proud of the fact that they are the sixth-best hospital in America. There are 985 beds of which over 100 are devoted to critical care. It is privately run by a board of trustees and does not have official links with any medical school. Students are therefore a bit of a novelty and get treated pretty well. The critical care unit boasts, with some justification, that they provide some of the best care of acute medical and surgical care anywhere and the hospital has an 'international' feel that is unusual and distinctive for a hospital in the Midwest.

O Elective notes: There are many serious and interesting cases. As a student in critical care you can get to insert CVP lines and Swan–Ganz catheters. It's a work hard, play hard environment. In neurology you are expected to get involved and do consults. You'll also do admissions. These consults and admissions become *your* patients and you're responsible for information-gathering and presenting them on ward rounds. A few reports show that some teams are not all that friendly.

Accommodation: Is free and pretty good (single rooms with shower and toilet between two. In the past they have even contributed towards your plane ticket ($200 voucher with $70 deducted for rent)!

Oklahoma

University of Oklahoma College of Medicine

PO Box 26901, Oklahoma City, Oklahoma 73190, USA Tel: (405) 271 2331 Fax: 271 3032 www.ouhsc.edu

This very modern college offers teaching centres in Oklahoma City and Tulsa. In Oklahoma City, the college has a 200-acre complex with 17 public and private institutions making up the Oklahoma Health Center.

Oregon

Oregon Health Sciences School of Medicine

3181 SW Sam Jackson Park Road, Portland, Oregon 97201 3098, USA Tel: (503) 494 2998 Fax: 494-3400 www.ohsu.edu/

The school was founded in 1887 and is situated on a 100-acre campus in Sam Jackson Park overlooking the city and only one and a half miles from the business centre. The two hospitals on site provide 509 beds. The Child Development and Rehab Center and Crippled Children's Division are also on site. The **VA** (563 beds) is also affiliated. Like much of America, an elective here can be hard work.

Accommodation: In the University halls of residence (708 SW Sam Jackson Rak Road) (cheap and convenient). For exploring outside Portland you really need a car.

Pennsylvania

Jefferson Medical College of Thomas Jefferson University

1025 Walnut Street, Philadelphia, Pennsylvania 19107, USA Tel: (215) 955 6983 Fax: 923 6939 www.tju.edu/

Founded in 1824, teaching is at the Thomas Jefferson University Hospital (111 South 11th Street, Philadelphia, PA 19107 Tel: 215 955 6000, a regional trauma and spinal injuries centre with specialities such as liver transplantation and AIDS) and 15 associated hospitals. The college is developing research opportunities.

MCP Hahnemann University School of Medicine

2900 Queen Lane, Philadelphia, Pennsylvania 19129, USA Tel: (215) 991 8100 Fax: 843 1766 www.mcphu.edu

When founded in 1850 MCP was the first medical school for women but became co-ed in 1969. It still seeks diverse students. The Hahnemann University is a private institution. The college uses a large network of hospitals, including **Hahnemann University Hospital** (Broad and Vine Streets, Philadelphia, PA 19102 Tel: 215 762 7000, 618 beds). HUH has high-tech specialities such as cardiac transplantation as well as a level one trauma centre and aeromedical transport programme.

Pennsylvania State University College of Medicine

PO Box 850, Hershey, Pennsylvania 17033, USA Tel: (717) 531 8755 Fax: 531 6225. www.collmed.psu.edu

The Medical College was founded after a generous grant from the Hershey Foundation in 1963. The college utilizes the Pennsylvania State University Hospital. The 550-acre campus is in hills eight miles from the capital, Harrisburg, and has the 504-bed **Milton Hershey Medical Center** with a Children's Hospital, Emergency Department (level one adult and paed trauma centre) and rehab hospital. There is a helipad for LIFE LION aeromedical service.

University of Pennsylvania School of Medicine

Philadelphia, Pennsylvania 19104–6056, USA Tel: (215) 898 8001 Fax: 573 6645 www.med.upenn.edu/

Founded in 1765, the school claims to be

the first medical school in the US and was founded by Benjamin Franklin. It's well-known as one of the Ivy League Universities. Hospitals affiliated include **University of Pennsylvania Hospital**, the **VA**, the **Children's Hospital of Philadelphia**, **Phoenixville and Pennsylvania** hospitals and the **Presbyterian Medical Center**.

University of Pittsburgh School of Medicine

Scaife Hall, Pittsburgh, Pennsylvania 15261, USA Tel: (412) 648 9891/9040 Fax: 648 8768 http://www.dean-med.pitt.edu/

The School (founded 1886) is in the Oakland district of Pittsburgh and uses the huge **University of Pittsburgh Medical Center** which has: UPMC Presbyterian and Shadyside hospitals and a number of speciality hospitals. Nine community hospitals are associated. It also uses the **Children's Hospital of Pittsburgh** and the **VA Medical Center**.

Temple University School of Medicine

3400 N Broad Street, Philadelphia, Pennsylvania 19140, USA Tel: (215) 707 3656 Fax: 707 6932
www.temple.edu/medschool/

The School, situated with Temple Hospital, was founded in 1901. Clinical teaching is at the **New Temple University Hospital**, the **New Temple University Children's Medical Center**, **Albert Einstein Medical Center** and 23 other centres.

POPULAR HOSPITALS IN PENNSYLVANIA:

Hospital of the University of Pennsylvania

Spruce Street, Philadelphia, PA 19104–6021, USA.

The hospital: Being the main hospital for the University of Pennsylvania it is busy and has all specialities.

O Elective notes: Whatever department you work in, be prepared to work very hard. Cardiothoracic surgery is busy with ward rounds at 5.30 am and theatre starting at 8 am. Excellent if you like cardiothoracic surgery, not good if you wanted a holiday. Other departments are a bit more relaxed than this. Write to the Office of International Relations 1007 Blockley Hall, 423 Guardian Drive, Philadelphia PA 19104-6021.

Accommodation: May be arranged for $500+ a month (£375). Stay in International House, it's friendly.

Veterans Administration Medical Centre

University Avenue, Philadelphia, Pennsylvania, USA.

The hospital: Also associated with the University of Pennsylvania and has most general specialities.

O Elective notes: Again, be prepared to work incredibly hard (5.45 am ward rounds in general surgery). There is a fantastic amount of responsibility, but occasionally students have felt they were treated poorly and not enjoyed the long days.

Pittsburgh Medical School

(See address above.)

Full details of this incredibly expensive elective can be found on the web (where there is an application form for the truly rich). Quoting from their web site: there is a non-refundable application fee $50. Tuition expense (flat rate for 4–8 weeks) is $2100. They then estimate monthly expenses (including rent at $595) to total another $1074. You've therefore spent $3224 and you haven't even bought your airline ticket. This can really only be described as criminal since their students can visit hospitals in Europe and Australia for free (including free rent). Ask your Dean to write and say that your hospital will charge their students silly figures too. Surf the net ... find the department you want to do an elective in and apply directly. See Harvard for more tips on how to get around stupid fees. You have to ask yourself, if they are really making it that awkward, do you really want to go there?

Puerto Rico

Universidad Central del Caribe School of Medicine

PO Box 60-327, Bayamón, Puerto Rico 00960–6032, USA Tel: (787) 740 1611 Fax: 269 7550 www.uccaribe.edu

Founded in 1976 the School uses the **Dr Ramón Ruíz Arnau University Hospital** as its principle teaching hospital in the city of Bayamón.

Ponce School of Medicine

PO Box 7004, Ponce, Puerto Rico 00732, USA Tel: (787) 840 2511 Fax: 840 9756.

Initially the Catholic University of Puerto Rico School of Medicine, the name changed in 1980. **Damas Hospital** (356 beds) is the main teaching hospital. **La Playa Diagnostic Center**, **Ponce District Hospital** (550 beds), **Dr Pila Hospital** (160 beds) and **St Luke's Hospital** (160 beds) are also used. In San Germán, the **Concepcíon Hospital** (188 beds) and the **Yauco Regional Hospital** (140 beds) are also linked.

University of Puerto Rico School of Medicine

PO Box 365067, San Juan, Puerto Rico 00936–5067, USA. Tel: (787) 758 2525 Fax: 282 7117.

Founded in 1949, the University School of medicine is affiliated with the Puerto Rico Medical Center and the Hospital Consortium. It is based next to the University District Hospital.

Rhode Island

Brown University School of Medicine

97 Waterman St, Providence, Rhode Island 02912–9706, USA Tel: (401) 863 2149 Fax: 863 2660 www.brown.edu

The school (which unusually has an eight-year college and medical course) is affiliated with **Rhode Island Hospital** (with 719 beds the largest hospital in the state, also with trauma facilities). **Bradley** (child psychiatric centre), **Butler** (psychiatric), **Miriam** (247-bed general hospital with research), **Memorial** (294-bed general/rehab hospital), **Women** (obstetrics) and **Infants** and the local **VA** hospitals are also associated. For electives there are no tuition fees and malpractice insurance is around $70.

South Carolina

Medical University of South Carolina College of Medicine

171 Ashley Avenue, Charleston, South Carolina 29425, USA Tel: (803) 792 3283 Fax: 792 3764 http://www2.musc.edu

The oldest medical school in the South was founded in 1824 and hospitals utilized include the **Medical University Hospital**, **Children's Hospital**, the **Storm Eye Institute**, **Psychiatric Institute** and **Hollings Cancer Center** which make up the MUSC Medical Center. The **Charleston Memorial**, **VA Hospitals** and local hospitals are also linked.

University of South Carolina School of Medicine

Columbia, South Carolina 29208, USA Tel: (803) 733 3325 Fax: 733 3328 www.med.sc.edu

The School is relatively new (1974) and is on a newly renovated 93-acre campus. The **Palmetto Richland Memorial Hospital** (649 beds), **William Hall Psychiatric Hospital** (270 beds), **Dorn Veterans Hospital** (530 beds), **Moncrief Army Hospital** and others are the main teaching sites.

South Dakota

University of South Dakota School of Medicine

414 East Clark Street, Vermillion, South Dakota 57069, USA Tel: (605) 677 5233 Fax: 677 5109 www.usd.edu/med/som

Initially (1907) the school only had a basic sciences course, but it now has three clinical sites (Yankton, Sioux Falls and Rapid City). Its prime objective is to create primary care doctors for South Dakota.

Tennessee

East Tennessee State University James H Quillen College of Medicine

PO Box 70580, Johnson City, Tennessee 37614 0580, USA Tel: (423) 439 6221 Fax: 439 8206 http://qcom.etsu.edu

Situated in a large metropolitan area of Tennessee, Quillen (founded 1978) uses a number of hospitals (many rural) to specialize in training primary care physicians. Hospitals in Johnson City (the medical center), Kingsport, Bristol and Elizabethton provide 3000 beds to the school.

Meharry Medical College School of Medicine

1005 DB Todd Boulevard, Nashville, Tennessee 37208, USA Tel: (615) 327 6204 Fax: 327 6568 www.mmc.edu

Meharry, when founded in 1876, was designed to educate freed slaves and the poor. Today the school provides excellent training for African Americans and other minorities. The **Metropolitan Nashville General Hospital**, **Blanchfield Community**, **York VA** and **Murfreesboro VA** hospitals are affiliated.

University of Tennessee Memphis College of Medicine

790 Madison Avenue, Memphis, Tennessee 38163–2166, USA Tel: (901) 448 5559 Fax: 448 1740 www.utmem.edu/medicine

Founded in 1851, **The University of Tennessee Bowld Hospital, St Jude Children's Hospital, Baptist Memorial Hospital**, the **VA** and **LePasses Rehabilitation Center** make up the 6000 beds on the 41-acre campus.

Vanderbilt University School of Medicine

209 Light Hall, Nasville, Tennessee 37232–0685, USA Tel: (615) 322 2145 Fax: 343 8397 www.mc.vanderbilt.edu/medschool/

The school is on the Vanderbilt campus and uses 5000 beds in a number of hospitals.

Texas

Baylor College of Medicine

1 Baylor Plaza, Houston, Texas 77030, USA Tel: (713) 798 4451 Fax: 798 5563 www.bcm.tmc.edu

Founded in 1900, Baylor moved to Houston in 1943. It is one of the medical schools in the huge 356-acre Texas Medical Center in Houston containing 13 hospitals and four nursing schools providing 4200 beds in the pleasant south-west area of Houston.

Texas A&M University System Health Science Center College of Medicine

159 Joe Reynolds Medical Building, College Station, Texas 77843–1114, USA Tel: (409) 845 7743 Fax: 845 5533 http://hsc.tamu.edu

This large university (founded in 1971) has one of the top five research budgets of the US. The Central Texas Medical Center on campus consists of a number of hospitals and clinics. It also uses **Teague Veteran's Center** in Temple, Texas, **Driscoll Children's Hospital** in Corpus Christi, Texas and others. In total there are 1976 beds with a 2 million outpatient turnover.

Texas Tech University Health Sciences Center School of Medicine

3601 4th Street, Lubbock, Texas 79430, USA Tel: (806) 743 2297 Fax: 743 2725 www.ttuhsc.edu

The school, established in 1969, uses hospitals in Lubbock (the main campus), Amarillo and El Paso. These with other community hospitals provide 2900 beds.

University of Texas Southwestern Medical Center at Dallas Southwestern Medical School

5323 Harry Hines Boulevard, Dallas, Texas 75235–9096, USA Tel: (214) 648 6776/5617 Fax: 648 3289 www.swmed.edu

Founded in 1943, the 100-acre campus just north of Dallas offers good facilities. **Parkland Memorial**, **Lipshy University** and **Presbyterian Hospitals** along with the **Children's medical Center**, **Baylor University Medical Center**, **St Paul Medical Center**, **Texas Scottish Rite Hospital for Children** and the **Southwestern Institute of Forensic Sciences** are all affiliated.

University of Texas Medical School at Galveston

Ashbel Smith Building, Galveston, Texas 77555–1317, USA Tel: (409) 772 3517 Fax: 772 5753 www.utmb.edu

Established in 1891, the medical branch uses eight hospitals (providing 923 beds), the **Marine Biomedical Institute**, the **Institute for the Medical Humanities** and the **Shriners Burns Institute**.

University of Texas Houston Medical School

PO Box 20708, Houston, Texas 77225, USA Tel: (713) 500 5116 Fax: 500 0604 www.med.uth.tmc.edu

The **Hermann Hospital** (650 beds) is the main hospital in the Texas Medical Center in Houston. The school (founded 1969) makes use of this and many other institutions in the centre. Other hospitals include the **University of Texas**, **Anderson Cancer Center**, **Southwest Memorial Hospital**, **St Joseph** and **Lyndon Baines Johnson Hospitals**.

University of Texas Medical School at San Antonio

Health Sciences Center at San Antonio, 7703 Floyd Curl Drive, San Antonio, Texas 78284–7702, USA Tel: (210) 567 2665 Fax: 567 2685 www.uthscsa.edu

Founded in 1959, the school's main hospitals include the University hospital and health centre and Murphy VA. Affiliated hospitals include **Wilford Hall USAF Hospital**, the **Aerospace Medical Division of USAF**, **Brooke Army Hospital**, **Baptist Memorial Hospital** and **Santa Rosa Medical Center**.

POPULAR HOSPITALS IN TEXAS:

Texas Medical Center

Houston, Texas, USA.

The centre: The world's largest medical centre. With 42 institutions it is said to have 100,000 visitors a day. It has many world-leading pioneers and even the smallest speciality is catered for. There is a free bus service around the centre although a car is really needed to get around Houston. Of note: the Ben Taub is the county hospital providing free care to those without insurance. **The Hermann Hospital** (6411 Fannin, Houston, Texas 77030) has a busy ER (but with not as much trauma as say Washington or New York). The **Methodist Hospital** is a private hospital with advanced neurosurgery. There is also the **Texas Children's Hospital**. **The Texas Heart Institute** (at St Luke's Episcopal Hospital, PO Box 20345, Houston 77225–0345, Texas) has good elective reports. It is a (non-profit) private institution founded in 1962 and claims to be the largest cardiovascular centre in the world. The first heart transplant in the US and the first artificial heart were implanted here. No fee is charged and malpractice insurance is not required. Contact The Surgical Associates of Texas PA, Texas Heart Institute. The affiliates with each medical school are listed above.

Accommodation: The various medical schools or institutions normally help out, but if you have major problems contact: University Housing, 7900 Cambridge, Houston, Texas 77054 Tel: 713 792 8112 or Texas Women's University, Director of Housing, 1130 MD Anderson Blvd, Houston, Texas 77030 Tel: 713 794 2157. Linda Vista Apartments 1303, Eaton Street, Houston, Texas comes recommended (cost $500/month).

Veterans Affairs Medical Center

2002 Holcombe Boulevard, Houston, Texas 77030, USA.

The hospital: A busy general hospital also in Houston.

O Elective notes: Prepare to work hard. For example, general and vascular surgery have ward rounds at 6 am and the day finishes at 7 pm. There's also a 6 am ward round on Saturday. Elective students are integrated into the local student programme. The theatre time is excellent . . . students are allowed to scrub up and close the abdomen. Minor procedures can also be performed under supervision. The staff and students are extremely friendly. If you can take long days, this is a good experience.

Note: To organize this you have to apply to the Baylor College of Medicine . . . early.

Accommodation: Arranged through Baylor and is very good.

Utah

University of Utah School of Medicine

50 North Medical Drive, Salt Lake City, Utah 84132, USA Tel: (801) 581 7498 Fax: 585 3300 http://medstat.med.utah.edu/som

Established in 1904, the school is part of a multi-faculty university using its own **University Hospitals, Howard Hughes Medical Institute, Utah Genome Center, Utah Cancer Center, Moran Eye Center** and other specialized institutions.

Vermont

University of Vermont College of Medicine

Burlington, Vermont 05405, USA Tel: (802) 656 2154 www.med.uvm.edu

Burlington on the eastern shores of Lake Champion is the home to Vermont (established 1822). It uses **Fletcher Allen Health Care's Medical Center Hospital** (500 beds) on campus.

Virginia

Eastern Virginia Medical School of the Medical College of Hampton

721 Fairfax Avenue, Norfolk, Virginia 23507–2000, USA Tel: (757) 446 5812 Fax: 446 5896 gopher://picard.evms.edu/1

EVMS is a community-based teaching institution founded in 1973. It aims to produce top-notch primary care doctors. Using 33 community-based institutions it provides healthcare for a third of Virginia. On Campus is **Sentara Norfolk General Hospital**, the tertiary referral centre.

Virginia Commonwealth University School of Medicine

PO Box 980565, Richmond, Virginia 23298–0565, USA Tel: (804) 828 9629 Fax: 828-1246 www.vcu.edu

The school (founded 1838) is very near the governmental area of downtown Richmond and therefore centrally located. It has an excellent clinical research center (MCV) and a 1000-bed hospital on the main campus with the largest neonatal ICU and emergency room in Virginia. It also uses 800 beds at a new VA hospital.

University of Virginia School of Medicine

Charlottesville, Virginia 22908, USA Tel: (804) 924 5571 Fax: 982 2586 www.med.virginia.edu/home.html

The school (founded in 1825) is situated with the University hospital in the grounds of the University. The medical centre has 552 beds with seven separate ITUs. In total there are 27,000 inpatients/year. It is also associated with the **Veteran Affairs Medical Center** (Roanoke–Salem Program, VAMC), Medical Service (111), 1970 Roanoke Boulevard, Salem, Virginia 24153). This has some good elective reports especially for ICU.

Washington

University of Washington School of Medicine

Health Sciences Center, Seattle, Washington 98195–6340, USA Tel: (206) 543 7212
www.washington.edu/medical/som/

The school was established in 1945 and uses a number of hospitals.

Note: The Children's hospital refuses to take elective students.

POPULAR HOSPITALS IN SEATTLE:

Harborview Medical Center

325 Ninth Avenue, Seattle, Washington 98104 2499, USA Tel: (206) 731 3263 Fax: (206) 731 3563.

The hospital: Has the only level one trauma centre for a large area of north-west USA. There is plenty of trauma (RTAs, stabbings). Other specialities are also provided.

O Elective notes: ER shifts are 12 hours long. Lots of experience and procedures. The paramedics are some of the best in the world.

West Virginia

Marshall University School of Medicine

1600 Medical Center Drive, Huntingdon, West Virginia 25701 3655, USA Tel: (304) 691 1600.

Marshall has been committed since its foundation in the early 1980s to encouraging primary healthcare physicians and a community-based course is used. An ambulatory care centre, the VA and rural clinics are utilized. The **Marshall University Medical Center** has medicine (including cardiovascular), O&G, paeds, and surgery departments. There is also a large forensic science programme.

West Virginia University School of Medicine

Health Sciences Center, PO Box 9815. Morgantown, West Virginia 26506, USA Tel: (304) 293 3521 Fax: 293 7968
www.hsc.wvu.edu/som/

Although basic sciences have been taught since the turn of the century, the school has only been clinical in the last half. The **Ruby Memorial** (400 beds), **Chestnut Ridge Psychiatric** (80 beds) and **Mountainview Rehabilitation Hospital** (80 beds) are affiliated.

Wisconsin

Medical College of Wisconsin

8701 Watertown Plank Road, Milwaukee, Wisconsin 53226, USA Tel: (414) 456 8246
www.mcw.edu/medschool/

The school (originating from the turn of the century) is in the Milwaukee Regional Medical Center. Affiliated hospitals include the **Froedtert Memorial Lutheran Hospital** (469 beds with cancer, transplant, trauma and neuro centres), **Children's Hospital of Wisconsin** (222 beds, 24 PICU) and the **Zablocki VA** providing over 7000 beds in total.

University of Wisconsin Medical School

Medical Sciences Center, 1300 University Avenue, Madison, Wisconsin 53706, USA Tel: (608) 263 4925 Fax: 262 2327
www.biostat.wisc.edu

The University of Wisconsin Center for Health Sciences houses the medical school (founded 1907), University Hospital and Clinics on its campus in Madison.

SOMETHING DIFFERENT:

Forensic medicine

America is a pretty good place to do forensic medicine. It's not all murders as you might expect, but there is a great deal more than in Europe, Oz or NZ. Africa does have high violence and murder rates, but there isn't the system to investigate it.

For these reasons, America is ideal. In a land where medical care costs a small fortune, you'll be pleased to know that everyone has the right to a free autopsy if the family wishes. There are a number of places to look for information. A good place to start is to visit: www.criminalistics.com/gadprog.htm This lists all institutions with a forensic science programme for example the **Marshall University Forensic Science Programme** (1542 Spring Valley Drive, Huntington, West Virginia 25755–9310 Tel: 304-696-7394 http://meb.marshall.edu/forensic). The most popular elective destination for forensic medicine is New York.

The Office of the Chief Medical Examiner

520 First Avenue, New York NY 10016, USA.

The office: The OCME investigates sudden, unexpected, suspicious and violent deaths as well as fatalities in special legally defined circumstances such as in public institutions, occupational diseases, communicable diseases that are a threat to public health and those who die from diagnostic or therapeutic procedures. Of the 10 million living in New York, 70,000 deaths occur per annum, half of which get referred to the OCME.

Elective notes: If you've got a strong stomach and are genuinely interested this is an excellent place to do an elective. There are opportunities to go out to the scene of death and to court.

Note: After getting the OK from the OCME you have to go through the NYU.

Accommodation: NYU can offer accommodation in NY for a hefty $500/week. There are plenty of hostels.

Skiing

Let's face facts ... most people are just looking for an excuse to have a holiday. What better way to have one than to cleverly disguise a skiing holiday as working for a medical ski patrol. You must, of course, be a very good skier already. There are a number of institutions, especially in the Rockies, that will take medical students, and the web (*search under skiing*) is a good place to start. Write to them all and see who replies. If you have no luck you can still go to a hospital (*see* Colorado for examples) with skiing nearby. A ski patrol that comes highly recommended is:

Eldora Ski Patrol

Eldora Mountain Resort, Eldora, Colorado, USA. (Write to the Ski Patrol Director.)

The patrol: Eldora is a small resort at 10,000 ft one hour from Denver. Day trippers come from Denver and Boulder to ski here. Approximately eight patrollers ensure that the slopes are safe in the morning and then attend to the injured during the day. Trauma due to falling and colliding is common, as is Acute Mountain Sickness.

Vail Valley Medical Center

Vail, Colorado, USA.

Vail is one of the largest ski areas in America with 8000 skiers on the slope a day and 30 patrollers. Because of its size Vail has its own hospital (with CT and MRI) in the village. There are opportunities here to both go on the slopes and work in a fully equipped hospital.

NASA

NASA has become an increasingly popular elective destination. There are many different places within the organization where medics can work and do research. The people who work of them are generally incredibly friendly and enthusiastic. NASA is also desperately trying to promote a good public image and increase awareness of the need for space research. This is making it very student friendly. Now is an excellent time to try to get out there. From the author's own personal experience, the simplest way to organize something is to go to Mediline, type in NASA and Gravity (for example) and see what you get. If you have any specific interests, put them in the search as well. This will churn out the names of people doing research and the addresses they are at. You can then either write to them or dial international directory enquires and get the fax number. You will be surprised at the response. Alternatively, visit NASA's homepage http://www.nasa.gov/ and search for people that way. Whatever, apply very very early as it's becoming popular and there is quite a bit of paperwork to get a J1 Visa and the necessary passes for NASA bases.

Today, only a few specific NASA centres can cater for medics. Universities are now doing some of the research instead. In brief, the main places for medical/space physiology research are:

Johnson Space Center

2101 NASA Road 1, Houston, Texas, USA
Tel: 281 483 0123 www.jsc.nasa.gov/

Johnson is about 20 miles south-east of downtown Houston. It is where the Shuttle is controlled from, but more importantly for medics, it is where a great deal of the medical research pertaining to space flight is done. It is also the main centre for astronaut selection which also involves thorough medical examinations. Excellent information regarding their research is available on the web.

NASA Ames Research Centre

Moffett Field, CA 94035, USA Tel: 650 604 5000 http://www.arc.nasa.gov/

If you're wanting to combine working with NASA with being in California (just up the bay from San Francisco), Ames is ideal. Recently, however, the space physiology department has started to move to University College San Diego.

Kennedy Space Center

Merrit Island, Florida, USA
http://www.ksc.nasa.gov/ksc.html

Although Kennedy Space Centre is the launch site for the Shuttle, it has transferred much of its medical research over to Johnson.

There are a number of other centres, including **Langley** in Virginia and the **Stennis Space Center**, but they deal more with flight testing and aeronautics. You may be able to get more advice from the NASA headquarters in Washington http://www.hq.nasa.gov/ If you're really desperate, jump ship and try Star City (the Russian equivalent!).

Bermuda

Population: 60,000
Language: English
Capital: Hamilton
Currency: Dollar
Int Code: +1

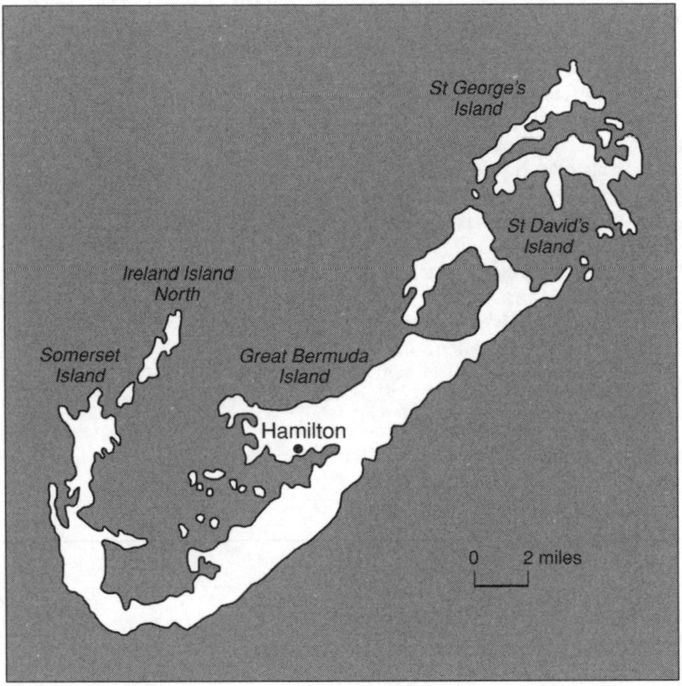

The 138 islands which comprise Bermuda lie in the North Atlantic, 568 miles due east of the nearest land at Cape Hatteras in North Carolina. Together they form an area of just over 20 square miles. Of the 60,000 who live there, 60% are black, the remainder being of mixed race or white (British or Portuguese descent). The numbers swell by half a million when the tourists arrive. It has been a British Crown colony since 1612 and is now a tourist and tax haven. Bermuda has one of the highest incomes per capita in the world and a recent campaign by the former leader to gain independence from the UK was firmly rejected.

Bermuda has two hospitals: the King Edward VII Memorial Hospital (KEMH), a general hospital, and St Brendan's, a psychiatric unit.

✪ Climate:
Normally mild and humid due to the Gulf Stream, but hurricanes can cause havoc between June and November.

The King Edward VII Memorial Hospital
PO Box HM 1023, Hamilton, Bermuda HM DX.

The hospital: Officially opened in the 1960s and, with extensions, now has 323 beds. There are six wards (two general surgical, two general medical, one maternity and one children's) plus an extended care and intensive care unit. It is well-equipped with a CT scanner. There is one junior doctor (often a SHO from the UK) who looks after each ward, but it is the GPs who are actually responsible for their patients while in hospital and therefore visit at least once every day. The healthcare system is insurance-based like that in the USA. There are many conditions to see here, but HIV is extremely common.

Accommodation: Has previously been provided free. Apply early as the KEMH can only accept three students simultaneously and gives priority to Bermudans. Write to the Bermuda Hospitals Board at the above address.

St Brendan's Hospital
PO Box 501 DV, Devonshire, Bermuda.

The hospital: St Brendan's is the only psychiatric hospital in Bermuda. The population is generally affluent with very low unemployment. This is reflected here as even chronic schizophrenics manage to hold down jobs. There are two-hour teaching sessions a week but the doctors give informal teaching.

Canada

Population: 29.5 million
Languages: English and French
Capital: Ottawa
Currency: Canadian dollar
Int Code: +1

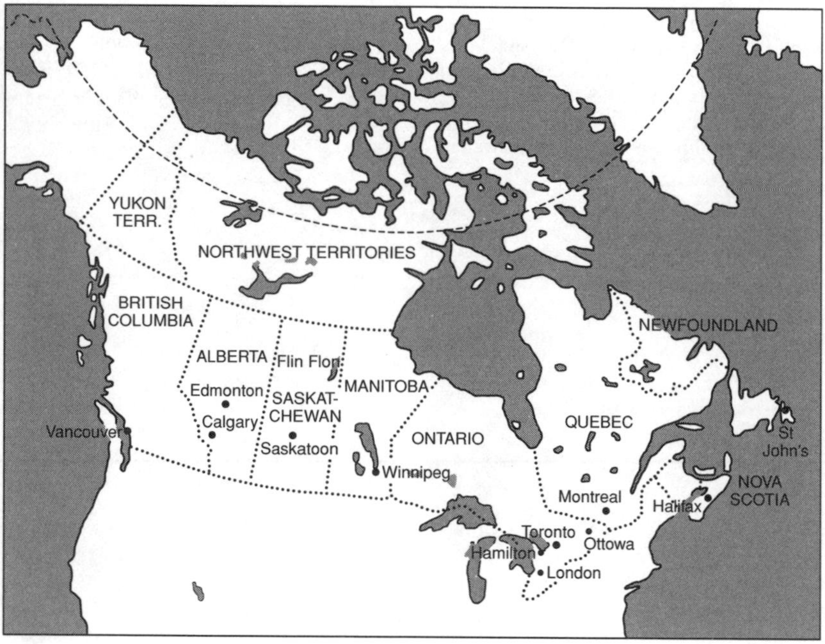

The world's second-largest country, Canada, stretches across five time zones and is made up of ten provinces and two territories. Forty per cent of the population is British in origin, 27% French, 20% from other European countries and only 4% are indigenous. Because of its size, Canada has had to develop a good transportation system. The rail and road systems reach far into the north.

Medicine:
A National Insurance scheme provides state health service for the entire population. However, approximately 25% chose to use private healthcare. As with many developed nations, the costs of newer treatments and an ageing population is putting a strain on the system. The doctor:patient ratio is one per 455. The typical big Western killers – heart, respiratory diseases and cancers – bump most people off.

All medical students have a degree before starting med school. Many also have a PhD. Because of this their first preclinical years are very clinically orientated and then they do only two clinical years. The students have patients to look after and hence elective students will too. This is why malpractice insurance is vital.

Climate and crime:
Cold. In the South (Vancouver) it is cold, but can occasionally get warm. In the north (Ellesmere Island) it is polar and consistently freezing. Canada has a much better crime record than neighbouring USA. This is mostly attributable to strict gun laws and safer cities.

Visas and work permits:
British citizens do not need a visa to stay in Canada for up to six months as a tourist; however, you may be asked to prove sufficient funds and a return ticket on arrival. Those studying (including medical students) do need to get authorisation from the Canadian High Commission. To work you need employment authorization from the High Commission before you leave your country. An agreement exists whereby if in full-time education and aged 18–30, you may be allowed to work temporarily if returning to full-time education. For both electives and work, you will be required to have a medical. The medical has to be done by an approved GP (costing around £60, but plead poverty of course). You'll also need a CXR and syphilis screen (£15). To try to save some cash: see if your hospital can do the CXR and visit your local STD clinic (paper bag on head) to get a free VDRL blood test. The reports of these then need to be sent to the Canadian High Commission who then write a letter of facilitation saying you are fit to work in Canada. It must be presented to the Canadian Immigration Officer upon arrival. Also ask your host hospital what they need. They may want a doctor's certificate saying what vaccinations you have had, in which case get it done whilst having your medical.

Note: Quebec has similar but separate immigration procedures (*see* Section 3: The Appendix).

If you're wanting to work in Canada you can write directly to hospitals and hence addresses have been included. Community hospitals are often desperate for staff. You will need to contact the appropriate medical board for the area to get registration. This can be a problem in some areas due to complete American style rules that can't be bent. For example, you may just want to do A&E or you may be a specialist in a specific field. If you haven't done four weeks of paeds or O&G though your application may be refused. This is because they have to so these subjects in their residency year. You can argue till blue in the face, but some of the boards will stick by their guns. Try to ask the hospital offering work to help you out.

MALPRACTICE INSURANCE:

For electives firstly find out if the host institution covers you as it would their own students. They may charge you for this or recommend a broker. Ask your defence union/protection society whether they cover you. They may for electives (e.g. the MDDUS does) but they probably won't for working. If they can, ask your host institution whether they accept their cover. If not contact **The Canadian Medical Protection Association** (CMPA), PO Box 8225, Stn T, Ottawa, Canada Tel: 613 725 2000 Fax: 613 725 1300.

USEFUL ADDRESSES

For French speakers:

Association des médicins de langue française du Canada, 8355 boul Saint-Laurent, Montréal, PQ H2P 2Z6, Canada Tel: 514 388 2228 www.amlfc.com
Collège des Médecins www.cmq.org

There are 16 medical schools in Canada, they are listed under each region.

British Columbia

VANCOUVER:

With a population of 1.8 million, Vancouver is a great city with loads to see and do. Stanley Park, Chinatown and Downtown must all be visited. (Steer clear of E. Hastings which is a bit dodgy.) The other great boon for skiers is Whistler, only two hours away.

University of British Columbia

Address at Point Grey Campus: Faculty of Medicine, 317–2194 Health Sciences Mall, Vancouver, British Columbia, Canada V6T 1Z3 Tel: (604) 822 2421 Fax: (604) 822 6061 www.med.ubc.ca
Address at Vancouver Hospital: Faculty of Medicine, Deans Office, Vancouver Hospital and Health Sciences Centre 3250–910 West 10th Avenue, Vancouver, BC Canada V5Z 4E3 Tel: (604) 875 4500 Fax: (604) 875 5611.

Founded in 1950, the faculty uses the on-site **Vancouver Hospital** and **Health Sciences Centre** (with 240 acute beds, 300 extended care beds and 60 psychiatric beds), **St Paul's Hospital** and **Children's and Women's Health Centre** of BC.

The University can arrange electives in any of the hospitals in British Columbia (write to the Clinical Clerkship Elective Programme at the Vancouver Hospital address); however, note that they recently placed restrictions on elective students visiting their main teaching hospitals (Vancouver Hospital – UBC Site and Oak Site, St Paul's, BC's Children's Hospital, BC. Women's and Sunnyhill). You can still apply, but they may not accept you to these teaching centres (some people have phoned directly to find a couple of spaces available. It's worth a try). They will try to put you in a community hospital: Burnaby, Chilliwack General, Dawson Creek and District, Delta, Fort St John General, GR Baker Memorial, Greater Victoria, Kelowna General, Kimberley and District, Kitimat General, Kootenau Lake District, Maple Ridge, Matsqui-Suma-Abbotsford General, Mills Memorial, Nanaino Regional General, Peace Arch District, Penticton Regional, Powell River General, Prince George Regional, Prince Rupert Regional, Queen Charlotte Islands General, Queen Victoria, Richmond, Royal Inland, St Joseph's General, St Mary's, St Vincent's, Surrey Memorial, Trail Regional, Vernon Jubilee, Victoria General, West Coast General, WCB Rehab Centre, United Church of Canada: Bella Coola General, RW Large Memorial, Wrinck Memorial Hospitals.

UBC charges around $250 (£110) elective fee, but that includes malpractice insurance. They have previously helped with accommodation for those in Vancouver, but it is not great value. Most students either stay in youth hostels (HI Downtown recommended)) or in the YMCA/YWCA costing about £400 for seven weeks. Shaughnessy Village (1125 West 12th Avenue (604) 736 5511) is also recommended. Community Hospitals all provide lodgings.

Vancouver General Hospital and Health Sciences Centre

899 West 12th Avenue, Vancouver V5Z 1M9 Tel: (604) 875 4111
www.vanhosp.bc.ca

The hospital: When it first opened in 1886, Vancouver hospital was a nine-bed tent used to treat injured railway workers. Now it is split over four sites: **Vancouver General Hospital**, **UBC**

Hospital, GF Strong Rehab Centre and **George Pearson Centre**. Today this totals 1900 beds. Vancouver General Hospital is a large, modern friendly hospital providing virtually every speciality bar paeds and maternity. Trauma, burns, MS, sports medicine, transplants, epilepsy surgery and brain/ spinal cord injury are just a few of its specialized services.

O Elective notes: Students are responsible for patients they clerk in, organizing CTs, taking bloods etc. It's a busy place. Teaching, however, often ends up cancelled. In neurology, the twice-daily rounds mean you may be there until 7 or 8 pm. Cadiothoracics has good reports. For forensics, see the end of this section.

St Paul's Hospital

1081 Burrard Street, Vancouver, BC, V6Z 1Y6, Canada.

The hospital: As one of the main hospitals affiliated with the University of British Columbia, this is a busy hospital situated in downtown Vancouver. It is particularly known for cardiology and pathology. It also receives all the major trauma.

O Elective notes: The ER is a great place for an elective. This is very near the YMCA.

BC Children's Hospital

Vancouver BC, Canada Tel: (604) 875 2345
www.childhosp.bc.cs/Childrens/bcch.HTM

The hospital: A very friendly 242-bed hospital catering for children up to 16 years of age throughout BC. It has all paeds specialities. It is also a teaching and research centre. The cardiology department has had good elective reports.

St Vincent's Hospital

744 West 33rd Avenue, Vancouver, British Columbia U52 2K4, Canada.

The hospital: A friendly community hospital. It is a peripheral hospital with mainly geriatrics and psychiatry specialities. There is a small ER open from 8 am to 8 pm.

O Elective notes: Although some have found being the only student in the OR good for teaching, others have found it incredibly dull and had wished they had chosen somewhere more central. For specialities such as orthopaedics, urology, ophthalmology and cardio thoracic surgery you need to visit St Paul's Hospital. To do an elective here you still need to apply through the UBC.

BC Women's Hospital and Health Centre

4500 Oak Street, Vancouver, British Columbia V6H 3N1, Canada
www.childhosp.bc.ca/womens/

The hospital: Vancouver's specialist maternity hospital.

Sunnyhill Health Centre for Children

3644 Slozan St Vancouver, BC V5M 3E8, Canada Tel: (604) 434 1331.

The hospital: A centre for children with developmental disabilities.

COMMUNITY HOSPITALS IN BC:

To do electives in these you should apply through UBC.

Note: if it's skiing you're after, snow usually settles between November and March.

Kootenay Lake District Hospital

3 View Street, Nelson, British Columbia, Canada V1L 2V1.

The hospital: It is small and very friendly seeing a lot of skiing accidents. It's very busy as the next nearest hospital is over 100 miles away. Nelson is a small town of 10–15,000 people in BC, approximately 600 km east of Vancouver. It is situated on the shore of Kootenay Lake amidst the Kootenay Mountains (at 3,000 feet) and was a common destination for the hippies and draft dodgers of the 1970s. Many of these people are still here along with the more recent influx of New Age people, altogether making Nelson a very colourful and active community. It is also a beautiful place to visit. Skiing (£12/day) is some of the best. From May water sports on the lake take over.

O Elective notes: It is a popular destination for Canadian as well as foreign elective students. Many specialities are catered for, but you are free to do as you please. There is no schedule, but the informal teaching is good. The ER and internal medicine are recommended. The staff are very friendly giving you an ample social life and opportunities to explore the beautiful scenery.

Accommodation: Basic but with beautiful mountain views. Both it and food are currently free although this may change soon. Don't panic though, there is a good youth hostel in town.

Dawsons Creek and District Hospital

816–103rd Avenue, Dawsons Creek, BC VIG 2GI, Canada.

The hospital: A small friendly DGH, (18 hours by coach from Vancouver, two hours by plane) serving the population in Dawson (11,000) and surrounding areas. It has surgery, medicine, O&G, and psychiatric wards as well as an ER. Some of the cases in the ER are due to the social antagonism within the community (esp. native Indians). There is a large GP input into the hospital.

O Elective notes: You can do as much or as little as you want.

Kimberley and District Hospital

260 Fourth Avenue, Kimberley, BC VIA 2R6, Canada.

The hospital: A small GP-run hospital with 35 beds. It is 35 miles from the nearest speciality hospital. Six GPs run the clinics from 10 am to 5 pm and also run the hospital. They do their own deliveries, including C-sections. In the ski season (Feb/March) there are plenty of orthopaedic injuries from the ski slope 5 min away. A few specialists visit to do clinics.

O Elective notes: This is a good place to learn a lot and there is plenty of experience. It is frowned on if you don't turn up but days off for skiing are encouraged. The nearest airport is Cranbrook.

Trail Regional Hospital

1200 Hospital Bench Trail V1R 4M1, BC, Canada.

The hospital: Pretty small but medicine, surgery, paeds, A&E, anaesthetics are all catered for.

O Elective notes: You can do whatever you want; the doctors are pleased to have a student about. It's in the middle of nowhere and can get a bit lonely. Pretty easy to get to the ski hills though.

Accommodation: And food are free.

Vernon Jubille Hospital

31st Street, Vernon, BC, Canada Tel: 250 549 5225.

The hospital: A medium-sized DGH with ER, major specialities and family practice.

O Elective notes: Good practical teaching. No other students around. Flexible timetable (good skiing nearby).

Royal Inland Hospital

Kamloops, BC, Canada.

The hospital: Is a nice clean hospital in the centre of Kamloops.

O Elective notes: Unfortunately it is a fairly small city but there are excellent ski resorts nearby. Friendly doctors who let you do what you want. Advised to go with friend.

Accommodation: A good room with phone. Food in the canteen is reasonable.

Chilliwack General Hospital

45600 Menholm Road, Chilliwack, BC V2P 5J4, Canada.

The hospital: A medium-sized, mainly GP-run hospital. There are some permanently employed specialists who mostly work in A&E. Chilliwack is a nice town about an hour from the nearest ski slopes.

Surrey Memorial Hospital

13750 96th Avenue, Surrey, BC V3V 1Z2, Canada.

The hospital: Is a community hospital and there are rarely students. It's a friendly place with good teaching.

FORENSIC MEDICINE:

Dept of Forensic Pathology

1st Floor Laurel Pavillion, Vancouver Hospital Health Services CTR, 855 West 12th Avenue, Vancouver BC, V5Z 1M9, Canada.

Forensic medicine at the hospital comes thoroughly recommended. The chap in charge is very friendly. Most work is finished by 2–3 pm giving you the evenings free. Hob-nob with the police and try to get a day with them. Students can help in about 3–4 autopsies/day.

Alberta

CALGARY:

Calgary is a fairly large city ... most of which seems to have been built for the 1988 winter Olympics. Banff National Park in the heart of the Rockies is only one and a half hours away. The pubs and clubs shut at 2 am and hence there's a good night life.

University of Calgary

Faculty of Medicine, 3330 Hospital Drive, NW Calgary, Alberta, Canada T2N 4N1
Tel: (403) 220 4262
www.med.calgary.ca/ume/infoda.html

The Medical Faculty was founded in 1970 and is situated in the Calgary Health Sciences Centre. They can arrange electives in Calgary's hospitals. There's a charge of around $200. The only Calgary hospital to provide accommodation is the Foothills. Previously students have stayed in University digs (around $300/month), handy for Downtown.

Alberta Children's Hospital

1820 Richmond Road SW, Calgary, Alberta T2T 5C7, Canada.

The hospital: A fairly large, modern hospital. It's the paeds tertiary referral hospital for Alberta and hence has all specialities. It's a 10–15 minutes' bus ride from downtown Calgary.

O Elective notes: The staff and other medical students are very welcoming. They organize the programme for you ... a typical rotation being one week emergency, one week neonatology and four weeks general. They do expect you to work, but as a student you are given quite a lot of responsibility.

Accommodation: None is available in the hospital. You can stay at the Foothills Hospital, a 10–15-minute bus ride away.

Calgary General Hospital

841 Centre Ave East, Calgary, Alberta T2E 0A1, Canada.

The hospital: Is one of Calgary's main hospitals and was sited on two sites, Bar Valley and Peter Longheed, but recently the Bar Valley site has been closing. The ER is a busy department seeing many acute surgical and medical emergencies; however, most trauma goes to Calgary's other main hospital, the Foothills.

O Elective notes: As a student in ER you are given a rota with different supervisors. You are never expected to work overnight.

Accommodation: Cannot be provided in the hospital; however, if you apply to the Foothills hospital you can stay there.

Foothills Hospital

1403–29 St NW, Calgary, Alberta T2N 2T9, Canada.

The hospital: A large, well-equipped friendly hospital. It has many specialities including Calgary's trauma department.

O Elective notes: You can do as much or as little as you want. Trauma comes highly recommended.

Accommodation: Basic ... no cooking facilities and no sheets or pillows provided, but cheap. It is in the Foothills grounds, great as you can lie in before work, but you are a fair way out from the nightlife. The public transport is good, but you'll need to get a taxi back from the night clubs.

FORENSIC MEDICINE:

Office of the Chief Medical Examiner
6070 Bowness Road NW, Calgary, Alberta T3B 3R7, Canada.
Forensic medicine: There are plenty of autopsies and court visits. The offices are very friendly and work is usually finished by the early afternoon and the staff positively encourage you to go out and see Calgary and the Rockies.

University of Alberta
Faculty of Medicine, Medical Sciences Building, Edmonton, Alberta, Canada T6G 2H7 Tel: (780) 492 9524
Fax: (780) 492 9531.
Founded in 1913 the University campus has the Walter Mackenzie Health Sciences Centre on site. The University also uses the **Royal Alexandra, Alberta, Glenrose, Edmonton General, Misericordia, Grey Nuns** and **Charles Camsell** hospitals as well as the **Cross Cancer Institute**. It is not a common elective destination for students from the UK. Write to the school for elective opportunities in any of their hospitals.

Saskatchewan

University of Saskatchewan
College of Medicine, Health Sciences Building, 107 Wiggins Road, Saskatoon, Saskatchewan, Canada S7N 5E5
Tel: (306) 966 8554. Fax: (306) 966 6164
www.usask.ca/medicine
Established in 1926, clinical teaching is now carried out at the **Royal University Hospital, St Paul's** and **Saskatoon City Hospitals** in Saskatoon and the **Plains Health Centre** and **General Hospital** in Regina.

Manitoba

University of Manitoba
Faculty of Medicine, 753 McDermot Avenue, Winnipeg, Manitoba Canada R3E 0W3 Tel: (204) 789 3569 Fax: (204) 789 3929.
The College was founded in 1883 and today is situated opposite the Winnipeg Health Sciences Centre (which is separate from the rest of the University). Within the Health Sciences Centre there are children's, adult's, women's, respiratory and rehab hospitals totalling over 1000 beds. Other hospitals used include: **Boniface General Hospital** (900 beds), **Misericordia** (409 beds), **Seven Oaks** (336 beds), **Deer Lodge Veterans** (500 beds), **Grace** (306 beds) and **Victoria** hospitals (254 beds).

Flin Flon General Hospital
Flin Flon, Manitoba, Canada R8A 1N2.
The hospital: Flin Flon is a mining town that lies between the provinces of Manitoba and Saskatchewan. It is a small northern Canadian town, with a total population of 15,000 (including the neighbouring native Canadian reserves). The hospital has 100 beds and is staffed by ten doctors. It is well equipped with two theatres, an X-ray and ultrasound department, an ITU and emergency room. Each of the doctors is employed by the regional health authority and works both as a specialist and as a GP in the town. Two to three times a week they fly out to native Canadian reserves in northern Saskatchewan. The clinics here can be a real eye-opener as there are terrible political problems. They are forced to live in very poor conditions on designated reserve land. Alcohol and drug abuse are huge problems and the clinics are very busy.
O Elective notes: A typical day starts with a ward round reviewing any patients admitted in the night and then going to theatre. There could be specialist or minor surgical procedures to get involved in. The afternoon is usually spent in a clinic in the town or flying to

clinics north. Your help is greatly appreciated here. When on call there are many opportunities to perform procedures such as chest drains etc.

The coldest time is from January through to March where the temperatures range from 0 to –37 ºC. Winter activities include ice fishing, ice hockey, ski-dooing, curling etc. There's plenty to do in the days, but at night ... the nearest cinema is one and a half hours away and the nearest city (Winnipeg or Saskatoon) about eight hours away.

Ontario

TORONTO:

Toronto is a pleasant lively modern city with skyscrapers, a beautiful harbour, museums, ice-rinks and good restaurants. CN Tower and a Blue Jays game must be done.

University of Toronto

Faculty of Medicine, Toronto, Ontario, Canada M5S 1A8 Tel: (416) 978 2717 Fax: 971 2163.
http://utll.library.utoronto.ca/www/medicine/ume.htm

This large faculty is associated with eight teaching hospital units: Those on University Avenue include: **The University Health Network** (Toronto General (which has merged with Toronto Western) and Princes Margaret), **The Hospital for Sick Children** and **Mount Sinai**. Others are **St Michael's**, **Toronto Rehab Institute**, **Sunnybrook** and **Women's College Health Sciences Centre**, **Clarke Institute of Psychiatry** and **Baycrest Centre for Geriatric Care**.

To do an elective anywhere in Toronto you should first write to The Visiting Electives Co-ordinator, Room 2124, Medical Sciences Building, Faculty of Medicine, University of Toronto, 1 King's College Circle, Toronto, Ontario, Canada M5S 1A8 Tel: 416 978 2691 Fax: 416 971 2163.

Elective information is on the university web site. They charge between C$216 for one to two weeks up to C$432 for eight-week long electives. You MUST apply at least four months before the proposed elective date or they'll fine you another C$50. Then add on a bit for malpractice insurance (around C$100 per four weeks, this can be arranged through the University). Do not pay for insurance until they have confirmed your elective. APPLY EARLY ... especially if you want to do something popular (e.g. trauma).

Then, if you're needing accommodation try **Student Housing** (Koffler Student Centre, University of Toronto, 214 College Street, M5T 1R2 Tel: (416) 978 8045). Many stay at **Tartu College** (310 Bloor St W, Toronto, Ontario M5S 1W4 Tel: 416 925 9405 Fax: 416 925 2295). Another place to try is 'Toronto General Hospital Residence' (90 Gerrard St Wst, Toronto, Ontario M5G 1J6 Fax: 416 340 3923). This costs about $200/week. Some have saved money by getting right out of town (50-min train ride from centre) to Hospitality York, York University, 4200 Keele St, North York, Ontario (only £6/night). If really stuck try **Toronto Tourist Information**, Toronto Eaton Centre, 1 Dundas Street West, M5G 1Z3, Canada.

Warning: You may be expected to work quite hard in Toronto. Here electives can make up to 50% of Canadian students' study and therefore are considered an integral part of the course. They may not understand that it's supposed to be a cleverly disguised holiday.

The University Health Network comprises Toronto General, Toronto Western, and Princes Margaret Hospitals. All are in downtown and on www.uhealthnet.on.ca

Toronto General Hospital

200 Elizabeth Street, University Avenue, Toronto, Canada Tel: (416) 340 3131.

The hospital: A huge teaching hospital with numerous specialities including heart disease, transplantation, tropical disease, eating disorders and a busy emergency department treating 30,000 a year. The hospital has had some pretty amazing firsts including the development of insulin, invention of the pacemaker and world's first single and double lung transplants. It has Canada's largest HIV clinic and first eating disorders clinic.

O Elective notes: Early starts 7.30 am so try to get accommodation near by.

Toronto Western Hospital

399 Bathurst Street, Toronto, Canada
Tel: (416) 603 5801.

The hospital: Is doing a great deal of research into brain, spinal cord and PNS, lung and vision diseases. It has a busy Emergency Department seeing 40,000/year.

Princess Margaret Hospital

610 University Avenue, Toronto, Ontario Canada M5G 2M9 Tel: (416) 946 2000.

The hospital: With its research arm, the Ontario Cancer Institute, it is regarded as one of the top cancer centres in the world. It is a beautiful, well-equipped hospital with very friendly and good teaching staff.

The Hospital for Sick Children

555 University Avenue, Toronto, Canada M5G 1X8.

The hospital: The Hospital for Sick Children ('Sick Kids') is one of the largest paeds academic health science centres in the world. It is a very modern (opened 1993) and well-equipped tertiary referral institution for the whole of the Toronto–Ontario area. As such it sees a wide variety of rare diseases. The entrance hall has fluffy toys and a Disney store and patients have their own rooms.

O Elective notes: Highly recommended if you are interested in paeds. Apply over a year in advance. There are some excellent teachers (esp. cardiology). Bear in mind that subjects like infectious diseases are mainly ward work while cardiology has many more outpatient clinics. Students tend to be taught rather than given house officer jobs. When applying you have to select a subspeciality from adolescent medicine, cardiology, genetics, emergency, endocrinology, GI and nutrition, haematology, hepatology, infectious diseases, neonatology, neurology, perinatology, respiratory medicine or rheumatology.

Accommodation: In a building just across the road from the hospital. It costs C$150 per week. The hospital can provide you with details.

St Michael's Hospital

30 Bond Street, Toronto, Ontario M5B 1W8 Tel: (416) 360 4000 Fax: (416) 864 5870.

The hospital: Is part of the University of Toronto and has the busiest of the three emergency departments in the city.

O Elective notes: In the ER hours are fairly flexible and offers excellent experience: clerking patients, doing the preliminary investigations and suturing. Teaching is good, but staff are often too busy.

Queens Street Mental Health Centre

1001 Queen St West, Toronto, Ontario, Canada.

The hospital: Toronto's main psychiatric facility. An elective here is very supervisor-dependent. As with most psychiatry, admissions can take a great deal of time and unless you get good teaching you may get bored.

Sunnybrook and Women's College Health Sciences Centre

Toronto, Ontario, Canada
www.sunnybrook.utoronto.ca

The hospital: Has 1300 beds and was originally for veterans but now is an acute care civilian hospital.

St Joseph's Health Centre

30 The Queensway, Toronto, Ontario, Canada M6R 1B5.

The hospital: Two km away from downtown with a good transport system (buses, street cars and a subway). Although not the largest hospital in Toronto it has the main specialities and

offers good opportunities to see and assist in general surgery and a busy ER.
Accommodation: The residences are sparse and basic (C$25/week), but it's easy to get into the city centre.

HAMILTON:

Hamilton is a large town between Toronto and Niagara Falls. The town has a large industrial base and is therefore not the prettiest town in Canada.

McMaster University

Health Sciences Centre, 1200 Main Street West, Hamilton, Ontario, Canada L8N 3Z5
Tel: (905) 525 9140. Fax: (905) 527 2707
www.fhs.mcmaster.ca/mdprog

The University offers an undergraduate medical programme and postgraduate medical education. The clinical components of their undergraduate course occur in the McMaster Division of the Hamilton Health Sciences Corporation and other hospitals in Hamilton.

St Peter's Hospital

Mapel Wood Road, Hamilton, Ontario, Canada.
The hospital: One of the teaching hospitals in Hamilton.
O Elective notes: Good for care of the elderly. You can use McMasters facilities. You really need a car to get around from here though.

St Joseph's Hospital

50 Charlton Avenue, Hamilton, Ontario L8N 4A6, Canada.
The hospital: Most specialities are available.
O Elective notes: Some have found it a bit isolated and lonely.

Hamilton Psychiatric Hospital

100 West 5th Street, Hamilton, Ontario L8N 3K7, Canada.
The hospital: The psychiatry is practised with a great deal of compassion and innovation. As a quaternary referral centre (affiliated with McMaster University) a great deal of pathology is there to be seen.
Accommodation: Cheap, comfortable and convenient and organized by McMaster University.

University of Ottawa

Faculty of Medicine, 451 Smyth Road, Ottawa, Ontario, Canada K1H 8M5 Tel: (613) 562 5409 Fax: (613) 562 5420.

Within the University are the faculty of medicine and schools of nursing and human kinetics. Due to a change in policy, since December 1997, the University of Ottawa no longer accepts foreign elective students.

The University of Ottawa serves three hospitals in Ottawa, one is **Ottawa Civic Hospital** (1053 Carling Avenue, Ottawa, Ontario K1Y 4E9). This is both English- and French-speaking.

Queen's University

Faculty of Health Sciences School of Medicine, Kingston, Ontario, Canada K7L 3N6
Tel (613) 533 2542 Fax: 533 6884
http://meds.queensu.ca/medicine/calendar/toc.html

Founded in 1854 the University campus is in Kingston on Lake Ontario. The three major hospitals (currently in process of reforms) are the **Kingston General Hospital** (for acute inpatient care), the **Hotel Dieu Hospital** (for ambulatory care) and **St Mary's of the Lake Hospital** (for elderly, rehab and palliative care).

Kingston General Hospital

76 Stuart Street, Kingston, Ontario K7L 2V7, Canada.
The hospital: A large teaching hospital on the North Shore of Lake Ontario about three hours by train from Toronto and Montreal. The senior staff are friendly and encourage evidence-based medicine.
O Elective notes: Sign-in rounds occur daily and you'll be given patients to assess. It can be very hard work and the finalists will spend most of the time in

the library rather than coming out to play. This is a great elective and you will learn a lot (especially cardiology). However, it's not so great if you really just want to travel and see Canada.

University of Western Ontario

Faculty of Medicine and Dentistry, Medical Sciences Building, London, Ontario, Canada N6A 5C1 Tel: (519) 661 3744 Fax: (519) 661 3797 www.med.uwo.ca

The Medical Faculty has been around since 1882. It's a private University based in London, Ontario and uses a number of local hospitals.

Quebec

MONTREAL:

A great city with much to do in June/July and August. In the winter it goes down to –20°C, so don't go then if you don't like the cold. This is arguably the most beautiful time of the year though. There is also a jazz festival as an added incentive. It helps to be able to speak some French as about half the population is French-speaking.

The two universities in Montreal are **McGill** (English-speaking) and **Université de Montréal** (French-speaking). Beware of going to a French-speaking hospital, as the French is slightly different to European and you may get problems.

McGill University

Faculty of Medicine, 3655 Drummond Street, Montreal, Quebec, Canada H3G 1Y6 Tel: (514) 398 3517 Fax: (514) 398 4631 (http://www.mcgill.ca/)

McGill came about in 1811 when James McGill bequeathed his estate. With the Montreal General Hospital, the medical school was set up and became the first medical faculty in Canada in 1821. Today it has grown considerably and uses the **Montreal Children's**, **Montreal General**, **Montreal Neurological**, **Sir Mortimer B Davis–Jewish General**, **Shriner's Crippled Children's**, **Douglas** and **Royal Victoria** hospitals. Many hospitals outside Quebec are also associated. Instruction in McGill institutions is in English.

Apply to McGill for electives at any of their institutions. They can also help out with accommodation. Try to stay at the McGill-affiliated Halls of Residence … the order of preference is:

- Royal Victoria College ($50 (£25)/week)
- Montreal Diocesan College
- Presbyterian College

They are all near University Street. Neither of the last two are religious places! You'll get to meet more people at these places.

Royal Victoria Hospital

Avenue Des Pins Ouest (or 687 Pine Avenue), Montreal, Quebec H3A 1A1, Canada.

The hospital: Is huge and the main hospital for McGill University medical school. The renal department is world-renowned and the teaching is excellent. It's very friendly both among staff and other students. There is a very team-based approach to medicine. Nearly all specialities are catered for. English is used most commonly.

○ Elective notes: There are good reports from the cardiology and general medicine departments. If doing obs and gynae, medical students take it in turn to be on call at nights and catch deliveries. Apply early, it's popular.

Montreal General Hospital/ Hôpital General de Montreal

1650 Cedar Avenue, Montreal, Quebec, Canada H3G 1A4 Tel: (514) 9376011.

The hospital: Hosts many specialities and has a busy ER.

○ Elective notes: There are many opportunities for practical procedures and the teaching is very good. Medical intensive care comes recommended.

Montreal Neurological Institute and Hospital
3801 University Street, Montreal, Quebec H3A 2B4, Canada
http://www.mcgill.ca/mni/
The hospital: Is the place to do neurology in Canada and has a worldwide reputation. Its long history includes the development of the EEG. This is a very friendly place. The hospital is central and so clubs and bars are near by.
O Elective notes: At 8 am there is a signing-in session where interesting cases are presented. Then there is a teaching ward round. The rest of the day you're admitting patients and following them around the hospital. It can be very hard work but comes thoroughly recommended by all who have been there.

Sir Mortimer B Davis–Jewish General Hospital
3755 Cote St Catherine Road, Montreal, Quebec H3T 1EZ, Canada Tel: 514 30 8222 Fax: 514 340 7510 (675 beds).

Université de Montréal
School of Medicine, PO Box 6128, Station Centre-Ville, Montreal, Quebec, Canada H3C 3J7 Tel: (514) 33 6265 Fax: (514) 343 6629 http://medes3.med.umontreal.ca
The medical school was founded in 1843 and today uses 14 teaching hospitals and research centres. Note: All instruction is in FRENCH.

QUEBEC MEDICAL SCHOOLS OUTSIDE MONTREAL:

Université Laval
Faculty of Medicine, Ste-Foy, Quebec, Canada G1K 7P4 Tel: (418) 656 2131 Fax: (418) 656 2733 www.ulaval.ca
Established in 1852 by Royal Charter, the University uses its health sciences centre and an affiliated hospital for its teaching.

University of Sherbrooke
Faculty of Medicine, Sherbrooke, Quebec, Canada J1H 5N4 Tel: (819) 564 5208 Fax: (819) 564 5378 www.usherb.ca
This relatively new faculty (admitting since 1966) is entirely FRENCH-speaking. It is multi-disciplinary with a faculty of nursing. Its Health Sciences Centre includes a 700-bed teaching hospital. Twelve other hospitals are also used.

Nova Scotia

Halifax has a population of 700,000 but has four Universities. This is therefore very much a student city.

Dalhousie University
Faculty of Medicine, 5849 University Avenue, Halifax, Nova Scotia, Canada B3H 4H7 Tel: (902) 494 1620 Fax: (902) 494 8884 www.mcms.dal.ca
e-mail: medical.communications@dal.ca
The faculty, founded in 1868, covers the three Maritime Provinces of Canada (Nova Scotia, New Brunswick and Prince Edward Island) with a population of 1.7 million. The teaching hospitals total 2300 beds.

The major teaching hospitals used include:

- **The Queen Elizabeth II Health Sciences Centre** in the heart of Halifax (including Camp Hill, Victoria General, Nova Scotia Rehab and New Halifax Infirmary). This is the major referral centre for Maritime Canada www.qe2-hsc.ns.ca
- **The IWK Grace Health Centre**
- The **Nova Scotia** (Psychiatric) Hospital
- **St John Regional Hospital** a large modern hospital in New Brunswick

To do electives in these write to the University. Previously they have been awkward about malpractice insurance though their position may have changed.

The Victoria General Hospital
Halifax, Nova Scotia, Canada.
The hospital: Is the largest teaching hospital in Nova Scotia with a full range of medical specialities and research facilities. It is in downtown Halifax next to the children and maternity hospitals, a stone's throw from the medical campus.

Newfoundland

Newfoundland, right in the far east of Canada, has a population of 500,000, most of whom live in St John's. St John's itself is built around a pleasant harbour.

Memorial University of Newfoundland

Faculty of Medicine, St John's, Newfoundland, Canada A1B 3V6 Tel: (709) 737 6615 Fax: 737 5186 www.med.mun.ca/med/

Founded in 1925, Memorial is the only University in Newfoundland. The Health Sciences Centre includes the general hospital with 530 beds. A number of other hospitals in St John's are also used. To do an elective in these hospitals you'll need to apply to the university. They have a fee of around C$100 and can provide malpractice cover for around C$137.

Memorial University Hospital

St John's, Newfoundland A1B 3V6, Canada.

The hospital: Provides nearly all specialities, but the **Grace Hospital** provides obstetric care and the **Charles Janeway Children's Hospital** (Pleasantville, St John's) provides paediatric care. These hospitals provide tertiary referral care for a massive area up to Labrador and hence rescue flights are common. Soon the Janeway and Grace will close and everything will be at the Mem.

Charles S Curtis Memorial Hospital

Grenfell Regional Health Services, St Anthony, Newfoundland, Canada A0K 4S0 Tel: 709 454 3333 Fax: 709 454 2052.

The hospital: In St Anthony (population 3200), the healthcare is very much GP ('family medicine') orientated. The GPs run clinics in the hospital and admit directly. Once in they can then direct patient's care. The hospital has 60 beds and six ITU beds. Family practice also covers obs, gynae and emergency medicine. The CCMH covers a large area ... the northern Newfoundland Peninsula, coastal Quebec and southern Labrador. Due to the great distances, flying is an integral part of medical practice, bringing in patients from far out nursing stations or taking more serious ones to St Johns. The obstetrics department receives on average 250 deliveries a year and, with the gynae unit, has two antenatal and two general outpatient clinics a week.

O Elective notes: This is an incredibly popular destination for students and hence the length of this section. As a student you go out to the local communities for clinics and are involved with the hospital carc. You thcrcforc gct a grcat deal of experience in a number of specialities and in the hospital you are given a great deal of responsibility. In surgery you effectively work as a JHO. Here they actually NEED you and you become a valued member of the team. There is a rota (no more then 1:3) for on-call where the medical students cover the entire hospital and admit in the A&E. If doing surgery, you are the assistant. Don't go here if you don't like being isolated.

Note: In obs and gynae there have apparently been some problems between staff (nursing and medical) and students as sometimes a bit too much is expected of them and there is not much teaching. The others are great though.

St Anthony is a town where cod fishing and moose hunting are the topics of the day and the locals really do wear red and black lumberjack shirts. The population is rapidly diminishing as people move to the cities. There is high unemployment (20%) since cod fishing (their main industry) was made illegal in 1992 to preserve fish stocks. In the winter there are whales, icebergs and moose to see and the opportunity to try 'ski-dooing'. You can also visit the only Viking settlement in North America (*L'Anse Aux Meadows*). In July and August it can be warm (20 ºC), but fog is still common. During Jan–March it is very cold with snow storms. Many festivals occur in the summer. Corner Brook is the nearest town (six hours in the car) and Gros Morne National Park is great for hiking. The local ice rink does not hire skates and there are no commercial ski-hire businesses. Transport is also a major problem.

Accommodation: Currently accommodation, food and money towards your airfare (Can$1000) are provided by CCMH (if you stay for eight weeks); however, this is in the process of changing. The accommodation was with other elective students (there are no resident students) and very friendly.

NON-GOVERNMENTAL ORGANIZATIONS

***Acord**
Francis House, Francis Street, London SW1P 1DQ or Dean Geadley House, 52 Horseferry Road, London SW1P 2AF Tel: 020 7227 8600.

Action Against Hunger
Sally Tillett, 1 Catton Street, London WC1R 4AB Tel: 020 7831 5858 Fax: 020 7831 4259.

Action Against Disability
Tracey Mole, Regional Rehab Centre, Hunters Road, Newcastle upon Tyne NE2 4NR.

Action Health
Kate Graham, The Gate House, 25 Gwydir Street, Cambridge CB1 2LO Tel: 01223 460853 Fax: 01223 460853.
Sends professional volunteers to India, Tanzania and Uganda to train local people in inexpensive, effective healthcare skills. They provide costs but you must be between 24–60, have skills and work for a minimum of six months. They provide costs.

Action on Disability and Development
Richard Stowell, 23 Lower Keyford, Frome, Somerset BA11 4AP.

ActionAid
Akila Kassam, Hamlyn House, MacDonald Road, London N19 5PG.

Africa Evangelical Fellowship
Sheila McMillan, 6 Station Court, Station Approach, Borough Green, Sevenoaks, Kent TN15 8AD.

* = They only tend to send very experienced health workers.

Africa Inland Mission
Peter MacLure, 2 Vorley Road, Archway, London N19 5HE Tel: 020 7281 1184 Fax: 020 7281 4479.

Agency for Personal Service (APSO)
30 Fitwilliam Square, Dublin 2, Ireland Tel: +353 1 661 4411 Fax: +353 1 661 4202.
This is the central organization for all of Ireland's NGOs.

American Refugee Committee
2244 Nicolette Avenue, Suite 250, Minneapolis MN 55404, USA Tel: +1 612 872 7060 Fax: +1 612 872 4309.

AMREF
Alexander Heroys,
11 Old Queen Street, London SW1H 9LA.

Baptist Missionary Society
Sian Williams, PO Box 49, Baptist House, 129 Broadway, Didcot, Oxon OX11 8XA Tel: 01235 512 077 Fax: 01235 511 265.

British Executive Service Overseas (BESO)
David Lewis, 164 Vauxhall Bridge Road, London SW1V 2RB.

British Council
Dr Douglas Buchanan, Bridgewater House, 58 Whitworth Street, Manchester M1 6BB.

British Nepal Medical Trust
Mrs Gay Peck, Stafford House, 16 East Street, Tonbridge TN9 1HG or 130 Vale Road, Tonbridge, Kent TN9 1SP Tel: 01732 360284 Fax: 01732 363876.

***British Red Cross Society**
Joan Coyle, 9 Grosvernor Crescent, London SW1X 7EJ Tel: 020 7235 5454.

CAFOD
Martin Kelly, 2 Romero Close, Stockwell Road, London SW9 9TY.

Calcutta Rescue Fund
Ruth Catty, PO Box 52, Brentford, Middlesex TW8 0TF.

***Care International UK**
Elaine Smart, Tower House, 8–14 Southampton Street, London WC2E 7HA Tel: 020 7379 5247.

Children's Aid Direct
Alison Sidwell, 12 Portman Road, Reading, Berks RG30 1EA Tel: 0118 584 000 Fax: 0118 958 8988.

Christian Aid
Wendy Spink, PO Box 100, London SE1 7RT.

Christian Medical Fellowship
Dr David Clegg, 157 Waterloo Road, London SE1 8XN Tel: 020 7928 4694.

Christian Outreach Relief and Development (CORD)
Kay Bugg, 1 New Street, Leamington Spa, Warwicks CV31 1HP Tel: 01926 315301.

Christians Abroad
Chris Hiscock, 1 Stockwell Green, London SW9 9HP Tel: 020 7346 5951 Fax: 020 7346 5955.

Christoffel Blindenmission
Bill McAllister, Orwell House, Cowley Road, Cambridge CB4 4WY or Nibelungenstrasse 124, D-6140 Bensheim 4, Germany Tel: +48 62511310 Fax: +49 6251131165.

Church of Scotland World Mission
Rev Ray Gaston, 121 George Street, Edinburgh EH2 4YN.

Church Missionary Society (CMS)
Stuart Buchanan, Partnership House, 157 Waterloo Road, London SE1 8UU Tel: 020 7928 8681 Fax: 020 7401 2910.

* = They only tend to send very experienced health workers.

Commonwealth Society for the Disabled
Brigadier JA Davis, Dilke House, Malet Street, London WC1E 7JA.

Concern Universal
Pam Morris, 17a New Road Avenue, Chatham, Kent ME4 6BA.

Concern Worldwide UK
Valerie Sullivan, 47 Frederick Street, Belfast BT1 2LW or 248/250 Lavender Hill, London SW11 1LJ Tel: 020 7738 1033 Fax: 020 7738 1032.

Crown Agents
Mr Richard Faulkner, St Nicholas House, St Nicholas Road, Sutton SM1 1EL.

***Department for International Development (DFID)**
Mrs Jackie Kirwan, Abercombie House, Eaglesham Road, East Kilbride G75 8EA or 94 Victoria Street, London SW1E 5JL Tel: 020 7917 0107 Fax: 020 7917 0174.

East European Partnership
Debbie Epstien, Carlton House, 27A Carlton Drive, London SW15 2BS Tel: 020 8780 2841 Fax: 020 8780 9592.

Edinburgh Medical Missionary Society
Mr Robin Arnott, Executive Director, 7 Washington Lane, Edinburgh, EH11 2HA.

Emmanuel Hospital Association
Mr Paul East, European Fellowship, PO Box 43, Sutton SM2 5WL.

Goal UK
Heather Kerr, c/o Mean Road, London W3 8AN or PO Box 19, Dun Loaghaire, Co Dublin, Ireland Tel: +252 1 280 9779 Fax: +353 1 280 9215.

Handicap International
14 Avenue Bethelot, 69361 Lyon, France Tel: +334 78697979 Fax: +334 7869 7994.

Hands Around the World
Dr David Steiner, The Old Vicarage, Christchurch Nr. Colefor, Glos GL16 7NS.

Healthnet International
Singel 540, 1017 Amsterdam, Netherlands Tel: +31 20 420 1115 Fax: +31 20 420 1503.

Health Projects Abroad
Mr Simon Headington, PO Box 24, Bakewell, Derbyshire DE45 1ZW.
They work with communities in Tanzania giving training beforehand. They want people aged 18–28 and say that no skills are required, but medics and engineers must have three years experience!

Health Unlimited
Jo MacKenzie, Prince Consort House, 27–9 Albert Embankment, London SE1 7TS Tel: 020 7582 5999 Fax: 020 7582 5900.

***Helpage International**
Mr James Davidson, 67–74 Saffron Hill, London EC1N 8QX Tel: 020 7404 7201.

HMD International
Mr Philip Garvin, 27a Pembridge Villas, London W11 3EP.

ICD
Maureen O'Sullivan, Unit 3, Canonbury Yard, 190a New North Road, London N1 7BJ.

Institute for Health
Mr Ken Grant, Development Sector, 27 Old Street, London EC1V 9HL.

International Care and Relief
Terri Lewis, PO Box 180, 16 St John's Hill, Sevenoaks, Kent TN13 3NR.

International Child Care Trust
Mr P Beanlands, Unit 3L, Leroy House, 436 Essex Road, London N1 3QP.

* = They only tend to send very experienced health workers.

International Corporation for Development
Unit 3, Canonbury Yard, 190a New North Road, London N1 7BJ Tel: 020 7354 0883 Fax: 020 7359 0017.

International Health Exchange
Mr Patrick Brooks, 134 Lower Marsh Road, London SE1 7AE Tel: 020 7620 3333 www.ihe.org.uk e-mail info@ihe.org.uk

International Medical Corps
Mr Ivan Tomlin, 3 Anselm Road, Hatch End, Pinner HA5 4LH.

International Nepal Fellowship
Mr John Reynolds, 69 Wentworth Road, Harborne, Birmingham B17 9SS Tel: 0121 427 8833 Fax: 0121 428 3110.

International Rescue Committee
122 East 42nd Street, 12th Floor, New York, NY 10168–1289, USA Tel: +1 212 551 3000 Fax: +1 212 551 3180.

International Rescue Corps
Mr Willie McMartin, 8 Kings Road, Grangemouth, Stirlingshire FK3 9BB.

International Voluntary Service Inc
1424 16th Street, NW Suite, 504, Washington DC, 20036, USA.

Interserve
Ruth Millson, Personnel Director, 325 or 186 Kennington Park Road, London SE11 4QH Tel: 020 7735 8227 Fax: 020 7587 5362.

Karim Rida Said Foundation
Marieke Bosman, 7th Floor, Berkley Square, London W1X 6LS.
LEPRA Faifax House, Causton House, Colchester CO1 1PU.

Leprosy Mission
Sue Slatter, Goldhay Way, Orton Goldhay, Peterborough, PE2 5GZ Tel: 01733 370505.

Leprosy Mission International
Rose Barrett, 80 Windmill Road, Brentford, Middlesex TW8 0QH.

Ludhiana British Fellowship
Margaret Smith, 157 Waterloo Road, London SE1 8UU Tel: 020 7928 1173.

Marlborough Brandt Group
Mr Ken Wright, 1a London Road, Malborough SN8 1PH.

MAP
Suliman Mleahat, 33a Islington Park Street, London N1 1QB.

***Marie Stopes International**
Fiona Fraser 153–7 Cleveland Street, London W1P 5PG/Bruce Mackay, 62 Grafton Way, London W1P 5LD Tel: 020 7574 7423.

MEDAIR
Mrs Kay Pither, 13 Highfield Oval, Ambrose Lane, Harpenden AL5 4BX.

Médecins du Monde UK
11 Sovereign Close, Sovereign Court, London E1 9HW Tel: 020 7488 4888.
Will take medics for as little as three months.

Médecins sans Frontières UK
Gabriella Breebaart, 124–32 Clerkenwell Road, London EC1R 5DL Tel: 020 7713 5600 Fax: 020 7713 5004.
MSF is the world's largest independent organization for emergncy medical relief operating in over 60 countries where there have been either natural or man-made disasters. They want skilled medical and technial people over 25 for a minimum of nine months. The cost to the volunteer is nil.

Medical Aid for Iraq
Heidi Phillips, Unit 16, Foundation House, 38 Kingsland Road, London E2 EDQ.

Medical Aid for Palestinians (MAP)
33a Islington Park Street, London N1 1QB Tel: 020 7226 4114 Fax: 020 7226 0880.

Medical Emergency Relief International (MERLIN)
Bryony Glenn, 14 David Mews, London W1M 1HW Tel: 020 7487 2505 Fax: 020 7487 4042.

Medical Missionaries for Mary
Dr Moira O'Donohue, 66 Newland Street, Silvertown, London E16 2HN.

Mercy Corps Europe/Scottish European Aid
11 Grovelands Avenue, Swindon, Wilts SN1 4ET Tel: 01793 486 036 Fax: 01793 643 383.

Methodist Church Overseas Division
Rev Winston Graham, Overseas Division, 25 Marylebone Road, London NW1 5JR Tel: 020 7486 5502 Fax: 020 7487 4042.

Mid Africa Ministry
Owen Davies, Partnership House, 157 Waterloo Road, London SE1 8UY Tel: 020 7928 8681 Fax: 020 7401 2910.

Mines Advisory Group
Mike Watson, 54a Main Street, Cockermouth, Cumbria CA13 9LU.

Murabinda Hospital
John Connolly, c/o 6 Park Grove, Frizinghall, Bradford BD9 4JY.

Nepal Leprosy Trust
James Lowether, 15 Duncan Road, Richmond, Surrey TW9 2JD.

One World Action
Hazel Plunkett, Bradley's Close, White Lion Street, London N1 9PF.

Options
Katie Chapman, 6 Grafton Mews, London W1P 5LF.

***Oxfam**
Goldie Prince, 274 Banbury Road, Oxford OX2 7DZ Tel: 01865 311311 Fax: 01865 312380.

Plan International
Mary Mackenzie, Chobham House, Christchurch Way, Woking GU21 1JG.

Population Concern
Wendy Thomas, Director, 178–202 Great Portland Street, London W1N 5TB.

Power
Michael Boddington, 14 Western Road, Henley on Thames, Oxfordshire RG9 1JL.

Project Hope
Deborah Machaneck, Wilson Building, Stockley Park West, Uxbridge UB11 1BT.

Quaker Peace and Service
Pauline Leader, Friends House, Euston Square, London NW1 2BJ.

Raleigh International
Alison Bolton, 27 Parsons Green Lane, London SW6 4HZ.
This is a youth development charity organizing community and environmental expeditions around the world. Applicants are usually aged between 17 and 25 (over 25 are staff). The time taken is usually three months and you do have to raise some funds.

Relief Fund for Romania
Edward Parry 54–62 Regent Street, London W1R 5PJ.

Rescue and Preparedness in Disasters (RAPID)
27 Aleyn Way, Baldock, Hertfordshire SG7 6SU Tel: 01462 637266.

Rotary Doctor Bank of GB and Ireland
Alan Thomas, Morawelon, St Hilary, Cowbridge CF71 7DP.

Ryder Cheshire Foundation
(for physiotherapists) Simon Hardwick, Poleshill Cottage, Langford Budville, Wellington, Somerset TA21 0RX Tel/Fax: 01823 672271.

* = They only tend to send very experienced health workers.

Salvation Army
Health Services, 101 Queen Victoria Street, PO Box 249, London EC4 4EP Tel: 020 7332 0101 Fax: 020 7236 4981.

Sandy Gall's Afghanistan Appeal
Mrs Eleanor Gall, PO Box 145, Tonbridge, Kent TN11 8SA.

***Save The Children Fund**
Leonie Lonton, 17 Grove Lane, Camberwell, London SE5 8RD Tel: 020 7703 5400 Fax: 020 7703 2278.

Scottish Churches World Exchange
Lynn Whitehead, 7 Randolf Crescent, Edinburgh EH3 7TH.

Scottish European Aid
John Musson, 5 Lemington Terrace, Edinburgh, EH10 4JW.

Skillshare Africa
Mr Dave Harries, 3 Belvoir Street, Leicester LE1 6SL or 126 New Walk, Leicester LE1 7JA Tel: 116 254 1862 Fax: 01160 254 2614.
This group tries to transfer skills to those in Africa. You should be aged between 21 and 63 and although costs are covered, the minimum length of time is two years.

Southeast Asian Outreach
John Heard, 90 Windmill Street, Gravesend, Kent DA12 1LH.

St Andrew's Evangelical Mission
126 Ealing Road, Brentford, Middlesex TW8 0LD.

St Mary's Hospital
Trevor Lines, Human Resources, Praed Street, London W2 1NY.

Tear Fund
Anthea Fisher, 100 Church Road, Teddington, Middlesex TW11 8QR Tel: 020 8977 9144.

Terre des Hommes
PO Box 388, 1000 Lausanne, Switzerland.

The Halo Trust
Susan Mitchell, 804 Drake House, Dolphin Square, London SW1V 3NA.

The Ockenden Venture
Constitution Hill, Woking, Surrey GU22 7UU.

THET
Professor Eldryd Parry, 1 Park Square West, London NW1 4LJ.

Trocaire
169 Booterstown Avenue, Blackrock, Co Dublin, Ireland Tel: 353 1 288 5385.

Ugandan Society for Disabled Children
145a London Road, Kingston upon Thames, Surrey KT2 6NH.

***UNICEF UK**
55 Lincolns Inn Fields, London WC2 Tel: 020 7405 5592.

United Nations Association International Service (UNAIS)
Stella Hobbs, Suite 3a, Hunter House, 57 Goodramgate, York YO1 2LS Tel: 01904 647799 Fax: 01904 652 353.
This group works with locally managed initiatives in Bolivia, Brazil, Burkina Faso, Mali and the West Bank and Gaza Strip. Primary healthcare is a particular priority. You must be over 18; two years are usually required but costs are covered.

United Nations Volunteers (UN)
Palais des Nations, 1211 Geneva, Switzerland Tel: +41 22 985850.

* = They only tend to send very experienced health workers.

United Society for the Propagation of the Gospel (USPG)
Partnership House, 157 Waterloo Road, London SE1 8XA Tel: 020 7928 8681 Fax: 020 7928 2371.

URBANAID
79 Amsterdam Road, London Yard, London E14 3UU Tel: 020 7515 7366.

Valley Mission Project
12 Fishers Lane, Chiswick, London W4 1RX.

Volunteer Missionary Movement
Matthew Brambach/Monica Pereira, 1 Stockwell Green, London SW9 9JF Tel: 020 7737 3678 Fax: 020 7346 5955.
This ecumenical organization recruits and prepares volunteers for a number of skills in Africa and Central America. You must be over 24 and commitment of two years is normally required.

VSO
John Nurse, 317 Putney Bridge Road, London SW15 2PN.
VSO now take medics for as little as three months.

Wateraid
Mrs Suba Shivanathan-Beast, Prince Consort House, 27–9 Albert Embankment, London SE1 7UB Tel: 020 7793 4500.

World Church and Mission
8 Tavistock Place, London WC1H 9RT.

Worldvision UK
Cliff Eaton, World Vision House, 599 Avebury Boulevard, Milton Keynes MK9 3PG Tel: 01908 841014.

World Exchange
St Colm's International House, Inverleith Terrace, Edinburgh EH3 5NS Tel: 0131 315 4444.

***World Health Organization**
Personnel Officer, Avenue Apia 20, 1211 Geneva 27, Switzerland.

World Service Enquiry
Tel: 020 7346 5950.
This organization provides vocational information both to Christians and non-Christians. They have information on voluntary and paid opportunities short (from two weeks) or long-term in aid, development and mission agencies. They catered for the skilled and unskilled over 18.

Youth Vision with a Mission
Graham Fawcett, Highfield Oval, Ambrose Lane, Harpenden AL5 4BX.

ELECTIVE AND TRAVEL BURSARIES

AH Bygott Undergraduate Scholarships (for London medical/dental students only doing electives in public health) makes awards of up to £750. Contact: the Secretary to the Academic Trust Funds Committee, University of London, Senate House (Room 234), Malet Street, London WC1E 7HU Tel: 020 7862 8041 Fax: 020 7862 8042. L.West@acadmic.lon.ac.uk.

Note: They also give one £1500 award for postgrads for research work, including travel in public health and related subjects.

The Alchemy Foundation, Trevereux Manor, Limpsfield Chart, Oxted, Surrey RH8 0TL.

Anglo-Israel Association, 9 Bentinck Street, London W1M 5RP Tel: 020 7486 2300 Fax: 020 7935 4690. Wyndham Deedes Memorial Travel Scholarship is open to graduates or senior students who travel to Israel to study an aspect of Israel life (economical, cultural, scientific etc.). Each scholarship is valued up to £2000. You must stay at least six weeks and write 5000 words.

Association of Anaesthetists of Great Britain and Ireland, Honorary Secretary, 9 Bedford Square, London WC1B 3RA. Offers prizes for essays written.

British Association of Forensic Medicine, Department of Forensic Pathology, The Medico-Legal Centre, Watery Street Sheffield S3 7ES Tel: 0114 2738721. Offers a prize (awarded retrospectively) of around £200 for the best elective report on a project undertaken in forensic medicine. Needs to be a scientific-type presentation of around 2000 words.

The British Association of Plastic Surgeons at the Royal College of Surgeons, 35–43 Lincoln's Inn Fields, London WC2A 3PN. They have four annual elective grants of around £350. Applications in the form of a letter giving an itinerary and costs, together with a brief CV should be submitted to the Chairman of the Education and Research Sub-Committee. A report is required three months after return. (Closing date is end of January.)

British Federation of Women Graduates, 28 Great James Street, London WC1N 3ES Tel: 020 7404 6447 Fax: 020 7404 6505. They have previously helped with living expenses.

British Geriatrics Society for the Health of the Aged, 1 St Andrew's Place, Regents Park, London NW1 4LB. Offers awards of up to £500 to UK medical students doing electives concerned with health/health care of old age.

The British Medical and Dental Student's Trust, The Secretary, Mackintosh House, 120 Blythswood Street, Glasgow, G2 4EA Tel: 0141 221 5858 Fax: 0141 228 1208. They give a number of awards often around the £150–£600 mark.

The British Nutrition Foundation, High Holborn House, 52–4 High Holborn, London WC1V 6RQ Tel: 020 7404 6504 Fax: 020 7404 6747 www.nutrition.org.uk run the following two schemes: **The Nestlé Bursary Scheme**. Since 1978, the *BNF* and Nestlé Charitable Trust have aimed to 'help medical students to undertake an elective concerned with nutritional problems encountered in the Third World, associated with adults in apparent health and disease states, including the special areas of maternal health and infant nutrition'. Twelve bursaries of up to £500 are available. A report is required five months after return. **The Dennis Burkitt Study Awards**. Also run by the *BNF* (in conjunction with Kellogg's). The ten awards (a tribute to Burrkitt as in lymphoma and research into diet and worldwide disease) are for students of medicine, nutrition science and related subjects who undertake studies into food and nutrition, especially in developing countries. Awards of up to £750 are made.

British Society for Haematology, Scientific Secretary, 2 Carlton House Terrace, London, SW1Y 5AF. Eight scholarships are awarded to medical students wishing to do an elective project involving haematology. Each is a maximum of £600. Send a letter outlining the project and costs, a letter from the Dean and host institution.

Cancer Research Campaign, 10 Cambridge Terrace, London NW1 4JL. Gives ten bursaries of £500 each to UK medical students doing an elective involving the prevention, detection, treatment or management of cancer.

Child Health Research Appeal Trust, The Institute of Child Health, University of London, 30 Guildford Street, London, WC1N 1EH. Five awards of £125/week are offered nationally for those undertaking epidemiological, psychiatric or community based clinical work in the UK only. Apply to the Registrar.

The Clegg Scholarship, *BMJ*, BMA House, Tavistock Square, London WC1H 9TR. This is for an elective with the *BMJ* to learn about medical journalism. Write to Luisa Dillner at this address.

The Commonwealth Foundation Medical Elective Bursaries offers awards for senior medical students doing electives in developing Commonwealth countries. They are not available for Australia, the UK, Canada and New Zealand. Approximately 50 awards of up to £1000 are offered for tenure in May. You should apply via your Dean before January. A report is required on return. Countries covered include: AFRICA: Botswanna, Cameroon, Gamba, Ghana, Kenya, Lesotho, Malawi, Mauritius, Mozambique, Namibia, South Africa, Swaziland, Tanzania, Uganda, Zambia, Zimbabwe. CARIBBEAN: Belize, Dominica, Grenada, Guyana, Jamaica, St Lucia, St Vincent, Trinidad and Tobago. ASIA: Bangladesh, India, Malaysia, Pakistan, Singapore, Sri Lanka. PACIFIC: Fiji, Kiribati, Nauru, Papua New Guinea, Solomon Islands, Tonga, Tuvalu, Vanuatu, Western Samoa. The award is given on (i) the feasibility and scientific merit of the attachment proposed and its usefulness to the student and receiving institution and (ii) the educational record and motivation of the student.

Eating Disorders Association, Sackville Place, 44 Magdalen Street, Norwich, Norfolk NR3 1JU. Offers prizes for essay writing.

The Edward Boyle Memorial Trust offers six elective bursaries of up to £500. A separate application is not required if applying to the Commonwealth Foundation.

Faculty of Public Health Medicine of the Royal Colleges of Physicians of the UK, 4 St Andrew's Place, London NW1 4LB. Offer the Cochrane Prize for UK medical students doing an educational activity in public health.

Israel Medical Association, 22 Macheson Road, London NW3 2LU Tel: 020 7267 6784. Awards eight £300 awards to medical students doing electives in a hospital in Israel. Include your CV, a proposal of what you are doing and a letter from your host. An alternative address is Dr Lionel Balfour-Lynn, 120 Harley St, London W1N 1AG.

Kabi Pharmacia Elective Grant, Kabi Pharmacia Ltd, Knowhill, Milton Keynes MK5 8PH. They make six awards of £250 for those doing electives in developing countries. Awards are made on the basis of a written application of no more that 400 words. Write to Dr Richard Wild, Haderburg, Medical Director at the above address.

LEPRA (The British Leprosy Relief Association), Fairfax House, Causton Road, Colchester, Essex CO1 1PU Tel: (01206) 5662286 Fax: (01206) 762151. Offers awards for essays.

Leukaemia Research Fund, 43 Great Ormond Street, London WC1N 3JJ Tel: 020 7405 0101 Fax: 020 7242 2488. They make five awards of up to £600 for electives allied to the study of haematological malignancy.

The Lord Mayor's 800th Anniversary Awards Trust, 401 Salisbury House, London Wall, London EC2M 5RR Tel: 020 7638 8358 Fax: 020 7638 9681. They have previously given awards to medical students going on elective. Preference is given to those who have a connection with the City of London. Applicants need to be aged between 17 and 25 and grants are normally around £500.

Medical Research Council, 20 Park Crescent, London W1N 4AL Tel: 020 7636 5422 Fax: 636 3427. The MRC runs the 'Rogers Fund Elective Period in the Tropics'.

Medical Women's Federation Student Elective Bursaries, 62 Denbigh Street, London SW1V 2EX. One award of £300 is made to a London student studying maternal or child health in a developing country. Submit a CV and project outline to Dr J Wells.

The Medicine Group and The Glaxo Wellcome Medical Fellowship, The Medicine Group (Journals) Ltd, Freespost, Elective Grant Co-ordinator, Publishing House, 62 Stret Street, Abingdon, Oxon OX14 3BR Tel: (01235) 555770 Fax: (01235) 554691. Annually (on 31 March) awards one £400 prize to an applicant from each UK medical school for an elective in the following 12 months. One top award of £1000 is given. Send a CV a comprehensive description of your proposed elective and reasons for doing it, confirmation from your host (if available) and name of two referees (Dean and a Consultant).

The Mental Health Foundation, 20/21 Cornwall Terrace, London NW1 4QL Tel: 020 7535 7400 Fax: 020 7535 7474 www.mentalhealth.org.uk For electives in psychiatry (may require essay). Eight awards of up to £400 are made.

Milupa Student Elective Grant Fund, Milupa Ltd, Milupa House, Uxbridge Road, Hillingdon, Middlesex UV10 0NE. Ten awards of up to £500 are given nationally for an elective with research into paediatric nutrition. Write to the Managing Director (Mr T Bell).

The National Birthday Trust Fund, 27 Sussex Place, Regent's Park, London NW1 4SP. Provides two awards of £250 for those doing electives in obstetrics or neonatology.

Newby Trust Limited, Hill Farm, Froxfield, nr Petersfield, Hampshire GU32 1BQ.

Pathological Society of Great Britain and Ireland, The Education Secretary, The Royal College of Pathologists, 2 Carlton House Terrace, London SW1Y 5AF. Awards up to £50/week for a maximum of 12 weeks. It needs a report within three months of return. £150 is given to the best.

The Renal Association, Triangle House, Broomhill Road, London SW18 4HX Tel: 020 8875 2413 Fax: 020 8877 9308. Gives four bursaries of £250 for medical students doing an elective in which renal medicine is a significant component.

The Royal College of General Practitioners. Offers elective prizes for primary care/GP electives.

Royal College of Obstetricians and Gynaecologists, 27 Sussex Place, Regent's Park, London NW1 4RG Tel: 020 7262 5425 Fax: 020 7723 0575. Offer prizes for students showing the greatest understanding of a clinical problem in O&G. Maximum 3000-word case history.

Royal College of Surgeons of England, Preiskel Elective Prize in Surgery, Research and Audit Board, 35/43 Lincoln's Inn Fields, London WC2A

3PN Tel: 020 7312 6672 Fax: 020 7831 5741 arakababoo@rcseng.ac.uk. Gives awards of between £500 and £1000 for students wishing to pursue a career in surgery who do a surgical elective in the developing world. Send six copies of: your CV, details of the proposed project, a letter from the Dean and a letter from the surgeon at the host institution. Write to Mr Martyn Coomer.

The Royal Society of Medicine, Section of the History of Medicine, 1 Wimpole Street, London W1M 8AE Tel: 020 7290 2985 Fax: 020 7290 2989. They offer the Norah Schuster Prize to preclinical, clinical and dental students.

Royal Society of Tropical Medicine and Hygiene, Manson House, 26 Portland Place, London W1N 4EY Tel: 020 7580 2127 Fax: 020 7436 1389. Gives £300 for an account of any work carried out by a medical student of any nationality during an elective in a tropical/developing county. It is awarded on originality and contribution to knowledge/understanding of tropical diseases.

St Francis Leprosy Guild, 21 The Boltons, London SW10 9SU. Has previously given elective awards of up to £600 for those doing electives involving leprosy.

The Scottish Eastern Association of the Medical Women's Federation, (Contact Dr JW Keeling, Pathology Department, Royal Hospital for Sick Children, 2 Rillbank Crescent, Edinburgh EH9 1LF). Open to female medical students in Aberdeen, Dundee and Edinburgh (gives £200 twice a year).

Sir John Cass's Foundation, PO Box 853, 31 Jewry Street, London EC3N 2HA Tel: 020 7480 5884. They can offer awards to students who have been residents in inner London for the last three years and who are under 25.

The Society of Occupational Medicine, 6 St Andrew's Place, Regent's Park, London NW1 4LB Tel: 020 7486 2641 Fax: 020 7486 0028. The Thackrah Award for Undergraduate Study of occupational medicine is offered at up to £1000 for research or an elective in occupational medicine. It is funded by Nestlé UK.

The Vandervell Foundation, Bridge House, 181, Queens Street, London EC4 4DD Tel: 020 7248 9045.

Wellbeing (The Health Research Charity for Women and Babies), 27 Sussex Place, Regent's Park, London NW1 4SP Tel: 020 722 5337 Fax: 017 724 7725. They run the National Birthday Trust Fund that each year gives two bursaries of £250 to elective students studying obs or neonatal paeds.

The Winston Churchill Memorial Trust, 15 Queen's Gate Terrace, London SW7 5PR Tel: 020 7584 9315 Fax: 020 7581 0410 www.wcmt.org.uk Set up to commemorate Winston Churchill, the trust offers around 100 awards a year (totalling around £500,000). Each year they produce a leaflet suggesting categories to apply for. They can be very broad e.g. '*Health Promotion for Young People*', '*Leadership in the Community*'. Any medical staff could therefore apply if doing anything that is either personally or community-enhancing.

Other bursaries that are available only through your clinical school registry are:

Churchill Livingston Student Bursary. One award of £1000 for an essay.

Clinical Endocrinology Trust Elective Bursaries. Ten £500 awards are made nationally.

Cow and Gate Prize. Medical schools (Dept of Paedictrics) often have information on a number of their prizes.

Dr Robert Malcolm Trust Awards. A £300 award is available for every medical school.

The Royal College of Physicians, Oscar Reginald Lewis Wilson Scholarship. A £250 award is awarded to an applicant from each medical school that is British or a member of the Commonwealth. Applications are viewed in terms of a proposed project and the financial situation of the student.

The University of London Convocation. Two awards of variable amounts are made per school.

Wellcome Trust. Student elective prizes. Open to UK medical students who must do a research project under supervision in any discipline bar cancer. One-third of awards are for tropical medicine. Up to £1000 can be given for personnel support and up to £600 for the costs of the project. Nominations are only accepted from the Dean of your medical school (or director of overseas Wellcome Trust). Each school has a quota of awards and a 1500-word essay is required on return. Wellcome ask that this is applied for via your Dean. Do not contact them directly.

Contact addresses for Wellcome Trust Overseas Units:

KENYA

Dr W Watkins, Wellcome Trust Laboratories, PO Box 43640, Nairobi, Kenya Tel: +254 (2) 711673.

THAILAND AND VIETNAM

Paul Hogben, Grants Administrator, Nuffield Department of Clinical Medicine Room 5803, John Radcliffe Hospital, Headington, Oxford OX3 9DU.

EMBASSIES AND HIGH COMMISSIONS

The following section contains pretty comprehensive lists of Embassies in the UK, Australia and America. Occasionally, embassies move or change phone number. If you have any problems either (i) look in the phone book, (ii) do a search on the net or (iii) visit www.tagish.co.uk which has some of the major embassies listed.

EMBASSIES IN THE UK

Afghanistan: Embassy of the Islamic State of Afghanistan, 31 Princes Gate, London SW7 1QQ Tel: 020 7589 8891/020 7589 8892 Fax: 020 7589 3452.

Albania: Embassy of the Republic of Albania, 4th Floor, 38 Grosvenor Gardens, London SW1W 0EB Tel: 020 7730 5709 Fax: 020 7730 5747.

Algeria: Algerian Embassy, 54 Holland Park, London W11 3RS Tel: 020 7221 7800 Fax: 020 7221 0448 e-mail: mail@admi.freeserve.co.uk www http://www.personal.u-net.com/~consalglond/

Angola: Angolan Embassy, 98 Park Lane, London W1Y 3TA Tel: 020 7495 1752 Fax: 020 7495 1635.

Argentina: Embassy of Argentina, 65 Brook Street, London W1Y 1YE Tel: 020 7318 1300 Fax: 020 7318 1301 e-mail: blj@atina.ar www http://www.argentine-embassy-uk.org/

Armenia: Embassy of the Republic of Armenia, 25a Cheniston Gardens, London W8 Tel: 020 7938 5435.

Australia: Australian High Commission, Australia House, The Strand, London WC2B 4LA Tel: 020 7379 4334 Fax: 020 7240 5333
www http://www.australia.org.uk/
Australian Consulate (Immigration Managed Post) Chatsworth House, Lever Street, Manchester M1 2DL Tel: 0161 228 1344 Fax: 0161 236 4074.

Austria: Austrian Embassy and Consular Section, 18 Belgrave Mews West, London SW1X Tel: 020 7235 3731.

Azerbaijan: Republic Embassy of Azerbaijan, 4 Kensington Court, London W8 Tel: 020 7938 3412.

Bahamas: The Bahamas High Commission, 10 Chesterfield Street, London W1X Tel: 020 7408 4488.

Bahrain: Embassy of the State of Bahrain, 98 Gloucester Road, London SW7 Tel: 020 7370 5132.

Bangladesh: The Bangladesh High Commission, 28 Queens Gate, London SW7 Tel: 020 7584 0081.

Barbados: Barbados High Commission, 1 Great Russell Street, London WC1 Tel: 020 7631 4975.
Belarus: Embassy of the Republic of Belarus, 6, Kensington Court, London W8 5DL Tel: 020 7937 3288. Fax: 020 7361 0005.
Belgium: Belgian Embassy, 103 Eaton Square, London SW1W 9AB Tel: 020 7470 3700 Fax: 020 7259 6213 www http://www.belgium-embassy.co.uk/
Belize: Belize High Commission, 22 Harcourt Houses, 19 Cavendish Square, London W1M Tel: 020 7499 9728.
Benin: Benin Consulate, Dolphin House, 16 The Broadway, Stanmore, Middlesex HA7 4DW Tel: 020 8954 8800 Fax: 020 8954 8844.
Bermuda: The Bermuda Society and Secretariat, Five Trees Wood Lane, Stanmore HA7 Tel: 020 8954 0652.
Bolivia: Bolivian Embassy, 106 Eaton Square, London SW1W 9AD Tel: 020 7235 4248 or 020 7235 4255 (Consulate) Fax: 020 7235 1286.
Bosnia and Herzegovina: Embassy of Bosnia and Herzegovina, 320 Regent Street, 4th Floor, London W1R 5AB Tel: 020 7255 3758 Fax: 020 7255 3760.
Botswana: Botswana High Commission, 6 Stratford Place, London W1N 9AE Tel: 020 7499 0031.
Brazil: Brazilian Embassy, 32 Green Street, London W1Y 4AT Tel: 020 7499 0877 Fax: 020 7493 5105 www http://www.brazil.org.uk/
Brunei: Brunei Darussalam High Commission, 19–20 Belgrave Square, London SW1X Tel: 020 7581 0521.
Bulgaria: Embassy of the Republic of Bulgaria, 186–8 Queens Gate, London Tel: 020 7584 9400.
Cameroon: Cameroon Embassy, 84 Holland Park, London W11 Tel: 020 7727 0771.
Canada: Canadian High Commission, 1 Grosvenor Square, London W1X 0AB Tel: 020 7258 6600 Fax: 020 7258 6333 www http://www.canada.org.uk/
Caribbean: Eastern Caribbean Commission, 10 Kensington Court, London W8 Tel: 020 7937 9522.
Cayman Islands: Cayman Islands Government Office in the UK, 6 Arlington Street, London SW1A 1RE. Tel: 020 7491 7772 Fax: 020 7491 7944.
Chile: Chilean Embassy, 12 Devonshire Street, London W1N Tel: 020 7580 6392.
China: Embassy of the People's Republic of China, 31 Portland Place, London W1N 3AG Tel: 0891 990909 or 020 7631 1430. **Manchester:** Denison House, 49 Denison Road, Manchester M14 5RX Tel: 0161 224 8672. **Edinburgh:** 43 Station Road, Edinburgh EH12 7AF Tel: 0131 316 4789 www http://www.chinese-embassy.org.uk
Colombia: Colombian Embassy, 3 Hans Crescent, London SW1X Tel: 020 7589 9177.
Congo (Democratic Republic of): Congolese Embassy, 26 Chesham Place, London SW1X 8HH Tel: 020 7235 6137 Fax: 020 7235 9048 or 12 Caxton Street, London SW1H Tel: 020 7222 7575.
Costa Rica: Costa Rican Embassy, Flat 1, 14 Lancaster Gate, London W2 Tel: 020 7706 8844.
Cote d'Ivoire: Embassy of the Republic Cote d'Ivoire, 2 Upper Belgrave Street, London SW1 Tel: 020 7235 6991.
Croatia: Embassy of the Republic of Croatia, 21 Conway Street, London W1P Tel: 020 7387 1144.
Cuba: Commercial Office of the Cuban Embassy, 167 High Holborn, London WC1V Tel: 020 7240 2488.
Cyprus: Cyprus High Commission, 93 Park Street, London W1Y Tel: 020 7499 8272.
Czech Republic: Czech Embassy, 26 Kensington Palace Gardens, London W8 4QY Tel: 020 7243 1115/020 7243 7900 Fax: 020 7727 9654.
Denmark: Royal Danish Embassy, 55 Sloane Street, London SW1X 9SR Tel: 020 7333 0200 Fax: 020 7333 0270 www http://www.denmark.org.uk/ **Danish Consulate in Edinburgh:** 4 Royal Terrace, Edinburgh Tel: 0131 556 4263.
Dominica: Dominican High Commission, 1 Collingham Gardens, London W8 Tel: 020 7370 5194.
Ecuador: Embassy of Ecuador, Flat 3b, 3 Hans Crescent, London SW1X Tel: 020 7584 1367.

Egypt: Embassy of the Arab Republic of Egypt, 2 Lowndes Street, London SW1X Tel: 020 7235 9719.
El Salvador: Embassy of El Salvador, Tennyson House, 159 Great Portland Street, London W1N Tel: 020 7436 8282.
Eritrea: Consulate of the State of Eritrea, 96 White Lion Street, London N1 Tel: 020 7713 0096.
Estonia: Estonian Embassy, 16 Hyde Park Gate, London SW7 5DG Tel: 020 7589 3428 Fax: 020 7589 3430 e-mail: loa@estonia.gov.uk www http://www.estonia.gov.uk/
Ethiopia: Ethiopian Embassy, 17 Princes Gate, London SW7 Tel: 020 7589 7212.
Europe: Commission of the European Communities, 8 Storeys Gate, London SW1P Tel: 020 7973 1992.
Fiji: Embassy of Fiji, 34 Hyde Park Gate, London SW7 Tel: 020 7584 3661.
Finland: Finnish Embassy, 38 Chesham Place, London SW1X 8HW Tel: 020 7838 6200 Fax: 020 7235 3680 e-mail: sanomat.lon@formin.fi www http://www.finemb.org.uk/
France: French Embassy, 23 Cromwell Road, London SW7 2EL Tel: 020 7201 1000/ 020 7838 2055 Fax: +44 020 7201 1004 www http://www.ambafrance.org.uk/ http://fr-inst.gov.uk
Gabon: Gabonese Embassy, 27 Elvaston Place, London SW7 Tel: 020 7823 9986.
Gambia: Gambia High Commission, 57 Kensington Court, London W8 Tel: 020 7937 6316.
Georgia: Georgian Embassy, 3 Hornton Place, Kensington, London W8 Tel: 020 7937 8233.
Germany: German Embassy, 23 Belgrave Square, London SW1X Tel: 020 7824 1300 Fax: 020 7824 1435 e-mail: mail@german-embassy.org.uk www http://www.german-embassy.org.uk/
Ghana: High Commission for Ghana, 104 Highgate Hill, London N6 Tel: 020 8342 8686.
Greece: Consulate General of Greece, 1a Holland Park, London W11 Tel: 020 7221 6467.
Guatemala: Embassy of Guatemala, 13 Fawcett Street, London SW10 Tel: 020 7351 3042. Fax: 020 7376 5708.
Guyana: Guyana High Commission, 3 Palace Court, Bayswater Road, London W2 4LP Tel: 020 7229 7684/8 Fax: 020 7727 9809.
Honduras: Embassy of Honduras, 115 Gloucester Place, London W1H 3PJ. Tel: 020 7486 4880 Fax: 020 7486 4550.
Hungary: Embassy of Hungary, 35B Eaton Place, London SW1X 8BY Tel: 020 7235 2664 Fax: 020 7235 8630 (Visa line: 0891 171 204).
Iceland: Icelandic Embassy, 1 Eaton Terrace, London SW1W Tel: 020 7590 1100 Fax: 020 7730 1683.
India: High Commission of India, India House, Aldwych, London WC2B Tel: 020 7836 8484. www http://www.hcilondon.org/ **Consulate General of India, Glasgow** Fleming House, 6th Floor, 134 Renfrew Street, Glasgow G3 7ST Tel: 0141 331 0777 Fax: 0141 331 0666 e-mail: cgiglasgow@btinternet.com
Indonesia: Indonesian Embassy, 38 Grosvenor Square, London W1X Tel: 020 7499 7661.
Iran: Embassy of Iran, 16 Princes Gate, London SW7 Tel: 020 7225 3000.
Iraq: Iraqi Embassy, 21 Queens Gate, London SW7 Tel: 020 7584 7141.
Ireland: Embassy of Ireland, 17 Grosvenor Place, London SWIX 7HR Tel: 020 7235 2171 Fax: 020 7245 6961.
Israel: Israeli Embassy, 2 Palace Green, London W8 4QB Tel: 020 7957 9500 Fax: 020 7957 9555 e-mail: isr-info@dircon.co.uk www http://www.israel-embassy.org.uk/london/
Italy: Italian Embassy, 14 Three Kings Yard, London, London W1Y 2EH Tel: 020 7312 2200 Fax: 020 7312 2283. 24-hour information line 0891 600340 (50p/minute). e-mail: emblondon@embitaly.org.uk www http://www.embitaly.org.uk/ **Edinburgh Consulate General,** 32 Melville Street, Edinburgh EH3 7HA Tel: 0131 226 3631/0131 220 3695 Fax: 0131 2266260 **London Consulate General**, 38 Eaton Place, London SW1X 8AN Tel: 020 7235 9371 Fax: 020 7823 1609
Jamaica: Jamaican High Commission, 1–2 Prince Consort Rd, London SW7 2BZ

Tel: 020 7823 9911 Fax: +44 020 7589 5154 e-mail: jamhigh@jhcuk.com www http://www.jhcuk.com/
Japan: Embassy of Japan, 101–4 Piccadilly, London W1V 9FN Tel: 020 7465 6500 Fax: 020 7491 9347 e-mail: info@embjapan.org.uk www http://www.embjapan.org.uk/
Jordan: Embassy of the Hashemite Kingdom of Jordan, 6 Upper Phillimore Gardens, London W8 7HB Tel: 020 7937 3685 Fax: 020 7937 8795 www http://www.jordanembassyuk.gov.jo/
Kazakstan: Embassy for the Republic of Kazakstan, 33 Thurloe Square, London SW7 Tel: 020 7581 4646.
Kenya: Kenya High Commission, 45 Portland Place, London W1N Tel: 020 7636 2371.
Korea: Embassy of the Republic of Korea, 4 Palace Gate, London W8 5NF Tel: 020 7581 0247/020 7581 3330 (Visa Section) Fax: 020 7581 8076 or 60 Buckingham Gate, London SW1 Tel: 020 7227 5500.
Kuwait: Embassy of the State of Kuwait, 2 Alberts Gate, London SW1X Tel: 020 7590 3400.
Kyrgz Republic: Kyrgz Republic Embassy, 119 Crawford Street, London W1H 1AF Tel: 020 7935 1462 Fax: 020 7935 7449 e-mail: embassy@kyrgyz-embassy.org.uk www http://www.kyrgyz-embassy.org.uk/
Latvia: Latvian Embassy, 45 Nottingham Place, London W1M 3FE Tel: 020 7312 0040 Fax: 020 7312 0042 e-mail: latemb@dircon.co.uk
Lebanon: Lebanese Embassy, 21 Kensington Palace Gardens, London W8 Tel: 020 7229 7265.
Lesotho: The High Commission of the Kingdom of Lesotho, 7 Chesham Place, Belgravia, London SW1 8HN Tel: 020 7235 5686.
Liberia: Liberian Embassy, 2 Pembridge Place, London W2 Tel: 020 7221 1036.
Libya: Libyan Interests Section, 119 Harley Street, London Tel: 020 7486 8250.
Lithuania: Embassy of the Republic of Lithuania, 84 Gloucester Place, London W1H Tel: 020 7486 6401.
Luxembourg: Luxembourg Embassy, 27 Wilton Crescent, London SW1X Tel: 020 7235 6961.
Macedonia: Embassy of the Republic of Macedonia, 10 Harcourt House, 19a Cavendish Square, London W1M 9AD Tel: 020 7499 5152 Fax: 020 7499 2864.
Madagascar: Consulate of the Republic of Madagascar, 16 Lanark Mansions, Pennard Road, London W12 Tel: 020 8746 0133.
Malawi: Malawian Embassy, 33 Grosvenor Street, London W1X 0DE Tel: 020 7491 4172 Fax: 020 7491 9916.
Malaysia: The Malaysian Embassy, 45 Belgrave Square, London SW1 8QT Tel: 020 7235 8033.
Malta: Malta High Commission, Malta House, 36–8 Piccadilly, London W1V Tel: 020 7292 4800.
Mauritius: Mauritius High Commission, 32 Elvaston Place, London SW7 Tel: 020 7581 0284.
Mexico: Mexican Embassy, 42 Hertford St, London W1Y 7TF Tel: 020 7499 8586 Fax: 020 7495 4035 e-mail: mexuk@easynet.co.uk www http://www.demon.co.uk/mexuk/
Consular Section: 8 Halkin St, London SW1X 7DW Tel: 020 7235 6393 Fax: 020 7235 5480 e-mail: consullondon@easynet.co.uk
Monaco: The Consulat Général de Monaco, 4 Cromwell Place, London SW7 2JE Tel: 020 7225 2679 Fax: 020 7581 8161.
Mongolia: Mongolian Embassy, 7 Kensington Court, London W8 Tel: 020 7937 5238.
Morocco: Moroccan Embassy, 49 Queens Gate Gardens, London SW7 Tel: 020 7581 5001.
Mozambique: Mozambique High Commission, 21 Fitzroy Square, London W1 Tel: 020 7383 3800.
Myanmar: Embassy of the Union of Myanmar, 19a Charles Street, London W1X Tel: 020 7499 8841.
Namibia: Namibian High Commission, Centre Link, 34 South Molton Street, London W1Y 2BP Tel: 020 7344 9706 Fax: 020 7409 7306 or 6 Chandos Street, London W1M 0LQ Tel: 020 7636 6244 Fax: 020 7637 5694.

Nepal: Royal Nepalese Embassy, Visa Section, 12A Kensington Palace Gardens, London W8 4QU Tel: 020 7229 1594 Fax: 020 7792 9861.
Netherlands: The Royal Netherlands Embassy, 38 Hyde Park Gate, London SW7 Tel: 020 7590 3200.
New Zealand: New Zealand High Commission, New Zealand House, The Haymarket, London SW1Y 4TQ Tel: 020 7930 8422 (Chancery), 020 7973 0366, 020 7973 0370 (Immigration/visas), 020 7930 8422/020 7839 4580 (Consular/passports), 020 7973 0363/020 7839 8929 (Tourism).
Nicaragua: Nicaraguan Consulate, 58 Kensington Church Street, London W8 Tel: 020 7938 2373.
Nigeria: The Nigeria High Commission, 56–7 Fleet Street, London EC4Y 1BT Tel: 020 7353 3776 Visa Department: Tel: 020 7353 3776 Ext 227–229 Fax: 020 7353 4352 or Nigeria House, 9 Northumberland Avenue, London WC2N Tel: 020 7839 1244.
Norway: Royal Norwegian Embassy, 25 Belgrave Square, London SW1X 8QD Tel: 020 7591 5500 Fax: 020 7245 6993 e-mail: morten@embassy.norway.org.uk www http://www.norway.org.uk
Oman: Embassy of the Sultanate of Oman, 167 Queens Gate, London SW7 Tel: 020 7225 0001.
Pakistan: High Commission for Pakistan, (Medical Division) 36 Lowndes Square, London SW1X 9JN Tel: 020 7664 9200 Fax: 020 7664 9224.
Panama: Embassy of Panama, 48 Park Street, London W1Y Tel: 020 7493 4646 Consulate: 40 Hertford Street, London Tel: 020 7409 2255.
Papua New Guinea: PNG High Commission: Visa Section, PNG High Commission, 14 Waterloo Place, London SW1Y 4AR Tel: 020 7930 0922/6.
Paraguay: The Embassy of Paraguay, Braemar Lodge, Cornwall Gardens, London SW7 4AQ Tel: 020 7937 1253/6629 Fax: 020 7937 5687.
Peru: The Peruvian Consulate General, 52 Sloane Street, London SW1X 9SP Tel: 020 7235 6867 Fax: 020 7823 2789.
Philippines: Philippines Embassy, 9a Palace Green, London W8 4QE Tel: 020 7937 1600 Fax: 020 7937 2125.
Poland: Embassy of Poland, Chancery, 47 Portland Place, London W1N 4JH Tel: 020 7580 4324 Fax: 020 7323 4018 www http://www.poland-embassy.org.uk/
Edinburgh Consulate General: 2 Kinner Road, Edinburgh EH3 5PE Tel: 0131 552 0301 Fax: 0131 552 1086.
Portugal: Portuguese Embassy, 11 Belgrave Square, London SW1X Tel: 020 7235 5331.
Qatar: Qatar Embassy, 30 Collingham Gardens, London SW5 Tel: 020 7370 6871.
Romania: Embassy of Romania, 4 Palace Green, London W8 Tel: 020 7937 9666.
Russian Federation: Russian Federation Embassy, 13 Kensington Palace Gardens, London W8 4QX Tel: 020 7229 3628/9 Fax: 020 7727 8624/5 020 7299 5804.
Russian Federation Consulate: 5 Kensington Palace Gardens, London W8 4QS Tel: 020 7229 8027 Recorder Visa Message: 0891 171271 Fax: 020 7229 3215 **Russian Federation Consulate in Edinburgh:** Tel: 0131 225 7098 Fax: 0131 225 9587.
Rwanda: Embassy of the Republic of Rwanda, 58–9 Trafalgar Square, London WC2N Tel: 020 7930 2570.
Saudi Arabia: Royal Embassy of Saudi Arabia, 119 Harley Street, London W1N Tel: 020 7935 9931.
Senegal: Senegalese Embassy, 11 Phillimore Gardens, London W8 7QG Tel: 0207 937 0925 or 020 7937 0926 Fax: 020 7937 8130 or 39 Marioes Road, London W8 Tel: 020 7938 4048.
Seychelles: Seychelles Embassy, PO Box 4PE, 2nd Floor, Eros House, 11 Baker Street, London W1M 1FE Tel: 020 7224 1660 Fax: 020 7487 5756 www http://www.seychelles.uk.com/
Sierra Leone: Sierra Leone High Commission, 33 Portland Place, London W1N Tel: 020 7636 6483.
Singapore: The Singapore High Commission, 9 Wilton Crescent, London SW1X 8RW Fax: 020 7245 6583 or 020 7235 8315.
Slovakia: Embassy of the Slovak Republic, 25 Kensington Palace Gardens,

London W8 4QY Tel: 020 7243 0803 Fax: 020 7727 5824.

Slovenia: Embassy of Slovenia; Cavendish Court, 11–15 Wigmore St, London W1H 9LA Tel: 020 7495 7775 Fax: 020 7495 7776 e-mail: slovene-embassy.london@virgin.net www http://www.embassy-slovenia.org.uk/

South Africa: South African Embassy, South Africa House, Trafalgar Square, London WC2N 5DP Tel: 020 7930 4488 Fax: 020 7925 0367.

Spain: Spanish Consulate General at 20 Draycott Place, London SW3 2RZ Tel: 020 7589 8989. The Spanish Embassy, 39 Chesham Place, London SW1X 8SB.

Sri Lanka: High Commission of the Democratic Socialist Republic of Sri Lanka, 13 Hyde Park Gardens, London W2 2LU Tel: 020 7262 1841–6 Fax: 020 7262 7970 e-mail: lancom@easynet.co.uk www http://ourworld.compuserve.com/homepages/lanka/

Swaziland: Kingdom of Swaziland High Commission, 20 Buckingham Gate, London SW1E Tel: 020 7630 6611.

Sweden: Embassy of Sweden, Consular Section, 11 Montagu Place, London W1H 2AL Tel: 020 7724 2101/020 7917 6400 Fax: 020 7917 6475/020 7917 6476 e-mail: embassy@swednet.org.uk www http://www.swedish-embassy.org.uk/embassy/index.html

Switzerland: Swiss Embassy, 16–18 Montagu Place, London W1H 2BQ Tel: 020 7616 6000 Fax: 020 7724 7001 e-mail: vertretung@lon.rep.admin.ch www http://www.swissembassy.org.uk/

Syria: Syrian Embassy, 8 Belgrave Square, London SW1X Tel: 020 7245 9012.

Tanzania: Tanzania High Commission, 43 Hertford Street, London W1Y 8DB Tel: 020 7499 8951 Fax: 020 7491 9321 e-mail: Balozi@tanzania-online.gov.uk www http://www.tanzania-online.gov.uk

Thailand: Royal Thai Embassy, 29–30 Queen's Gate, London SW7 5JB Tel: 020 7589-2944 Fax: 020 7823-9695 e-mail: dx42@cityscape.co.uk www http://thaidip.mfa.go.th/london/

Tonga: Tonga High Commission, 36 Molyneux Street, London W1H 6AB Tel 020 7724 5828 Fax 020 7723 9074.

Trinidad and Tobago: Trinidad and Tobago High Commission, 42 Belgrave Square, London SW1X Tel: 020 7245 9351.

Tunisia: Tunisian Embassy, 29 Princes Gate, London SW7 1QG Tel: 020 7584 8117 Fax: 020 7225 2884.

Turkey: Turkish Embassy, 43 Belgrave Square, London SW1X 8PA Tel: 020 7393 0202 Fax: 020 7393 0066 e-mail: info@turkishembassy-london.com www http://www.turkishembassy-london.com/

Turkish Consulate: www http://www.turkconsulate-london.com/

Turkmenistan: Embassy of Turkmenistan, 2nd Floor, 14 Wells Street, London W1 Tel: 020 7255 1071.

Uganda: Ugandan High Commission, Uganda House, 58–9 Trafalgar Square, London WC2N 5DX Tel: 020 7839 5783 Fax: 020 7839 8925.

Ukraine: Embassy of Ukraine, 78 Kensington Park Road, London W11 Tel: 020 7727 6312.

United Arab Emirates: Embassy of the United Arab Emirates, 30 Princes Gate, London SW7 Tel: 020 7589 3434.

Uruguay: Uruguayan Consulate, 140 Brompton Road, London SW3 Tel: 020 7589 8735.

USA: American Embassy, 24 Grosvenor Square, London W1A 1AE Tel: 020 7499 9000 Fax: 020 7894 0699 www http://www.usembassy.org.uk/

Consulates: Belfast Tel: 028 328 239 Fax: 028 224 8482 **Edinburgh** 3 Regent Terrace, Scotland, EH7 5BW Tel: 0131 556 8315 Fax: 0131 557 6023.

Uzbekistan: Uzbekistan Embassy, 41 Holland Park, London W11 Tel: 020 7229 7679.

Venezuela: Venezuela Embassy, Consular Section: 56 Grafton Way, London W1P 5LB Tel: 020 7387 6727 Fax: 020 7383 3253 e-mail: venezlon@venezlon.demon.co.uk www http://www.venezlon.demon.co.uk/

Vietnam: Vietnam Embassy, 12 Victoria Road, London W8 Tel: 020 7937 3174.

Yemen: Embassy of the Republic of Yemen, 57 Cromwell Road, London SW7 Tel: 020 7584 6607.

Zaire: Diplomatic Mission of the Republic of Zaire, 26 Chesham Place, London SW1X Tel: 020 7235 6137.

Zambia: Zambian High Commission, 2 Palace Gate, London W8 5NG Tel: 020 7589 6655 Fax: 020 7581 1353.
Zimbabwe: The High Commission of the Republic of Zimbabwe, Zimbabwe House, 429 Strand, London WC2R 05A Tel: 020 7836 7755 Fax: 020 7379 1167.

EMBASSIES IN AUSTRALIA

Afghanistan: Consulate of the Islamic State of Afghanistan, PO Box 88 Canberra 2601 Tel: 02 629 8024.
Argentina: Argentina Embassy, 1 Alfred Street, Piso 13, Suite 1302, Gold Fields House, Circular Quay, Sydney 2000 NSW Tel: 02 9251 3402 Fax: 02 9251 3405 e-mail: mail@consarsydney.org.au www: http://www.consarsydney.org.au/ Embassy of Argentina, MLC Tower Philip, Canberra Tel: 6282 4555.
Austria: Austrian Embassy, 12 Talbot Forest Tel: 02 6295 1533 Fax: 02 6239 6751.
Bangladesh: Bangladesh High Commission, 35 Endeavour Red Hill Tel: 02 6295 3328.
Belgium: Belgian Embassy, Arkana Street Yarralumla ACT 2600, Canberra Tel: 02 6273 2501 Fax: 06 273 33 92 **Consulate General**: 12a, Trelawney Street, Woollahra, Sydney NSW 2025 Tel: 02 9327 8377 Fax: 02 9328 7924.
Bosnia and Herzegovina: Embassy of the Republic of Bosnia and Herzegovina, 15 State Circle Forest, Canberra Tel: 02 6239 5955.
Brazil: Brazilian Embassy, 19 Forster Crescent, Yarralumla Act 2600, Canberra Tel: 02 6273 2372 Fax: 02 6273 2375 www http://people.interconnect.com.au/~aasbrem/emb.htm **Consular Section** 19 Forster Crescent, Yarralumla Act 2600, Canberra Tel: 02 6273 4837, Fax: 02 6273 4837.
Burma: National Coalition Government of the Union of Burma, PO Box 2024, Queanbeyan NSW 2620 Tel: 02 6297 7734 see Myanmar.
Cameroon: Consulate of the Republic of Cameroon, 65 Bingara Road, Beecroft, New South Wales 2119 Tel: 02 9876 4544 Fax: 02 9869 2470 e-mail: consular@tig.com.au www http://www.cameroonconsul.com/
Canada: Canadian Embassy, Level 5, Quay West, 111 Harrington St., Sydney NSW W2000 Tel: 02 364 3050 Fax: 02 364 4099. **High Commission** of Canada, Yarralumla, Commonwealth Avenue Tel: 02 6273 3844 Fax: 02 6273 3285 (Visa nos Tel: (02) 9364 3050 Fax: (02) 9364 3099).
Chile: Chilean Embassy, 10 Culgoa Circuit, O'Malley 2606 ACT. Postal address: PO Box 69 Monaro Crescent ACT 2603, Canberra Tel: 02 6286 2430 e-mail: echileau@dynamite.com.au www http://www.netinfo.com.au/chlle/
Consulates: Sydney: 8th Floor, National Mutual Centre, 44 Market Street Sydney NSW 2000 Tel: 02 9299 2533 Fax: 02 9299 2868. **Melbourne:** Level 43, Nauru House, 80 Collins Street, Melbourne VIC 3000 Tel: 03 9654 4479 Fax: 03 9650 8290 e-mail: cgmelbau@magna.com.au
China: Embassy of the Peoples Republic of China, 15 Coronation Drive, Yarralumla, Canberra Tel: 02 6273 4780.
Colombia: Embassy of Colombia, 101 Northbourne Avenue, Turner, Canberra ACT 2612 Tel: 02 6257 2027.
Croatia: Embassy of the Republic of Croatia, 14 Jindalee Crs, O'Mally, Canberra Tel: 02 6286 6988.
Cyprus: Cyprus High Commission, 30 Beale Crescent, Deakin, Canberra Tel: 02 6281 0834.
Czech Republic: Czech Embassy, 38 Culgoa Circuit, O'Maly, Canberra ACT 2606 Tel: 02 6290 1386 Fax: 02 6290 0006.
Denmark: Danish Embassy, 15 Hunter, Yarralumla, Canberra Tel: 02 6273 2195 Fax: 02 6273 3864. Danish Consulate General, Gold Fields House, 1 Alfred St, Circular Quay, Sydney NSW 2000 Tel: 02 9247 2224 Fax: 02 9251 7504 e-mail: dkconsul@dkconsul-sydney.org.au www http://www.dkconsul-sydney.org.au/
Egypt: Embassy of the Arab Republic of Egypt, 1 Darwin Ave, Yarralumla, Canberra Tel: 02 6273 4437.

European Union: Delegation of the European Commission, 18 Arkana, Yarralumla Tel: 02 6271 2777 Fax: 02 6273 4445 e-mail: australia@ecdel.org.au www http://www.ecdel.org.au/

Fiji: Embassy of the Republic of Fiji, 19 Beale, Deakin, Canberra Tel: 02 6239 6872 or 97 Mugga Way, Red Hill, Canberra Tel: 02 6260 5115.

Finland: Finnish Embassy, 10 Darwin Avenue, Yarralumla, Canberra ACT 2600 Tel: 02 6273 3800 Fax: 02 6273 3603 e-mail: sanomat.can@formin.fi www http://www.finland.org.au/ **Consulates: Sydney:** 537 New South Head Road, Double Bay NSW 2028 Tel: 02 9327 7904 Fax: 02 9327 7528 e-mail: finconsul@hartingdale.com.au

France: French Embassy, 6 Perth Avenue, Yarralumla ACT 2600 Tel: 02 6216 0100 Fax: 02 6216 0156 e-mail: embassy@france.net.au www http://www.france.net.au/frames_eng.html

Germany: Embassy of the Federal Republic of Germany, 119 Empire Cct, Yarralumla, Canberra Tel: 02 6270 1911.

Greece: Greek Consulate General, Stanhill House 34 Queens Road, Melbourne 3004 Tel: 03 9866 4524, 03 9866 4525 Fax: 03 9866 4933 or Embassy of Greece, Cnr Turrana and Empire Cct, Yarralumla Tel: 6273 3011.

Hungary: Hungarian Embassy, 17 Beale Crescent, Deakin, Canberra Tel: 02 6282 3226.

India: High Commission of India, 3 Moonal Place, Yarralumla, Canberra Tel: 02 6273 3999.

Indonesia: Indonesian Embassy, 8 Darwin Ave, Yarralumla, Canberra Tel: 02 6273 3222 or 6250 8600. **Consulates: Adelaide:** Tel: 08 8223 6535 **Darwin:** Tel: 089 8981 9352 **Melbourne:** Tel: 03 9690 7811 **Perth:** Tel: 09 9219 8212. **Sydney**: Tel: 02 93449933.

Iran: Embassy of the Islamic Republic of Iran, 25 Culgoa Cct, O'Maly Tel: 6290 2421 Fax: 6290 2431.

Iraq: Embassy of Republic of Iraq, 48 Culgoa Cct, O'Maly, Canberra Tel: 02 6286 1333.

Ireland: Embassy of Ireland, 20 Arkana Street, Yarralumla ACT 2600 Tel: 06 273 3022, 06 273 3201 Fax: 06 273 3741.

Israel: Israeli Embassy, 6 Turrana Street, Yarralumla, Canberra ACT 2600 Tel: 02 62731309/0 Fax: 06 2734273 e-mail: Isremb.Canberra@U030.Aone.Net.Au **Consulate:** 37 York Street, Sydney 2000 Tel: 02 2647933 Fax: 02 2902259.

Italy: Italian Embassy, 12 Grey Street Deakin ACT 2600, Canberra Tel: 06 2733333 Fax: 02 62734223 e-mail: italembassy@netinfo.com.au **Consulates: Melbourne:** 509, St Kilda Road, Melbourne VIC 3004 Tel: 03 8675744 Fax: 03 8663932 www http://www.iicmelau.org/iicmel/ **Sydney:** Level 43 'The Gateway', 1 Macquarie Place, Sydney NSW 2000 Tel: 02 3927900 Fax: 02 2524830 www http://www.geocities.com/Baja/Dunes/3023/ **Adelaide:** Glynde SA 5070 Tel: 08 3370777 Fax: 08 3651540 **Brisbane:** AMP Place, 10 Eagle Street, 14' Level, Brisbane 4000 Tel: 07 32298944 Fax: 32298643 **Perth:** 31 Labouchere Road, South Perth, WA 6160 Tel: 09 3678922, 09 3673603 Fax: 09 4741320 e-mail: italcons@ca.com.au

Japan: Embassy of Japan, 112 Empire Cct, Yarralumla, Canberra Tel: 02 6273 3244.

Jordan: Embassy of the Hasemite Kingdom of Jordan, 20 Roebuck, Red Hill, Canberra Tel: 02 6295 9951.

Kenya: Kenya High Commission, 33 Ainslie Avenue, Canberra City, Canberra Tel: 02 6247 4788.

Korea: Embassy of the Republic of Korea, 113 Empire Cct, Yarralumla, Canberra Tel: 02 6273 3044.

Kuwait: Kuwait Military Liasion Office, 37 Culgoa Cct, O'Maly, Canberra Tel: 02 6286 2516.

Laos: Embassy of Laos Peoples Democratic Republic, 1 Dalman Crs, O'Maly, Canberra Tel: 02 6286 6933.

Lebanon: Embassy of Lebanon, 27 Endeavour Red Hill, Canberra Tel: 02 6295 7378.

Malaysia: Malaysian High Commision, 7 Perth Avenue, Yarralumla, Canberra Tel: 02 6273 1543.

Malta: Malta High Commission, 261 La Perouse, Red Hill, Canberra Tel: 02 6295 1586 **Consulate General** of Malta, Level 5, 343 Little Collins Street, Melbourne 3000 Tel: 03 9670 8427 Fax: 03 9670 9451

e-mail: maltacg@alphalink.com.au www http://www.vu.edu.au/malta/

Mauritius: Mauritius High Commission, 2 Beale Crescent, Deakin, Canberra Tel: 02 6281 1203.

Mexico: Embassy of Mexico, 14 Perth Ave, Yarralumla, Canberra Tel: 02 6273 3963.

Myanmar: Embassy of the Union of Myanmar, 22 Arkana, Yarralumla, Canberra Tel: 02 6273 3811.

Netherlands: Embassy of the Netherlands, 120 Empire Cct, Yarralumla, Canberra Tel: 02 6273 3111 Fax: 02 6273 3206.

New Zealand: New Zealand High Commission, Commonwealth Avenue, Canberra ACT 2600 Tel: 02 6270 4211 Fax: 02 6273 3194 **Consulates:** Watkins Place Building, 288 Edward Street (GPO Box 62) Brisbane, Queensland 4001 Tel: 07 221 9933 Fax: 07 229 7495 **Melbourne:** 60 Albert Road, South Melbourne, Victoria 3205 Tel: 03 9696 0501 Fax: 03 9696 0391 **Sydney:** Level 14, Gold Fields Building, 1 Alfred Street, Circular Quay (GPO Box 365), Sydney NSW 2000 Tel: 02 247 1999 Fax: 02 247 1754.

Nigeria: Nigeria High Commission, 7 Terrigal Cct, O'Maly, Canberra Tel: 02 6286 1322 Fax: 02 6286 5332 e-mail: nigeria_act@netinfo.com.au

Norway: Embassy of Norway, 17 Hunter, Yarralumla, Canberra Tel: 02 6273 3444 or 80 Mugga Way Red Hill, Canberra Tel: 02 6295 1048.

Pakistan: High Commission for Pakistan, 4 Timbarra Crs, O'Maly, Canberra Tel: 02 6290 1676.

Palestine: Palestinian Delegation, 19 Carnegie Crescent, Narbndh, Canberra Tel: 02 6925 0222.

Royal Embassy of Cambodia, 5 Canterbury Crescent, Deakin, Canberra Tel: 02 6273 1259/1154 Fax: 02 6273 1053.

Papua New Guinea: High Commission of Papua New Guinea, 39–41 Forster Crescent, Yarralumla, Canberra Tel: 02 6273 3322 Fax: 02 6273 3732.

Peru: Embassy of Peru, 43 Culgoa Cct, O'Maly, Canberra Tel: 02 6290 0922.

Philippines: Embassy of the Philippines, 1 Moonah Place, Yarralumla, Canberra Tel: 02 6273 2535 Fax: 02 6273 3984.

Poland: Embassy of the Republic of Poland, 6 Turrana, Yarralumla, Canberra Tel: 02 6273 1208.

Portugal: Embassy of Portugal, 23 Culgoa Cct, O'Maly, Canberra Tel: 02 6290 1733.

Romania: Embassy of Romania, 4 Dalman Crs, O'Maly, Canberra Tel: 02 6286 2343.

Russian Federation: Russian Federation Embassy, 78 Canberra Avenue, Griffith, Canberra ACT 2603 Tel: 06 295 9033, 06 295 9474.

Saudi Arabia: Embassy of Saudi Arabia, 8 Culgoa Cct, O'Maly Tel: 02 6286 2099.

Singapore: High Commission of Singapore, 17 Forster Crescent, Yarralumla, Canberra Tel: 02 6273 3944 Fax: 02 6273 3260 e-mail: singaporehc@u030.aone.net.au

Slovakia: Embassy of the Slovak Federal, 47 Culgoa Cct, O'Mly, Canberra Tel: 02 6290 1516.

Slovenia: Embassy of Slovenia, Level 6, 60 Marcus Clarke Street Postal address: PO Box 284 Civic Square, Canberra ACT 2601 Tel: 02 6243 4830 Fax: 02 6243 4827 e-mail: embassyofslovenia@webone.com.au www http://slovenia.webone.com.au/

Solomon Islands: Solomon Islands High Commission, 19 Napier Close, Deakin, Canberra Tel: 02 6282 7030.

South Africa: High Commission of South Africa, State Circle, Yarralumla, Canberra Tel: 02 6273 2424.

Spain: Embassy of Spain, 15 Arkana, Yarralumla, Canberra Tel: 02 6273 3555.

Sri Lanka: Sri Lankan High Commission, 35 Empire Circuit, Forrest, Canberra 2603 Tel: 06 2397041 06 2397042 Fax: 06 2396166 e-mail: slhc@atrax.net.au www http://slhccanberra.webjump.com/

Sweden: Embassy of Sweden, Turrana St, Yarralumla, Canberra Tel: 02 6270 2700.

Switzerland: Embassy of Switzerland, 7 Melbourne Ave Forest, Canberra Tel: 02 6273 3977.

Thailand: Royal Thai Embassy, 111 Empire CCT Yarralumla 2600, Canberra Tel: 06 273 1149 Fax: 06 273 1518 e-mail: Thai@csccs.com.au www http://www.geocities.com/CapitolHill/7789/

Turkey: Turkish Embassy, 60 Mugga Way, Red Hill, Canberra 2603 ACT Tel: 02 62 95 02 27/28 Fax: 02 62 39 65 92 e-mail: turkembs@ozemail.com.au www http://www.ozemail.com.au/~turkembs/ **Consulates: Sydney:** 66 Ocean Street, Woollahra, Sydney NSW 2025 Tel: 029 327 6629 Fax: 029 362 4730 e-mail: dtsid@adcom.com.au www http://www.adcom.com.au/dtsid/
United Kingdom: British High Commission, Consular Section, SAP House Akuna Street (cnr Bunda Street) Tel: 1902 941 555, 1900 920 273 (both have recorded info), 02 6270 6666 (General Enquires) Fax: 1902 941 600 or 02 6273 3236 Alternatively: British High Commission, Commonwealth Avenue, Yarralumla, Canberra ACT 2600 Tel: 02 6270 6666 Fax: Chancery: 02 6270 6653 Information: 02 6270 6606 www http://www.uk.emb.gov.au/ **Canberra: Passport/Visa/Consular Section**: Level 10 CBS Tower, Canberra City ACT 2601 Tel: 02 6257 2434 (Passports), 02 6257 1982 (Entry Clearances) Fax: 02 6257 5857 **British Consulates: Adelaide:** (22nd Floor), 25 Grenfell Street, Adelaide SA Tel: 08 212 7280, 08 212 7281 Fax: 08 212 7283 **Brisbane:** Level 26, Waterfront Place, 1 Eagle Street, Brisbane, Queensland 4000 Tel: 07 3236 2575/77/81 Fax: 07 3236 2576 **Melbourne:** 17th Floor, 90 Collins Street, Melbourne, Victoria 3000 Tel: 03 9650 2990 Fax: 03 9650 2990 **Perth:** Level 26, Allendale Square, 77 St George's Terrace, Perth, WA 6000 Tel: 09 221 5400 Fax: 09 221 2344 **Sydney:** Level 16, The Gateway, 1 Macquarie Place, Sydney Cove, Sydney 2000, NSW Tel: 02 247 7521 Fax: 02 251 6201.
Uruguay: Embassy of the Uruguay Chancery, 24 Brisbane Avenue, Brtn, Canberra Tel: 02 6282 4800.
USA: Embassy of the United States of America, 21 Moonah Place, Yarralumla, Canberra ACT 2600 Tel: 02 6270 5000 Fax: 02 6270 5970, 02 6270 5940 e-mail: usiscanb@ozemail.com.au www http://www.usis-australia.gov/embassy.html **Consulate Generals: Melbourne:** Level 6, 553 St. Kilda Road, Melbourne Tel: 03 9526-5900 www http://www.ozemail.com.au/~usaemb/melbourne/ **Sydney**: Level 59, MLC Centre, 19–29 Martin Place, Sydney NSW 2000 Tel: 02 9373 9200 (Reception), Fax: 02 9373 9107 www http://www.ozemail.com.au/~usaemb/sydney/ **Perth:** 16 St Georges Terrace, Perth WA 6000 Tel: 08 9231 9400 Fax: 08 9231 9444 www http://www.ozemail.com.au/~usaemb/perth/
Venezuela: Embassy of Venezuela, 5 Culgoa Cct, O'Maly, Canberra Tel: 02 6290 2900 e-mail: venezuela@linkpro.com.au www http://www.linkpro.com.au/venezuela/
Vietnam: Embassy of the Socialist Republic of Vietnam, 6 Timbara Crs, O'Maly, Canberra Tel: 02 6286 6059.
Yugoslavia: Embassy of Federal Republic of Yugoslavia, 11 Nuyts Red Hill, Canberra Tel: 02 6295 1458.

EMBASSIES IN THE USA

Afghanistan: Embassy of the Republic of Afghanistan, 2341 Wyoming Ave, NW, Washington DC 20008 Tel: 202 234 3770 Fax: 202 328 3516.
Albania: Embassy of the Republic of Albania, 2100 S Street, NW, Washington DC 20008 Tel: 202 223 4942 Fax: 202 628 7342.
Algeria: Embassy of the Democratic and Popular Republic of Algeria, 2118 Kalorama Road NW, Washington DC 20008 Tel: 202 265 2800 Fax: 202 667 2174 e-mail: embalgus@cais.com www http://www.algeria-us.org/
Angola: Embassy of Angola, 1615 M Street, NW Suite 900, Washington DC 20036 Tel: 202 785 1156 Fax: 202 785 1258 e-mail: angola@angola.org www http://www.angola.org/
Antigua and Barbuda: Embassy of Antigua and Barbuda, 3216 New Mexico Avenue, NW, Washington DC 20016 Tel: 202 362 5122 Fax: 202 362 5225.

Argentina: Embassy of the Argentine Republic, 1600 New Hampshire Avenue, NW, Washington DC 20009 Tel: 202 238 6400 Fax: 202 332 3171 e-mail: embajadaargentina@worldnet.att.net www http://www.embassyofargentina-usa.org/
Armenia: Embassy of the Republic of Armenia, 2225 R Street, Washington DC 20008 Tel: 202 319 1976 Fax: 202 319 2982 www http://www.armeniaemb.org/
Australia: Embassy of Australia, 1601 Massachusetts Avenue, NW, Washington DC 20036 Tel: 202 797 3000 Fax: 202 797 3168 www http://www.austemb.org/
Austria: Embassy of Austria, 3524 International Court, NW, Washington DC 20008 Tel: 202 895 6700 Fax: 202 895 6750.
Azerbaijan: Embassy of the Republic of Azerbaijan, 927 15th Street, NW, Suite 700, Washington DC 20035 Tel: 202 842 0001 Fax: 202 842 0004 e-mail: azerbaijan@tidalwave.net www http://www.azembassy.com/
Bahamas: Embassy of the Commonwealth of the Bahamas, 2220 Massachusetts Avenue, NW, Washington DC 20008 Tel: 202 319 2660 Fax: 202 319 2668.
Bahrain: Embassy of the State of Bahrain, 3502 International Drive, NW, Washington DC 20008 Tel: 202 342 0741 Fax: 202 362 2192 e-mail: info@bahrainembassy.org www http://www.bahrainembassy.org/
Bangladesh: Embassy of the People's Republic of Bangladesh, 2201 Wisconsin Avenue, NW, Suite 300, Washington DC 20007 Tel: 202 342 8372 Fax: 202 333 4971 e-mail: BanglaEmb@aol.com www http://members.aol.com/banglaemb/index.html
Barbados: Embassy of Barbados, 2144 Wyoming Avenue, NW, Washington DC 20008 Tel: 202 939 9200 Fax: 202 332 7467.
Belarus: Embassy of the Republic of Belarus, 1619 New Hampshire Avenue, NW, Washington DC 20009 Tel: 202 986 1604 Fax: 202 986 1805.
Belgium: Embassy of Belgium, 3330 Garfield Street, NW, Washington DC 20008 Tel: 202 333 6900 Fax: 202 333 3079 e-mail: washington@diplobel.org www http://www.diplobel.org/usa/default.htm
Belize: Embassy of Belize, 2535 Massachusetts Avenue, NW, Washington DC 20008 Tel: 202 332 9636 Fax: 202 332 6888.
Benin: Embassy of the Republic of Benin, 2737 Cathedral Avenue, NW, Washington DC 20008 Tel: 202 232 6656 Fax: 202 265 1996.
Bhutan: Embassy of Bhutan, (Consulate-General) 2 UN Plaza, 27th Floor, New York NY 10017 Tel: 212 826 1919 Fax: 212 826 2998.
Bolivia: Embassy of Bolivia, 3014 Massachusetts Avenue, NW, Washington DC 20008 Tel: 202 483 4410 Fax: 202 328 3712.
Bosnia and Herzegovina: Embassy of Bosnia and Herzegovina, 2109 E Street NW, Washington DC 20037 Tel: 202 337 1500 Fax: 202 337 1502 e-mail: Embofbih@aol.com www http://www.bosnianembassy.org/
Botswana: Embassy of Botswana, 1531-3 New Hampshire Avenue, NW, Washington DC 20036 Tel: 202 244 4990 Fax: 202 244 4164.
Brazil: Embassy of Brazil, 3006 Massachusetts Avenue, NW, Washington DC 20008 Tel: 202 238 2700 Fax: 202 238 2827 e-mail: scitech@brasil.emb.nw.dc.us www http://www.brasil.emb.nw.dc.us/
Brunei: Embassy of Brunei, Watergate, Suite 300, 2600 Virginia Avenue, NW, Washington DC 20037 Tel: 202 342 0159 Fax: 202 342 0158.
Bulgaria: Embassy of the Republic of Bulgaria, 1621 22nd Street, NW, Washington DC 20008 Tel: 202 387 7969 Fax: 202 234 7973 e-mail: bulgaria@access.digex.net www http://www.bulgaria-embassy.org
Burkina Faso: Embassy of Burkina Faso, 2340 Massachusetts Avenue, NW, Washington DC 20008 Tel: 202 332 5577 Fax: 202 265 6972.
Burundi: Embassy of the Republic of Burundi, 2233 Wisconsin Avenue, NW, Suite 212, Washington DC 20007 Tel: 202 342 2574 Fax: 202 342 2578.
Cameroon: Embassy of the Republic of Cameroon, 2349 Massachusetts Avenue,

NW, Washington DC 20008 Tel: 202 265 8790 Fax: 202 387 3826.

Canada: Embassy of Canada, 501 Pennsylvania Avenue, NW, Washington DC 20001 Tel: 202 682 1740 Fax: 202 682 7726 www: http://www.cdnemb-washdc.org/

Cape Verde: Embassy of the Republic of Cape Verde, 3415 Massachusetts Avenue, NW, Washington DC 20007 Tel: 202 965 6820 Fax: 202 965 1207 e-mail: cvefont@sysnet.net www http://www.capeverdeusembassy.org/

Central African Republic: Embassy of the Central African Republic, 1618 22nd Street, NW, Washington DC 20008 Tel: 202 483 7800 Fax: 202 332 9893.

Chad: Embassy of the Republic of Chad, 2002 R Street, NW, Washington DC 20009 Tel: 202 462 4009 Fax: 202 265 1937 e-mail: info@chadembassy.org www http://www.chadembassy.org

Chile: Embassy of Chile, 1732 Massachusetts Avenue, NW, Washington DC 20036 Tel: 202 785 1746 Fax: 202 887 5579.

China: Embassy of the People's Republic of China, 2300 Connecticut Ave, NW, Washington DC 20008 Tel: 202 328 2500 Fax: 202 588 0032 e-mail: webmaster@china-embassy.org www http://www.china-embassy.org/

Colombia: Embassy of Colombia, 2118 Leroy Place, NW, Washington DC 20008 Tel: 202 387 8338 Fax: 202 232 8643 e-mail: webmaster@colombiaemb.org www http://www.colombiaemb.org/

Comoros: Embassy of the Federal and Islamic Republic of the Comoros, 336 East 45th, 2nd Floor, New York NY 10017 Tel: 212 972 8010.

Congo: Embassy of the Republic of Congo, 4891 Colorado Avenue, NW, Washington DC 20011 Tel: 202 726 5500 Fax: 202 726 1860 Embassy of the Democratic Republic of Congo, 1800 New Hampshire Avenue, NW, Washington DC 20009 Tel: 202 234 7690 Fax: 202 237 0748.

Costa Rica: Embassy of Costa Rica, 2114 S Street, NW, Washington DC 20008 Tel: 202 234 2945 Fax: 202 265 4795 www http://www.costarica.com/embassy/

Cote d'Ivoire: Embassy of the Republic of Cote d'Ivoire (Ivory Coast), 2424 Massachusetts Avenue, NW, Washington DC 20008 Tel: 202 797 0300.

Croatia: Embassy of the Republic of Croatia, 2343 Massachusetts Avenue, NW, Washington DC 20008 Tel: 202 588 5899 Fax: 202 588 8936 e-mail: croatia@mail.idt.net www http://idt.net/~croatia/

Cuba: Cuba Interests Section, 2630 and 2639 16th Street, NW, Washington DC 20009 Tel: 202 797 8518.

Cyprus: Embassy of the Republic of Cyprus, 2211 R Street, NW, Washington DC 20008 Tel: 202 462 5772 Fax: 202 483 6710.

Czech Republic: Embassy of the Czech Republic, 3900 Spring of Freedom Street, NW, Washington DC 20008 Tel: 202 274 9100 Fax: 202 966 8540 e-mail: washington@embassy.mzv.cz www http://www.czech.cz/washington/

Denmark: Royal Danish Embassy, 3200 Whitehaven Street, NW, Washington DC 20008 Tel: 202 234 4300 Fax: 202 328 1470 e-mail: ambadane@erols.com www http://www.denmarkemb.org/

Djibouti: Embassy of the Republic of Djibouti, 1156 15th Street, NW, Suite 515, Washington DC 20005 Tel: 202 331 0270.

Dominica: Embassy of the Dominican Republic, 1715 22nd Street, NW, Washington DC 20008 Tel: 202 332 6280 Fax: 202 265 8057 e-mail: embdomrepusa@msn.com www http://www.domrep.org/

Ecuador: Embassy of Ecuador, 2535 15th Street, NW, Washington DC 20009 Tel: 202 234 7200 www http://www.ecuador.org/

Egypt: Embassy of the Arab Republic of Egypt, 3521 International Court, NW, Washington DC 20008 Tel: 202 966 6342.

El Salvador: Embassy of El Salvador, 2308 California Street, NW, Washington DC 20008 Tel: 202 265 9671 e-mail: cbartoli@elsalvador.org www http://www.elsalvador.org

Equatorial Guinea: Embassy of Equatorial Guinea, 1721 I Street NW, Suite 400, Washington DC 20006 Tel: 914 738 9584.

Eritrea: Embassy of Eritrea, 1708 New Hampshire Ave, NW, Washington DC 20009 Tel: 202 319 1991 Fax: 202 319 1304 e-mail: veronica@embassyeritrea.org
Estonia: Embassy of Estonia, 2131 Massachussets Avenue, NW, Washington DC 20008 Tel: 202 588 0101 Fax: 202 588 0108 www http://www.estemb.org/
Ethiopia: Embassy of Ethiopia, 2134 Kalorama Road NW, Suite 1000, Washington DC 20008 Tel: 202 234 2281 Fax: 202 483 8407 e-mail: ethiopia@tidalwave.net www http://www.ethiopianembassy.org/
Fiji: Embassy of Fiji, 2233 Wisconsin Avenue, NW, Suite 240, Washington DC 20007 Tel: 202 337 8320 Fax: 202 337 1996 e-mail: fijiemb@earthlink.net
Finland: Embassy of Finland, 3301 Massachusetts Avenue, NW, Washington DC 20008 Tel: 202 298 5800 Fax: 202 298 6030 e-mail: info@finland.org www http://www.finland.org/
France: Embassy of France, 4101 Reservoir Road, NW, Washington DC 20007 Tel: 202 944 6000 Fax: 202 944 6072 www http://www.info-france-usa.org/
Gabon: Embassy of the Gabonese Republic, 2034 20th Street, NW, Suite 200, Washington DC 20009 Tel: 202 797 1000 Fax: 202 332 0668.
Gambia: Embassy of the Gambia, 1155 15th Street, NW, Suite 1000, Washington DC 20005 Tel: 202 785 1399 e-mail: gamembdc@gambia.com www http://www.gambia.com/index.html
Georgia: Embassy of the Republic of Georgia, 1511 K Street, NW, Suite 400, Washington DC 20005 Tel: 202 393 5959 Fax: 202 393 4537 e-mail: 73324.1007@compuserve.com www http://www.steele.com/embgeorgia/
Germany: Embassy of Germany, 4645 Reservoir Road, NW, Washington DC 20007 1998 Tel: 202 298 4000 Fax: 202 298 4249 or 333 2653 www http://www.germany-info.org/
Ghana: Embassy of Ghana, 3512 International Drive NW, Washington DC 20008 Tel: 202 686 4520 e-mail: hagan@cais.com www http://www.ghana-embassy.org/
Greece: Embassy of Greece, 2221 Massachusetts Avenue, NW, Washington DC 20008 Tel: 202 939 5800 www http://www.greekembassy.org/
Grenada: Embassy of Grenada, 1701 New Hampshire Ave, NW, Washington DC 20009 Tel: 202 265 2561.
Guatemala: Embassy of Guatemala, 2220 R Street, NW, Washington DC 20008 Tel: 202 745-4952 Fax: 202 745 1908 e-mail: Embaguat@sysnet.net www http://www.mdngt.org/agremilusa/embassy.html
Guinea: Embassy of the Republic of Guinea, 2112 Leroy Place, NW, Washington DC 20008 Tel: 202 483 9420.
Guinea-Bissau: Embassy of the Republic of Guinea-Bissau, 918 16th Street, NW (Mezzanine Suite), Washington DC 20006.
Guyana: Embassy of Guyana, 2490 Tracy Place, NW, Washington DC 20008 Tel: 202 265 6900 e-mail: guyanaem@erols.com www http://www.wam.umd.edu/~swi/embassy.htm
Haiti: Embassy of the Republic of Haiti, 2311 Massachusetts Avenue, NW, Washington DC 20008 Tel: 202 332 4090 Fax: 202 745 7215 www http://www.haiti.org/embassy/
Honduras: Embassy of Honduras, 3007 Tilden Street, NW, Washington DC 20008 Tel: 202 966 7702.
Hungary: Embassy of the Republic of Hungary, 3910 Shoemaker Street, NW, Washington DC 20008 Tel: 202 362 6730 Fax: 202 686 6412 www http://www.hungaryemb.org/
Iceland: Embassy of Iceland, 1156 15th Street, NW, Suite 1200, Washington DC 20005 1704 Tel: 202 265 6653 Fax: 202 265 6656 e-mail: icemb.wash@utn.stjr.is www http://www.iceland.org/
India: Embassy of India, 2107 Massachusetts Avenue, NW, Washington DC 20008 Tel: 202 939 7000 www http://www.indianembassy.org/
Indonesia: Embassy of the Republic of Indonesia, 2020 Massachusetts Avenue, NW, Washington DC 20036 Tel: 202 775 5200 www http://kbri.org/
Iran: Iranian Interests Section, 2209 Wisconsin Avenue NW, Washington DC

20007 Tel: 202 965 4990 www http://www.daftar.org/default_eng.htm
Iraq: Iraqi Interests Section, 1801 P Street, NW, Washington DC 20036 Tel: 202 483-7500 Fax: 202 462 5066
Ireland: Embassy of Ireland, 2234 Massachusetts Avenue, NW, Washington DC 20008 Tel: 202 462 3939 www http://www.irelandemb.org/
Israel: Embassy of Israel, 3514 International Drive, NW, Washington DC 20008 Tel: 202 364 5500 Fax: 202 364 5423 e-mail: ask@israelemb.org www http://www.israelemb.org/
Italy: Embassy of Italy, 1601 Fuller Street, NW, Washington DC 20009 Tel: 202 328-5500 Fax: 202 462 3605 www http://www.italyemb.nw.dc.us/italy/index.html
Jamaica: Embassy of Jamaica, 1520 New Hampshire Avenue, NW, Washington DC 20036 Tel: 202 452 0660 Fax: 202 452 0081 e-mail: emjam@sysnet.net www http://www.caribbean-online.com jamaica/embassy/washdc/
Japan: Embassy of Japan, 2520 Massachusetts Avenue NW, Washington DC 20008 Tel: 202 238 6700 Fax: 202 328 2187
www http://www.embjapan.org/
Jordan: Embassy of the Hashemite Kingdom of Jordan, 3504 International Drive, NW, Washington DC 20008 Tel: 202 966 2664 Fax: 202 966 3110 www http://www.jordanembassyus.org/
Kazakhstan: Embassy of the Republic of Kazakhstan, 1401 16th Street, NW, Washington DC 20036 Tel: 202 232 5488.
Kenya: Embassy of Kenya, 2249 R Street, NW, Washington DC 20008 Tel: 202 387 6101 Fax: 202 462 3829 e-mail: info@kenyaembassy.com www http://www.kenyaembassy.com/
Korea: Embassy of the Republic of Korea, 2450 Massachusetts Avenue, NW, Washington DC 20008 Tel: 202 939 5600 www http://www.koreaemb.org/
Kuwait: Embassy of the State of Kuwait, 2940 Tilden Street, NW, Washington DC 20008 Tel: 202 966 0702.
Kyrgyz: Embassy of the Kyrgyz Republic, 1732 Wisconsin Avenue, NW, Washington DC 20007 Tel: 202 338 5141 Fax: 202 338 5139 e-mail: Embassy@kyrgyzstan.org www http://www.kyrgyzstan.org/
Laos: Embassy of the Lao People's Democratic Republic, 2222 S Street, NW, Washington DC 20008 Tel: 202 332 6416 Fax: 202 332 4923 www http://www.laoembassy.com/
Latvia: Embassy of Latvia, 4325 17th Street, NW, Washington DC 20011 Tel: 202 726 8213 Fax: 202 726 6785 e-mail: latvia@ambergateway.com www http://www.latvia-usa.org/
Lebanon: Embassy of Lebanon, 2560 28th Street, NW, Washington DC 20008 Tel: 202 939 6300 Fax: 202 939 6324 e-mail: EmbLebanon@aol.com www http://www.erols.com/lebanon/
Lesotho: Embassy of the Kingdom of Lesotho, 2511 Massachusetts Avenue, NW, Washington DC 20008 Tel: 202 797 5533.
Liberia: Embassy of the Republic of Liberia, 5201 16th Street, NW, Washington DC 20011 Tel: 202 723 0437.
Lithuania: Embassy of Lithuania, 2622 Sixteenth Street, NW, Washington DC 20009 4202 Tel: 202 234 5860 Fax: 202 328 0466 e-mail: admin@ltembassyus.org www http://www.ltembassyus.org/
Luxembourg: Embassy of Luxembourg, 2200 Massachusetts Avenue, NW, Washington DC 20008 Tel: 202 265 4171.
Macedonia: Embassy of the Republic of Macedonia, 3050 K Street, NW, Suite 210, Washington DC 20007 Tel: 202 337 3063 Fax: 202 337 3093 e-mail: rmacedonia@aol.com
Malawi: Embassy of Malawi, 2408 Massachusetts Avenue, NW, Washington DC 20008 Tel: 202 797 1007.
Malaysia: Embassy of Malaysia, 2401 Massachusetts Avenue, NW, Washington DC 20008 Tel: 202 328 2700.
Mali: Embassy of the Republic of Mali, 2130 R Street, NW, Washington DC 20008 Tel: 202 332 2249 Fax: 202 332 6603 e-mail: info@maliembassy-usa.org www http://www.maliembassy-usa.org
Malta: Embassy of Malta, 2017 Connecticut Avenue NW, Washington DC 20008 Tel: 202 462 3611.
Marshall Islands: Embassy of the Republic of the Marshall Islands, 2433

Massachusetts Avenue, NW, Washington DC 20008 Tel: 202 234 5414 Fax: 202 232 3236 e-mail: info@rmiembassyus.org www http://www.rmiembassyus.org/usemb.html
Mauritania: Embassy of the Islamic Republic of Mauritania, 2129 Leroy Place, NW, Washington DC 20008 Tel: 202 232 5700 Fax: 202 232 5701.
Mauritius: Embassy of Mauritius, 4301 Connecticut Avenue, NW, Suite 441, Washington DC 20008 Tel: 202 244 1491 Fax: 202 966 0983 www http://www.idsonline.com/usa/embasydc.html
Mexico: Embassy of Mexico, 1911 Pennsylvania Avenue, NW, Washington DC 20006 Tel: 202 728 1600 www http://www.embassyofmexico.org/
Micronesia: Embassy of the Federated States of Micronesia, 1725 N Street, NW, Washington DC 20036 Tel: 202 223 4383.
Moldova: Embassy of the Republic of Moldova, 2101 S Street, NW, Washington DC 20008 Tel: 202 667 1130/31/37 Fax: 202 667 1204 e-mail: embassy@moldova.org www http://www.moldova.org/
Mongolia: Embassy of Mongolia, 2833 M Street NW, Washington DC 20007 Tel: 202 333 7117 www http://members.aol.com/monemb/
Morocco: Embassy of the Kingdom of Morocco, 1601 21st Street, NW, Washington DC 20009 Tel: 202 462 7979.
Mozambique: Embassy of the Republic of Mozambique, 1990 M Street, NW, Suite 570, Washington DC 20036 Tel: 202 293 7146.
Myanmar: Embassy of the Union of Myanmar, 2300 S Street, NW, Washington DC 20008 Tel: 202 332 9044.
Namibia: Embassy of the Republic of Namibia, 1605 New Hampshire Avenue, NW, Washington DC 20009 Tel: 202 986 0540.
Nepal: Embassy of Nepal, 2131 Leroy Place, NW, Washington DC 20008 Tel: 202 667 4550.
Netherlands: Embassy of the Netherlands, 4200 Linnean Avenue, NW, Washington DC 20008 Tel: 202 244 5300 Fax: 202 362 3430 www http://www.netherlands-embassy.org/
New Zealand: Embassy of New Zealand, 37 Observatory Circle, Washington DC 20008 Tel: 202 328 4800 Fax: 202 667 5227 e-mail: nzemb@dc.infi.net www http://www.emb.com/nzemb/
Nicaragua: Embassy of Nicaragua, 1627 New Hampshire Avenue, NW, Washington DC 20009 Tel: 202 939 6570 Fax: 202 939 6542 e-mail: embanic_usa@amdyne.net www http://members.aol.com/embanic1/
Niger: Embassy of the Republic of Niger, 2204 R Street, NW, Washington DC 20008 Tel: 202 483 4224.
Nigeria: Embassy of the Federal Republic of Nigeria, 1333 16th Street, NW, Washington DC 20036 Tel: 202 986 8400 Fax: 202 775 1385 www http://tribeca.ios.com/~n123/
Norway: Royal Embassy of Norway, 20 34th Street, NW, Washington DC 20008 Tel: 202 333 6000 www http://www.norway.org/
Oman: Embassy of the Sultanate of Oman, 35 Belmont Road, NW, Washington DC 20008 Tel: 202 387 1980.
Pakistan: Embassy of the Islamic Republic of Pakistan, 15 Massachusetts Avenue, NW, Washington DC 20008 Tel: 202 939 6200 e-mail: info@pakistan-embassy.com www http://www.pakistan-embassy.com/
Panama: Embassy of the Republic of Panama, 2862 McGill Terrace, NW, Washington DC 20008 Tel: 202 483 1407.
Papua New Guinea: Embassy of Papua New Guinea, 1779 Massachusetts Ave, NW, Suite 805, Washington DC 20036 Tel: 202 745 3680 Fax: 202 745 3679 e-mail: Kunduwash@aol.com www http://www.pngembassy.org
Paraguay: Embassy of Paraguay, 2400 Massachusetts Avenue, NW, Washington DC 20008 Tel: 202 483 6960.
Peru: Embassy of Peru, 1700 Massachusetts Avenue, NW, Washington DC 20036 Tel: 202 833 9860 Fax: 202 659 8124 e-mail: peru@peruemb.org www http://www.peruemb.org
Philippines: Embassy of the Philippines, 1600 Massachusetts Avenue, NW, Washington DC 20036 Tel: 202 467 9300 Fax: 202 467 9417 www http://us.sequel.net/RPinUS
Poland: Embassy of Poland, 2640 16th

Street, NW, Washington DC 20009 Tel: 202 234 3800 Fax: 202 328 6271e-mail: embpol@dgs.dgsys.com www http://www.polishworld.com/polemb/

Portugal: Embassy of Portugal, 2125 Kalorama Road, NW, Washington DC 20008 Tel: 202 328 8610 Fax: 202 462 3726 e-mail: portugal@portugalemb.org www http://www.portugalemb.org/

Qatar: Embassy of the State of Qatar, 4200 Wisconsin Ave, NW, Suite 200, Washington DC 20016 Tel: 202 274 1600 Fax: 202 237 0061.

Russia: Embassy of the Russian Federation, 2650 Wisconsin Avenue, NW, Washington DC 20007 Tel: 202 298 5700 Fax: 202 298 5749 www http://www.russianembassy.org

Rwanda: Embassy of the Republic of Rwanda, 1714 New Hampshire Avenue, NW, Washington DC 20009 Tel: 202 232 2882 Fax: 202 232 4544 www http://www.rwandemb.org/

Saint Kitts and Nevis: Embassy of Saint Kitts and Nevis, 3216 New Mexico Avenue, NW, Washington DC 20016 Tel: 202 833 3550 www http://www.stkittsnevis.org/

Saint Lucia: Embassy of Saint Lucia, 3216 New Mexico Avenue, NW, Washington DC 20016 Tel: 202 364 6792/93/94/95 Fax: 202 364 6723.

Saint Vincent and the Grenadines: Embassy of Saint Vincent and the Grenadines, 3216 New Mexico Avenue, NW, Washington DC 20016 Tel: 202 364 6730 Fax: 202 364 6736.

Saudi Arabia: Royal Embassy of Saudi Arabia, 601 New Hampshire Avenue, NW, Washington DC 20037 Tel: 202 337 4076 e-mail: info@saudiembassy.net www http://www.saudiembassy.net/

Senegal: Embassy of the Republic of Senegal, 2112 Wyoming Avenue, NW, Washington DC 20008 Tel: 202 234 0540.

Seychelles: Embassy of the Republic of Seychelles, 800 Second Avenue, Suite 400, Washington DC 10017 Tel: (212) 687 9766.

Sierra Leone: Embassy of Sierra Leone, 1701 19th Street, NW, Washington DC 20009 Tel: 202 939 9261 www http://amenhotep4.virtualafrica.com/slmbassy/

Singapore: Embassy of the Republic of Singapore, 3501 International Place, NW, Washington DC 20008 Tel: 202 537 3100 Fax: 202 537 0876 e-mail: singemb@bel-latlantic.net www http://www.gov.sg/mfa/washington/

Slovakia: Embassy of the Slovak Republic, 2201 Wisconsin Avenue, NW, Suite 250, Washington DC 20007 Tel: 202 965 160 Fax: 202 965 5166 e-mail: svkemb@concentric.net www http://www.slovakemb.com/

Slovenia: Embassy of the Republic of Slovenia, 1525 New Hampshire Avenue, NW, Washington DC 20036 Tel: 202 667 5363 Fax: 202 667 4563 www http://www.embassy.org/slovenia/

South Africa: Embassy of South Africa, 3051 Massachusetts Avenue, NW, Washington DC 20008 Tel: 202 232 4400 Fax: 202 265 1607 e-mail: safrica@southafrica.net www http://www.southafrica.net/

Spain: Embassy of Spain, 2375 Pennsylvania Avenue, NW, Washington DC 20037 Tel: 202 452 0100 Fax: 202 833 5670 www http://www.spainemb.org/information/

Sri Lanka: Embassy of Sri Lanka, 2148 Wyoming Avenue, NW, Washington DC 20008 Tel: 202 483 4025–28 Fax: 202 232 7181 and 202 483 8017 e-mail: slembasy@clark.net www http://www.slembassy.org

Sudan: Embassy of the Republic of the Sudan, 2210 Massachusetts Avenue, NW, Washington DC 20008 Tel: 202 338 8565 Fax: 202 667 2406 e-mail: info@sudanembassyus.org www http://www.sudanembassyus.org/

Surinam: Embassy of the Republic of Surinam, 4301 Connecticut Avenue, NW, Suite 460, Washington DC 20008 Tel: 202 244 7488 Fax: 202 244 5878.

Swaziland: Embassy of the Kingdom of Swaziland, 3400 International Drive, NW, Washington DC 20008 Tel: 202 362 6683 Fax: 202 244 8059.

Sweden: Embassy of Sweden, 1501 M Street, NW, Washington DC 20005 Tel: 202 467 2600 Fax: 202 467 2656 www http://www.swedenemb.org/

Switzerland: Embassy of Switzerland, 2900 Cathedral Avenue, NW, Washington

DC 20008 Tel: 202 745 7900 Fax: 202 387 2564 www http://www.swissemb.org/

Syria: Embassy of the Syrian Arab Republic, 2215 Wyoming Avenue, NW, Washington DC 20008 Tel: 202 232 6313 Fax: 202 234 9548.

Taiwan: Republic of China on Taiwan, 4201 Wisconsin Avenue, NW, Washington DC 20016 Tel: 202 895 1800 Fax: 202 966 0825.

Tanzania: Embassy of the United Republic of Tanzania, 2139 R Street, NW, Washington DC 20008 Tel: 202 939 6125 Fax: 202 797 7408.

Thailand: Royal Thai Embassy, 1024 Wisconsin Avenue, NW, Suite 401, Washington DC 20007 Tel: 202 944 3600 Fax: 202 944 3611 e-mail: thai.wsn@thaiembdc.org www http://www.thaiembdc.org/

Togo: Embassy of the Republic of Togo, 2208 Massachusetts Avenue, NW, Washington DC 20008 Tel: 202 234 4212 Fax: 202 232 3190.

Tonga: Embassy of the Kingdom of Tonga (Based in London) c/o Tonga High Commission, 36 Molyneux Street, London W1H 6AB Tel: 020 7724 5828 Fax: 020 7723 9074.

Trinidad and Tobago: Embassy of the Republic of Trinidad and Tobago, 1708 Massachusetts Avenue, NW, Washington DC 20036 Tel: 202 467 6490 Fax: 202 785 3130.

Tunisia: Embassy of Tunisia, 1515 Massachusetts Avenue, NW, Washington DC 20005 Tel: 202 862 1850.

Turkey: Embassy of the Republic of Turkey, 1714 Massachusetts Avenue, NW, Washington DC 20036 Tel: 202 659 8200 Fax: 202 659 0744 www http://www.turkey.org/turkey/

Turkmenistan: Embassy of Turkmenistan, 2207 Massachusetts Avenue, NW, Washington DC 20008 Tel: 202 588 1500 Fax: 202 588 0697 e-mail: turkmen@earthlink.net www http://www.embassyofturkmenistan.org

Uganda: Embassy of the Republic of Uganda, 5911 16th Street, NW, Washington DC 20011 Tel: 202 726 7100 Fax: 202 726 1727 e-mail: ugaembassy@rocketmail.com www http://www.ugandaweb.com/ugaembassy/

Ukraine: Embassy of Ukraine, 3350 M Street, NW, Washington DC 20007 Tel: 202 333 7507 Fax: 202 333 7510 e-mail: infolook@aol.com www http://www.ukremb.com/

United Arab Emirates: Embassy of the United Arab Emirates, 1255 22nd Street, NW, Suite 700, Washington DC 20037 Tel: 202 955 7999.

United Kingdom: Embassy of the United Kingdom of Great Britain and Northern Ireland, 3100 Massachusetts Ave, NW, Washington DC 20008 Tel: 202 588 6500 Fax: 202 588 7870 www http://www.britainusa.com/bis/embassy/embassy.stm

Uruguay: Embassy of Uruguay, 2715 M Street, NW, 3rd Floor, Washington DC 20007 Tel: 202 331 1313 Fax: 202 331 8142 e-mail: uruguay@embassy.org www http://www.embassy.org/uruguay/

Uzbekistan: Embassy of the Republic of Uzbekistan, 1746 Massachusetts Avenue, NW, Washington DC 20036 Tel: 202 887 5300 Fax: 202 293 6804 www http://www.uzbekistan.org/

Venezuela: Embassy of the Republic of Venezuela, 1099 30th Street NW, Washington DC 20007 Tel: 202 342 2214 Fax: 202 342 6820 e-mail: embavene@dgsys.com www http://www.embavenez-us.org/

Vietnam: Embassy of the Socialist Republic of Vietnam, 1233 20th Street NW, Suite 400, Washington DC 20037 Tel: 202 861 0737 Fax: 202 861 0917 e-mail: vietnamembassy@msn.com www http://www.vietnamembassy-usa.org/

Western Samoa: Embassy of Western Samoa, 800 Second Avenue, Suite 400D, New York NY 10017 Tel: (212) 599 6196.

Yemen: Embassy of the Republic of Yemen, 2600 Virginia Avenue, NW, Suite 705, Washington DC 20037 Tel: 202 965 4760 Fax: 202 337 2017 e-mail: info@yemenembassy.org www http://www.yemenembassy.org

Yugoslavia: Embassy of the Former S F Republic of Yugoslavia, 2410 California Street, NW, Washington DC 20008 Tel: 202 462 6566 e-mail: yuembassy@compuserve.com www http://ourworld.compuserve.com/homepages/yuembassy/

Zambia: Embassy of the Republic of Zambia, 2419 Massachusetts Avenue, NW, Washington DC 20008 Tel: 202 265 9717.
Zimbabwe: Embassy of the Republic of Zimbabwe, 1608 New Hampshire Avenue, NW, Washington DC 20009 Tel: 202 332 7100 www http://www.zimweb.com/ Embassy/ Zimbabwe/

Travel vaccinations

Polio and tetanus boosters are recommended for all countries listed, but see item marked†

Destination	Typhoid	Hepatitis A	Diphtheria	Tuberculosis	Hepatitis B	Rabies	Men. meningitis	Yellow fever	Jap B enceph	Tick-borne encephalitis	Malaria risk
Antigua & Barbuda	S	R	S	S	S						
Argentina	R	R	S	S	S	S					✓
Armenia	R	R	S	S	S	S				S	
Azerbaijan	R	R	R	S	S	S				S	✓
Bahamas	S	R	S	S	S						
Bangladesh	R	R	S	S	S	S			S		✓
Barbados	S	R	S	S	S						
Belarus	S	R	R	S	S	S				S	
Belize	R	R	S	S	S	S					✓
Bermuda	S	R	S	S	S						
Bolivia	R	R	S	S	S	S		R			✓
Bosnia	R	R	S	S	S	S				S	
Botswana	R	R	S	S	S	S					✓
Brazil	R	R	S	S	S	S	S	S			✓
Brunei	R	R	S	S	S	S			S		
Cayman Islands	S	R	S	S	S						
Chile	R	R	S	S	S	S					
China	R	R	S	S	S	S			S		✓
Colombia	R	R	S	S	S	S		R			✓
Cook Islands	R	R	S	S	S						
Croatia	R	R	R	S	S	S				S	
Cuba	R	R	S	S	S	S					
Czech Republic	S	S								S	
Dominican Republic	R	R	S	S	S	S					✓
Ecuador	R	R	S	S	S	S		R			✓
Fiji	R	R	S	S	S						
Gambia	R	R	S	S	S	S	S	R			
Ghana	R	R	S	S	S	S	S	M			✓
Grenada	S	R	S	S	S	S					
Guatamala	R	R	S	S	S	S					✓
Guyana	R	R	S	S	S	S		R			✓
Haiti	R	R	S	S	S	S					✓
Honduras	R	R	S	S	S	S					✓
Hong Kong	S	S	S	S	S						✓
India	R	R	S	S	S	S			S		✓
Israel	S	R	S	S	S						
Jamaica	S	R	S	S	S						
Japan									S		

†The Americas are now polio-free and boosters may be omitted for short-term travellers

Key to immunisation recommendations

M = immunisation mandatory

R = immunisation recommended as risk of infection is substantial

S = immunisation sometimes recommended

Vaccines recommended in some circumstances S are for more than three visits in a year, or a stay of more than three months in a rural area, or if the traveller is in a high-risk occupation. Seek specialist advice for complex itineraries.

NB Receiving country outside a yellow fever zone may require a valid yellow fever certificate from travellers going through yellow fever countries.

No vaccines recommended

There are no particular health or vaccine recommendations for the following countries, but check that travellers to these and all other countries have their tetanus and polio immunisations up to date.

Australia
Austria✣
Azores
Belgium
Canada
Canary Islands*
Corfu*
Corsica
Crete*
Cyprus*
Denmark
Falkland Islands
Finland✣
France
Germany✣
Gibraltar
Greece*
Greenland
Hawaii
Hungary✣
Ibiza*
Iceland
Ireland
Italy*
Luxembourg
Madeira*
Majorca*
Malta*
Minorca*
Monaco
New Zealand
Netherlands
Norway✣
Portugal*
Sardinia
Spain*
Sweden✣
Switzerland✣
USA

*Longer-term travellers should also consider hepatitis A immunisation.

✣Longer-term travellers should also consider tick-borne encephalitis immunisation.

Polio and tetanus boosters are recommended for all countries listed, but see item marked†

Destination	Typhoid	Hepatitis A	Diphtheria	Tuberculosis	Hepatitis B	Rabies	Men. meningitis	Yellow fever	Jap B enceph	Tick-borne encephalitis	Malaria risk
Jordan	R	R	S	S	S	S	S				
Kenya	R	R	S	S	S	S	S	R			✓
Lesotho	R	R	S	S	S						
Macedonia	R	R	S		S	S				S	
Madagascar	R	R	S	S	S	S					✓
Malawi	R	R	S	S	S	S	S				✓
Malaysia	R	R	S	S	S	S			S		✓
Maldives	R	R	S	S	S	S					
Mauritius	R	R	S	S	S	S					✓
Mexico	R	R	S	S	S	S					✓
Mozambique	R	R	S	S	S	S	S				✓
Namibia	R	R	S	S	S	S	S				✓
Nepal	R	R	S	S	S	S	S		S		✓
Nicaragua	R	R	S	S	S	S					✓
Nigeria	R	R	S	S	S	S	S	R			✓
Pakistan	R	R	S	S	S	S			S		✓
Papua New Guinea	R	R	S	S	S						✓
Paraguay	R	R	S	S	S	S					✓
Peru	R	R	S	S	S	S		R			✓
Philippines	R	R	S	S	S	S			S		✓
Poland		S				S				S	
Puerto Rico	R	R	S	S	S	S					
Romania	R	R	R	S	S	S				S	
Russian Federation	R	R	R	S	S	S				S	
St Lucia	S	R	S	S	S						
Samoa	R	R	S	S	S						
Seychelles	R	R	S	S	S	S					
Singapore	S	S		S	S						
Slovakia	S	S	S							S	
Solomon Islands	R	R	S	S	S						✓
South Africa	R	R	S	S	S	S					✓
Sri Lanka	R	R	S	S	S	S			S		✓
Swaziland	R	R	S	S	S	S					✓
Tanzania	R	R	S	S	S	S	S	R			✓
Thailand	R	R	S	S	S	S			S		✓
Tobago	S	R	S	S	S	S		R			
Trinidad	S	R	S	S	S	S		R			
Turkey	S	R	S	S	S	S					✓

†The Americas are now polio-free and boosters may be omitted for short-term travellers

Key to immunisation recommendations

M = immunisation mandatory
R = immunisation recommended as risk of infection is substantial
S = immunisation sometimes recommended

Vaccines recommended in some circumstances S are for more than three visits in a year, or a stay of more than three months in a rural area, or if the traveller is in a high-risk occupation. Seek specialist advice for complex itineraries.

NB Receiving country outside a yellow fever zone may require a valid yellow fever certificate from travellers going through yellow fever countries.

No vaccines recommended

There are no particular health or vaccine recommendations for the following countries, but check that travellers to these and all other countries have their tetanus and polio immunisations up to date.

Australia
Austria✥
Azores
Belgium
Canada
Canary Islands*
Corfu*
Corsica
Crete*
Cyprus*
Denmark
Falkland Islands
Finland✥
France
Germany✥
Gibraltar
Greece*
Greenland
Hawaii
Hungary✥
Ibiza*
Iceland
Ireland
Italy*
Luxembourg
Madeira*
Majorca*
Malta*
Minorca*
Monaco
New Zealand
Netherlands
Norway✥
Portugal*
Sardinia
Spain*
Sweden✥
Switzerland✥
USA

*Longer-term travellers should also consider hepatitis A immunisation.
✥Longer-term travellers should also consider tick-borne encephalitis immunisation.

Polio and tetanus boosters are recommended for all countries listed, but see item marked†

Destination	Typhoid	Hepatitis A	Diphtheria	Tuberculosis	Hepatitis B	Rabies	Men. meningitis	Yellow fever	Jap B enceph	Tick-borne encephalitis	Malaria risk
Uganda	R	R	S	S	S	S	S	R			✓
Uruguay	R	R	S	S	S	S					
Vanuata	R	R	S	S	S						✓
Venezuela	R	R	S	S	S	S		R			✓
Zambia	R	R	S	S	S	S	S	S			✓
Zimbabwe	R	R	S	S	S	S					✓

†The Americas are now polio-free and boosters may be omitted for short-term travellers

Key to immunisation recommendations

M = immunisation mandatory

R = immunisation recommended as risk of infection is substantial

S = immunisation sometimes recommended

Vaccines recommended in some circumstances S are for more than three visits in a year, or a stay of more than three months in a rural area, or if the traveller is in a high-risk occupation. Seek specialist advice for complex itineraries.

NB Receiving country outside a yellow fever zone may require a valid yellow fever certificate from travellers going through yellow fever countries.

No vaccines recommended

There are no particular health or vaccine recommendations for the following countries, but check that travellers to these and all other countries have their tetanus and polio immunisations up to date.

Australia	Ibiza*
Austria✥	Iceland
Azores	Ireland
Belgium	Italy*
Canada	Luxembourg
Canary Islands*	Madeira*
Corfu*	Majorca*
Corsica	Malta*
Crete*	Minorca*
Cyprus*	Monaco
Denmark	New Zealand
Falkland Islands	Netherlands
Finland✥	Norway✥
France	Portugal*
Germany✥	Sardinia
Gibraltar	Spain*
Greece*	Sweden✥
Greenland	Switzerland✥
Hawaii	USA
Hungary✥	

*Longer-term travellers should also consider hepatitis A immunisation.

✥Longer-term travellers should also consider tick-borne encephalitis immunisation.

Authors

Dr Michael Jones, associate specialist, and

Dr Philip Welsby, consultant physician, Regional Infection Unit, Western General Hospital, Edinburgh

We thank TRAVAX, an information service provided by the Scottish Centre for Infection and Environmental Health for access to its database in compiling this chart.

TRAVAX can be accessed via the internet (http://www.axl.co.uk/scieh) or in viewdata format on PCs. For travel or other TRAVAX queries phone 0141-300 1130.

While every effort is made to ensure that this information is correct, the compilers and Pulse cannot accept responsibility for the consequences of errors. © PULSE 2000

Reproduced from *Pulse*, January 22, 2000, with permission.

Note: Up-to-date information on vaccinations **must** be obtained before you travel.

Index

Arnold and Mark Wilson would value your comments on this book. Please feel free to contact us at:
www.medicsworldwide.com
e-mail: updates@medicsworldwide.com

Or fill in the form below and return it to
Arnold, 338 Euston Road, London NW1 3BH, UK

NAME ....

PERMANENT ADDRESS ....
....
....

E-MAIL ADDRESS ....

MEDICAL SCHOOL ....

YEAR OF STUDY (ie 3rd/4th) ....

COUNTRIES VISITED ....

SPECIFIC COMMENTS (PLEASE CONTINUE OVERLEAF)

Would you be interested in being approached for comments for the next edition?

Yes ❑
No ❑